RECENT PROGRESS IN

MICROBIOLOGY

VIII

Recent Progress in

MICROBIOLOGY

SYMPOSIA HELD AT THE VIII INTERNATIONAL

CONGRESS FOR MICROBIOLOGY

MONTREAL 1962

Under the auspices of the
International Association of Microbiological Societies
I A M S
and the
Canadian Society of Microbiologists
Société canadienne des Microbiologistes

With an ADDENDUM (in English and French) on the
STRUCTURE OF IAMS

Editor: N. E. GIBBONS

UNIVERSITY OF TORONTO PRESS

PREFACE

THIS VOLUME contains the papers presented in the thirteen symposia at the VIII International Congress for Microbiology, in Montreal, August 20–24, 1962, as well as the main papers given in the panel discussions on industrial microbiology. It has been given the same title as the volume for the Stockholm Congress, in the hope that a more uniform series of publications of the Congresses for Microbiology may thus be started.

Planning the programme of an international congress is somewhat akin to crystal-ball gazing—trends have to be assessed several years in advance to ensure topical subjects at congress time. The programme committee chose very wisely and most of the symposia are up-to-date accounts of important developments.

Some of the symposia were planned to cover aspects of microbiology which had not been covered in recent Congresses for Microbiology. This was the basis for the symposia in Agricultural Microbiology, chosen after consultation with specialists in many countries, and the Panel Discussions in Industrial Microbiology, the topics for which were chosen by workers in industry.

In most instances the symposium was organized by its chairman. There was thus considerable variation in the number of speakers and the time allotted to each. This left the editor with the problem of deciding whether to insist that all papers be of comparable length, as originally intended, or to allow some freedom. Actually it has been necessary to exercise our own judgment and there is considerable variation in length of papers.

Congresses also have their formal, social and business aspects. The volume would not be complete without the Presidential Addresses given at the opening ceremonies. Dr. S. Mudd, President of IAMS, recalls the changes in microbiology during his lifetime and points out some of the resulting responsibilities. Dr. E. G. D. Murray, President of the Congress, also mentions the changing outlook on science.

And finally, the official deliberations of the Congress and the Structure of IAMS are set forth in an Addendum.

The Organizing Committee of the Congress wishes to thank all those who made the Congress and this volume possible, particularly the chairmen and the speakers. It is also grateful for the assistance provided in many ways by the federal, provincial and municipal governments, and by numerous scientific and commercial organizations. The editor wishes to thank the authors who eased his task with well-prepared manuscripts and those who accepted so graciously his criticisms and demands.

N. E. G.

CONTENTS

VIROLOGY

Veuillez transmettre mes voeux les plus cordiaux aux délégués du Congrès International de Microbiologie.

Le Canada est honoré de recevoir ce Congrès, dont le but est d'approfondir les connaissances scientifiques dans plusieurs domaines.

Au nom de Sa Majesté La Reine Elizabeth II, je souhaite la bienvenue à ceux qui viennent de l'étranger, et assure tous les délégués d'un accueil chaleureux.

juillet 1961.

Please convey my warmest
greetings to all those attending the 8th
International Congress for Microbiology.

It is an honour for Canada
to receive an assembly, whose discussions
will advance the cause of science in many
vital fields.

On behalf of Her Majesty
Queen Elizabeth II, I welcome those members who came from overseas, and wish to
all the fullest measure of success.

July, 1961.

The Organizing Committee of the Congress is particularly grateful to the following organizations, whose contributions were used exclusively for the partial support of some of the symposia published in this Volume.

THE COUNCIL FOR INTERNATIONAL ORGANIZATIONS OF MEDICAL SCIENCES (CIOMS)

THE INTERNATIONAL UNION OF BIOLOGICAL SCIENCES (IUBS)

THE NATIONAL SCIENCE FOUNDATION through
THE AMERICAN INSTITUTE OF BIOLOGICAL SCIENCES (AIBS)

(A complete list of donors is given on p. 685.)

PRESIDENTIAL ADDRESSES

to the members of the VIII International Congress for Microbiology
delivered at the Opening Ceremonies held in the Grand Salon,
Queen Elizabeth Hotel, Montreal, August 19, 1962

MICROBIOLOGICAL RESEARCH: A STUDY IN EMERGING SOPHISTICATION

STUART MUDD

President of IAMS

FORTY-ODD YEARS AGO, when microbiologists of my generation were making their first professional contacts with the microscopic forms of life, microbiology was passing from its vigorous and creative youth into a maturity which is proving equally creative, but creative in quite different ways. Bacteriology had had its golden age of discovery, in which the infectious agents of most of the bacterial diseases had been identified and cultivated. The basic reactions of immunology had been described and applications begun in the diagnosis, prevention and treatment of infectious diseases. A *contagium vivum fluidum* had been separated by filtration by Iwanowski and Beijerinck, a viral agent of foot-and-mouth disease disclosed by Loeffler and Frosch and of yellow fever by Walter Reed and colleagues. Industrially important products—ethyl alcohol, acetic acid, lactic acid—had been shown to be producible by the action of micro-organisms. Many facts concerning the enrichment of the soil, as in the nitrogen cycle, had been worked out.

However, it is not my purpose today to review the splendors of the past accomplishments of microbiology. Rather, I would call to your attention aspects of the maturing of microbiology as a science. This is indeed a story of emerging sophistication.

Within the years of our professional activity we have seen microbiology emerge from descriptive bacteriology, mycology, and protozoology, to become a major segment of biology in general. Included, of course, are the viruses, obligate parasites in the twilight zone between organized cells and cell organelles, whose study is telling us much new about the least common denominators of life processes and about the essentials of interaction between living forms.

In *Morphology* we have progressed from Gram's stain and the staining of spores, capsules and flagella to study of ultrathin sections by electron microscopy. The internal organization of the microbial cell is revealing complexity and order at the macromolecular level which promise better understanding of the significance of organization within more complex cells.

In *Cell Physiology* we have advanced from "cultural reactions" to elucidation of aspects of the biochemical dynamics of the cell, including many general pathways of degradation and biosynthesis. The fact that reactions within a bacterial population can be studied statistically, that effective techniques are available for producing and investigating biochemical mutants, and the versatility, adaptability and general manipulatability of bacteria have made them enormously useful to biochemists and cell physiologists.

In *Genetics* we have progressed from a dreary succession of monotonous fissions to analysis of the essentials of genetic continuity, genetic recombination and segregation. We can now study the sex lives of bacteria, which makes things considerably more interesting in the laboratory. Much of the nascent understanding of DNA and RNA synthesis, of the code and mechanisms by which genetic information is transmitted from nuclear DNA through RNA to govern ribosomal synthesis of enzymes and other proteins, is being derived from bacterial models. In the as yet only dimly discerned mechanisms of DNA replication in bacteria and of virus multiplication there is a beginning of understanding of the essentials of genetic continuity and change, more general and more basic than the tribal rituals of Meiosis and Mitosis.

Of applications of microbiology in agronomy and in industry I will not venture to speak as an amateur in the presence of so many highly qualified professionals.

In *Pathogenesis* we have progressed from the description of infectious agents as the *causes* of disease to recognition of infectious disease as essentially a struggle between the biological systems of host and parasite, with the complex interplay of survival mechanisms of both systems critical for the outcome. We have learned something of useful intervention in the struggle between host and parasite and something of the limitations imposed by toxicity, specificity and hypersensitivity. We have learned something of intervention in infection by chemotherapeutic means and by the antibiotic agents elaborated by micro-organisms themselves. We have a very great deal more to learn about the micro-parasites and their products, and even more to learn about the constitutional factors and mechanisms involved in host resistance to the micro-parasites.

With the emergence of *exobiology* as a special field, microbiologists are becoming concerned with the possibilities of detecting microscopic unicellular life in meteoric dust in space and in due course on the moon and planets. They are concerned with the effects of highly energetic ionizing particles (protons and stripped atomic nuclei of billions of electron-volt energies) on the viability and mutation rates of micro-organisms. The earth's magnetic field is of 0.4 gauss intensity and that of the moon is believed to be only 1×10^{-4} gauss. It is possible that intense magnetic fields (100–1,000 gauss) may be employed to deflect cosmic radiations in space travel. Therefore, microbiologists are becoming interested in the possible effects of magnetic fields of reduced and of augmented intensity and of weightlessness on cellular activity.

As professional microbiologists we can contribute to human resources through the activities of the microscopic forms of life which are our special province. Our little friends of course contribute to the dissolution of the flora and fauna that have died, and so to the renewal of life. They fix the nitrogen of the air; they bring about many fermentations and many syntheses which add to human resources. We may look to yeasts and algae as considerable sources of food. Increasing understanding of the physiology, biochemistry and genetics of the micro-parasites and of their interaction with macro-organisms has enormously reduced the incidence of disease, and application of this growing understanding will continue to do so. In these matters we, as microbiologists, can take just pride.

I say *pride*, however, certainly not complacency or even *unreserved satisfaction*. For there is another side. In the development of civilization certain steady states have obtained between fertility on the one hand and mortality on the other. The recent advances of medicine, in particular medical microbiology and immunology and their applications, have resulted in a profound disequilibrium between fertility and mortality. In consequence populations are growing at a crisis rate, at a rate out of all proportion to any possible rate of increment of human resources of food or living space. In so far as we increase the expectancy of life without taking into account our excessive capacity for multiplication we contribute to a profound disturbance of the ecology of man. I do not wish to offend the sensibilities of any religious faith. Actually, informed persons of all religious faiths are aware of this problem. Differences between faiths are in principle at least differences in regard to ways by which the problem can be met, and these I do not propose to discuss.

The atomic scientists, who have been instrumental in bringing all civilization—indeed all higher forms of life—into terrible jeopardy, have felt a profound concern for the consequences of their work and have made themselves, through the Bulletin of the Atomic Scientists and in other ways, a powerful constructive force. Those of us in particular who are medical microbiologists have contributed toward the present profound disequilibrium between population growth and world resources. I earnestly hope that we as citizens can do as well as the Atomic Scientists in making understood the potentially disastrous consequences of this disturbance of human ecology and in supporting the necessary corrective programs in our respective countries.*

---

*A formal policy statement of the American Public Health Association, adopted in October, 1959, is relevant: "There is today an increase of population which threatens the health and well-being of many millions of people. In many areas of the world substantial population increase means malnutrition and outright starvation. In other areas it may mean increased stress in family life, reduction of educational opportunity and the retardation of the industrial development on which a nation's rising standard of living depends. No problem—whether it be housing, education, food supply, recreation, communication, medical care—can be effectively solved today if tomorrow's population increases out of proportion to the resources available to meet those problems. . . .

"The Public Health profession has long taken leadership in defeating disease, disability, and death. It must now assume equal leadership in understanding public health implications of population imbalance and in taking appropriate action."

It is good that we can meet together here, as scientists and as citizens of many nations, and can consider in friendliness and objectivity these matters which concern us all. In this respect we are functioning, as your great Canadian psychiatrist and humanist, Dr. Brock Chisholm, has so strongly urged us to function, as *members of the human species*. It is within our capacities as scientists and as citizens to contribute to the coming to terms of the human species with its environment and with itself. The fossil beds of the world bear eloquent testimony to the extinction of thousands of species which have failed to come to terms with their environments. And let us remember that to solve the problems upon which the survival and the good life for man depend, we do not have geologic time. Never before has the rate of change in human ecology been so great; never before have goodwill among men and clear-sighted vision and action been so urgently necessary.

OPENING OF THE CONGRESS

E. G. D. MURRAY

The Honourable Dr. A. Couturier (Minister of Health of the Province of Quebec); Dr. R. F. Farquharson (representing the Government of Canada); Monsieur R. Bourret (representing the City of Montreal); Dr. Stuart Mudd (President of IAMS); Professor Sven Gard (President of the VII International Congress); Professor E. H. Garrard (President of the Canadian Society of Microbiologists); Distinguished Guests and the Officers and Members of this VIII International Congress for Microbiology; Ladies and Gentlemen:

I wish to thank His Excellency the Governor General of Canada for his graceful Message of Welcome; and to thank the distinguished representatives of the Government of Canada, of the Government of the Province of Quebec, and of the City of Montreal for the welcome they have brought to us. We are grateful, too, to Dr. Stuart Mudd, President of IAMS, for his address, given with the authority of the highest officer of the International Association, which directs the regulation, promotes the interests, and safeguards the representations of microbiology by securing the co-operation of microbiologists of all countries to these ends. IAMS is also the mouthpiece of Microbiology in the Councils of the International Scientific Unions and the organizations responsible to the United Nations Organization.

An assemblage such as this, of distinguished scientists earnestly concerned with a subject of vague meaning to the general public, should excite some curiosity about its purpose and nature. So, in making a declaration to open the Congress, it seems well advised to avoid both misunderstanding and apathy by a brief statement of our intentions. Therefore I ask the members of the Congress to be patient with what is obvious to them and allow me to make a brief statement for public information.

The Congress is a means of bringing together the delegates of the world-wide Member Societies to effect the business of the International Association, and the carefully organized scientific sessions are for the exchange of knowledge and opinions among scientists intimately concerned with the immediate problems of microbiology.

Microbiology is a comprehensive term which implies the study of everything to do with microscopic life, whether it be of animal forms (such as protozoa) or of plant forms (such as yeasts, moulds and algae) or of bacteria and viruses.

These studies comprise the activities and processes of diverse, abundant and universal minute forms of life, both free-living and parasitic, independently of whether they are indifferent to man's estate, whether they are injurious to other forms of life by disease or destructiveness, or whether they provide substances or conditions essential to the very life of other living beings and to the progress of human industry and welfare.

The recognition of microscopic life and the understanding of it we have gained so far have given man his most influential modifying power over his environment, and that has now created new and sometimes formidable problems and is giving a new dimension to human history in the making.

F. W. Andrewes said, in his Linacre Lecture (1926), "Of all the teeth in the terrible comb with which Nature sorts out the inefficient, disease is one of the most formidable." The younger people of today, even those whose study is infectious disease, do not properly appreciate the change accomplished during the past fifty years by the reduction of incidence and mortality of infections. By this interference, it almost seems that natural selection has been displaced by artificial selection and we might wonder whether we have the wisdom and the courage to cope with the emergency.

In recent years Science has noticeably become the tool of politics and the handmaid of industry, and in the popular mind this seems to be over-shadowing its true purpose. In reality, Science is the history of the intellectual adventures of inquiring minds in search for perfect understanding of whatever happens in Nature. The method is inherent in the pertinaceous questions what, where, when, how, and, above all, that most difficult question, why. That intensely human Welsh poet Dylan Thomas perceptively complained that he was given a book that told him everything about the wasp except why; and it is sadly true that the best excuse we could give him is to be found in the words of the sixteenth-century philosophical poet, Sir John Davies,

> Skill comes so slow and life so fast doth fly,
> We learn so little and forget so much.

Ladies and Gentlemen, you yourselves are the Congress, and the Canadian Society of Microbiologists has done everything it can to provide the opportunity for you to make the business and scientific proceedings a success. We hope you will find the amenities conducive to your purpose and to geniality, so that you will take home pleasant memories of Canada.

Les microbiologistes de qualité ici assemblé ne manquèrent pas de remarquer que la Société canadienne de Microbiologistes a fait le mieux possible de subvenir aux besoins de ce Congrès. C'est pour nous un grand plaisir de vous faire accueil, et nous vous souhaitons les souvenirs les plus agréables de votre séjour.

Dès aujourd'hui, Mesdames et Messieurs les congressistes, c'est à vous d'entrer en jeu pour assurer le succès du Congrès, et de faire valoir les délibérations scientifiques. Il ne me reste maintenant que de déclarer le Congrès en session.

I wish to thank everyone for participating in this formal opening of the VIII International Congress for Microbiology, which I now declare officially in session.

SYMPOSIUM I

MEMBRANE PERMEATION

Chairman: KENNETH McQUILLEN

WOUTERA van ITERSON
Membranous Structures in Micro-organisms

E. KODICEK
Aspects of the Constitution of Bacterial Membranes

A. KEPES
Permeases: Identification and Mechanism

ROY J. BRITTEN
The Mechanism of Pool Formation in *Escherichia coli*

CHAIRMAN'S REMARKS

KENNETH McQUILLEN

Sub-Department of Chemical Microbiology
Department of Biochemistry
University of Cambridge, Cambridge, England

THE PASSAGE OF SUBSTANCES into and out of micro-organisms is obviously of great importance but little is known of the mechanisms involved. The localization, anatomy and molecular biology of the barriers to free interchange are being actively investigated. Only a few years ago the very existence in bacteria of a cytoplasmic membrane (plasma membrane) separate and separable from the cell wall was controversial. Now from some species it is possible to prepare walls and membranes which are free from contamination by the other. Much is known about the chemistry of cell walls from some species: much less about cytoplasmic membranes. This symposium attempts to review aspects of the nature of these membranes and of permeation mechanisms with which they are associated.

The techniques of electron microscopy have developed rapidly and Dr. van Iterson describes how they can now reveal a complexity in bacterial cell structure which was not envisaged even quite recently. However, it is important when discussing comparative morphology to bear in mind differences in size between plant and animal cells as compared with bacterial cells. Mitochondria from higher organisms have about the same dimensions as entire cells of many micro-organisms. Nevertheless, membranes of similar structure and thickness can be seen at the periphery of the cytoplasm of most kinds of cell. It is likely that they form an important osmotic barrier but it is an oversimplification to consider the protoplast to be only a semipermeable bag surrounding cytoplasm in which particles float in a solution of small molecules and soluble proteins. Some micro-organisms possess complex membranous organelles which seem to originate by invagination of the cytoplasmic membrane. They may be concerned in secretion of walls and/or membranes, or with terminal oxidation reactions, or with reorganization of nuclear material during sporulation and they may have affinities with mitochondria and with endoplasmic reticulum.

Professor R. G. E. Murray reported the occurrence of elaborate membranous structures in the cytoplasm of certain micro-organisms and Dr. Giesbrecht and Dr. Toennies indicated that the amount of membranous material per cell was variable over a wide range depending on the conditions of culture.

Such methods as exist for the separation of cell membranes (or fractions believed to be derived from membranes) yield material which is predominantly lipoprotein in character. Dr. Kodicek discusses the constitution of membranes and attempts to relate it to their functions which probably comprise both metabolic and permeation mechanisms of many kinds—simple, facilitated and exchange diffusion, active transport, etc. Some or all of the protein component may be enzyme-like and both protein and lipid (largely phospholipid) may act as carriers for specific metabolites. The existence in several bacterial species of phosphatidylglycerols to which amino acids may be bound (transiently?) is intriguing. It is also somewhat surprising to find in closely related strains of *Bacillus megaterium* that the membrane lipid in one contains no nitrogen and is largely cardiolipin-like polyphosphatidic acid whereas in another it is mainly phosphatidylethanolamine. The fatty acids components are also of interest and it is clear that further investigations of membrane lipids should prove a fruitful field for study. The facility with which a membrane composed of lipid and protein might alter its structure in response to external stimuli might be invoked to explain permeation mechanisms, many of which are highly specific.

The concept of permeases developed at the Institut Pasteur by Monod and his co-workers is discussed by Kepes. Permeases were postulated as a class of proteins resembling enzymes, located in the cytoplasmic membrane and involved in specific transport systems—initially for sugars and amino acids and later for many other substances. The model system now put forward to account for a variety of experimental observations ranging from genetics, nutrition and physiology to enzymology, active accumulation and leakage, involves both a protein permease and a carrier molecule. This model (related to one proposed by Mitchell) is somewhat similar to that described by Dr. Britten, which is based on data accumulated at the Department of Terrestrial Magnetism, Carnegie Institution of Washington. But there are differences between Paris and Washington and Dr. Britten discusses alternative models with respect to amino acid uptake by *Escherichia coli*. It appears that precursors of proteins and nucleic acids may exist in physically separate compartments which do not allow of rapid mixing and/or in chemically different forms which again do not readily interchange. Thus there seems to be more than one kind of amino acid "pool" and similarly with nucleic acid precursor "pools." Exogenous material may bypass one such "pool" on its way to end-product. It is apparent that we know little of the physico-chemical organization of compounds in the "juice" of microbial cells.

It was unfortunate that illness prevented Dr. Peter Mitchell from contributing to this symposium. He presents a third point of view in controversies over membrane permeation and sums up his position by saying "it turns out that all 'active transport' processes must be primarily caused by enzyme systems for which substrate accessibility is spatially anisotropic." Hence his use of the term "vectorial metabolism" as opposed to "scalar metabolism." Hence his preoccupation with the localization and orientation of metabolic systems in cell membranes.

The existence of these membranes is now well established; something is known about their chemistry; enzyme activities are associated with, if not an integral part of, them; many permeation studies have been made on whole cells. Perhaps the time has come when the behaviour of artificial and reconstructed membranes should be explored. It might be possible to test some of Kodicek's notions about the properties of lipids and it would be exciting to try to incorporate enzymes and carriers, oriented in a specific manner, as Mitchell has suggested.

MEMBRANOUS STRUCTURES IN MICRO-ORGANISMS

WOUTERA VAN ITERSON

Laboratory of Electron Microscopy
University of Amsterdam
Amsterdam, The Netherlands

SOME FIVE YEARS AGO there still existed a tendency to regard the anatomy of bacteria and blue-green algae as being so primitive that it would be of no interest whatsoever to study their morphology for parallels to cells in higher stages of evolution. Since 1958, when better methods of fixation and embedding for electron microscopy came into use (Ryter & Kellenberger, 1958), this attitude has changed radically. It is now becoming most fascinating to consider the various cell constituents of micro-organisms in the light of comparative morphology, but we are still very much in the beginning.

Electron microscopy (e.m.) in recent years has made us aware of a great resemblance in the general ultrastructural pattern of animal and plant cells. Plate I is an attempt to design a basic cell scheme for both cell types. Assuming the length of the complete animal or plant cell to amount to about 15 μ, we drew more or less to scale two bacterial halves, i.e., of a gram-positive bacterium of the type of *Bacillus subtilis* and of a gram-negative photosynthetic organism of the type of *Rhodospirillum rubrum*; in addition, a swollen element of *Proteus* and a Pleuropneumonia-like organism. In the scheme principal membranous cell constituents are shown.

Originally in the common practice of fixation for e.m. with buffered OsO_4 and embedding in methacrylate mixtures, membranes appeared as single dense lines. But under certain incompletely understood conditions of fixation and staining, as, for example, with $KMnO_4$, or simply using higher e.m. resolution sometimes in combination with embedding in araldite or vestopal, a triple-layered structure appears in the membranes. This structure was found to be so universal in nature that Robertson (1959) ventured to introduce the term "unit membrane" for such a triple-layered unit. It is now commonly agreed (Stoeckenius, 1960) that this image of two dense layers with a lighter interzone may be interpreted as one bimolecular leaflet of lipid some 40–60 A thick, covered on both sides by a protein layer of a minimum thickness of about 10 A (Finean, 1961). In the dehydrated state the lipoprotein layer would thus have a thickness in the range 50–100 A.

Every cell is secluded from its environment by a layer of supposedly selective permeability; in bacteria this is usually called the osmotic barrier. An animal tissue cell is bounded by its cell membrane only; a plant cell has

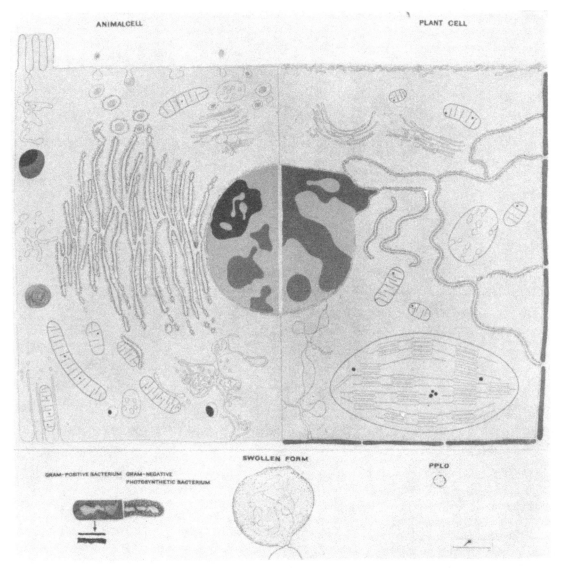

ANIMAL CELL

PLANT CELL

SWOLLEN FORM

PPLO

GRAM-POSITIVE BACTERIUM GRAM-NEGATIVE
PHOTOSYNTHETIC BACTERIUM

PLATE I. Diagram representing various cell types, drawn to scale to show their membranous constituents. In the large cells the nuclear envelope consists of two membranes, the outer one being continuous with the membranes composing the endoplasmic reticulum. Most of the elements seclude their content with a single membrane, but the structure of the mitochondria and the chloroplast in the large cells is based on double membranes.

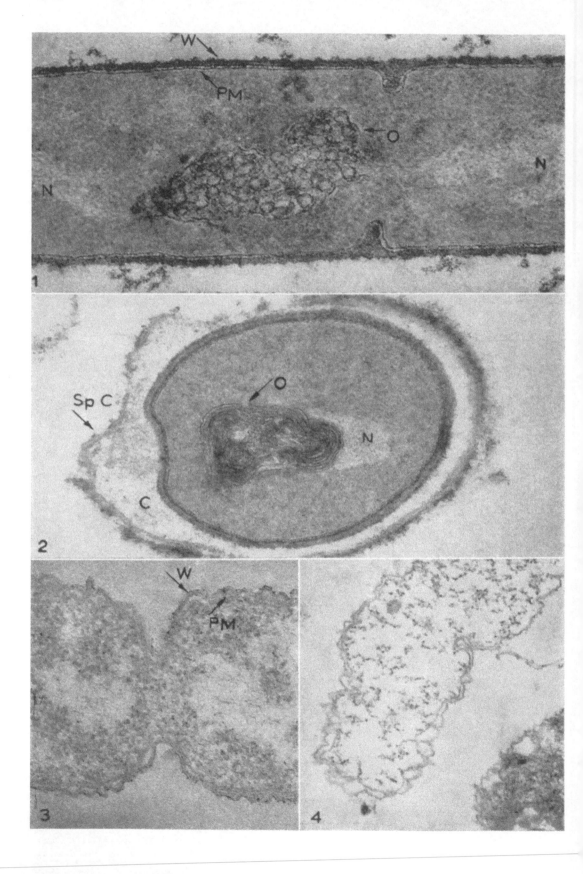

a similar boundary and in addition a cell wall. All free-living micro-organisms have a rigid or semi-rigid envelope which apparently maintains their shape and size. When such a wall is removed or weakened, bacteria can grow to impressive dimensions. This is illustrated in the scheme by a copy of an electron micrograph of a swollen form of *Proteus* found in a culture treated with penicillin. Since the diameter of the body is 4–5 times the width of the normal cell the cytoplasmic boundary may increase in area and also be endowed with considerable elasticity.

Inside the large cells there are various entities of specialized cellular function, enclosed in at least one membrane interposing a barrier between their interior and the cellular milieu. Biochemical data indicate, among other things, that in the living state assemblies of specific enzymes may be integrated in these barriers of hydrated lipoprotein, and that, besides allowing for the passage of solutes and for other functions, these membranes may serve as the structural basis for various energy transfer processes as in respiration, photosynthesis, impulse transmission, etc.

There are separate entities such as secretion or pinocytosis vesicles which seclude their contents with a single membrane. The fine structure of mito-chondria and plastids appears to be based on double membranes, i.e., on two unit membranes, the principle of which might be that a third phase can be secluded from both the interior and the cytoplasmic phase. Besides separate elements there are others bearing a more or less continuous char-acter like the endoplasmic reticulum (ER). This system of tubules, vesicles or flattened cisternae is believed to be continuous from the perinuclear space all the way to the periphery of the cell, if not beyond this. Robertson (1959) regards the ER as an elaborate infolding of the cell's surface, while Porter (1961) likes to think of the membranes as "derivatives or extensions of the nuclear envelope." Because of the intimate association of the inner nuclear membrane with the chromatin, Porter regards the ER as "the formerly invisible purveyor of genetic information from nucleus to cytoplasm."

One glance at the over-all sizes of the elements of the large cells, as com-pared with the dimensions of the microbial cell, should show the futility of expecting in it similar elements just evolved on a smaller scale. We even know of minute cocci that are several times smaller than the average mito-chondrion (Van Iterson & Ruys, 1960). Notably, the respiratory and photo-synthetic apparatus in the bacteria and blue-green algae cannot be identical

PLATE II. FIG. 1, *Bacillus subtilis*; × 140,000. An organelle (O) composed of vesicles is in contact with nucleoplasm (N). The solid cell wall (W) is contiguous with the plasma membrane (PM). FIG. 2, *Bacillus subtilis*; × 95,000. Cell from a late phase of spore germination. A membranous organelle (O) extends into the nuclear area (N). Around the cell are remains of the spore coat (Sp.C.) and the cortex (C). FIG. 3, *Hemophilus influenzae*; × 105,000. In this gram-negative organism the cell wall (W) appears as a thin sinuous integument separate from the triple-layered plasma membrane (PM). The cell division appears to proceed by a simple process of constriction, without formation of a cell plate. FIG. 4, Autolysed cell of *Proteus vulgaris*; × 55,000. The sinuosity of the cell wall is preserved in this dead cell. Note the presence of two separate integuments.

to those in large cells. Only the building units on the macromolecular scale, in particular the lipoprotein membranes, may sometimes be comparable (cf. Mitchell, 1959).

Several types of bacteria have now been observed to possess membranes in their cytoplasm; the most elaborate systems so far known probably occur in the Actinomycetes. In a micrograph of *Actinomyces bovis*, made by Dr. Mercedes Edwards from the New York State Department of Health, the triple structure of the plasma membrane is clearly revealed by special staining with chromyl chloride. Glauert (1959, 1960) concluded from her enlightening electron micrographs that such membranes seem reminiscent of ER because of their continuity with the plasma membrane. As mentioned before, in Porter's conception of ER it is the continuity with the nuclear envelope that counts. Although in bacteria and blue-green algae a nuclear envelope is missing altogether, this does not preclude intimate association of membrane systems with chromatin mass, as we see in Plate II, Fig. 1, 2.

These examples have been chosen from gram-positive bacteria. Concentrating on the comparative morphology of the various types of bacteria, I started wondering whether one might distinguish intrinsic structural differences between the gram-positive and the gram-negative bacteria. As far as the limited amount of data permits any conclusions to be drawn, these differences seemed to concern the relationship between cell wall and plasma membrane, the cell division, and the presence or absence of organized membranous organelles of a particular type. These differences will be illustrated by the next figures.

There is still some reluctance to ascribe to gram-negative bacteria a plasma membrane separate from the cell wall, although Kellenberger (1958) demonstrated in *E. coli* a dense line representing this layer. In Fig. 3 of the gram-negative bacterium *Hemophilus influenzae* we see that after Kellenberger fixation the cell wall appears as a thin sinuous structure, separate from the triple-layered plasma membrane. Even after autolysis the sinuosity of the cell wall can be preserved (Fig. 4). Cell division in *Hemophilus* (Fig. 3) and in *Proteus* appears to proceed by cell constriction followed by fission (for *E. coli* cf. Conti, 1962). No particular organelles have been found, therefore the cell pattern of the gram-negatives seems to be the more remote from the complicated cell scheme.

PLATE III, FIG. 5, *Proteus vulgaris*; × 95,000. Normal cell from 6 hr aerated liquid culture. The sinuous cell wall is separate from the plasma membrane. In the cell wall three denser tortuous lines can be distinguished. FIG. 6a, *Proteus vulgaris* treated with penicillin; × 45,000. Note in this spheroplast the straightening of the plasma membrane (PM), the rounding-off of the cytoplast and the loosening of the cell wall (W). FIG. 6b, Detail of Fig. 6a; × 120,000. As a result of the penicillin treatment in the cell wall (W) only two dense layers are now apparent (cf. Fig. 5). There are flocks adhering to the wall. FIG. 7, *Proteus vulgaris* treated with penicillin; × 50,000. Note the appearance of membrane-bounded vacuoles (V) in the cytoplast. FIG. 8, *Proteus vulgaris* treated with penicillin; × 49,000. Small elements containing cytoplasm are isolated from the cytoplast (arrows).

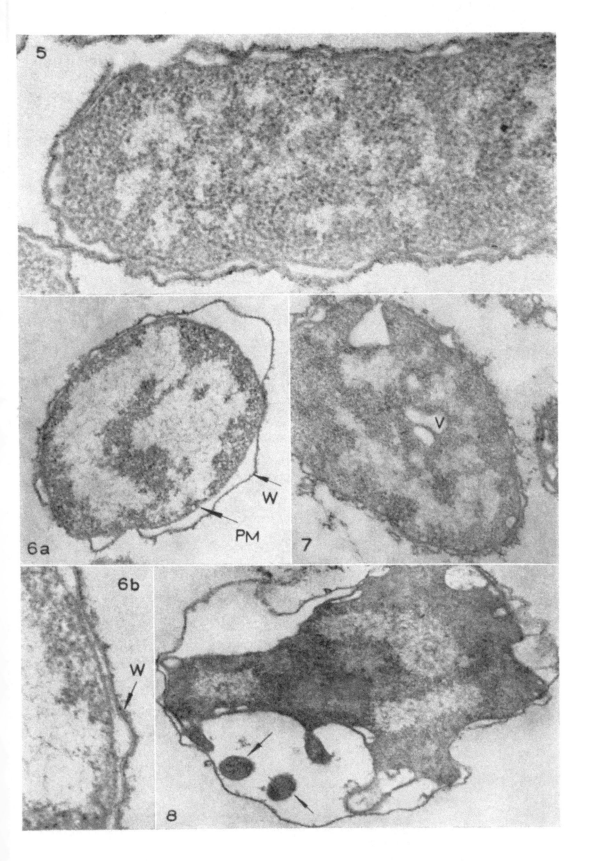

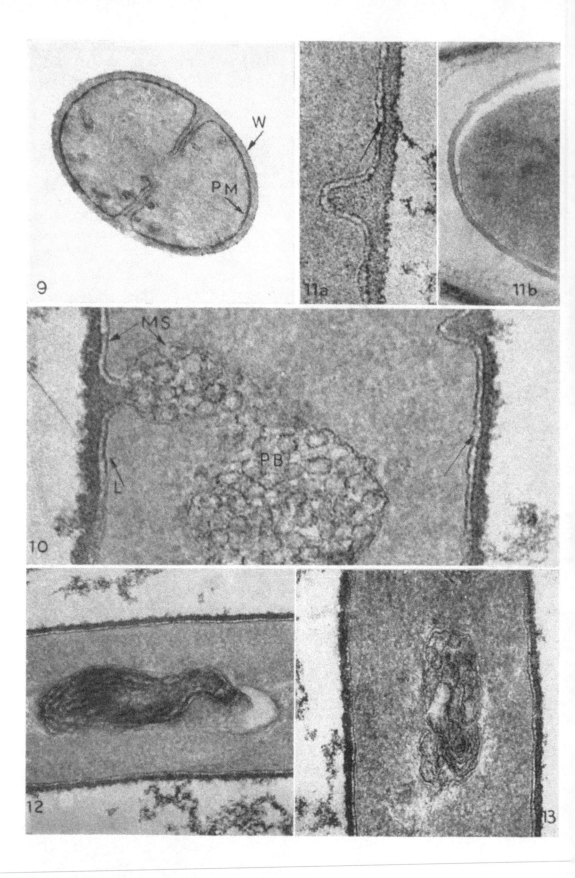

An experiment that might be interesting to mention here is our study of the influence of penicillin on *Proteus vulgaris*. In the cell wall of the normal cell (Plate III, Fig. 5), with some effort, three lines can be distinguished, which do not seem to be parallel layers but to follow tortuous courses. When penicillin is added to such a *Proteus* culture (Fig. 6a) we notice straightening of the plasma membrane, rounding-off of the cytoplast and fusion of the nuclear areas (cf. Tulasne, *et al.*, 1962). The loose wall may have lost some material, since in Fig. 6b it partly shows only two parallel dark lines with small flocks adhering. Although penicillin inhibits cell wall synthesis, this need not influence the formation of membranes because membrane-bounded spaces appear, either empty (Fig. 7) or enclosing some cytoplasmic material (Fig. 8). We wonder whether the elements isolated from the main cytoplast in Fig. 8, if they contained nucleoplasm and cytoplasm in the right proportions, would remain viable—in other words, could become L forms.

With regard to the differences between the gram-positive and the gram-negative bacteria, we observed that in the gram-positive bacteria a thick cell wall covers the plasma membrane smoothly and completely (see Plate IV, Fig. 9, *Micrococcus albus*). We even got the impression that both integuments are structurally united and this might explain why in general gram-positives are less readily plasmolysed than the gram-negatives (A. Fischer, 1903). Division in the *Micrococcus* (Fig. 9) appears to be accomplished by the development of a circular septum consisting of the double cell wall lined on its four sides with the plasma membrane. The latter is seen to form invaginations into the cytoplasm, which may develop into organelles; these we observed occasionally to be in contact with the nucleoplasm (Van Iterson, 1960). In several species typical organelles, called peripheral bodies by Chapman and Hillier (1953), seemed involved in the division process. Fig. 10 of *B. subtilis* shows such a body to be integral with

PLATE IV, FIG. 9, *Micrococcus albus*; × 77,000. In this gram-positive bacterium the heavy cell wall (W) is contiguous with the plasma membrane (PM). The cell division appears to be initiated by the development of a circular septum comprising the two prospective cell walls. The plasma membrane also lines the new walls and forms invaginations into the cytoplasm. FIG. 10, *Bacillus subtilis*; × 200,000. A peripheral body (PB) is seen to be integral with the ingrowing cross wall. It appears to be composed of vesicles bounded by one dense line. The body is enveloped in a dense sheet (MS) seen to be continuous with what the author has interpreted (1961) as the inner layer of the plasma membrane. The outer layer would then coincide with the dense line (arrow) adjacent to the cell wall material. Along the inner dense line there is sometimes a light zone (L). FIG. 11a, b, *Bacillus subtilis*; (a) × 190,000, (b) × 120,000. The relation of the plasma membrane to the cell wall in this gram-positive bacterium might be analysed when the cytoplast retracts from the cell wall. In Fig. 11a the plasma membrane crudely tears off along the lighter zone in between the two dense lines (arrow Fig. 11a). FIG. 12, *Bacillus subtilis*; × 70,000. In the cell center there is a whirl of concentric membranes clearly of the unit membrane type. FIG. 13, *Bacillus subtilis*; × 130,000. The organelle appears composed of both lamellae and vesicles. Figure 9 was originally published in Proc. Eur. Reg. Conf. on Electron Microscopy, Delft 1960, 2: 763; Figs. 10, 12 and 13 were originally published in J. Biophys. Biochem. Cytol. 1961, 9: 183 as Figs. 13, 3 and 5 resp.

the ingrowing septum; it appears composed of vesicles bounded by one delicate dense line. Centrally the vesicle cluster appears in contact with nucleoplasm. Both the peripheral body and the developing cross wall have a common boundary, seen as a delicate line, which I interpreted as a continuation of the inner dense layer of the triple-structured plasma membrane. The outer dense layer I believed to coincide with the dense line immediately adjacent to the cell wall material (see Fig. 11a). However, at some sites along the inner dense line a light zone can be distinguished, and Glauert (1961) believes that the plasma membrane comprises this light zone with, as outer boundary, the layer we interpreted as inner dense layer. In Fitz-James's opinion (1960) our inner dense line represents the middle layer of the membrane, described by him as "a dense backbone line bordered by two lighter zones." These three views are summarized in text Fig. 1. I do not

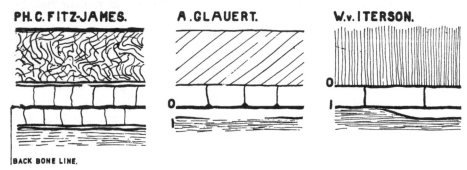

PH. C. FITZ-JAMES.   A. GLAUERT.   W.v. ITERSON.

BACK BONE LINE.

Text FIG. 1. Diagram showing the interpretations of the delineation of the plasma membrane by three authors.

think they should be taken too seriously because the membrane readily forms supplementary layers; also, the picture obtained depends a good deal on the technique used and on the image formation of the e.m. The behaviour of the structure on separation from the wall could supply some information. However, Fig. 11b might be interpreted in support of all three theories. The more delicate separation effected with ether by Robinow (1962) resulted in typical unit membranes.

Apart from organelles consisting of vesicles (Figs. 1, 10) systems of unit membranes may occur (Figs. 2, 12). Such whirls as in Fig. 12 of *B. subtilis*

PLATE V, FIG. 14, *Bacillus subtilis*; × 45,000. The electron opaque sites have been produced by the reduction of tellurite in the living cell. The organelle appears quite black. FIG. 15, *Proteus vulgaris*; × 70,000. At arrows there is gain in contrast resulting from the reduction of tellurite. FIG. 16a, b, Large and small particle fractions obtained from *Azotobacter agilis*; × 70,000. (a) Large particle fractions precipitated at 7,000–12,000 g; (b) Small particle fraction precipitated at 12,000–17,000 g mainly containing small membranous structures and ribosomes. FIG. 17, *Azotobacter agilis*; × 110,000. The membrane-bounded vesicles (V) might well be the same membranous structures as seen in Fig. 16b. FIG. 18, *Rhodospirillum rubrum*; × 111,000. The membranous vesicles in this organism are known to carry the photosynthetic pigments. In this partly autolysed cell some indications are found that the membranes are interconnected with the plasma membrane (arrows).

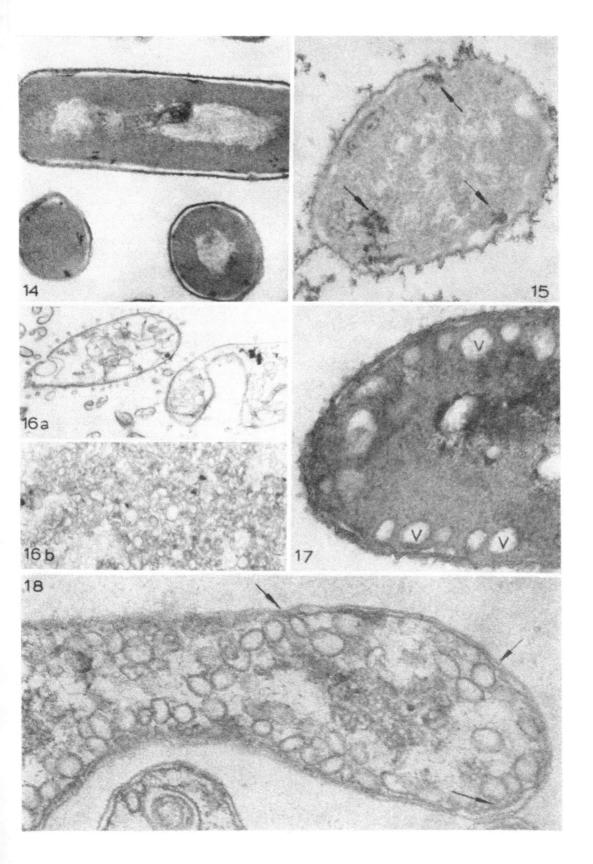

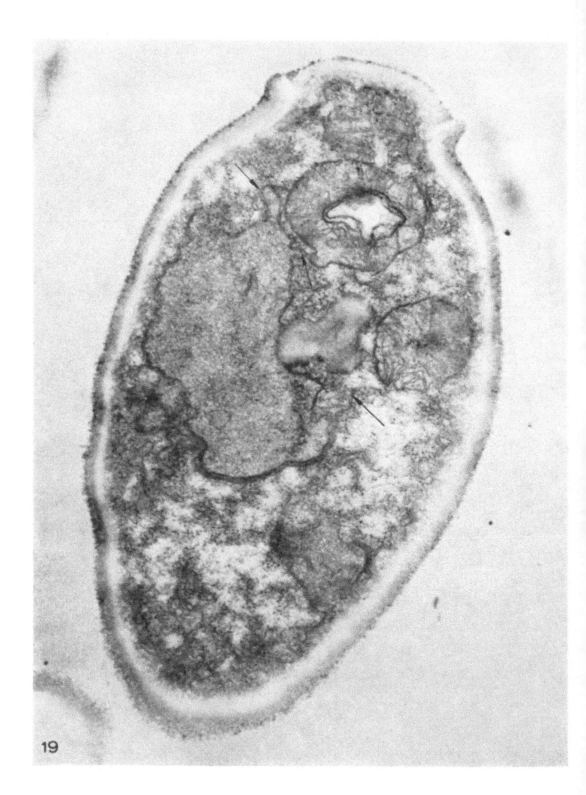

19

are reminiscent, for example, of structures described for *Plasmodium berghei* (Rudzinska, 1959) or for the anaerobically cultured yeast cell (Linnane, 1962), where they are supposed to possess mitochondrial functions. Possibly transitions occur between membranes and vesicles (Fig. 13), so that they may belong together. Organelles either consisting of vesicles or tubules or forming more or less elaborate systems of unit membranes have been reported for Actinomycetes (e.g., Stuart, 1959; Glauert, 1959–60; Hagedorn, 1959), Mycobacteria (e.g., Shinohara, 1958; Zapf, 1958; Koike, 1961), bacilli (e.g., Giesbrecht, 1960; Van Iterson, 1961), cocci and other gram-positive bacteria.

In the light of comparative morphology, what may be the significance of the membranous structures in bacteria? Shinohara *et al.* (1958), Kawano (1960), Giesbrecht (1960) and other authors consider them equivalent to mitochondria. However, the structure of true mitochondria is based on double membranes. Decisive in the evaluation of the character of the structures is their physiological activity. Mudd (1956) in particular has advocated that in bacteria oxidative-reductive events are localized in granules, whereas most authors follow Weibull (1953) in taking the plasma membrane as the locus of respiratory enzymes. There are two approaches to a decision in this controversy (Marr, 1960):

The first is direct cytochemistry. According to Barnett and Palade (1957) potassium tellurite, added to living cells, will accept electrons from respiratory enzyme systems. In Plate V, Fig. 14, of *B. subtilis* treated this way, the plasma membrane certainly did not gain in electron opacity owing to tellurite reduction, but the reaction products appear restricted to small areas, some connected perhaps with the insertion of the flagella or with the development of a cross wall; the organelles often seem darker than usual. In the gram-negative *Proteus* (Fig. 15) the gain in contrast with tellurite appears associated with details in the cytoplasmic fine structure (cf. Nermut, 1960).

The other approach to the localization of respiratory enzymes is analytical morphology. Recently Robrish and Marr (1962) published micrographs of fractions of *Azotobacter agilis* in which these enzymes were recovered in the large particle fraction, composed of all membranous structures of different shapes and sizes when centrifuged down after osmotic shock. Concurrently Mrs. G. Pandit-Hovenkamp prepared two fractions of the same organism, one (Fig. 16a) containing the cell walls, the largest membranes and some smaller ones, the other being composed of only very small membranous structures and ribosomes (Fig. 16b). Her small particle fraction had the higher specific activity of DPNH—oxidase and the higher P/O ratio obtained with DPNH oxidation. It should now be investigated whether after a better

PLATE VI, Fig. 19, *Pichia membranaefaciens*; × 56,000. In this yeast cell the nuclear envelope appears to continue as the outer composite membrane of the mitochondria. This is seen at the arrows at the upper mitochondrion and less clearly at the lower mitochondrion.

separation of the larger and the smaller membranes the latter display more respiratory activity, since they need not be fragments of the plasma membrane but may be integral elements of the living cell, as is borne out by Fig. 17. However, it is dangerous to draw any general conclusions about gram-negative bacteria from experiments with *Azotobacter*, since the amount of membranous vesicles seen in this organism is quite exceptional. We wonder whether the vesicles play a part in the nitrogen fixation process. The vesicles resemble those found by Vatter and Wolfe (1958) and others in *Rhodospirillum rubrum* and other photosynthetic bacteria. But in *Rhodospirillum* (Fig. 18) they undoubtedly represent the bacterial equivalents of plastids, called chromatophores by Pardee (1952) or grana by Thomas (1952). We wonder whether they are the functional equivalents of the grana discs or lamellae of the plastids of the larger cells. Lamellae bearing the photosynthetic pigments do occur in some bacteria and in the blue-green algae. There are some indications in partly autolysed *Rhodospirillum* cells that the vesicles and the plasma membrane are interconnected.

One might be tempted to conclude that in bacteria the various membranous structures, having functions analogous to those in the large cells, are derivatives of the plasma membrane. In addition for some of these organelles an obvious stage of contact with the nucleoplasm was demonstrated. Little is known about the origin of the membranous entities like the mitochondria in the large cells. Looking for stages intermediate in evolution we found in a yeast cell (Plate VI, Fig. 19) an instance in which the mitochondrial boundary appears to form a continuum with the nuclear envelope, which would define it as ER. This phenomenon emphasizes once again how numerous the potentialities of membranes are, the most conspicuous being marked structural and functional specialization and the attaining of relative independence, so striking in the higher stages of evolution.

ACKNOWLEDGMENTS

The author's thanks are due to Mr. W. Leene, Mr. J. L. F. Gerbrandij, Mr. H. van Heuven, Miss G. R. van Rhijn, Miss J. C. Kielich, Mrs. J. van den Berg-Koremans, Miss P. van Dillen, Mr. J. L. van Rij and Mr. N. Koster for their share in the work.

REFERENCES

Barnett, R. J., and G. E. Palade. 1957. Histochemical demonstration of the sites of activity of dehydrogenase systems with the electron microscope. J. Biophys. Biochem. Cytol. 3: 577–588.

Chapman, G. B., and J. Hillier. 1953. Electron microscopy of ultra thin sections of bacteria. I. Cellular division in *Bacillus cereus*. J. Bacteriol. 66: 362–373.

Conti, S. F., and M. E. Gettner. 1962. Electron microscopy of cellular division in *Escherichia coli*. J. Bacteriol. 83: 544–550.

Finean, J. B. 1961. Chemical ultrastructure in living tissues. Ed. by I. Newton Kugelmass. Charles C. Thomas, Springfield, Ill. U.S.A.

Fischer, A. 1903. Vorlesungen über Bakterien. Fischer, Jena.

Fitz-James, P. C. 1960. Participation of the cytoplasmic membrane in the growth and spore formation of bacilli. J. Biophys. Biochem. Cytol. 8: 507–528.

Giesbrecht, P. 1960. Ueber "organisierte" Mitochondrien und andere Feinstrukturen von *Bacillus megaterium*. Zentr. Bakteriol. Parasitenk., Abt. I., Orig. *179*: 538–582.

Glauert, A. M., and D. A. Hopwood. 1959. A membranous component of the cytoplasm in *Streptomyces coelicolor*. J. Biophys. Biochem. Cytol. *6*: 515–516.

Glauert, A. M., and D. A. Hopwood. 1960. The fine structure of *Streptomyces coelicolor*. J. Biophys. Biochem. Cytol. *3*: 479–488.

Glauert, A. M., E. M. Brieger and J. M. Allen. 1961. The fine structure of vegetative cells of *Bacillus subtilis*. Exptl. Cell Res. *22*: 73–85.

Hagedorn, H. 1959–60. Elektronenmikroskopische Untersuchungen an *Streptomyces griseus* (Krainsky). Zentr. Bakteriol. Parasitenk. *113*: 234–253.

Iterson, W. van. 1960. Membranes, particular organelles and peripheral bodies in bacteria. Proc. Eur. Reg. Conf. on Electron Microscopy, Delft 1960, *2*: 763–768.

Iterson, W. van. 1961. Some features of a remarkable organelle in *Bacillus subtilis*. J. Biophys. Biochem. Cytol. *9*: 183–192.

Iterson, W. van, and A. C. Ruys. 1960. On the nature of P.P.L.O. II. Electron microscopy. Antonie van Leeuwenhoek *26*: 9–22.

Iterson, W. van, and A. C. Ruys. 1960. The fine structure of the Mycoplasmataceae (Micro-organisms of the Pleuropneumoniae Group = PPLO). J. Ultrastructure Research *3*: 282–301.

Kawano, A. 1960. Studies on the fine structure of tubercle bacilli. Shikoku Acta Medica, supplement, *16*: 683–699.

Kellenberger, E., and A. Ryter. 1958. Cell wall and cytoplasmic membrane of *Escherichia coli*. J. Biophys. Biochem. Cytol. *4*: 323–326.

Koike, M., and K. Takeya. 1961. Fine structures of intracytoplasmic organelles of mycobacteria. J. Biophys. Biochem. Cytol. *9*: 597–608.

Linnane, W., E. Vitols and P. G. Nowland. 1962. Studies on the origin of yeast mitochondria. J. Cell. Biol. *13*: 345–354.

Marr, A. G. 1960. Localization of enzymes in bacteria. *In* The Bacteria, ed. I. C. Gunsalus and R. Y. Stanier, *1*: 443–465. Academic Press, New York.

Mitchell, P. 1959. Structure and function in micro-organisms. Biochem. Symp. *16*: 73–93.

Mudd, S. 1956. Cellular organization in relation to function. Bacteriol. Rev. *20*: 268–271.

Nermut, M. V. 1960. Ueber die Lage der Tellurit-Reduktionsorte in Zellen von *Proteus vulgaris*. Zentr. Bakteriol. Parasitenk., Abt. I. Orig. *178*: 348–356.

Pardee, A. B., H. K. Schachman and R. Y. Stanier. 1952. Chromatophores of *Rhodospirillum rubrum*. Nature *169*: 282–283.

Porter, K. R. 1961. The ground substance: observations from electron microscopy. *In* The Cell, ed. J. Brachet and A. E. Mirsky, *2*: 621–675. Academic Press, New York and London.

Robertson, J. D. 1959. The ultrastructure of cell membranes and their derivatives. Biochem. Symp. *16*: 3–43.

Robinow, C. F. 1962. On the plasma membrane of some bacteria and fungi. Circulation *26*: 1092–1104.

Robrish, S. A., and A. G. Marr. 1962. Location of enzymes in *Azotobacter agilis*. J. Bacteriol. *83*: 158–168.

Rudzinska, M. A., and W. Trager. 1959. Phagotrophy and two new structures in the malaria parasite *Plasmodium berghei*. J. Biophys. Biochem. Cytol. *6*: 103–112.

Ryter, A., and E. Kellenberger. 1958. Etude au microscope électronique de plasmas contenant de l'acide désoxyribonucléique. Z. Naturf. *13b*: 597–605.

Shinohara, Ch., K. Fukushi and J. Suzuki. 1958. Mitochondrial structure of *Mycobacterium tuberculosis* relating to its function. Japan. J. Electron Microscopy *6*: 47–52.

Stoeckenius, W. 1960. Osmium tetroxide fixation of lipids. Proc. Eur. Reg. Conf. on Electron Microscopy, Delft 1960, 2: 716–720.

Stuart, D. C. 1959. Fine structure of the nucleoid and internal membrane systems of Streptomyces. J. Bacteriol. *78*: 277–281.

Thomas, J. B. 1952. A note on the occurrence of grana in algae and in photosynthesizing bacteria. Proc. Ned. Ac. Wetensch. *55*, series C: 207–208.

Tulasne, R., R. Minck and A. Kirn. 1962. Etude comparative, au microscope électronique, d'un *Proteus* et des formes L des types A et B correspondantes. Ann. Inst. Pasteur *102*: 292–299.

Vatter, A. E., and R. S. Wolfe. 1958. The structure of photosynthetic bacteria. J. Bacteriol. *75*: 480–483.

Weibull, C. 1953. Characterization of the protoplasmic constituents of *Bacillus megaterium*. J. Bacteriol. *66*: 692–702.

Zapf, K. 1959. Vergleichende Untersuchungen zur Morphologie und Zytologie des *Mycobacterium tuberculosis* (BCG). Zentr. Bakteriol. Parasitenk. *174*: 253–263.

ASPECTS OF THE CONSTITUTION OF BACTERIAL MEMBRANES

E. KODICEK

Dunn Nutritional Laboratory
University of Cambridge and Medical Research Council
Cambridge, England

THE STUDIES of Mitchell (1953, 1954) have demonstrated the existence of an osmotic barrier, situated at the periphery of the bacterial cytoplasm but inside the cell wall, which regulates the exchange of matter between the interior of the bacterial cell and the external medium surrounding it. Information about the nature of this barrier could only be obtained after the important discovery that the bacterial cell wall of *Bacillus megaterium* can be removed by controlled treatment with lysozyme without lysis of the bacterial cytoplasm (Tomcsik & Guex-Holzer, 1952; Weibull, 1953). This stabilization of the naked protoplast could be achieved by treating the cells in a medium of high osmotic pressure, thus substituting for the cell wall. After transfer into a medium of low osmotic pressure, the spherical protoplasts burst and the cytoplasm was extruded leaving as a residue spherical, membranous "ghosts." From further studies (for literature see McQuillen, 1960) it became evident that the protoplasts derived from gram-positive bacteria are surrounded by a protoplasmic membrane that displayed the essential characteristics of a semipermeable structure (Weibull, 1955, 1958). Only a few bacterial species have been shown so far to be amenable to such a lysozyme treatment. The resulting "ghosts" represent the nearest approach to a pure membrane fraction that is at present possible. They very often contain granules that may be, but many probably are not, directly related to the membrane. There is thus a possibility of contamination derived from the cytoplasm and it is important to scrutinize analytical figures with this in view. For instance, small amounts of nucleic acids have been found in "ghosts" prepared from *B. megaterium* (Weibull & Bergström, 1958) but it appears that they are cytoplasmic contaminants. Some organisms which are not converted into true protoplasts may be also disrupted by various means as discussed by McQuillen (1960) and Marr (1960). The resulting particulate fraction will include the cytoplasmic membrane but can be heavily contaminated with other constituents of the bacterial cell or, on the other hand, may have lost some of the constituents normally associated with the cytoplasmic membrane.

We have attempted to prepare by various techniques protoplasts of *Lactobacillus casei*, but were not successful (Thorne & Kodicek, 1962a); the cells were therefore fractionated by differential centrifugation after being ultrasonically disrupted according to Mitchell & Moyle (1951) and a fraction was obtained which contained the membrane. I shall refer to it later. There is no doubt that lactobacilli have a distinct membrane and numerous associated membranous organelles (mesosomes), as described by Fitz-James (1960) for *Bacillus medusa* and *B. megaterium*, and by Glauert, Brieger and Allen (1961) for *Bacillus subtilis*. Electron micrographs of sectioned *L. acidophilus* (Glauert, Thorne & Kodicek, unpublished results) (Plate I) show a similar picture, but also the presence of a thick wall that is at least 40–50 mμ thick, twice the thickness of the wall of *B. subtilis* at a similar state of growth.

Suitable procedures have been devised to produce osmotically labile spheroplasts from gram-negative bacteria, but in view of the complex structure of their cell wall, the "ghost" fraction contains some lipoprotein of the wall as well as membrane. Hence, analyses and conclusions based on them as to the structure of the cytoplasmic membrane are bound to be only approximate. I intend therefore to deal only with investigations on gram-positive bacteria.

The semipermeable membrane consists mainly of a lipoprotein, as we shall see presently, and constitutes about 8–15 per cent of the dry weight of the bacterial cell. It has to withstand great osmotic pressures that have been calculated by Mitchell (1961a) to be sometimes as great as 20 atmospheres. The non-rigid membrane appears to be about 8 mμ thick (Thorsson & Weibull, 1958; Fitz-James, 1960) when measured *in situ*, while the membrane of the "ghosts" seems to be thicker, about 15 mμ, indicating that some exogenous material may still be adhering.

The dimensions are similar to those postulated for membranes of animal cells, but it would be an oversimplification to compare a mammalian cell with a bacterial cell. Not only are the dimensions vastly different, since the bacteria are comparable in size to mitochondria, but also the functional parameters are different. In many animal cells substances have to be transported across an oriented membrane into the cytoplasm; they then cross the interior metabolic compartments to be transferred by an exit mechanism across an oppositely oriented membrane into the extracellular environment. The situation in micro-organisms is simpler, in that substances entering the bacterial cell are metabolized and/or incorporated, but are not carried across the cytoplasm to be excreted for the benefit of other cells as in the animal cell population. This permits a relatively simpler definition of the function of the bacterial cytoplasmic membrane.

THE FUNCTION OF THE CYTOPLASMIC MEMBRANE

The semipermeable cytoplasmic membrane is by virtue of its constitution eminently suitable to support some if not all forms of transport mechanisms that have been proposed for the movement of electrolytes, non-electrolytes,

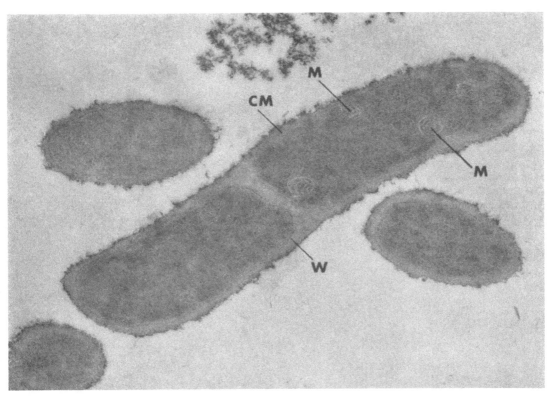

Plate I. Electron micrograph of a thin section of *L. acidophilus* (grown for 16 hr). The organisms have an unusually thick cell wall (W). Numerous mesosomes (M) are associated with the cytoplasmic membrane (CM) (Glauert, Thorne & Kodicek, unpublished results). × 60,000.

molecules or groups of molecules across cell membranes, namely: simple diffusion, solvent drag, diffusion restricted by membrane charge, diffusion restricted by a lipid barrier, facilitated diffusion, exchange diffusion and active carrier transport. Pinocytosis and phagocytosis, in animal cells, complete the list (Park, 1961). Some of these proposals are self-explanatory; diffusion restricted by a charge involves the movement of small anions, such as chloride, through positively charged aqueous channels; diffusion restricted by a lipid carrier would be concerned with the penetration of molecules of appropriate solubility characteristics that can dissolve first in the lipid and then in the aqueous phase. No pores are required in this instance. Facilitated diffusion (or mediated transport) is concerned with the accelerated transfer of molecules that combine reversibly with a carrier, mainly by hydrogen-bonding (Danielli, 1954), and this complex oscillates by thermal agitation between the surfaces to release or pick up molecules on either side; structural and steric factors are involved that provide hydrogen-bonding groups and proton conductors. Although no metabolic energy is required, this mechanism may result in transport against a concentration gradient if the penetrating molecule is continuously removed intracellularly either by being metabolized or by being converted into a bound form, or if there is a counterflow of a transport competitor. Exchange diffusion defines a mechanism in which the carrier can cross the membrane only in the complexed form. Net transport does not occur since, for each molecule moved inside, a similar molecule must be moved outside. If labelled substrates are being studied, this can give the erroneous impression of accumulation. In "active carrier transport" a concentration gradient is established requiring free energy such as that derived from the action of enzymes. The process is of great importance and permits the cell to concentrate substances from a relatively poor environment and to develop membrane potentials that can be as great as 50–70 mv (Kleinzeller, 1961).

I am afraid that this enumeration does not do justice to the complicated phenomena that occur in membranes. One cannot dissociate transport processes from the inherent metabolism of the membrane and of the cytoplasm with which it is closely associated. The cytoplasmic membrane should not be considered only as an organ of transport, but also as an integral part of the metabolism of the cell. Any alteration in the transport will affect the metabolism and any change in metabolism will cause a change in transport. This has been well expressed by Mitchell (1961b) in his concept of vectorial metabolism.

Transport and Metabolism

The presence of cytochromes and enzymes of the respiratory chain in membrane fractions (Storck & Wachsman, 1957; Weibull, Beckman & Bergström, 1959; Mitchell, 1959; Marr, 1960) provides important support to this thesis showing the possibility of a close structural and anatomical relationship between transport and metabolism. Subsequent contributors will deal with this problem in greater detail. Recently, adenosine triphosphate-cleaving enzymes have been found predominantly in the bacterial membrane, of *B. megaterium* (Weibull, Greenawalt & Löw, 1962; Greenawalt, Weibull & Löw, 1962) and of *Streptococcus faecalis* (Abrams, McNamara & Johnson, 1960). This finding of adenosine triphosphatase in the cell membrane emphasizes the interdependence of active transport and energy-rich phosphate bond metabolism. In this connection it may be of interest to note that adenosine triphosphatase has also been found in isolated cell membranes of red blood cells (Clarkson & Maizels, 1952; Post, Merritt, Kinsolving & Albright, 1960), of striated muscle (McCollester & Randle, 1961), of rat liver cells (Emmelot & Bos, 1962) and in membrane-derived material of the microsomal fraction of brain tissue (Hanzon & Toschi, 1960).

Abrams & McNamara (1962) found in the cytoplasmic membrane of metabolically lysed protoplasts of *S. faecalis* (ATCC No. 9790) a poly-nucleotide phosphorylase that produced polyadenylic acid and polyuridylic acid from adenosine diphosphate and uridine diphosphate, respectively, according to the equation:

$$n \, \text{ADP} \underset{}{\overset{\text{Mg}^{++}}{\rightleftharpoons}} \text{polyadenylic acid} + n \, \text{P}_i.$$

Little or no activity was in the soluble fraction, so that the presence of the polynucleotide phosphorylase in the membrane ghosts could not be due to contamination. The enzyme is thought of as a degradative enzyme, but on this assumption it is difficult at present to assess the significance of its localization in membranes.

Biosynthetic Mechanisms

A number of laboratories have provided evidence that some constituents of bacterial cell membranes, namely phospholipids, are involved in the uptake of amino acids (Hunter & Goodsall, 1961; Silberman & Gaby, 1961; Hill, 1962; Macfarlane, 1962a) and also in protein synthesis (Hunter, Brookes, Crathorn & Butler, 1959; Brookes, Crathorn & Hunter, 1959a; Godson & Hunter, 1961; Godson, Hunter & Butler, 1961; Hunter & Godson, 1961). Similar findings have been reported in mammalian cells for the incorporation of amino acids into liver phospholipids (Gaby & Silberman, 1960; Barnabei & Ferrari, 1961) and the possible involvement of lipids in protein synthesis has been studied in hen oviduct (Hendler, 1958, 1959a, b, 1960, 1962). The conclusion of Hendler was not confirmed by Haining, Fukui and Axelrod (1960) who failed to find any relationship between incorporation of amino acids into lipids and into protein of rat liver microsomes.

Some independent, though indirect evidence that there is a connection between lipid constituents of the cytoplasmic membrane and incorporation of amino acids and other substances is provided by the experiments of Dr. McQuillen and myself (see McQuillen, 1959) on the inhibitory effect of

TABLE 1

EFFECT OF LINOLEIC ACID AND VITAMIN D_2 ON THE UPTAKE
INTO "POOL" AND FIXATION OF ^{14}C-GLUTAMIC ACID BY *L. casei*

Linoleic acid µg/ml	Vitamin D_2 µg/ml	Counts/min		
		"Pool"	Fixed	Total
0	0	3600	1780	5380
5	0	4400	850	5250
10	0	5500	64	5564
5	20	3580	1640	5220
10	40	3840	1340	5180

Cells were incubated for 1 hr in glucose/phosphate containing
labelled glutamic acid ± linoleic acid ± vitamin D_2.
Similar results with ^{14}C-lysine and ^{14}C-arginine.

linoleic acid on the uptake of labelled compounds by *L. casei* and by
protoplasts of *B. megaterium*. A typical result is recorded in Table 1. While
the transport of amino acids was not impaired, as evidenced by the high
count in the "pool," the fixed fraction showed a great decrease in incorporation. We have suggested that the "pool" was perhaps not an obligatory stage
between exogenous substrate and fixed end-product. Linoleic acid might
penetrate into a lipid site (Kodicek, 1949, 1956) and uncouple transport
from biosynthetic systems that are located in or on the cytoplasmic membrane. Some of these interrelations are illustrated in Fig. 1.

Another synthetic mechanism that appears to be associated with the
cytoplasmic membrane has been studied by Markovitz and Dorfman (1962).
They report the synthesis of a capsular polysaccharide, hyaluronic acid, by
protoplast membranes of Group A Streptococcus. The preparations were
relatively free of nucleic acids and cell wall material, but the possibility
cannot be entirely discounted that the synthesizing activity is not only a

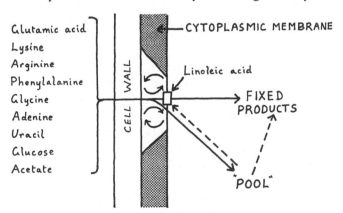

FIG. 1 Schematic interrelationship of systems studied with *L. casei*. Linoleic acid
inhibits incorporation of labelled substances into fixed products but has little or no
effect on uptake into "pool." Fixation may occur by a route independent of the "pool"
and this is closely integrated with transport mechanisms. The inhibition by linoleic
acid might occur at a site in the cytoplasmic membrane to uncouple the transport
from the subsequent synthetic reactions.

function of the membrane itself. The same considerations may apply to the finding of Brookes, Crathorn and Hunter (1959b) that peptide components of the cell wall of *B. megaterium* are synthesized at sites on or closely associated with the cytoplasmic membrane.

THE COMPOSITION OF THE CYTOPLASMIC MEMBRANE

Table 2 shows the composition of membranes of *B. megaterium, M. lyso-deikticus* and *Staph. aureus.* Despite the difference in species the distribution of the main constituents is fairly constant. The lipid component ranges from 18 to 37 per cent of the membrane dry weight; 50 to 80 per cent of the lipids

TABLE 2

COMPOSITION OF BACTERIAL MEMBRANES

(expressed as percentage of membrane dry weight)

	B. megaterium "M"[1]	"KM"[2]	*M. lysodeikticus*[3]	*Staph. aureus*[4] "Duncan"
Lipid:	18	—	28–37	22.5
neutral	—	12.9	9	—
phospholipid	—	10.0	28	(approx. 11.0)
Total P	1.3–1.6	0.4–1.8	1.2	1.7
Total N	10.6	12	8.4	9.5
Protein	67	75	50	41.0
Hexose	1–10	0.2–1.1	15–20	2.0

[1]Weibull & Bergström, 1958; Weibull, 1957.
[2]Yudkin, 1962.
[3]Gilby *et al.*, 1958; Macfarlane, 1961a.
[4]Mitchell & Moyle, 1951; Few, 1955.

are in the form of phospholipids. Proteins range from 50 to 75 per cent. A similar composition has been found in protoplast membranes of Group A streptococci by Freimer and Krause (1960). The amino acid composition (Gilby, Few & McQuillen, 1958; Weibull & Bergström, 1958) is fairly representative of normal proteins and enzymes that have been found in membranes (see Marr, 1960). An interesting finding is the large amount of mannose (15–20 per cent) in defatted membranes of *M. lysodeikticus* (Gilby *et al.*, 1958). The same sugar appears to be contained in a glycolipid complex, that yields on hydrolysis glycerophosphate, glycerol, mannose and fatty acids in molar ratio 1 : 1 : 1 : 4 (Macfarlane, 1961a). The occurrence of glucose in membranes of *B. megaterium* strain M (Weibull & Bergström, 1958) is less consistent, ranging from 1 to 10 per cent, and it was not found in strain KM (Yudkin, 1962).

Most of the nitrogen in membranes of *B. megaterium* strain M and of *M. lysodeikticus* can be accounted for by their protein content. In *B. mega-terium* strain KM (Yudkin, 1962) and in *Staph. aureus* (Few, 1955) high amounts of nitrogenous compounds are present in the membrane phospho-lipids while in the other bacterial membranes none were found, indicating that the high phosphorus content of these lipids must be due to the presence

TABLE 3

COMPOSITION OF MEMBRANE PHOSPHOLIPID

	B. megaterium[1] "M"	"KM"	M. lysodeikticus[2]	Staph. aureus[3]
Ethanolamine	0	+	0	+
Choline	0	0	0	0
Serine	0		0	+
Inositol	0		<1	
Nitrogen[4]	0	+	0	0.8
Phosphorus[4]	3.6	3.4	3.3–4.0	1.8

[1]Weibull, 1957; Yudkin, 1962.
[2]Gilby et al., 1958; Macfarlane, 1961a.
[3]Few, 1955: expressed as percentage of total lipid.
[4]Expressed as percentage of phospholipid.

TABLE 4

CHARACTERIZATION OF MEMBRANE PHOSPHOLIPIDS
(expressed as percentage of phospholipid)

	B. megaterium[1] "M"	"KM"	M. lysodeikticus[2]
Phosphatidic acids	90	—	68
Phosphatidylethanolamine	0	97	0
Phosphatidylinositol	0	—	5
Glycolipid complex (GP, G, mannose, fatty acid)	0	—	24

[1]Weibull, 1957; Yudkin, 1962.
[2]Macfarlane, 1961a.

of phosphatidic acids (Table 3). The occurrence of the various membrane phospholipids has been summarized in Table 4. The major part of the phospholipids in membranes of B. megaterium strain M and in M. lysodeikticus is in the form of phosphatidic acids. In the latter organism, cardiolipin-like diphosphatidylglycerol (G-P-G-P-G-lipid) and smaller amounts of mono-phosphatidylglycerol (G-P-G-lipid) have been isolated as the principal phospholipids (Macfarlane, 1961a, b). A similar result was obtained in Staph. aureus (Macfarlane, 1962b); on later investigation, it was found that the phosphatidylglycerol lipid contained about 60 per cent of amino acid esters (Macfarlane, 1962a). The other major phospholipid component of the M. lysodeikticus membrane is the glycolipid, mentioned earlier, that contains mannose. On the other hand, strain KM of B. megaterium seems to have almost all its phospholipid component as phosphatidylethanolamine, and small quantities of several amino acids were present (Yudkin, 1962).

The fatty acid composition of membranes from B. megaterium and M. lysodeikticus (Thorne & Kodicek, 1962b) is shown in Table 5. In both organisms, the major portion consists of branched-chain C_{15} acids; in M. lysodeikticus it is predominantly the anteiso-acid, 12-methyltetradecanoic acid (Macfarlane, 1961a). This is probably the main acid in Sarcina lipid (Akashi & Saito, 1960). In B. megaterium KM we have found equal amounts of the iso- and anteiso-acids, while Yudkin (1962) reports that the iso-acid,

TABLE 5

FATTY ACID COMPOSITION OF MEMBRANES FROM
B. megaterium KM AND *M. lysodeikticus*

Designation	Percentage composition	
	M. lysodeikticus	*B. megaterium*
14:br	1.1	3.0
14:0	0.8	2.6
15:br (iso)	}71.7	26.0
15:br (ante-iso)		28.9
15:0	1.5	2.9
16:br (iso)	0.6	1.3
16:br (ante-iso)	1.7	2.1
16:0	5.1	7.3
16:1	2.0	3.4
17:br (ante-iso)	3.3	2.6
17:1	0.6	1.3
18:0	2.3	2.6
18:1	2.4	8.8
20:1	1.2	0
21:0	0.4	2.0

13-methyltetradecanoic acid, predominates as it does in *B. subtilis* and *Bacillus natto* (Saito, 1960). The fatty acid composition of the neutral lipids was the same as that of the phospholipids (Yudkin, private communication).

The occurrence of branched-chain C_{15} fatty acids (with lesser amounts of C_{17} acids) is of interest in connection with the desired properties of an ideal semipermeable membrane. The branched chain fatty acids, which can originate from isoleucine and leucine (Lennarz, 1961), will resist being packed very closely in a surface film (Durham, 1955) and will thus give elasticity to a lamellar membrane, preventing its becoming rigid and brittle (Weitzel & Wojahn, 1951). These properties are highly desirable for a living membrane that is required to remain in a state of continuous transition.

The fatty acid composition of *L. casei* and of its "membrane" fraction, obtained by ultrasonic disruption and differential centrifugation (Thorne & Kodicek, 1962a), is shown in Table 6, together with that of membranes from striated muscles of the rat, prepared according to the method of McCollester (1962). It is apparent that the "membranes" of *L. casei* differ from whole cells by the significantly lower content of the C_{19}-propane acid, lactobacillic acid, and a somewhat higher proportion of the saturated fatty acids C_{14}, C_{16} and C_{18}. The principal components are palmitic, palmitoleic, vaccinic and lactobacillic acids and some branched fatty acids. Comparison of the membranes from *L. casei* and striated muscle show a remarkable similarity except that, instead of lactobacillic acid, linolenic acid was present in muscle membranes.

In none of the bacterial membranes nor in the muscle membrane did we find cholesterol. This agrees, for bacteria, with the negative findings of Weibull (1957) and of Fiertel and Klein (1959). Since lactobacilli have a

TABLE 6

FATTY ACID COMPOSITION OF LIPIDS FROM *L. casei*
AND MUSCLE MEMBRANES

Designation	*L. casei*[1]		Striated muscle[2] membranes %
	Whole cells %	"Membranes" %	
14:0	0.7	2.2	2.7
14:1	0	0.8	1.1
15:0	0.3	0.9	0.8
15:1	0	0	2.7
16:br (iso)	0.8	0.5	0
16:0	8.7	21.5	28.3
16:1	10.1	7.2	12.0
17:br (ante-iso)	0	1.1	0
17:0	0	1.6	0.7
17:1	2.0	4.5	1.7
18:br (iso)	0	1.1	0.9
18:0	1.4	6.8	8.5
18:1	26.1	21.7	20.8
18:2	0	0	13.6
19:br (ante-iso)	0	3.0	0
19:propane	49.4	16.6	0
21:0	0	8.3	0

[1]Thorne & Kodicek (1962b).
[2]Kodicek & McCollester (unpublished results).

specific requirement for mevalonic acid (MVA), a precursor of sterols, the possibility existed that MVA was converted into a substance which replaced sterols in bacteria. We have studied the fate of ^{14}C-MVA in lactobacilli (Thorne & Kodicek, 1962b, c, d), but although we found several labelled products, we have no evidence as yet of their localization in the cytoplasmic membrane.

Of the other unsaponifiable lipid constituents, carotenoids have been found in the cytoplasmic membrane of *B. megaterium* (Gilby *et al.*, 1958).

MOLECULAR BIOLOGY OF THE CYTOPLASMIC MEMBRANE

The significance of enzymes, be they permeases or those connected with the respiratory chain, will be dealt with by the subsequent contributors. I should like to discuss a different aspect of the same matter, namely, how far can molecular structure, particularly that of the lipid layer, affect the transporting function of membranes.

(1) Let us deal first with the lipid itself, which consists in the main of phospholipid. It is at present considered that the lipid layer forms a bimolecular leaflet with the hydrophobic ends of the molecules facing each other and the hydrophilic ends being arranged towards the protein layers between which the lipid is sandwiched and to which the hydrophilic groups are bound by ionic forces (Davson & Danielli, 1943) (Fig. 2a). A similar lamellar structure has been proposed by Stoeckenius (1959) on the basis of his electron microscope study of myelin figures. The only difference was

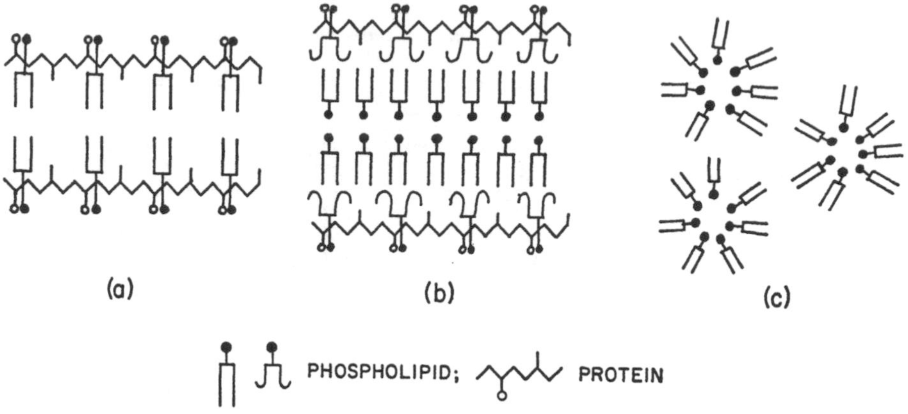

(a)   (b)   (c)

↑ ⌃ PHOSPHOLIPID; ∿∿ PROTEIN

FIG. 2. Schematic structure of cell membrane; (a) bimolecular leaflet of lipid according to Davson & Danielli (1943); (b) double bimolecular leaflet of lipid; phospholipid molecules nearest to the protein layer have the fatty acid chains bent back (according to Stoeckenius, 1959); (c) hexagonal phase of lipid, according to Luzzati & Husson, 1962; cylinders with hydrophilic groups of the lipid molecules facing inwards and forming a thin water channel.

that his smallest unit contained two bimolecular leaflets of lipid instead of one and, in its interior, contained a double layer of hydrophilic groups (Fig. 2b). To accommodate such a structure within a thickness of 8 mμ, as observed by him, he postulated that the hydrophobic side chains of the protein penetrate between the molecules of the lipid layer, forcing them apart and since these protein side chains are relatively short, the long fatty acid chains probably bend back to fill the gaps that would otherwise occur. Such a molecular arrangement would not be thicker than 8 mμ.

An arrangement of the bacterial membrane of the type described by Dourmashkin, Dougherty and Harris (1962) for animal cell membranes has not been observed so far. Dourmashkin *et al.* (1962) obtained an indentation of the membranes of red blood cells and of Rous sarcoma virus in a regular hexagonal form after treatment with saponin. The picture suggested that a lipid centre was surrounded by a ring of protein. This would imply that the lipid molecules are arranged as in a micelle with their hydrophilic groups facing the outside in the form of a globule or cylinder. No such arrangement has been found in bacterial membranes (Glauert & McQuillen, private communication, 1962), and electrophoretic studies of Few, Gilby and Seaman (1960) on protoplasts and membranes of *M. lysodeikticus* indicated that the lipid with groups of pK <1.0 was a component of the membrane but that it occupied an internal position sheathed by protein, as one would expect in a lamellar arrangement.

Another suggestion has been put forward by Luzzati and Husson (1962) on the basis of their studies of the structure of liquid-crystalline phases of lipid-water systems. Out of several possible structures, a natural phospholipid formed only two liquid-crystalline phases: a typical lamellar phase and a hexagonal phase which was a hexagonal array of cylinders, each cylinder being a thin water channel covered by the hydrophilic groups of the lipid molecules, facing inwards (Fig. 2c). A transition into a lamellar phase was effected by a lowering of the concentration of the phospholipid. Similar non-lamellar liquid-crystalline structures, if they existed *in vivo*, would have remarkable permeability properties. This would be particularly so if the lipoprotein could be in a state of phase transition depending on the concentration, temperature, electric potential and ion movement. All these parameters would cause drastic changes in the selective permeability of such a membrane.

If one adds to this the occurrence in the membrane of phosphatidic acids, in the form of phosphatidylglycerol (G-P-G) or diphosphatidylglycerol (G-P-G-P-G) which could combine reversibly with cations or amino acids, we have an extremely versatile phase system for the permeation of a great number of different molecules.

(2) The other aspect is the effect of the lipid constituents on the protein layer that is surrounding them and that consists of many active centres in the form of enzymes. I have previously suggested (Kodicek, 1949, 1956), on the basis of our studies with long-chain unsaturated fatty acids, that any alteration of the lipid structure by penetration of lipid molecules and consequent increased pressure will distort spatially the protein layer that is anchored with its hydrophobic groups in the lipid. This will produce a change in the spatial arrangement of the functional groups of enzymes and could be followed by changes in their activities. In a similar way, Strickland and Benson (1960) speculate about the potentialities of a diphosphatidyl-glycerol lipid that might be bonded to a membrane enzyme in such a way as to alter its structure and enzyme properties. The authors pointed out that "the hydrogen-bonding and ionic-bonding potentialities of G-P-G-P-G lipid are especially relevant since it can form two bonds, one with each of the two phosphate diesters."

This hypothetical picture of the function of membrane lipids is certainly oversimplified and any generalized molecular theory of transport will have to take into account the presence, in some instances, of glycolipids, of proteolipids and of small, but significant amounts of unsaponifiable matter of unknown function.

ACKNOWLEDGMENTS

I wish to thank Drs. A. M. Glauert, K. J. I. Thorne, M. G. Macfarlane, D. L. McCollester and M. D. Yudkin for allowing me to report some of the unpublished work. I am very grateful to Dr. K. McQuillen for helpful discussions and criticism.

REFERENCES

Abrams, A. and P. McNamara. 1962. Polynucleotide phosphorylase in isolated bacterial cell membranes. J. Biol. Chem. 237: 170–175.

Abrams, A., P. McNamara and F. B. Johnson. 1960. Adenosine triphosphatase in isolated bacterial cell membranes. J. Biol. Chem. *235*: 2639–3662.

Akashi, S. and K. Saito. 1960. A branched chain saturated C_{15}-acid (sarcinic acid) from *Sarcina* phospholipides and a similar acid from several microbial lipides. J. Biochem., Tokyo, *47*: 222–229.

Barnabei, O. and R. Ferrari. 1961. Incorporation of labelled amino acids into a lipid fraction of the isolated rat liver. Arch. Biochem. Biophys. *94*: 79–84.

Brookes, P., A. R. Crathorn and G. D. Hunter. 1959a. The incorporation of labelled amino acids into protein by the isolated cytoplasmic membrane of *Bacillus megaterium*. Biochem. J. *71*: 31P.

Brookes, P., A. R. Crathorn and G. D. Hunter. 1959b. Site of synthesis of the peptide component of the cell wall of *Bacillus megaterium*. Biochem. J. *73*: 396–401.

Clarkson, E. M. and M. Maizels. 1952. Distribution of phosphatases in human erythrocytes. J. Physiol. *116*: 112–128.

Danielli, J. F. 1954. Morphological and molecular aspects of active transport. Symp. Soc. Exptl. Biol. 8: 502–516.

Davson, H. and J. F. Danielli. 1943. The permeability of natural membranes, pp. 64–65. Cambridge University Press.

Dourmashkin, R. R., R. M. Dougherty and R. J. C. Harris. 1962. Electron microscopic observations on Rous sarcoma virus and cell membranes. Nature *194*: 1116–1119.

Durham, K. 1955. The interaction of monolayers of branched-chain fatty acids with calcium ions in the underlying solution. J. Applied Chem. 5: 686–692.

Emmelot, P. and C. J. Bos. 1962. Adenosine triphosphatase in the cell-membrane fraction from rat liver. Biochim. et Biophys. Acta 58: 374–375.

Few, A. V. 1955. Interaction of polymyxin E with bacterial and other lipids. Biochim. et Biophys. Acta *16*: 137–145.

Few, A. V., A. R. Gilby and G. V. F. Seaman. 1960. An electrophoretic study on structural components of *Micrococcus lysodeikticus*. Biochim. et Biophys. Acta 38: 130–136.

Fiertel, A. and H. P. Klein. 1959. On sterols in bacteria. J. Bacteriol. 78: 738–739.

Fitz-James, P. C. 1960. Participation of the cytoplasmic membrane in the growth and spore formation of bacilli. J. Biophys. Biochem. Cytol. 8: 507–528.

Freimer, E. H. and R. M. Krause. 1960. Chemical and immunological studies of protoplast membranes of *Group A Streptococci*. Fed. Proc. *19*: 244.

Gaby, W. L. and R. Silberman. 1960. The role of phospholipides in the metabolism of amino acids. II. The incorporation of leucine and tyrosine in liver phospholipides. Arch. Biochem. Biophys. 87: 188–192.

Gilby, A. R., A. V. Few, and K. McQuillen. 1958. Chemical composition of the protoplast membrane of *Micrococcus lysodeikticus*. Biochim. et Biophys. Acta 29: 21–29.

Glauert, A. M., E. M. Brieger and J. M. Allen. 1961. The fine structure of vegetative cells of *Bacillus subtilis*. Exptl. Cell Res. *22*: 73–85.

Glauert, A. M., K. J. I. Thorne and E. Kodicek. Unpublished results.

Godson, G. N. and G. D. Hunter. 1961. The role of phospholipids in protein biosynthesis. Biochem. J. 79: 37P.

Godson, G. N., G. D. Hunter and J. A. V. Butler. 1961. Cellular components of *Bacillus megaterium* and their role in protein biosynthesis. Biochem. J. *81*: 59–68.

Greenawalt, J. W., C. Weibull and H. Löw. 1962. The hydrolysis of adenosine triphosphate by cell fractions of *Bacillus megaterium*. II. Stimulation and inhibition of the enzymic activities. J. Biol. Chem. *237*: 853–858.

Haining, J. L., T. Fukui and B. Axelrod. 1960. Incorporation of amino acids into lipoidal material by microsomal and supernatant fractions of rat tissues. J. Biol. Chem. 235: 160–164.

Hanzon, V. and G. Toschi. 1960. Centrifugation of brain microsomes in a density gradient. Exptl. Cell Res. 21: 332–346.

Hill, P. B. 1962. Incorporation of orthophosphate into phospholipid by isolated membrane fractions of bacteria. Biochim. et Biophys. Acta 57: 386–389.

Hendler, R. W. 1958. Possible involvement of lipids in protein synthesis. Science 128: 143–144.

Hendler, R. W. 1959a. Passage of radioactive amino acids through "non-protein" fractions of hen oviduct during incorporation into protein. J. Biol. Chem. 234: 1466–1473.

Hendler, R. W. 1959b. Studies with lipid soluble amino acid complexes formed in hen oviduct during protein synthesis. Fed. Proc. 18: 245.

Hendler, R. W. 1960. Further studies with amino acid lipid complexes formed in hen oviduct during protein synthesis. Fed Proc. 19: 346.

Hendler, R. W. 1962. Further characterisation of amino acid-lipid complex from hen oviduct. Biochim. et Biophys. Acta 60: 90–97.

Hunter, G. D., P. Brookes, A. R. Crathorn and J. A. V. Butler. 1959. Intermediate reactions in protein synthesis by the isolated cytoplasmic-membrane fraction of Bacillus megaterium. Biochem. J. 73: 369–376.

Hunter, G. D. and G. N. Godson. 1961. Later stages of protein synthesis and role of phospholipids in the process. Nature 189: 140–141.

Hunter, G. D. and R. A. Goodsall. 1061. Lipo amino acid complexos from Bacillus megaterium and their possible role in protein synthesis. Biochem. J. 78: 564–570.

Kleinzeller, A. 1961. Discussion, in Membrane transport and metabolism, ed. A. Kleinzeller and A. Kotyk, p. 111. Academic Press, London, New York.

Kodicek, E. 1949. The effects of unsaturated fatty acids on gram-positive bacteria. Symp. Soc. Exptl. Biol. 3: 217–232.

Kodicek, E. 1956. The effect of unsaturated fatty acids, of vitamin D and other sterols on gram-positive bacteria. In Biochemical problems of lipids, ed. G. Popják and E. LeBreton, pp. 401–406. Butterworth Scientific Publications, London.

Lennarz, W. J. 1961. The role of isoleucine in the biosynthesis of branched-chain fatty acids by Micrococcus lysodeikticus. Biochem. Biophys. Res. Communications 6: 112–116.

Luzzati, V. and F. Husson. 1962. The structure of the liquid-crystalline phases of lipid-water systems. J. Cell Biol. 12: 207–219.

Macfarlane, M. G. 1961a. Composition of lipid from protoplast membranes and whole cells of Micrococcus lysodeikticus. Biochem. J. 79: 4P.

Macfarlane, M. G. 1961b. Isolation of a phosphatidylglycerol and a glycolipid from Micrococcus lysodeikticus cells. Biochem. J. 80: 45P.

Macfarlane, M. G. 1962a. Private communication.

Macfarlane, M. G. 1962b. Lipid components of Staphylococcus aureus and Salmonella typhimurium. Biochem. J. 82: 40P–41P.

Markovitz, A. and A. Dorfman. 1962. Synthesis of capsular polysaccharide (hyaluronic acid) by protoplast membrane preparations of Group A Streptococcus. J. Biol. Chem. 237: 273.

Marr, A. G. 1960. Enzyme localization in bacteria. Ann. Rev. Microbiol. 14: 241–260.

McCollester, D. L. and P. J. Randle. 1961. Isolation and some enzymic activities of muscle-cell membranes. Biochem. J. 78: 27P.

McCollester, D. L. 1962. A method for isolating skeletal-muscle cell-membrane components. Biochim. et Biophys. Acta 57: 427–437.

McQuillen, K. 1959.   Some aspects of bacterial structure and function: Observations on bacterial cell walls, protoplasts and spheroplasts together with a study of the effects of linoleic acid and vitamin D_2 on *Lactobacillus casei*. Fourth International Congress of Biochemistry, *13* (Colloquia): 406–429. Pergamon Press, London.

McQuillen, K. 1960.   Bacterial protoplasts. *In* The Bacteria, ed. I. C. Gunsalus and R. Y. Stanier, *1*: 249–359. Academic Press, New York.

Mitchell, P. 1953.   Transport of phosphate across the surface of *Micrococcus pyogenes*: Nature of the cell "inorganic" phosphate. J. Gen. Microbiol. *9*: 273–287.

Mitchell, P. 1954.   Transport of phosphate through an osmotic barrier. Symp. Soc. Exptl. Biol. *8*: 254–261.

Mitchell, P. 1959.   Biochemical cytology of micro-organisms. Ann. Rev. Microbiol. *13*: 407–440.

Mitchell, P. 1961a.   Discussion, *in* Membrane transport and metabolism, ed. A. Kleinzeller and A. Kotyk, p. 108. Academic Press, London, New York.

Mitchell, P. 1961b. Coupling of phosphorylation to electron and hydrogen transfer by a chain-osmotic type of mechanism. Nature *191*: 144–148.

Mitchell, P. and J. Moyle. 1951.   The glycerophospho-protein complex envelope of *Micrococcus pyogenes* strain Duncan. J. Gen. Microbiol. *5*: 981–992.

Park, C. R. 1961.   General aspects of transport phenomena. *In* Membrane transport and metabolism, ed. A. Kleinzeller and A. Kotyk, pp. 19–21. Academic Press, London, New York.

Post, R. L., C. R. Merritt, C. R. Kinsolving and C. D. Albright. 1960.   Membrane adenosine triphosphatase as a participant in the active transport of sodium and potassium in the human erythrocyte. J. Biol. Chem. *235*: 1796–1802.

Saito, K. 1960.   Bacterial fatty acids. Structure of subtilopentadecanoic and subtiloheptadecanoic acids. J. Biochem., Tokyo, *47*: 710–719.

Silberman, R. and W. L. Gaby. 1961.   The uptake of amino acids by lipids of *Pseudomonas aeruginosa*. J. Lipid Res. *2*: 172–176.

Strickland, E. H. and A. A. Benson. 1960. Neutron activation paper chromatographic analysis of phosphatides in mammalian cell fractions. Arch. Biochem. Biophys. *88*: 344–348.

Stoeckenius, W. 1959.   An electron microscope study of myelin figures. J. Biophys. Biochem. Cytol. *5*: 491–500.

Storck, R. and J. T. Wachsman. 1957.   Enzyme location in *Bacillus megaterium*. J. Bacteriol. *73*: 784–790.

Thorne, K. J. I. and E. Kodicek. 1962a. The metabolism of acetate and mevalonic acid by lactobacilli. III. Studies on the unsaponifiable lipids of *Lactobacillus casei* from mevalonic acid. Biochim. et Biophys. Acta *59*: 295–306.

Thorne, K. J. I. and E. Kodicek. 1962b. The metabolism of acetate and mevalonic acid by lactobacilli. IV. Analysis of the fatty acids by gas-liquid chromatography. Biochim. et Biophys. Acta *59*: 306–312.

Thorne, K. J. I. and E. Kodicek. 1962c. The metabolism of acetate and mevalonic acid by lactobacilli. I. The effect of acetate and mevalonic acid on growth. Biochim. et Biophys. Acta *59*: 273–279.

Thorne, K. J. I. and E. Kodicek. 1962d.   The metabolism of acetate and mevalonic acid by lactobacilli. II. The incorporation of [^{14}C] acetate and [^{14}C] mevalonic acid into the bacterial lipids. Biochim. et Biophys. Acta *59*: 280–294.

Thorsson, K. G. and C. Weibull. 1958.   Studies on the structure of bacterial L forms, protoplasts and protoplast-like bodies. J. Ultrastructure Res. *1*: 412–427.

Tomcsik, J. and S. Guex-Holzer. 1952.   Aenderung der Struktur der Bakterienwälle in Verlauf der Lysozym—Einwirkung. Schweiz. Z. Allgem. Pathol. u. Bakteriol. *15*: 517–525.

Weibull, C. 1953. The isolation of protoplasts from *Bacillus megaterium* by controlled treatment with lysozyme. J. Bacteriol. *66*: 688–695.

Weibull, C. 1955. Osmotic properties of protoplasts of *Bacillus megaterium*. Exptl. Cell Res. *9*: 294–304.

Weibull, C. 1957. The lipids of a lysozyme sensitive *Bacillus* species (Bacillus "M"). Acta Chem. Scand. *11*: 881–892.

Weibull, C. 1958. Bacterial protoplasts. Ann. Rev. Microbiol. *12*: 1–26.

Weibull, C., H. Beckman and L. Bergström. 1959. Localization of enzymes in *Bacillus megaterium*, strain M. J. Gen. Microbiol. *20*: 519–531.

Weibull, C. and L. Bergström. 1958. The chemical nature of the cytoplasmic membrane and cell wall of *Bacillus megaterium*, strain M. Biochim. et Biophys. Acta *30*: 340–351.

Weibull, C., J. W. Greenawalt and H. Löw. 1962. The hydrolysis of adenosine triphosphate by cell fractions of *Bacillus megaterium*. I. Localization and general characteristics of the enzyme activities. J. Biol. Chem. *237*: 847–852.

Weitzel, G. and J. Wojahn. 1951. Biochemie verzweigter Carbonsäuren. VII. Mitteilung. Darstellung der racemischen Monomethyl-stearinsäuren. Hoppe-Seyl. Z. physiol. Chem. *287*: 296–310.

Yudkin, M. D. 1962. Chemical studies of the protoplast membrane of *Bacillus megaterium* KM. Biochem. J. *82*: 40P.

PERMEASES: IDENTIFICATION AND MECHANISM

A. KEPES

Service de Biochimie Cellulaire
Institut Pasteur, Paris, France

THE MEMBRANE of the microbial cell is known to be very poorly permeable to highly hydrophilic substances. Most nutrients, sugars, organic acids and amino acids are of this class. This fact leads to the postulation of a great number of specialized mechanisms to account for the uptake of most nutrients which cannot flow through the membrane by purely physical forces.

A mechanism such as pinocytosis would account for a non-specific uptake of the solutes present in the environment even if the process is triggered by specific stimulatory agents, since the formation of a vesicle would inevitably include a random sample of the medium.

To explain the specific uptake of hydrophilic molecules from the medium, three different kinds of mechanisms can be *a priori* invoked.

The first would be a specific transport process either thermodynamically active or passive. It involves the binding of the transported molecule onto a specific site present in the surface structure of the cell and, as an ultimate result, the release of the unchanged transported molecule into the protoplasm as aqueous solute. When such a specialized system of transport includes a protein with a specific binding site for the transported substrate, it is defined as a permease system, the specific protein being the permease (Cohen & Monod, 1957).

A second mechanism used by cells to take up nutrients for which no specific transport mechanism exists, includes an enzyme either at the outer surface of the membrane or excreted into the medium, which breaks down the molecule to another form, for example, hydrolyses a disaccharide into two hexose molecules before the actual step of uptake (Sols & LaFuente, 1961). Such systems have been observed in yeast for disaccharides and the bacterial enzymes levan sucrase and dextran sucrase can be considered as fulfilling, among others, such a function. This mechanism is most common when large molecules, for example starch and proteins, serve as nutrients.

A third possibility is known as the group transfer (Mitchell, 1957), which includes one or several enzymes oriented in the cell membrane in such a way that the substrate binds to the active site on the external side and the product is released on the intracellular face. In the general case the product is different from the substrate. If the sequence of reactions is such that the final product is the same molecule as the first substrate, the system performs transport and is indistinguishable from a permease.

IDENTIFICATION OF BACTERIAL PERMEASES

The present paper deals only with permeases. All recognized permeases in bacteria (Table 1) perform active transport, but because of methodological difficulties in clearly establishing passive transport, the possibility of a number of passively transporting permeases cannot be ruled out. In such a case the intracellular concentration of the substrate could be much smaller than the concentration in the medium since metabolism tends to deplete the pool, and so the unchanged substrate might be difficult to identify.

TABLE 1
PERMEASES IDENTIFIED IN *E. coli*

Sugars	β-galactosides
	galactose
	maltose
	β-glucuronides
	α-glucosides (glucose)
Amino acids	Arginine, ornithine (lysine)
	Acetyl ornithine
	Phenylalanine (tyrosine)
	Methionine
	Valine, leucine, isoleucine
	Glycine, alanine, d-serine
	Histidine
	Proline
	Tryptophan
Ions	Potassium

In order to demonstrate that the permease controls the uptake of a given nutrient into the bacterial cell, one has to obtain experimental evidence: (a) that the unchanged substrate has been transported into the interior of the cell; (b) that a binding site exists which combines with the transported substrate; (c) that this binding site exhibits a specificity for the configuration of the substrate molecule and that it governs the uptake of substrate.

The experimental findings which help establish these points will be discussed in connection with two permeases; one is the β-galactoside permease, the experimental evidence for which is the most abundant, and the second the glucose permease which still raises some difficulties so that demonstration cannot be considered definitive.

THE β-GALACTOSIDE PERMEASE OF E. COLI

1.(a) The β-galactoside permease cannot accumulate its natural substrate lactose or ortho-nitrophenyl galactoside (ONPG), the chromogenic substrate widely used for β-galactosidase activity measurements, in the wild type of *Escherichia coli*. In fact these two galactosides are hydrolyzed in the protoplasm at such a high rate that the intracellular pool is depleted to nearly zero. But mutants unable to grow on lactose have been selected which are devoid of the capacity to synthesize β-galactosidase. These mutants, called Lac⁻ absolute, if properly induced, can accumulate lactose or ONPG far above the concentration in the medium.

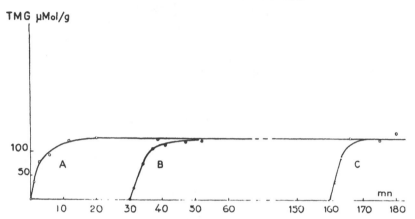

FIG. 1. Time course of uptake and exchange of methyl thiogalactoside (TMG) by a suspension of *E. coli* ML 308; temperature 15 C. Curve A: 10^{-3} M ^{14}C TMG added at time zero. Curves B and C: 10^{-3} M ^{12}C TMG added at time zero, and TMG ^{14}C at 30 and 160 min. Final concentration and specific activity of substrate is identical in all samples. Aliquots of 1 ml containing 180 μg dry cells were filtered on Millipore membrane filters and radioactivity was measured.

Beta-thiogalactosides which include an atom of sulphur in place of oxygen in the osidic linkage of galactosides, are not hydrolyzed by β-galactosidase. These analogues of the natural substrate (Rickenberg *et al.*, 1956) can be accumulated above the level in the external medium in the wild type, as in the Lac⁻ absolute mutants (Fig. 1). The accumulated substrate, either O-galactoside or thiogalactoside, can be extracted from the cell by mild procedures and characterized as the unchanged substrates. The finding by Sistrom (1958) that accumulated thiogalactosides contribute to the intracellular osmotic pressure in spheroplasts possessing the permease, supports the view that they are present in the protoplasm as chemically unchanged free solutes. This illustrates two conditions which favor accumulation of free substrate: one is a non-metabolizable analogue, the second is lack of active metabolic enzyme(s) as a result of mutation or in some other cases by the use of specific inhibitors.

(*b*) The level to which the galactoside is accumulated inside the cell by galactoside permease depends on the external concentration of substrate according to a Langmuir adsorption isotherm. If initial rates of uptake are measured, it is found that they depend on the external concentration according to the same law, which can be termed here the Michaelis law

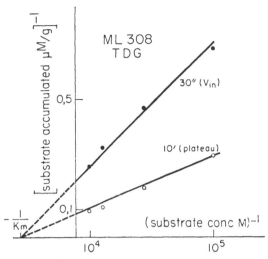

FIG. 2. Concentration dependence of the uptake of thio-di-galactoside (TDG) by *E. coli* ML 308. Reciprocal plot. The uptake in 30 sec after addition of the radioactive substrate is closely proportional to the initial rate of uptake. The uptake after 10 min measures the steady state accumulation.

(Fig. 2) (Kepes & Monod, 1957). The affinity constants K_m are the same for plateau values and initial velocities. The maximal accumulation obtainable with saturating concentrations of various substrates can differ as widely as 9 μmoles per gram dry weight for ONPG at 37° and more than 500 μmoles per gram for lactose at 4° (Table 2). Nevertheless, all galactosides and thiogalactosides compete with each other for the same system and can either completely displace a previously accumulated analogue or, if added before, completely prevent its uptake. The fact that neither the steady state accumulation level nor the initial velocity of uptake increases indefinitely with increasing concentrations of substrate, but tend to be saturated, as well as the competition of related molecules, at both of these stages, demonstrates the existence of a binding site which governs the rate limiting step of the uptake. Another proof of such a binding site and an identification of it as a part of a protein, derives from experiments with protein group reagents. Two classes of protein group reagents, namely SH reagents and reagents for amino groups, are inhibitory of permease activity. Inactivation can be demonstrated with parachloromercuri-benzoate, a typical SH reagent (Kepes, 1961), and with dinitrofluorobenzene, a typical amino reagent. If inactivation is tested with any of these reagents in the presence of a saturating concentration of thiodigalactoside, a strong protective effect is observed. This testifies that the protein group reagents bind at, or near, the specific site of substrate binding.

(c) The specificity of this structure responsible for galactoside accumulation and supported by a protein molecule is duly illustrated by the mutual competition of all β-thiogalactosides and by lack of competition of very

TABLE 2
Kinetic Parameters of β-Galactoside Permease

	Thiomethyl-galactoside	Thiodi-galactoside	Thiophenyl-galactoside	Lactose	O-nitrophenyl galactoside
Michaelis constant K_m (mole/liter)	5.10^{-4}	2.10^{-5}	$2.5 \quad 10^{-4}$	7.10^{-5}	10^{-3}
Capacity Y (μmole/g)	14 C 300 26 C 160 34 C 52	40	32	4 C 550 34 C 125	14 C 29 34 C 9
Time for half equilibrium $t^{\frac{1}{2}}$(min)	0.75	1.35	0.25	2.4	—
Maximal rate of uptake V_{in}^{max}(μmole/g/min)	148	20.4	86	158	—
Exit rate constant k_{ex}(ml/g/min)	0.82	0.59	2.7	—	—
Maximal concentration ratio G_{in}/G_{ex}	65	400	26	1950	—

Strain ML 308 was used for thiogalactosides TMG, TDG and TPG. Strain W2244 was used for lactose and ONPG. Temperature is 26 C unless otherwise stated. [14]C labelled TMG and lactose, ^{35}S labelled TPG and TDG are used. Incubation in growth medium with 50μg/ml chloromycetin added. At intervals 1 ml aliquots are pipetted on HA millipore filters previously covered with 6 ml ice cold mineral medium, vacuum filtered and rinsed twice with cold medium. Radioactivity is measured directly after drying in a thin window counter. Values are calculated from Lineweaver-Burk plots for K_m, V_{in} and Y, $t_{\frac{1}{2}}$ and k_{ex} from semilogarithmic plots. Maximal concentration ratio is Y/K_m/cell water/g dry wt. Cell water is assumed to be about 4 ml per gram. V^{max} and G_{in}/G_{ex} values for lactose are approximate extrapolations from experiments done at different temperatures. ONPG accumulation is measured at the steady state only by a spectrophotometric technique.

closely related molecules such as phenyl-thioglucoside. Another argument for the existence of such a specific structure comes from the finding of mutants devoid of permease. These mutants cannot grow on lactose and cannot accumulate thiogalactosides although they can be induced to synthesize a full complement of β-galactosidase which hydrolyzes lactose to glucose and galactose, both of which can support the growth of this bacteria. These mutants are called cryptic toward lactose (Cohen & Monod, 1957; Richenberg et al., 1956). The mutation to permeaseless did not impair any of the metabolic enzymes involved in lactose utilization, thus permease is distinct from metabolic enzymes. A further discrimination of β-galactoside permease from any other transport mechanism comes from the specific inducibility of its synthesis. As opposed to mutants of the structural genes, induced synthesis does not discriminate between galactoside permease and β-galactosidase, which are both induced in a coordinated way by the same inducers, but no other transport mechanism is induced or repressed under the same conditions (Stoeber, 1957; Horecker et al., 1960a).

2. *The a glucoside permease of E. coli.* It appears from the description below that *E. coli* possesses a distinct permease for a methyl glucoside. The discussion is primarily aimed to clarify its physiological role as the normal mechanism of glucose uptake.

(a) The existence of glucose permease in *E. coli* is based on the evidence of mutants observed by Doudoroff et al. (1949) which cannot grow on glucose, although they have normal hexokinase and glycolytic cycle enzymes. Halvorson et al. (1955) showed that these mutants cannot accumulate a methyl glucoside as the wild type does constitutively. a methyl glucoside is not metabolized by *E. coli* and its accumulation follows the same pattern as the accumulation of β-galactosides by the relevant permease. In contrast intracellular free glucose cannot be demonstrated since it is metabolized at a high rate by constitutive enzymes. No mutant devoid of metabolic enzymes for glucose has been isolated, presumably because such mutation would be lethal.

(b) The binding site responsible for a methyl glucoside accumulation is evidenced by its saturation and by the competitive effect of glucose. The Michaelis constant of glucose is very low. The K_m of a methyl glucoside is 10^{-4} M.

(c) The specific mutation observed by Doudoroff which impairs both glucose uptake and accumulation of a methyl glucoside provides good evidence for a common binding site with stringent stereospecificity. Moreover twelve independent clones of glucose positive transductants from the glucose negative strain recovered the ability to concentrate a methyl glucoside at the same time. Nevertheless, it is difficult to prove that this specific site plays the same role with glucose as with a methyl glucoside. Glucose is known to interfere with the functioning of several distinct permeases, either by speeding up the exit (Kepes, 1960; G. Ames, personal communication) or by providing an extra energy source (Britten & McClure, 1958).

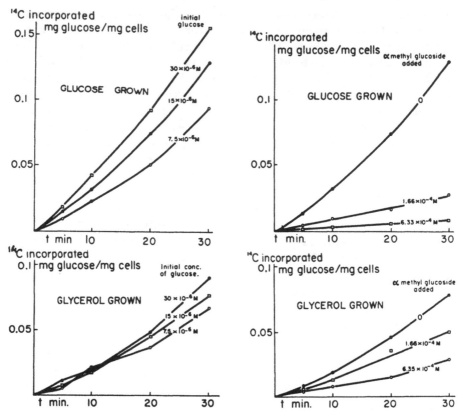

Fig. 3. Time course of incorporation of ^{14}C glucose by a growing culture of *E. coli* ML 308. Cultures were grown overnight on glycerol or glucose as sole carbon source respectively. They were harvested in the exponential growth phase and re-suspended in identical media containing ^{14}C glucose and ^{12}C glycerol. Aliquots were treated with cold trichloracetic acid and filtered on Millipore membranes. Glucose uptake is assumed to be rate-limiting for glucose incorporation. Note the very low concentrations of glucose used. The affinity for glucose and the competition of α-methyl glucoside are changed by the previous growth on glucose.

The competition of α methyl glucoside against glucose uptake could be demonstrated when using very low concentrations of glucose in highly diluted cell suspensions so that the concentration of glucose in the medium could be maintained approximately constant (Fig. 3). The competitive effect is observed to its full extent with the bacteria grown on glucose, but it is very slight if any with bacteria grown on glycerol. Still, the latter assimilate glucose at nearly the same initial rate as the former. This contradiction suggests that two different mechanisms exist for glucose uptake, a constitutive one which would be repressed by growth on glucose, and a second which would be induced under the same conditions. This second mechanism is susceptible to α methyl glucoside competition. This hypothesis is difficult to reconcile with the finding that α methyl glucoside is accumulated constitutively. The finding of two different mechanisms for uptake of the same nutrient is not unprecedented. G. Ames (personal communication) observed that histidine uptake in *Salmonella* has two components, one with a high affinity and a stringent specificity for histidine, and another with a low affinity which is susceptible to competition by several unrelated amino acids.

MECHANISMS

Very little is known about the mechanisms of permeases. The permease protein escapes isolation since no test is available once the bacterial cell is disrupted.

LOCATION OF THE PERMEASE SITE

β-galactoside permease effects transport at a rate which depends only on the extracellular concentration of substrate and not on the intracellular pool (Kepes & Monod, 1957) (Fig. 1). The same holds for methionine-permease and for valine-leucine-isoleucine-permease, i.e., turnover occurs at the same velocity as initial uptake (Kepes, 1961). This can be interpreted as showing that the rate limiting site is accessible to extracellular but not to intracellular substrate. The integrity of permease functions in lysozyme spheroplasts (Sistrom, 1958) shows that permease is not located in the rigid cell wall, but rather at the protoplasmic membrane.

ENERGY REQUIREMENT

When active transport is performed, its coupling with metabolic energy has to be postulated. This is often evidenced by the inhibitory effect of uncouplers of oxidative phosphorylation. An exception to this rule is the a methyl glucoside permease both in *E. coli* (Cohen & Monod, 1957) and in *Salmonella* (Engelsberg et al., 1961). Another evidence for energy requirement is the requirement of an external carbon source for the functioning of some permeases at full speed. But this requirement differs widely from one permease to another. For example, β-galactoside permease loses less than half of its activity after three hours starvation (Rickenberg et al., 1956; Koch, A. L., in press), whereas proline permease has its activity decreased by a factor of 12 under similar conditions (Britten & McClure, 1958). Thus, the energy for permease action can probably be derived from different primary energy sources in different cases. Extra oxygen uptake linked with the activity of β-galactoside permease (Kepes, 1957) supports the hypothesis that high energy phosphate bonds are involved since the data are consistent with the breakdown of one molecule of ATP per molecule of thiogalactoside transported, but the coupling of ATP breakdown with the actual transport does not seem necessary, since the uptake of ONPG, under conditions where it is hydrolyzed in the cell, is not significantly inhibited by uncouplers of oxidative phosphorylation. In this case, the energy can be derived from the concentration gradient which favors the inward flux. Still the uptake involves the permease, as can be shown by the unchanged competitive effect of different thiogalactosides under azide inhibition.

THE EXIT MECHANISM

When permease action results in accumulation of the substrate, a final steady state is reached where exit compensates for continuing uptake. With a given permease the relative velocities of entry and exit can differ widely so that the steady state level is widely different. This fact points to a certain degree of independence between entry and exit. The exit is a passive process; it is driven by the concentration difference, with first order kinetics (Koch, A. L., personal communication). Nevertheless, it cannot be visualized as a simple leakage by diffusion in view of its high temperature dependence in many cases, and in view of the changes of its first order rate constant under circumstances when no major physical change occurs in the membrane structure (Kepes, 1960). In some instances the exit process is negligibly small, for example in the maltose permease in *E. coli* (Wiesmeyer & Cohn, 1960) and in the case of glutamic acid accumulation in *Staphylococcus aureus* (Gale, 1954). Some inhibitors, such as parachloromercuribenzoate and formaldehyde, not only stop the uptake of β-galactosides but also slow down the exit process by a factor of 5 to 10.

EXISTENCE OF A CARRIER DISTINCT FROM THE PERMEASE

The peculiarities of the exit process lead to the postulation that exit is a carrier-mediated passive transport. The exit measured when entry is prevented by the absence of extracellular substrate is much slower than the exit in the steady state of accumulation. This suggests that the carrier for exit is partly supplied by the functioning of the uptake machinery. The question arises whether the carrier could be the permease itself. Several experimental findings argue against this hypothesis. First, in galactoside permease, the exit can be speeded up not only by the presence of a galactoside but also by the presence of such sugars as glucose, galactose and maltose when the bacteria have been grown on these respective carbon sources (Kepes, 1957, 1960). Glucose also speeds up the exit of galactosides in galactoside permeaseless mutants (Kepes, 1960), realizing a situation where glucose uptake actively drives galactoside out of the cell. A second argument that carrier is distinct from permease comes from the observation (Horecker *et al.*, 1960b) that the exit of galactose is strongly accelerated in bacteria grown on low concentrations of this sugar although the uptake machinery, the galactose permease, which is constitutive, is unchanged under these conditions.

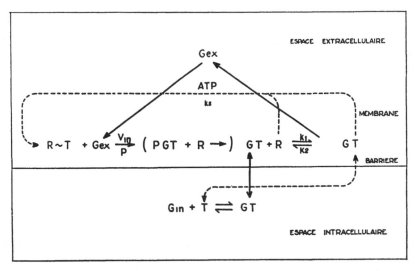

Fig. 4. A model for permease mechanism. A specific protein : permease (P) located in the membrane catalyzes a reaction with extracellular substrate (G_{ex}) to give a product (GT) represented as a substrate carrier compound. GT diffuses freely through the penetration barrier both ways and can dissociate at either side to give unchanged substrate. Active transport results from the higher energy content of the carrier in the permease catalyzed step, substantiated here as a high energy compound R ∼ T. This compound is synthesized at the expense of ATP.

A GENERAL MODEL

On the basis of the evidence, a permease system can best be visualized in the following way (Kepes, 1960) (Fig. 4). A specific permease protein P exists in the cell membrane with its active site oriented toward the medium. It catalyzes a reaction which results in the formation of a substrate carrier complex, GT. This complex is endowed with physical properties which enable it to cross the lipoid membrane freely. The complex dissociates on either side of the membrane releasing the free substrate. The rate of this dissociation can be different on the inner and outer surface, either by assuming a second enzyme on the inner face or by assuming a difference in the concentration of free carrier due to independent reactions. This general model can explain with small adjustments the known features of all identified permeases in *E. coli*.

REFERENCES

Britten, R. J. and F. T. McClure. 1958. *In* Carnegie Institution of Washington Yearbook 57.
Cohen, G. N. and J. Monod. 1957. Bacterial permeases. Bacteriol. Rev. *21*: 169–194.
Doudoroff, M., W. Z. Hassid, E. W. Putman, A. L. Potter and J. Lederberg. 1949. Direct utilization of maltose by *Escherichia coli*. J. Biol. Chem. *179*: 921–934.

Englesberg, E., J. A. Watson and P. A. Hoffee. 1961. The glucose effect and the relationship between glucose permease, acid phosphate and glucose resistance. Cold Spring Harbor Symposia on Quantitative Biology 26: 261–276.

Gale, E. F. 1954. The accumulation of amino acids within staphylococcal cells. *In* Active transport and secretion. Symp. Soc. Exptl. Biol. 8: 242–253.

Halvorson, H., W. Fry and D. Schwemmin. 1955. A study of the properties of the free amino acid pool and enzyme synthesis in yeast. J. Gen. Physiol. 38: 549–573.

Horecker, B. L., J. Thomas and J. Monod. 1960a. Galactose transport in *Escherichia coli*, I. J. Biol. Chem. 235: 1580–1585.

Horecker, B. L., J. Thomas and J. Monod. 1960b. Galactose transport in *Escherichia coli*, II. J. Biol. Chem. 235: 1586–1590.

Kepes, A. 1957. Metabolisme oxydatif lié au fonctionnement de la galactoside-perméase d'*Escherichia coli*. Comptes rendus 244: 1550–1553.

Kepes, A. 1960. Etudes cinétiques sur la galactoside-perméase d'*Escherichia coli*. Biochim. et Biophys. Acta 40: 70–84.

Kepes, A. 1961. *In* Biochemie des Aktiven Transports, p. 315. Springer Verlag.

Kepes, A. and J. Monod. 1957. Etude de fonctionnement de la galactoside-perméase d'*Escherichia coli*. Comptes rendus 244: 809–811.

Mitchell, P. 1957. A general theory of membrane transport from studies of bacteria. Nature 180: 134–136.

Rickenberg, H. V., G. N. Cohen, G. Buttin and J. Monod. 1956. La galactoside-perméase d'*Escherichia coli*. Ann. Inst. Pasteur 91: 829–857.

Sistrom, W. R. 1958. On the physical state of the intracellularly accumulated substrates of β-galactoside permease in *Escherichia coli*. Biochim. et Biophys. Acta 29: 579–587.

Sols, A. and G. La Fuente. 1961. *In* Membrane transport and metabolism, pp. 361–377. Czech. Acad. Sciences Publ., Prague and Academic Press, London.

Stoeber, F. 1957. Sur la β-glucuronide-perméase d'*Escherichia coli*. Comptes rendus 244: 1091–1094.

Wiesmeyer, H. and M. Cohn. 1960. The characterization of the pathway of maltose utilization by *Escherichia coli*. III. A description of the concentrating mechanism. Biochim. et Biophys. Acta 39: 440–447.

THE MECHANISM OF POOL FORMATION
IN *E. COLI*

ROY J. BRITTEN

Department of Terrestrial Magnetism
Carnegie Institution, Washington, D.C., U.S.A.

THE CENTRAL PROBLEM of this symposium is the nature of the mechanism by which small molecules are concentrated within living cells. Are the internally concentrated amino acids free or associated more or less strongly with macromolecules? Are there compartments within the cell? These questions are important to considerations of the permeation mechanisms themselves.

The work to be described here has been directed mainly towards an understanding of the function of the pool and its role in macromolecular synthesis. Naturally, then, the results which imply association of pool compounds with macromolecules have been emphasized and indications of complexity and multiplicity have been sought.

The term "pool" is here taken to mean collectively those compounds which may be extracted from the cell under conditions such that the macromolecules are not degraded, for example by brief exposure to 5 per cent trichloroacetic acid (TCA) at room temperature. The pool size is, for a given compound, simply the extractable quantity of that compound per unit mass of bacteria.

The experimental evidence concerning the formation and maintenance of proline pools in *E. coli* has been published in considerable detail (Britten and McClure, 1962). Therefore only the relevant conclusions will be summarized in tabular form (Tables 1, 2, and 3) with a minimum of comment in the text.

The experiments have been carried out with labelled amino acids and the membrane filter technique (Britten, Roberts and French, 1955). Pool sizes, rates of formation and exchange have been determined by careful analysis of the kinetics of incorporation of radioactivity into TCA-soluble (pool) and TCA-precipitable (protein) fractions in exponentially growing cells. The experiments have been principally carried out with proline; however, the generality of the conclusions has been checked with other amino acids.

I. SUMMARY OF THE FEATURES OF THE PROLINE POOL IN E. COLI

Observations relating to the maintenance of the pool have been listed in Table 1. They supply strong restrictions on models for the mechanism of

TABLE 1

STABILITY OF THE PROLINE POOL IN *E. coli*

Each of these conditions:	Leads to these results:
Absence of energy source Low temperature (0–5 C) Reduction of proline concentration	Suppresses increase of pool Maintains it at pre-established level Permits exchange at a rapid rate
However Osmotic shock Freezing Mild reagents or Small pH changes	lead to loss* of the pool

*Without necessarily interfering with the growth of the cells or their rapid recovery of normal growth rate after return to normal culture conditions.

the concentration process. Clearly the pool amino acid does not leave the cell promptly after removal of the conditions required for its rapid concentration. It thus appears that the pool size reaches a steady value as a result of a decrease in the inward flux of amino acid. If the steady state were reached as a result of outward flux rising to balance the large initial inward flux, then the conditions listed in Table 1 would cause a rapid loss from the pool. This feature sets severe restrictions on models of the concentration process.

Table 2 summarizes some evidence that there exist stereospecific sites which act as catalysts for the concentration of amino acids by the bacterial

TABLE 2

EVIDENCE FOR A CATALYTIC STEP IN THE AMINO ACID CONCENTRATING PROCESS

1. Isoleucine interferes with valine uptake at a concentration far below that which gives a maximum isoleucine pool.
2. Rate of pool formation is maximal at an external concentration far below that at which the pool size becomes maximal.
3. Exchange rate at 0 C is almost independent of external concentration but is proportional to pool size.

cell. Isoleucine and valine, when present at high external concentration, give rise to relatively large pools. Studies of the reciprocal inhibition of their uptake indicate that a common mechanism (Cohen and Rickenberg, 1956; Cohen and Monod, 1957) is apparently utilized. When the two amino acids are present at roughly equal concentrations their affinities for the common step in the concentration process are not very different. However when isoleucine is present at a concentration which yields only a small pool it nevertheless inhibits, by a factor of at least 50 (Britten and McClure, 1962, Fig. 7), the uptake of valine present at about 1/200 of the isoleucine concentration. Thus the common step in the concentration process is very nearly completely saturated with isoleucine. This demonstrates the existence of something equivalent to a catalytic site and further that this site is saturated at an external concentration far below that which gives a maximum pool.

Table 3 summarizes the evidence that there exists more than one component in the pool of a given amino acid. The observed time course of proline exchange at 0 C does not follow a simple exponential. When kinetic experiments covering a wide range of concentrations and pool sizes are examined, at least two components with widely different time constants can be resolved. Since the only process occurring is the trading of a labelled

TABLE 3
EVIDENCE FOR MORE THAN ONE COMPONENT IN THE POOL

1. Exchange at 0 C shows two components with widely different rates and sizes.
2. Curve for pool size as a function of external concentration (formation at 25 C) shows two components.
3. Small pools are specific while large pools are unspecific.

molecule in the pool for an unlabelled one in the environment, a simple exponential decay of pool radioactivity would result if there were a single component in the pool. Thus it may be concluded that there are at least two separate components.

The proline pool size is not proportional to the external concentration even at low concentrations, but the data fit a curve which is the sum of two classical adsorption isotherms. This evidence suggests the presence of two components, but does not prove it since it is not known on independent grounds that a single component follows a classical adsorption isotherm.

At low concentrations of proline the rate of uptake and the small pool size reached are not influenced by the presence of fifteen other amino acids, each at 100 times the proline concentration. However, the maximal proline pool reached at high concentrations of external proline is strikingly reduced in the presence of other amino acids. This is consistent with the presence of two components and even suggests that a different and less specific mechanism plays a role in the formation of large pools.

The two (or possibly more) components of the proline pool must be associated with the cell in different ways. If the pool were assumed to be in the form of unbound amino acid, then the existence of a second impermeable membrane would have to be postulated. In the carrier model described below the two components of the pool are assumed to be associated with two groups of sites having different affinities for the amino acid.

II. A CARRIER MODEL FOR THE AMINO ACID CONCENTRATION PROCESS

We have been led to postulate the major features of the carrier model since other proposed models lead to predictions which are inconsistent with the evidence concerning the amino acid pools in *E. coli*.

The fact that pools are maintained under adverse conditions (Table 1) where they might be expected to leak out, combined with other evidence, has led us to include the more or less labile binding of amino acids to sites as the major mechanism for maintaining the pool. The strong evidence that a catalytic site participates in pool formation has led us to include such an intermediate step in the formation of the site–amino acid complex (pool).

We have, therefore, postulated that the catalytic site is part of a molecule of moderate molecular weight termed the "carrier." The carrier molecule is assumed to be large enough to form a stereospecific complex with the amino acid but small enough to diffuse within the cell. The mobility of the carrier is necessary since there are few carriers to transfer amino acids to the many pool holding sites.

According to this model the pool is formed in the following way. An external amino acid (A) diffuses into the cell and collides with an unoccupied carrier (E) which is specific for the particular amino acid or class of amino acids. A complex is formed: $A + E \rightleftarrows \overline{AE}$. The complex diffuses through the cell and collides with an unoccupied site (R). In a reaction involving an energy donor, the amino acid is transferred from the carrier to the storage site: $R + \overline{AE} \rightarrow \overline{AR} + E$. In turn an unoccupied carrier may collide with an occupied site and remove the amino acid: $E + \overline{AR} \rightarrow \overline{AE} + R$. This reverse reaction reduces the quantity of free carrier as the pool ($\overline{AR}$) rises. In turn the net rate of reaction of carrier with free amino acid falls. Thus a steady value of the pool size is reached as a result of a decrease in the rate of uptake of free amino acid as indicated by the experimental evidence discussed at the beginning of section I.

In the detailed analysis of the model (Britten and McClure, 1962) it is assumed that amino acid associated with carrier is utilized for protein synthesis and a subsidiary reaction was proposed to control the rate of internal synthesis of the amino acid. Thus the concentrations of carrier-complex and free carrier determine not only the rate of incorporation of amino acid and the pool size but also the rate of internal synthesis.

III. THE PREDICTIONS OF THE CARRIER MODEL

Comparison of the results of the mathematical analysis of this model with the experimental evidence lies outside the scope of this discussion. It can only be stated that for proline all of the quantitative measurements of the rate of formation and pool size as well as rate of internal synthesis over a range of external concentration from 2×10^{-8} M to 5×10^{-4} M may be fitted to the model. The model is further consistent with the data on exchange at 25 and 0 C and with the measurements on the rate of loss from the pool. Most of the rate constants for the reactions shown above have been numerically evaluated (Britten and McClure, 1962).

The principal features of the model may be understood without mathematical analysis. Two distinct properties lead to maintenance of the pool when formation is suppressed (Table 1). We could assume the reverse reaction ($\overline{AR} + E \rightarrow \overline{AE} + R$) to be energy dependent and then clearly the pool would be maintained in the absence of glucose. Alternatively, we are at liberty to choose a small value for the constant k_2 (controlling the rate of dissociation of $\overline{AE}$ into A + E) without influencing other properties of the model, and then the loss rate under all conditions (short of damaging the cell) can be set as low as necessary. The choice of a small k_2 simply means that the carrier (or catalytic site) has a high affinity for the amino acid, and thus the amount of carrier complex will be saturated at low concentrations. This is consistent with the exchange rate and of the formation rate being maximal at low external concentrations.

Clearly the carrier plays the role of the catalytic site (Table 2) for pool formation. The external concentration at which it is saturated is essentially independent of the concentration at which either component of the pool is maximal. The existence of two components in the pool simply implies that there are two classes of sites (R and R') present in different quantities and with different reaction constants.

The evidence on exchange (Tables 1, 2, and 3) is explained if it is assumed that exchange may occur between free amino acids and those associated with the carrier but *not* between free amino acids and those associated with storage sites. Exchange must also occur between amino acids associated with sites and those associated with carriers without coupling to energy donors. Since it is probable that the former exchange rate is more rapid than the latter the specific radioactivity (in an exchange experiment with labelled amino acids) of amino acid associated with the carrier will always be close to that of the external amino acid.

Thus, since the amount of carrier complex is saturated, the exchange rate will be independent of the external concentration. The collisions between carrier complexes (constant specific activity and quantity) and site complexes control the rate of exchange which is therefore proportional to the number of site complexes and thus to the pool size.

The consistency of the predictions of this model with the evidence does not permit the assertion that the function of storage sites and carriers has been rigorously proved or that the function of an osmotic barrier has been demonstrated to be unimportant in the maintenance of the pool. All that can be said is that the reactions given above and the equations derived from them accurately describe the experimental data. Any model which gave essentially the same set of equations would also be satisfactory. An equivalent set of reactions might very well be derived from a model in which the underlying mechanisms were quite different.

IV. THE INCORPORATION OF NUCLEIC ACID BASES

Studies of the incorporation of labelled nucleic acid bases by growing *E. coli* (McCarthy and Britten, 1962; Buchwald and Britten, 1963) have shown the direct entry of radioactivity into ribonucleic acid (RNA) without delay by the large pools of nucleoside-phosphates. Since this behavior is very different from that of amino acids the observations will be briefly

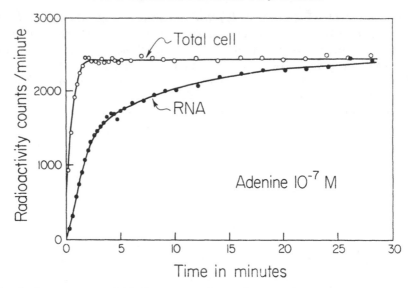

FIG. 1. Incorporation of 10^{-7} M 8-C^{14}-adenine by *E. coli* ML-30 growing at 37 C with a generation time of 51 min. Cell concentration 0.33 mg (wet) per ml. Open circles represent radioactivity of total cell samples collected by membrane filtration. Solid circles represent the radioactivity of RNA measured on samples collected by membrane filtration after treatment with 5 per cent TCA.

described, taking adenine as an example, and discussed in relation to the carrier model. Fig. 1 shows the incorporation into the pool and RNA of 8-C^{14}-adenine present at a relatively low concentration (10^{-7} M). The adenine is almost completely removed from the medium in about 1½ min. During this period radioactivity enters the RNA at a rate corresponding to about 40 per cent of the total rate of uptake by the cells. The time required to establish this rate is very short.

It is clear that there are large pools of adenine compounds in the cell. Therefore it appears that a special class of pool adenine compounds, present in small quantity, rapidly reach a specific radioactivity which is very much higher than the average and are effectively utilized for RNA synthesis. This class of compounds forms a bypass around the large pool for the entry of the exogenous base into RNA.

After 1½ min, when the adenine has been completely removed from the medium, the rate of incorporation of radioactivity into RNA falls although the cells continue to grow steadily. During this second phase radioactivity entering RNA must be drawn from various adenine compounds of the pool present in relatively large quantities and having a lower specific radioactivity. Fig. 2 is a semilogarithmic plot of the radioactivity of the pool during the period after the exogenous adenine has been exhausted. It is apparent that the decay of the pool radioactivity cannot be represented by a single exponential. This result implies either that there are a number of different adenine compounds in the pool with different turnover rates or

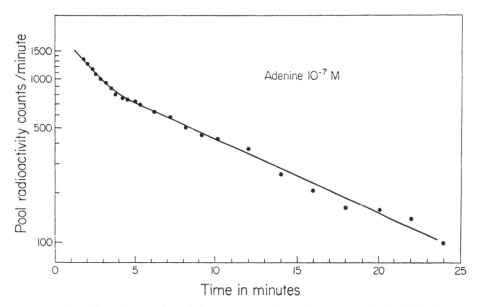

FIG. 2. Semi-logarithmic plot of the decay of the radioactivity of the C^{14}-adenine labelled pool. Data obtained from the experiment of Fig. 1 by subtracting the RNA radioactivity from the total cell radioactivity.

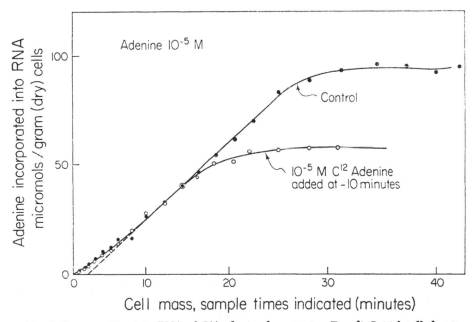

FIG. 3. Incorporation into RNA of C^{14}-adenine by growing *E. coli*. Initial cell density 0.42 mg (wet) per ml. Solid circles: 10^{-5} M C^{14}-adenine added at time zero. Open circles: 10^{-5} M C^{12}-adenine added at −10 min and carrier free C^{14}-adenine added at time zero. Incorporation of adenine into RNA (calculated from TCA precipitable radioactivity) plotted against a scale which is linear in cell mass. Sample times are indicated to permit estimation of the pool delay time.

that the principal pool compound utilized for RNA synthesis exists in several compartments or states of organization.

Fig. 3 shows the incorporation of C^{14}-adenine into the RNA at an external concentration (10^{-5} M) such that the exogenous adenine is not exhausted until after the specific radioactivity of the large pools has approached that of the tracer supplied. Initially, radioactivity is incorporated into RNA at about 40 per cent of the rate finally achieved, as expected from the operation of the bypass system. As the specific radioactivity of the major pool compounds rises, the rate of entry into RNA also rises.

The open circles on Fig. 3 represent the result of an experiment in which 10^{-5} M carrier C^{12}-adenine was added 10 min before the tracer. There is no indication of any difference between the two curves beyond that to be expected from the utilization of a certain fraction of carrier adenine before the tracer was added. There was, therefore, no detectable expansion of the pool of adenine compounds even at this relatively high concentration of external adenine.

From experiments of the type presented in Figs. 1 and 3 the fraction of the labelled base entering the cell which flows through the bypass system and the time constants for turnover of the major storage pools can be evaluated. Table 4 presents the results of such calculations based on

TABLE 4

BYPASS FLOWS AND TIME CONSTANTS

Base supplied	Uracil	Cytosine	Guanine	Adenine
Fraction of flow in bypass:				
Low concentration experiments[1]	.40	.45	.74	.4
High concentration experiments[2]	.37	.37	.68	.46
Pool time constant (minutes):				
Low concentration experiments[3]	10	21	2–6	2–12
High concentration experiments[4]	11	24	3.1	4

[1]From ratio of RNA incorporation rate to total cell incorporation rate.
[2]From ratio of initial RNA incorporation rate to final RNA incorporation rate.
[3]Time constant of exponential decay of pool radioactivity.
[4]Extrapolated delay time (corrected).

previously published data (McCarthy and Britten, 1962; Buchwald and Britten, 1963). These two parameters have been independently evaluated for experiments at low concentration (e.g., Fig. 1) and high concentration (e.g., Fig. 3). Their agreement gives strong support to the existence of the bypass process and indicates that the nucleoside-phosphate pools are not expanded in the presence of base supplements at high concentrations.

The differences and similarities between the observations of the behavior of amino acids and nucleic acid bases in *E. coli* may be summarized as follows: (1) The amino acids are not chemically converted to any great extent except in the usual pathways of amino acid synthesis but the bases are promptly converted to nucleoside phosphates. (2) Amino acid pools in the absence of supplement may be very small while the nucleoside-phosphate pools are large. (3) The amino acid pool size is responsive to the external concentration but the nucleoside phosphate pools are not influenced by the base concentration. (4) Amino acids may be taken up by the cell at ten times the rate required for protein synthesis while bases are not taken up at a greater rate than that required for formation of RNA. (5) Radioactivity from exogenous amino acids is diluted by the pool before entering protein while that from exogenous bases may bypass the nucleoside phosphate pools and enter RNA without delay. (6) Exchange plays an important role in the labelling of amino acid pools while it plays a negligible role in the labelling of the nucleoside phosphate pools. (7) Both amino acids and bases are taken up effectively at low concentrations. (8) Internal synthesis is effectively suppressed at moderate concentrations of the bases and certain of the amino acids. (9) Both are incorporated into macromolecules in the growing cell.

In spite of some striking differences in behavior, it is only necessary to alter a few of the reaction rate constants to make the predictions of the carrier model agree with the behaviour of nucleic acid bases. It is necessary to assume that the exogenous base forms a complex with the carrier, and at some unspecified stage in the process (before or after carrier complex formation) is converted to a nucleoside phosphate and ultimately to a form suitable for incorporation into RNA. If $\overline{AR}$ represents a large nucleoside-phosphate pool and the equilibrium for the reaction $\overline{AE} + R \rightleftarrows A\overline{R} + E$ is far to the right there will be little free R and a constant non-expandable pool will result. If, in addition, the rates in this reaction are not fast compared to the flow of material through the carrier complex ($\overline{AE}$) then this flow will bypass the large pool ($\overline{AR}$).

The fact that exogenous bases may be incorporated into RNA without entering the large nucleoside phosphate pools naturally raises the question of the state of organization of both the large pools and the molecules that follow the bypass route. It seems certain that only a small pool (equivalent to a few seconds supply) of compounds exists in a state which is suitable for incorporation into RNA, and that the exogenous bases are rapidly converted to this state.

The question remains open as to whether this state is simply the chemical form (for example a 5′ monophosphate) of the low molecular weight RNA precursor or is an association with an enzyme system or carrier in the sense of the carrier model. If the state is an association with the enzyme system for RNA synthesis, how is the RNA precursor molecule transported from the cell membrane to the site of synthesis without mixing with the large pools? It is conceivable that the site of RNA synthesis is in fact at the cell membrane but if it is not then a carrier molecule would have to be invoked.

VI. CONCLUSION

Over the past few years evidence has been accumulating which indicates that "the functional heterogeneity of intracellular pools" (Kipnis *et al.*,

1961) is of very general occurrence. Indications of the existence of heterogeneity have been found in practically every system that has been examined carefully.

Direct evidence of intracellular heterogeneity of amino acid pools has been published for yeast (Cowie & McClure, 1959; Kempner & Cowie, 1960; Halvorson & Cohen, 1958), for *E. coli* (Britten and McClure, 1962), for *Neurospora* (Zalokar, 1961), for the brain and liver (Waelsch, 1962; Garfinkel, 1962), for rat diaphragm and guinea pig lymph node cells (Kipnis *et al.*, 1961), for kidney cortex (Rosenberg *et al.*, 1962). There is some evidence of pool heterogeneity in plants (Steward, 1962; Aronoff, 1962; Matthews *et al.*, 1963). Further there is evidence for heterogeneity of the nucleic acid precursor pools in yeast (Cowie & Bolton, 1957), in *E. coli* (McCarthy & Britten, 1962; Buchwald & Britten, 1963), in *Euglena* (Britten, unpublished results) and in a subcellular system from *Pseudomonas* (Mizuno *et al.*, 1961). The greatest part of this evidence has come from the entry of labelled precursors into macromolecules where the kinetics imply that the major pools have been bypassed. However, in yeast (Cowie & McClure, 1959) a number of independent characteristics of two components of the amino acid pool have been studied. For *E. coli* the evidence cited in Table 3 shows that there are at least two major components in the pool.

In no case has the underlying cause of the heterogeneity of pools been shown. The obvious alternatives are: (1) chemical modification of the low molecular weight compounds themselves (possibly so labile as not to survive extraction); (2) the existence of physically distinct compartments separated by relatively impermeable membranes; (3) the binding of pool compounds to specific sites comparable to enzymatic sites but not necessarily catalyzing reactions; (4) the adsorption of pool compounds to macromolecular structures by relatively labile bonds of a more or less specific nature.

There can be no doubt that the phenomena represented by categories 1, 3 and 4 play a role for very small quantities of pool compounds. The question remains open for large pools, although sites equivalent to (3) or (4) are formally included in the carrier model. Physically distinct compartments (category 2) may be important in higher organisms and particularly in plants. They are difficult to visualize in micro-organisms, although the degree of complexity that can be observed is increasing (Van Iterson, see above, page 14).

Further progress in the understanding of the mechanism of pool maintenance may well rest on the development of experimental approaches to the following questions. How is the distinction maintained between the two or more fairly large components in the pool of yeast and bacteria? Are they chemically or physically separated? How is it possible, in the many systems where it has been observed, for exogenous compounds to reach the sites of macromolecular synthesis without entering the large pools? Can traces of special chemical forms or adsorbed states of compounds in the bypass route be extracted and recognized by their very high specific radio-activity in pulse experiments?

REFERENCES

Aronoff, S. 1962. Dynamics of amino acids in plants. *In* Amino acid pools. Elsevier Publishing Company, Amsterdam.

Britten, R. J. and F. T. McClure. 1962. The amino acid pool in *Escherichia coli*. Bacteriol. Rev. *26*: 292.

Britten, R. J., R. B. Roberts and E. F. French. 1955. Amino acid adsorption and protein synthesis in *Escherichia coli*. Proc. Natl. Acad. Sci. U.S. *41*: 863.

Buchwald, M. and R. J. Britten. 1963. Incorporation of ribonucleic acid bases into the metabolic pool and RNA of *E. coli*. Biophys. J. *3*: 155.

Cohen, G. N. and J. Monod. 1957. Bacterial permeases. Bacteriol. Rev. *21*: 169.

Cohen, G. N. and H. B. Rickenberg. 1956. Concentration spécifique réversible des amino acids chez *Escherichia coli*. Ann. Inst. Pasteur *91*: 693.

Cowie, D. B. and E. T. Bolton. 1957. The use of metabolic pools of purine compounds for nucleic acid synthesis in yeast. Biochim. et Biophys. Acta *25*: 292.

Cowie, D. B. and F. T. McClure. 1959. Metabolic pools and the synthesis of macromolecules. Biochim. et Biophys. Acta *31*: 236.

Garfinkel, D. 1963. Computer simulation of steady-state glutamate metabolism in rat brain. J. Theor. Biol. (in press).

Halvorson, H. O. and G. N. Cohen. 1958. Incorporation of endogenous and exogenous amino acids into yeast proteins. Ann. Inst. Pasteur *95*: 73.

Kempner, E. S. and D. B. Cowie. 1960. Metabolic pools and the utilization of amino acid analogs for protein synthesis. Biochim. et Biophys. Acta *42*: 401.

Kipnis, D. M., E. Reiss and E. Helmreich. 1961. Functional heterogeneity of the intracellular amino acid pool in mammalian cells. Biochim. et Biophys. Acta *51*: 519.

Matthews, R. E. F., E. T. Bolton and H. R. Thompson. 1963. Kinetics of labeling of turnip yellow mosaic virus with P^{32} and S^{35}. Virology *19*: 179.

McCarthy, B. J. and R. J. Britten. 1962. The synthesis of ribosomes in *E. coli*. I. The incorporation of C^{14}-uracil into the metabolic pool and RNA. Biophys. J. *2*: 35.

Mizuno, S., E. Yoshida, H. Takahashi and B. Maruo. 1961. Experimental proof of a compartment of "energy-rich" P in a subcellular system from *Pseudomonas*. Biochim. et Biophys. Acta *49*: 369.

Rosenberg, L. E., M. Berman and S. Segal. 1963. Studies of the kinetics of amino acid transport, incorporation into protein and oxidation in kidney cortex slices. J. Biol. Chem. (in press).

Steward, F. C. 1962. The free nitrogen compounds in plants considered in relation to metabolism, growth and development. *In* Amino acid pools. Elsevier Publishing Company, Amsterdam.

Waelsch, H. 1962. *In vivo* compartments of glutamic acid metabolism in brain and liver. *In* Amino acid pools. Elsevier Publishing Company, Amsterdam.

Zalokar, M. 1961. Kinetics of amino acid uptake and protein synthesis in *Neurospora*. Biochim. et Biophys. Acta *46*: 423.

SYMPOSIUM II

PROPERTIES OF ISOLATED
CELLULAR PARTICLES

Chairman: R. B. ROBERTS

G. ZUBAY

Physical and Chemical Properties of Particles

B. J. McCARTHY

Biosynthesis of Ribosomal and Complementary RNA in bacteria

S. SPIEGELMAN

The Use of DNA-RNA Hybridization as an Analytical Tool

G. von EHRENSTEIN

On the Biosynthesis of Hemoglobin in Reticulocyte Ribosomes

CHAIRMAN'S REMARKS

R. B. ROBERTS

Carnegie Institution of Washington
Washington, D.C., U.S.A.

THE FIELD OF INTEREST of this symposium is one of the most active areas of research. Accordingly, in inviting the speakers, it was not sufficient to find those who could report work already done. It was necessary to pick those who were most likely to carry out new and significant work during the intervening year. Success is evident, as the talks will describe experiments done since the invitations were issued.

A rapidly advancing field also implies a changing terminology. As new isolation procedures are brought into use and new methods for characterizing molecules become available new distinctions can be made. A few years ago RNA was RNA. Now many types of RNA can be recognized and names for these types have to be invented. Sometimes there are several names for the same molecule depending on whether the definition is an operational one or whether the function of the molecule is considered. It may therefore be useful to present a glossary of RNA terminology.

In extracts of cells (*E. coli*), we find two stable types of RNA which are the end product of synthesis. One is a class of relatively small molecules which is very familiar and well characterized. This was called soluble RNA or s-RNA since it does not spin down readily. It is also called acceptor RNA because it accepts amino acids, and transfer RNA because it can transfer amino acids to ribosomes during protein synthesis carried out *in vitro*. Finally, it is sometimes designated adaptor RNA. Molecules of this class are readily recognized by their small size ($\sim$ 85 nucleotides; 4S) and their composition.

The other class of stable RNA is found associated with protein in ribosomes.

TABLE 1
CELLULAR COMPONENTS OF *E. coli*

	S	% NA	Elutes from DEAE	Relative proportions
Ribosomes	30	65	.4 M NaCl	90
	50	65	.4 M NaCl	90
	70	65	.4 M NaCl	90
	100	65	.4 M NaCl	90
Neosome	$\sim$30	80	.5 M NaCl	7
	43	80	.5 M NaCl	7
Eosome	$\sim$14	100	.6 M NaCl	3
s-RNA	4	100	.5 M NaCl	10–20
DNA		100	.5 M NaCl	10–20

In addition, there are kinetically unstable forms which can be distinguished by chromatography or sedimentation. We designate these eosomes and neosomes, terms defined operationally but which suggest their roles as precursors of ribosomes. The characteristics of these different types are summarized in Table 1.

Treatment of the cell extracts with phenol releases the RNA from its association with protein and several classes can be distinguished, as shown in Table 2.

TABLE 2
RNA EXTRACTED BY PHENOL

	S	Composition	Features
s-RNA	4	High GC	AA accepter
Ribosomal RNA	23	High G	From 50S ribosomes
	16	High G	From 30S ribosomes
Eosomal RNA			
E_R	~8	High G	Unstable, transient
E_D	~8	Like DNA	Unstable, transient

These RNA's can also be defined in terms of functions, observed or hypothetical. The more frequently used definitions are listed in Table 3. As can be seen, the same RNA can be given several different names. The term messenger RNA often causes confusion. According to its original definition, it has three distinguishing features. At present, the term is frequently applied to rapidly labelled RNA of unobserved composition and function which would be more appropriately called nascent RNA.

We can only hope that definitions will become sharper, and the number of names will decrease as the field matures.

TABLE 3
DEFINITIONS OF VARIOUS RNA's

RNA	S	Composition	Kinetics	Function
s-RNA	4	High GC	Stable	Amino acid acceptor
Transfer, acceptor				
Ribosomal RNA	16, 23	Like ribosomes	Stable	Component of ribosomes
Informational RNA				Will form hybrid
Complementary RNA				
D-RNA		Like DNA		
Template RNA				Template for protein
ϕ RNA		Like DNA of ϕ		Formed after ϕ infection
Pulse RNA			Unstable	
Nascent RNA			Rapidly labelled	
Messenger RNA		Like DNA	Unstable	Template for protein

PHYSICAL AND CHEMICAL PROPERTIES
OF PARTICLES*

G. ZUBAY

Biology Department, Brookhaven National Laboratory
Upton, New York, U.S.A.

ELECTRON MICROSCOPY is invaluable in determining the organization of the bacterial cell. In Plate I we see an electron micrograph of a thin section of a single cell of *Escherichia coli*. There are three prominent regions: (1) the bacterial membrane, (2) the centrally located sparse region in which thin fibrils of DNA are located, and (3) the main body of the cell with densely packed particles. All the particles in the latter area are probably ribosomes. This paper will focus attention on the structure and function of ribosomes and nucleic acids directly involved in protein synthesis in *E. coli*. In Plate II a cell segment containing ribosomes is compared with a purified preparation of 70 Svedberg (S) and 100S ribosomes at the same magnification. Most ribosomes in the bacterium are similar in size to the 70S ribosome: further work on this point is in progress.

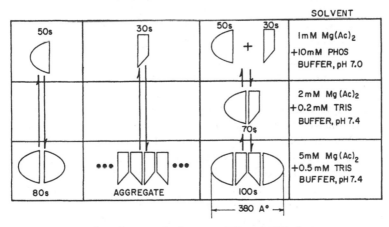

FIG. 1. The influence of solvent on 30S and 50S ribosomes.

In purified extracts the state of aggregation of the ribosomes is sensitive to the divalent cation concentration and ionic strength of the medium (1, 2). Fig. 1 summarizes information regarding the interaction of ribosomes. At low Mg^{++} concentration, one finds the ribosomes sedimenting as two

*Research carried out at Brookhaven National Laboratory under the auspices of the U.S. Atomic Energy Commission. The work discussed herein represents the joint effort of Dr. J. A. Bergeron and Dr. G. Zubay.

components, a 30S and a 50S component. If the magnesium is removed, these components break down irreversibly. On the other hand, if the Mg^{++} concentration is increased, the 50S and 30S particles interact to form a 70S component, which can dimerize to yield a 100S component. When the 50S particles are separated from the 30S, increasing the Mg^{++} concentration results in their dimerization to form an 81S component. The isolated 30S particles form aggregates of various lengths at high Mg^{++} concentration. These observations indicate that the 50S particle is monovalent, in that it has one face which can interact; whereas the 30S particle is bivalent, producing polymers when interacting with itself. Electron microscopy shows that when the two components are mixed, they preferentially interact with each other, and combination is made through only one of the interacting faces of the 30S particle. The approximate shapes of these ribosomes are indicated in Fig. 1. The 100S particle is composed of two 50S and two 30S particles. It has the general contour of a prolate ellipsoid with major and minor axes of 190 A and 75 A respectively. In the region between the 50S and 30S subunits, there is a groove-shaped cavity about 25 A across. The two interconnected 30S subunits have a wedge-shaped cavity on one side.

The 30S and 50S ribosomes are each composed of about two-thirds by weight RNA and one-third by weight protein (2). Kurland (3) has shown that the 30S ribosome contains a single molecule of RNA, while the 50S ribosome contains either one or two (3, 4). The average molecular weight of ribosomal protein is 25,000 (5) and from this it may be calculated that the 30S ribosome contains about 10 protein molecules, and the 50S ribosome about 25.

Biosynthetic studies of others (6–9) indicate a similarity in growth and development between ribosomes and some viral ribonucleoproteins, in that the large RNA molecule is fully formed before the small protein subunits cluster around it. Because of its net positive charge the protein interacts electrostatically with the RNA. Failure of concentrated salt solution to break the complex into its respective RNA and protein parts suggests that the RNA is effectively entrapped by the protein, and that the latter interacts with itself through hydrogen bonds and van der Waals forces so as to form a *loosely knit* network around the RNA. It is quite clear that the protein does not form a close packed shell around the RNA of the ribosome as it does in many simple viruses. Since I have labored this point previously (10), I shall not dwell on it here.

X-ray diffraction patterns obtained from ribosomal RNA contain the main elements of the double helical diffraction (11, 12) pattern, but without the same high degree of regularity suggested by DNA. Solution studies, too, suggest a double helical structure (12, 13), in that there is an increase in optical density at 260 mμ on heating, equal to two-thirds of that shown by DNA, and occurring over a broader range of temperature. These observations led us to the conclusion that the ribosomal RNA has an appreciable

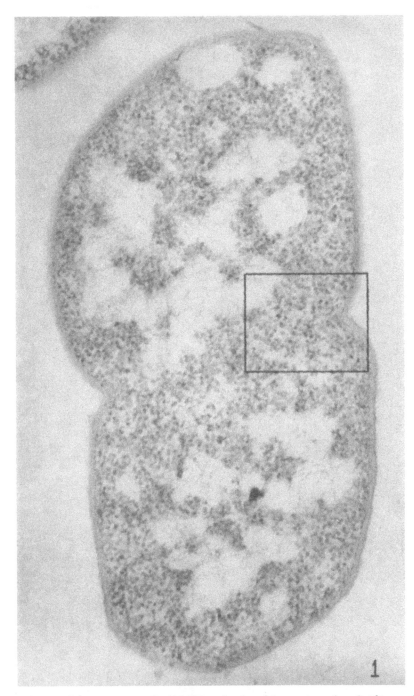

PLATE I. An electronmicrograph (86,000 ×) of a thin section of a dividing cell of *E. coli*. The organisms, from a log-phase culture, were fixed for two hours at 23 C in a medium containing 10 per cent formalin (pH 7), washed, repeated by centrifugation in fresh medium, postfixed for two hours at 23 C in Letterquist's 0.4 per cent osmium tetroxide solution (pH 7.4), washed again, and dehydrated down a temperature gradient to −25 C in an ethanol series containing 0.1 per cent uranyl nitrate, infiltrated with butyl methacrylate monomer and polymerized by γ radiation at −55 C. The organism, bounded by the cell wall and plasma membrane, consists of two main regions: the nucleoid, which contains ramifying filaments, and the cytoplasm which contains many small particles.

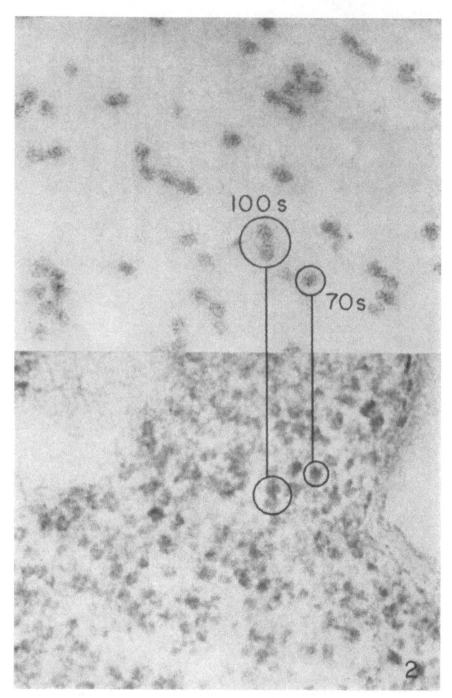

PLATE II. A comparison (300,000 ×) of isolated ribosomes of *E. coli* which have been fixed by formalin and stained with uranyl acetate and sprayed upon carbon film (from H. E. Huxley and G. Zubay) with the similarly fixed and stained cytoplasmic particles observed *in situ* (see inset Fig. 1 for lower magnification). The 100S type of configuration is very rarely observed, whereas the 70S type is very common. Given random orientation and the equivalence of images of 70S and 100S for planes other than the plane of section, the 100S type should be observed more frequently in sections if it is the usual rather than the unusual form.

amount of double helical structure with less regularity in the base pairing. We do not know the exact structure of ribosomal RNA. The most stable hydrogen bonds in RNA will probably be those formed between 6-keto and 6-amino bases (12), of which most naturally occurring RNA's have almost equal amounts. By a suitable arrangement of nucleotides along the poly-nucleotide chain, several different types of double helix may be formed as well as various complex folds and loops (14, 15). Hence, analogous to proteins, the primary structure in polynucleotides may be the most impor-tant factor in determining their secondary, as well as their tertiary, structure. The double helical structure of ribosomal RNA is preserved in the ribosome.

We come now to the question of how the structure of the ribosome is related to its function in protein synthesis. In studying this problem, one must be able to distinguish between the synthesis of ribosomal structural protein and nascent protein produced by the ribosome. McQuillen, Roberts and Britten (16) accomplished this in bacteria by very rapid pulse labelling experiments. This technique consists of labelling growing cells by the addi-tion of C^{14} amino acids, and stopping growth very soon thereafter. The cells are lysed, and macromolecular species are separated by centrifugation in a sucrose gradient, which stabilizes boundaries thus formed. After partial separation of discrete fractions, samples are taken from various depths in the centrifuge cell and analysed for nucleic acid and radioactivity. Experi-ments of this type suggest that most of the newly synthesized protein is associated with ribosomal components sedimenting at 70 S or faster. By lowering the Mg^{++} concentration to 10^{-4} M most of the ribosomes are broken down to 50S and 30S particles. *Nonetheless, the peak incorporation is still to be found in the 70S region.* This result has served as the basis for a good deal of further work. It has not yet been definitely established that this radioactive peak in the 70S region of the sucrose gradient is caused by a 70S ribosome with some nascent protein on it. However, assuming this is the case, we interpret this result to mean two things: only a small number of ribosomes have been caught in the process of protein synthesis, and these ribosomes do not dissociate as readily into their respective 50S and 30S subunits as do those ribosomes which are inactive. *Evidently there is some-thing additional holding them together.*

The techniques for studying protein synthesis *in vitro* in *E. coli* were soon to follow (17). Tissières, Schlessinger and Gros (18) found that *in vitro* only a small number of heavy ribosomes (10 per cent or less) have the *capacity* for amino acid incorporation. Most of the ribosomes have become damaged, so that they are unable to function properly, or lack an adequate supply of some essential nutrient to make them functional. Because of this, *in vitro* results are of less significance than the earlier *in vivo* experiments. Nevertheless, the same conclusion was reached—that the subunits of the active 70S particles are strongly bound together.

Good evidence exists that the structural ribosomal RNA does not act as a template in protein synthesis. Experiments on enzyme induction and virus infection suggest that the rate of production of a new RNA template for protein synthesis exceeds the average rate of synthesis of ribosomes (19). Further light has been shed on this problem from studies of the induction of RNA and protein synthesis in virus infected bacteria. These experiments were done using bacteriophage infected *E. coli*, in which most ribosomal RNA synthesis is inhibited, and the cell for the most part produces RNA similar in base composition to the bacteriophage DNA. This fraction of RNA is rapidly incorporated into the 70–100S particle fraction. It has been named messenger RNA since it is believed to carry, from the DNA, the genetic message necessary for the synthesis of bacteriophage protein. In these experiments of Brenner and co-workers (20), and Gros and co-workers (21), the binding of the messenger RNA did not affect the sedimentation rate or the density of the ribosomes. The messenger RNA either was of small molecular weight, or was replacing a molecule of equivalent size in the ribosome. More recent results of Risebrough, Tissières and Watson (22) indicate that in the earlier experiments there was a good deal of enzymatic degradation of the messenger RNA so that only a small part of it remained on the ribosomes. Indeed, it appears that messenger RNA is much more susceptible to enzymatic degradation and is therefore more exposed than the bulk of the ribosomal RNA. Experiments which avoid gross enzymatic damage suggest that the messenger RNA from phage has an average molecular weight of about 5×10^5, and that when attached to the ribosome it increases the average sedimentation rate by 20 per cent or more. The present picture of the ribosome, therefore, is that of a nonspecific ribonucleoprotein body which may or may not be transiently combined with a specific messenger RNA molecule. This means that most of the ribosomal RNA is "structural RNA" and does not code for the synthesis of protein.

The counterpart of these experiments has been carried out *in vitro*. By adding suitable purified messenger RNA to a cell free incubation mixture containing ribosomes, a large stimulating effect on amino acid incorporation can be achieved (23). The most exciting result in this area was the discovery of Nirenberg and Matthaei, that polyuridylic acid, acting like naturally occurring messenger RNA, stimulates specifically the synthesis of poly-phenylalanine (24). This system mimics the normal one in the ingredients required to produce peptide synthesis, and it has many advantages for purposes of investigation, since it is far simpler and isolation of a specific polypeptide has been demonstrated. Using this system, we have explored the question of which of the ribosomal species is responsible for protein synthesis (25). At one time or another, the 70S, the 85S, and the 100S ribosomes, or combinations thereof, have each been favored.

To determine if both the 50S and the 30S ribosomal components are necessary for polyphenylalanine synthesis, a preparation of unfractionated ribosomes was compared with fractionated preparations of 50S and 30S ribosomes. The results in Fig. 2 show that neither the 50S nor the 30S subunit alone is capable of stimulating polyphenylalanine synthesis. On the other

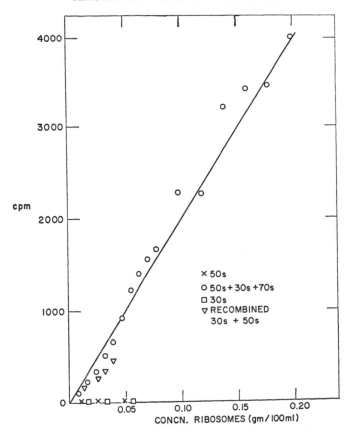

FIG. 2. Incorporation of phenylalanine as a function of ribosome concentration. Incubation mixture contains 0.09 M tris·HCl, pH 8.0, 9.5 mM Mg(Ac)$_2$, 0.45 M KCl, 5.4 mM mercaptoethanol, 0.9 mM ATP, 4.5 mM phosphoenolpyruvate, 18γ/ml pyruvate kinase, 93 γ/ml s-RNA (37), 2.15 mM GTP, .072 mM C^{14}-L-phenylalanine, sp. act. ~10 mc/mM, 29 γ/ml polyuridylic acid, <M.W.> ~150,000 and 0.05 ml/ml *E. coli* enzyme extract (36). Unfractionated ribosomes were prepared by the method of Tissières and Watson (37). 30S and 50S ribosomes were prepared by fractional ultracentrifugation and found to be 90 and 95 per cent pure by sedimentation analysis. The reaction mixture was incubated 30 min at 36 C. The hot trichloroacetic acid precipitable fraction was isolated according to the procedure of Siekevitz (38).

hand, the unfractionated ribosomes or recombined 50S and 30S ribosomes stimulate polypeptide synthesis, and the amount of incorporation is directly proportional to the quantity of ribosomes in the incubation mixture. Evidently both the 50S and the 30S ribosomes are indispensable to the process, and they probably combine when active in this role, since a linear dependence on concentration is indicated. Because 50S and 30S ribosomes can combine to form 70S or 100S ribosomes, it remained to be found which of these is active in protein synthesis. In Fig. 3 we see the results of incorporation studies where the state of aggregation of the ribosomes was controlled by varying the Mg^{++} concentration. It can be seen that phenylalanine incorporation begins around 5 mM Mg^{++} and reaches a peak at

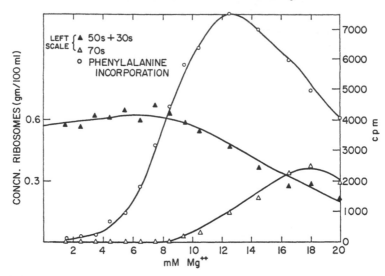

FIG. 3. Incorporation of phenylalanine and concentration of different ribosomes as a function of Mg++ concentration. Unfractionated ribosomes (Tissières and Watson (38)) were dialyzed against 0.01 M potassium phosphate + 0.001 M Mg(AC)₂, pH 7.0 for 12 hr at 5 C before use. The reaction mixture was incubated for 45 min at 36 C. Other incubation conditions are similar to those used in Fig. 1. Over the range of Mg++ concentrations studied, no 100S particles were observed.

12 mM, after which it falls off. In these experiments half of each assay mixture was used to measure the phenylalanine incorporation, and the other half was used directly for ultracentrifugation analyses in order to determine the amount of each ribosomal component. Between 5 mM and 8 mM Mg++ only about 1 per cent of the ribosomes appear in the 70S form. Thus the rise in phenylalanine incorporation precedes the rapid rise in 70S component. Evidently the potentially active 70S particles form first. The heterogeneity of ribosomes is further indicated by the fact that at any given Mg++ concentration a well-defined fraction of ribosomes interact to form 70S particles, and others do not. What is most striking is the fact that the 100S ribosomes do not form over the range of Mg++ concentration studied. As little as 1 per cent of the ribosomes in the 100S form would have been readily detectable. In 12 mM Mg++-tris buffer alone, the majority of the ribosomes are normally in the 100S form. Failure of the 100S ribosomes to form in the incubation mixture is caused by the presence of the other ionic ingredients. In the sucrose gradient experiments, an appreciable 100S component has usually been observed, and actually indicated by Riseborough, Tissières and Watson (22) as the primary ribosome involved in protein synthesis. Our observations show that the 100S particles must form after incubation as a result of diluting the incubation mixture with the sucrose solution. Because ribosomal components are quite sensitive to environment, future incorporation-sedimentation studies are contemplated on whole incubation mixtures without sucrose. Various sedimenting components could

be isolated by use of the partition cell. The results of the experiments just described argue that it is not necessary to have ribosomes in the 100S form for protein synthesis. We presume that the template function of polyuridylic acid in polyphenylalanine synthesis involves primarily its combination with a 70S ribosome. The polyuridylic acid we used had a weight average molecular weight of about 150,000 and could not change the sedimentation constant of the 70S ribosome by more than a few per cent. It seems highly likely that the 70S ribosome is a primary agent in protein synthesis.

We have previously suggested that the messenger RNA combines preferentially with one of the subunits in the 70S particle, and that the growing polypeptide chain is more closely associated with the other subunit (10). We should like to indicate a slight preference for the 30S subunit as being that to which the messenger RNA becomes attached. The 30S subunit alone contains a latent ribonuclease enzyme discovered by Elson (26). While adapter RNA does not turn over during protein synthesis (27), messenger RNA is often short lived (19). The function of this short life is probably to enable the cell to respond quickly to changing environment. If the need for a certain enzyme is ended, there are mechanisms which dictate that its messenger RNA no longer be produced, and that already existing messenger RNA will not survive for more than two or three minutes. In this respect, the *E. coli* system contrasts sharply with the reticulocyte system, where the function of the cell is to produce hemoglobin *ad infinitum*. Interestingly enough, we have detected less than 1/10,000th as much latent ribonuclease in reticulocyte ribonucleoprotein particles (28). To sum up, it seems likely that the latent ribonuclease in the 30S subunit relates to the short lifetime of *E. coli* messenger RNA, and that the messenger RNA might be directly associated with the 30S subunits, if it is to make contact with this enzyme at some stage.

We shall return to a detailed model for protein synthesis in a moment, but we must first consider the molecular structure of adapter RNA. Fig. 4

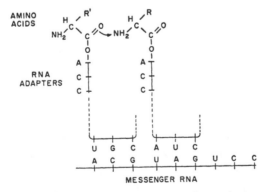

FIG. 4. The function of adapter RNA in protein synthesis. Amino acids are linked to specific adapter RNA's. These become transferred to the ribosome, where the adapter RNA's hydrogen-bond to complementary sites on the template. This places the amino acids in the proper juxtaposition for peptide synthesis.

indicates diagramatically the function of adapter RNA in protein synthesis. Amino acids are linked to specific adapter RNA's. These become transferred to the ribosome, where the adapter RNA's hydrogen bond to complementary sites on the template. This places the amino acids in the proper juxtaposition for peptide synthesis. The X-ray diffraction pattern of adapter RNA bears a strong resemblance to the diffraction pattern given by native sodium DNA (29). The orientation observed for the equatorial 23 A and meridional 3.3 A spacing strongly confirms the double helical nature of adapter RNA. The extreme sharpness of the main equatorial reflection indicates a regularity in packing between molecules only paralleled in nucleic acids by the best samples of DNA which have been studied by X-ray diffraction methods. Hyperchromasy studies suggest that adapter RNA maintains this double helical configuration in solution. The increase in optical density of purified leucine adapter RNA on heating is shown in Fig. 5. Also in this figure are the comparable melting curve for *E. coli*

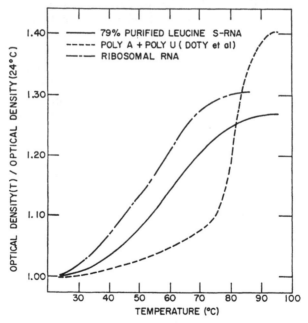

FIG. 5. The optical density at 260 mμ of various RNA's as a function of temperature. The results for the synthetic complex of polyadenylic acid polyuridylic acid are taken from reference 30.

ribosomal RNA, and the synthetic complex formed between high molecular weight polyadenylic acid and polyuridylic acid (30). The latter is believed to form a completely regularly base-paired double helix, indicated by the elevated and narrow range of temperature over which most of the melting occurs. Ribosomal RNA and adapter melt gradually over a broad range of temperature, and because of this we suggested that the base pairing was not completely regular as in DNA (29). Recently, Spencer and co-workers

(31) have succeeded in crystallizing a soluble RNA fraction from yeast, which they believe to be the adapter RNA. These results have led them to propose that yeast adapter RNA has completely regular DNA-type base pairing. The inconsistency of this proposal with the hyperchromasy data may result from the impossibility of detecting small irregularities in the base pairing by X-ray diffraction.

In solution the molecular weight of adapter RNA determined by ultracentrifugation techniques is about 24,000. There is correspondingly 1 nucleosidic terminal group/24,000 molecular weight units. Thus the double helix structure of the adapter RNA molecule must be formed by one polynucleotide strand interacting with itself. This led us to suggest two years ago (29) that the structure consists of a single polynucleotide chain with a bend approximately in the middle, and wound around itself in a helical manner. In this model for adapter RNA, the two halves of the chain are situated anti-parallel to each other so that hydrogen bonding between 6-amino and 6-keto bases could take place. The two halves of the adapter RNA double helix are each only about 30 nucleotides long.

These and other known properties of adapter RNA have been incorporated into the model illustrated in Fig. 6. All adapter RNA's have the terminal sequence: amino acid–adenylic acid–cytidylic acid–cytidylic acid on one end, and guanine on the other (32, 33, 34). Enzymatic degradation experiments (34) indicate that the AC terminal grouping is more susceptible to attack than the rest of the molecule, suggesting that this terminal grouping may be exposed as it would be if it were in the unpaired non-hydrogen bonded state. With 2 unpaired nucleotides on the amino acid end, the third nucleotide, which is a C, could make a DNA-type base pair with the G from the other end of the adapter RNA. In making the proposed bend in the middle of the adapter molecule a minimum three nucleotide residues must be placed in the unhydrogen-bonded condition, according to Fresco, Alberts, and Doty (15). These structural features can be correlated with the known function of adapter RNA in protein synthesis. The three unpaired nucleotides in the bend could conveniently serve as the coding trinucleotide sequence which is presumed to react by specific base pairing with the messenger RNA template. The unpaired AC grouping on the end, carrying the amino acid, may serve as an extendible arm, enabling the growing amino acids on adjacently adsorbed adapter RNA's to make adequate contact.

We are now in a position to consider a detailed stereochemical model for protein synthesis. The original adapter hypothesis put forward by Crick acknowledged the inability of structure-minded biochemists to conceive of a satisfactory template for protein synthesis, which involved the direct binding of amino acids by a template. It was proposed that the amino acids first become linked to specific trinucleotide adapters which are then absorbed to the template, followed by peptide synthesis. The weakness of this hypothesis—of which Crick was well aware—lay in the fact that

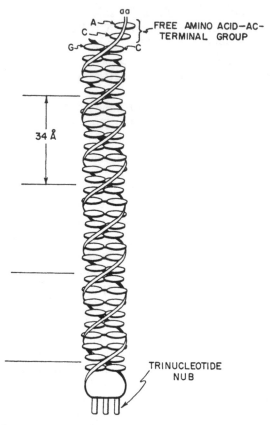

FIG. 6. Proposed structure for adapter RNA. A single polynucleotide chain interacts with itself by forming a bend near the middle. Hydrogen bonding takes place between the nucleotides from the two halves of the chain and results in the formation of a double helix structure. In the bend three bases of necessity are unpaired. The guanine from one end of the chain forms a DNA-type base pair with the cytosine third from the other end. This leaves two nucleotides on the end bearing the amino acid in the flexible state. The molecule is about 100 A long and 20 A wide.

adjacently adsorbed amino acid–trinucleotides are too far apart for the amino acid to make the necessary contact to become linked. The finding that adapter RNA's were actually fairly large macromolecules consisting of about 70 nucleotides, suggested a solution to this problem. The coding nucleotides could be bound to the template with the remainder of the molecule acting as a flexible extension.

There is good experimental evidence that the interaction between adapter RNA and messenger RNA involves DNA-type base pairing (35), but we fail to see how this type of interaction can involve the usual double helix formation between the two polynucleotides, and still produce a stereochemically sound structure which could serve as an intermediate in protein synthesis. A radically different structure is required. We are led to propose that DNA-type base pairing takes place between the coding

ADJACENTLY ADSORBED AMINO
ACID ADAPTER RNA MOLECULES

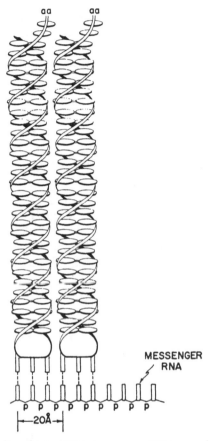

FIG. 7. Proposed structure for adapter RNA–messenger RNA complex. The polynucleotide chain of the messenger RNA is in the completely extended configuration with the bases situated on one side of the chain and the phosphate groups on the other side. The residue repeating distance is 6.8 A making the coding triplet repeating distance 20.4 A. The three alleged coding nucleotides in the adapter RNA adopt a similar extended configuration. The bases from the two polynucleotides interact producing a hydrogen bonded step ladder-like structure. Adjacently adsorbed adapter RNA's are nearly close packed. The necessary "reach" between amino acids is provided by the flexible AC terminal group.

nucleotides on the adapter RNA and the messenger RNA in the manner indicated in Fig. 7. The bases of the two molecules interact with the polynucleotide chain in the completely extended configuration so as to produce a hydrogen bonded stepladder-like structure analogous to the extended beta configuration in proteins. This is accomplished by orienting the polynucleotide chain of the messenger RNA in such a way that all the bases are situated on one side, and the phosphate groups on the other, with a residue repeating distance of 6.8 A along the chain. The three alleged coding nucleotides in the bend of the adapter RNA quite naturally adopt a similar extended configuration. The distance per three nucleotides along the extended messenger RNA would be 20.4 A, which is very nearly the distance of close approach of adjacent adapter RNA double helices. Amino acids on adjacent adapter molecules could not interact unless provided with a flexible extension, such as the postulated unpaired A-C terminal grouping of the RNA. Contact between adjacent amino acids must be so perfect that when adapter RNA's are hydrogen bonded to adjacent trinucleotides sites on the template, contact is possible, but if the adapter RNA should be displaced from adjacent sites by as little as one nucleotide, the contact between amino acids cannot be made. In order to achieve this degree of specificity, the effective length of the flexible extension of the adapter RNA molecule should be about 14 A. This would be provided by two nucleotides in an extended polynucleotide chain.

One limitation of the model is that it does not suggest a function for pseudouridylic acid known to occur uniquely in adapter RNA. It is also difficult to suggest the detailed role the ribosome might have in this template mechanism because little is known about its molecular structure. Evidence has been cited that the 70S ribosome is the active particle in

70s RIBOSOME

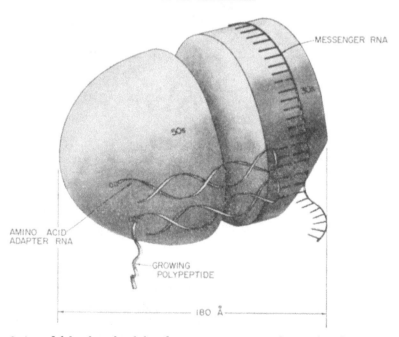

FIG. 8. A model for the role of the ribosome in protein synthesis. The ribosome provides a stabilizing surface for maintaining the messenger RNA in a configuration that would be thermodynamically unstable in solution and for maintaining the reacting adapter molecules in parallel register. Only part of the messenger RNA molecule can be bound at one time.

protein synthesis, and that during synthesis it is more firmly held together. It has also been suggested, very tentatively, that the messenger RNA might be bound to the 30S subunit when active. The site of binding must be chosen so that messenger RNA's of various sizes can be accommodated. Probably only part of the messenger is bound at one time as is suggested in Fig. 8. Adjacently adsorbed adapters might, for greater stabilization, be attracted to the outer surface of the 50S particle, and the polypeptide synthesis would thus be more closely associated with the 50S subunit. The function of the ribosome in this model is to provide a "stabilizing surface" for maintaining the messenger RNA in a configuration that would be thermodynamically unstable in solution and for maintaining the reacting adapter molecules in parallel register. The 50S and 30S subunits in the active particle would be more firmly held together than in the inactive 70S ribosome by virtue of the intersubunit linked adapter RNA which is connected to both the growing end of the polypeptide chain and the messenger RNA.

This investigation has attempted to link structural and biochemical information into a coherent pattern so as to produce a stereochemically sound model for the template mechanism involved in protein synthesis.

ACKNOWLEDGMENTS

We are grateful to Mr. Ken Hanson for his assistance in the construction of the molecular models, to Mr. Walter Geisbush for his assistance with the electron microscopy and to Mrs. Mac Zubay for her assistance with the manuscript.

REFERENCES

1. Tissières, A., J. D. Watson, D. Schlessinger, and B. Hollingworth. 1959. Ribonucleoprotein particles from Escherichia coli. J. Mol. Biol. 1: 221.
2. Huxley, H. E., and G. Zubay. 1960. Electron microscope observations on the structure of microsomal particles from Escherichia coli. J. Mol. Biol. 2: 10.
3. Kurland, C. G. 1960. Molecular characterization of ribonucleic acid from Escherichia coli ribosomes. I. Isolation and molecular weights. J. Mol. Biol. 2: 83.
4. Green, M. H., and B. D. Hall. 1961. A comparison of the native and derived 30S and 50S ribosomes of Escherichia coli. Biophys. J. 1: 517.
5. Waller, J. P., and J. I. Harris. 1961. Studies on the composition of the protein from Escherichia coli ribosomes. Proc. Natl. Acad. Sci. U.S. 47: 18.
6. Dagley, S., and J. Sykes. 1959. Effect of drugs upon components of bacterial cytoplasm. Nature 183: 1608.
7. Nomura, M., and J. D. Watson. 1959. Ribonucleoprotein particles within chloromycetin-inhibited Escherichia coli. J. Mol. Biol. 1: 204.
8. Kurland, C. G., M. Nomura and J. D. Watson. 1962. The physical properties of the chloromycetin particles. J. Mol. Biol. 4: 388.
9. Britten, R. J., B. J. McCarthy and R. B. Roberts. 1962. The synthesis of ribosomes in Escherichia coli. IV. The synthesis of ribosomal protein and the assembly of ribosomes. Biophys. J. 2: 83.

10. Zubay, G. 1962. The structure of nucleoproteins. *In* The molecular basis of neoplasia, p. 281. University of Texas Press, Austin.
11. Rich, A., and J. D. Watson. 1954. Some relations between DNA and RNA. Proc. Natl. Acad. Sci. U.S. *40*: 759.
12. Zubay, G., and M. H. F. Wilkins. 1960. X-ray diffraction studies on the structure of ribosomes from *Escherichia coli*. J. Mol. Biol. *2*: 105.
13. Schlessinger, D. 1960. Hypochromicity in ribosomes from *Escherichia coli*. J. Mol. Biol. *2*: 92.
14. Steiner, R. F., and R. F. Beers. 1961. Polynucleotides. Elsevier Publishing Co., Amsterdam, London, New York and Princeton.
15. Fresco, J. R., B. M. Alberts and P. Doty. 1960. Some molecular details of the secondary structure of RNA. Nature *188*: 98.
16. McQuillen, K., R. B. Roberts and R. J. Britten. 1959. Synthesis of nascent protein by ribosomes in *Escherichia coli*. Proc. Natl. Acad. Sci. U.S. *45*: 1437.
17. Lamborg, M. R., and P. C. Zamecnik, 1960. Amino acid incorporation into protein by extracts of *Escherichia coli*. Biochim. et Biophys. Acta *42*: 206.
18. Tissières, A., D. Schlessinger and F. Gros. 1960. Amino acid incorporation into protein by *Escherichia coli* ribosomes. Proc. Natl. Acad. Sci. U.S. *46*: 1450.
19. Jacob, F., and J. Monod. 1961. Genetic regulatory mechanisms in the synthesis of proteins. J. Mol. Biol. *3*: 318.
20. Brenner, S., F. Jacob and M. Meselson. 1961. An unstable intermediate carrying information from genes to ribosomes for protein synthesis. Nature *190*: 576.
21. Gros, F., H. Hiatt, W. Gilbert, C. G. Kurland, R. W. Risebrough and J. D. Watson. 1961. Unstable ribonucleic acid revealed by pulse labelling of *Escherichia coli*. Nature *190*: 581.
22. Risebrough, R. W., A. Tissières and J. D. Watson. 1962. Messenger-RNA attachment to active ribosomes. Proc. Natl. Acad. Sci. U.S. *48*: 430.
23. Matthaei, J. H. and Nirenberg, M. W. 1961. Characteristics and stabilization of DNAase-sensitive protein synthesis in *Escherichia coli* extracts. Proc. Natl. Acad. Sci. U.S. *47*: 1580.
24. Nirenberg, M. W. and J. H. Matthaei. 1961. The dependence of cell-free protein synthesis in *Escherichia coli* upon naturally occurring or synthetic polyribonucleotides. Proc. Natl. Acad. Sci. U.S. *47*: 1588.
25. Zubay, G. and J. Fresco. The effective ribosomal unit in protein synthesis. J. Mol. Biol. (in press).
26. Elson, D. and M. Tal. 1959. Biochemical differences in ribonucleoproteins. Biochim. et Biophys. Acta *36*: 281.
27. Hoagland, M. B. and L. T. Comly, 1960. Interaction of soluble ribonucleic acid and microsomes. Proc. Natl. Acad. Sci. U.S. *46*: 1554.
28. Zubay, G. Unpublished data.
29. Brown, G. L. and G. Zubay. 1960. Physical properties of the soluble RNA of *Escherichia coli*. J. Mol. Biol. *2*: 287.
30. Doty, P., H. Boedtker, J. R. Fresco, R. Haselkorn and M. Litt. 1959. Secondary structure in ribonucleic acids. Proc. Natl. Acad. Sci. U.S. *45*: 482.
31. Spencer, M., W. Fuller, M. H. F. Wilkins and G. L. Brown. 1962. Determination of the helical configuration of ribonucleic acid molecules by X-ray diffraction study of crystalline amino-acid-transfer ribonucleic acid. Nature *194*: 1014.
32. Hecht, L. I., M. L. Stephenson and P. C. Zamecnik. 1959. Binding of amino acids to the end group of a soluble ribonucleic acid. Proc. Natl. Acad. Sci. U.S. *45*: 505.

33. Zachau, H. G., G. Acs and F. Lipmann. 1958. Isolation of adenosine amino acid esters from a ribonuclease digest of soluble, liver ribonucleic acid. Proc. Natl. Acad. Sci. U.S. *44*: 885.
34. Preiss, J., M. Dieckmann and P. Berg. 1961. The enzymic synthesis of amino acyl derivatives of ribonucleic acid, IV. J. Biol. Chem. *236*: 1748.
35. Speyer, J. F., P. Lengyel, C. Basilio and S. Ochoa. 1962. Synthetic poly-nucleotides and the amino acid code. IV. Proc. Natl. Acad. Sci. U.S. *48*: 441.
36. Zubay, G. 1962. The isolation and fractionation of soluble ribonucleic acid. J. Mol. Biol. *4*: 347.
37. Tissières, A. and J. D. Watson. 1958. Ribonucleoprotein particles from *Escherichia coli.* Nature *182*: 778.
38. Siekevitz, P. 1952. Uptake of radioactive alanine in vitro into the proteins of rat liver fractions. J. Biol. Chem. *195*: 549.

THE BIOSYNTHESIS OF RIBOSOMAL AND COMPLEMENTARY RNA IN BACTERIA

B. J. McCARTHY

Department of Terrestrial Magnetism
Carnegie Institution of Washington
Washington, D.C.

THE BIOPHYSICS GROUP at the Department of Terrestrial Magnetism have been engaged upon studies of ribosome biosynthesis since 1957. Almost all of the information has been obtained from experiments in which bacteria have been labelled with one or more specific RNA or protein precursors for various periods of time and the cell extract is subsequently fractioned by a variety of procedures. This approach has indeed allowed the elucidation of the main sequence of steps in the assembly of ribosomes but has also provided much information relating to the synthesis and behavior of nucleic acid molecules other than ribosomal RNA. By combining the results obtained from different fractionation schemes it is possible to describe the flow of nucleotide material through the various types of molecule present in the cell, and to illuminate the complicated interrelationships which exist between precursor pools and polynucleotide, and between the synthesis of one type of polynucleotide molecule and another. As an adjunct to the studies of macromolecule synthesis a detailed study of base and nucleotide pools has been made. This has been described by R. J. Britten elsewhere at this Congress (page 49).

The experiments to be described result from the co-operation of the author with other members of the biophysics group, principally Drs. E. T. Bolton, R. J. Britten and J. E. Midgley.

I. THE SEQUENCE OF STEPS IN RIBOSOME BIOSYNTHESIS

The various stages in the assembly of ribosomes from RNA and protein can readily be shown by experiments in which samples of cell extracts are prepared and analysed from cells which have been labelled with C^{14}-uracil for various periods of time. A refinement of this technique involves the use of a second isotope P^{32} to label the cellular RNA randomly. In this case P^{32} as orthophosphate was supplied to exponentially growing cells of *E. coli* ML 30 for several generations. Subsequently C^{14}-uracil was supplied to the cells and samples taken at a series of times and chilled to 4 C by pouring over crushed frozen medium. The uniform P^{32} labelling of the RNA makes it possible to determine the specific radioactivity (that is, C^{14} radioactivity from uracil per unit total RNA) in any fraction free of lipid by means of a liquid scintillation counter. This leads to technical simplification and permits the analysis of smaller samples than possible by the use of ultraviolet absorption or chemical means.

The precursor stages in ribosome synthesis were first recognized by means of DEAE (diethylaminoethylcellulose) column analysis (McCarthy, Britten & Roberts, 1962). Fig. 1 shows the results of the DEAE column analysis of ribosomal pellets harvested from broken cells, prepared as described with the $MgCl_2$ concentration held at 10^{-2} M throughout. The existence of a sequence of stages is readily observed in the six parts of Fig. 1. At 25 sec all the radioactivity appears in a peak centered at fraction 28 (0.6 M NaCl).

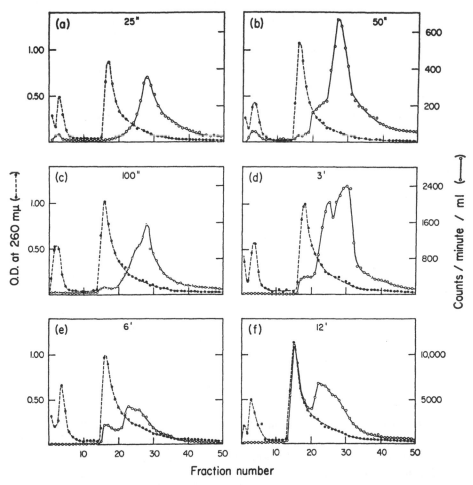

Fig. 1. Analysis of total ribosomal pellets (40K 240 minute pellets) on a DEAE cellulose column. Linear sodium chloride gradient from 0.2 M to 1.2 M in tris-HCl buffer 0.01 M containing $MgCl_2$ 0.01 M, pH 7.4. Salt gradient 0.004 M/ml. Volumes collected 3.6–3.8 ml: (a) 25-sec exposure to C^{14}-uracil, (b) 50 sec, (c) 100 sec, (d) 3 min, (e) 6 min, (f) 12 min.

At 50 sec and 100 sec a shoulder develops on the forward edge of the peak and becomes the dominant peak (fraction 23, 0.5 M NaCl) at 6 min. Meanwhile the radioactivity of the main peak of ribonucleoprotein (fraction 16, 0.4 M NaCl) remains at a very low level in the first three analyses, subsequently rising very rapidly in the period from 3 min to 12 min.

The quantitative analysis of this data has been described in detail elsewhere (McCarthy *et al.*, 1962), together with the theory underlying the procedures of data analysis (Britten & McCarthy, 1962) designed to test the existence of precuror product relationships between the three resolvable labelled objects and to measure the relative quantities of each.

It is, in fact, already apparent from inspection of the curves in Fig. 1 that precursor–product relationships exist. Thus at very early times all the newly formed RNA is present in the third peak, and a significant amount builds up in the middle peak only after that in the earliest component has levelled off. The radioactivity is found in the main ribosome peak only after much longer times, suggesting that RNA entering these objects, which represent the bulk of the ribosomal material as evidenced by the ultraviolet absorption, is delayed by passing through two precursor stages. For clarity and ease of discussion the two precursors have been named eosome and neosome in the order of their synthesis. As will be shown later these definitions do not rest solely upon their distinctive chromatographic behavior, for these objects can also be resolved from the bulk ribosomal material on the basis of their sedimentation coefficients.

Examination of the data in detail leads to the following quantities for the various precursors and products:

$$\rightarrow \text{ eosome } 2.7\% \rightarrow \text{ neosome } 6.8\% \rightarrow \text{ ribosome } 90.5\%$$

Fig. 2 shows the results of sedimentation analysis carried out on cells washed and broken in TCM buffer with 10^{-4} M $MgCl_2$ present throughout. This concentration of magnesium causes the ribosomes to dissociate to their 30S and 50S subunits, and allows the precursor stages to be resolved. At higher magnesium concentrations they are found in association with the large ribosomes. At 30 sec and at 1 min the C^{14} radioactivity appears almost entirely in a broad peak (eosome) at about 14S. At 2 min, two other peaks are clearly distinguishable, one associated with 30S ribosomes and another appearing between 30S and 50S at approximately 43S. Up to 4 min there is very little radioactivity to be associated with the 50S ribosome peak but between 4 and 10 min the radioactivity rises by a factor of about ten.

Close examination of this data and consideration of the flows of C^{14}-uracil in and out of the various components (McCarthy *et al.*, 1962) allows a correlation of the sedimentation with the chromatographic data. Thus it is immediately evident that the broad 14S peak is identical with the eosome peak in chromatography and similar quantities are obtained for each. The 43S component is certainly a representative of neosome material but seems to be only 5 or 6 per cent of the total ribosomal RNA. This and other

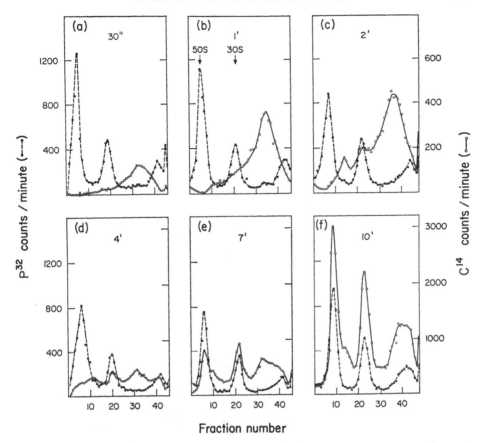

FIG. 2. Sedimentation analysis of six DNAase-treated total extracts made and centrifuged in tris-HCl 0.01 M, pH 7.4 $MgCl_2$ 10^{-4} M from cells steady-state-labelled with P^{32} given (a) 30-sec exposure to C^{14}-uracil, (b) 1 min, (c) 2 min, (d) 4 min, (e) 7 min, (f) 10 min. Centrifugation 175 min at 37,000 rpm 4 C. Samples analysed correspond to 0.5 mg dry weight of cells.

considerations lead to the conclusion that there must be also a neosome particle of 30S or less, part of which is a direct precursor to the 43S and part a precursor of 30S ribosomes. A summary of the cross connections between the two types of analysis is given by Britten, McCarthy and Roberts (1962).

These studies of the synthesis of the RNA portion of ribosomes provide only a few hints as to the concurrent synthesis of ribosomal protein, although the separation by chromatography itself reflects a different RNA/protein ratio in the three components. The step from 43S neosome to 50S ribosome involves both a change in sedimentation coefficient and a change in elution from DEAE cellulose, but no additional RNA is added. It seems quite obvious that this change is due to the addition of protein. The details of these concurrent processes are illustrated by similar experiments in which C^{14}-leucine is substituted as the pulse label for C^{14}-uracil (Britten et al.,

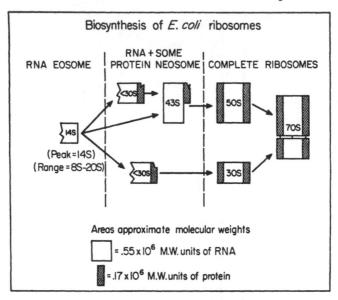

FIG. 3. The biosynthesis of ribosomes in *E. coli*. The open and shaded areas are proportional to weights of RNA and protein respectively.

1962). These experiments have already been reported in detail and it suffices merely to summarize the conclusions.

The final flow diagram, including both the RNA and the protein moieties of ribosomes, is shown in Fig. 3. The open and shaded areas are proportional to RNA and protein contents. Eosomes are shown as pure RNA since the protein content is certainly very low if not zero. The 30S and 43S neosome are shown with low protein content since it is clear that the conversion of neosome to ribosome involves only the addition of protein and that the greater part of the ribosomal protein is added in this step.

II. CHARACTERISTICS OF RAPIDLY LABELLED RNA

Published studies of rapidly labelled RNA contain two conflicting sets of observations. On the one hand it is evident from the kinetic studies of the flow of P^{32}-orthophosphate or C^{14}-uracil in and out of the 14S eosome fraction described above, that it can be considered predominantly, at least, as a precursor to the ribosomal RNA.

In Fig. 4 the time course of the entry of C^{14}-uracil into the 14S eosome fraction is plotted together with the radioactivity in ribosomal material including neosome and that in the total RNA. All the radioactivity initially enters the eosome and the curve levels off at 0.02 corresponding to 2 per cent of the total ribosomal RNA. The slope of the curve for ribosomes is essentially zero at zero time. Thus all the radioactivity entering ribosomes passes through the precursor eosome peak. Furthermore the ribosome curve falls

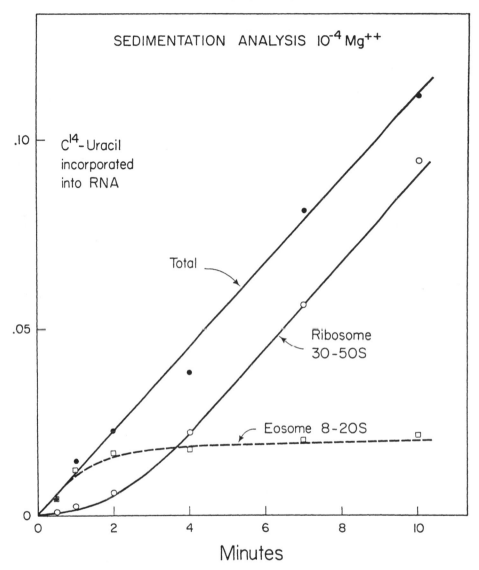

FIG. 4. The C[14]-uracil label incorporated into total RNA (●), the eosome region 8-20S (□), and the ribosome region (○), i.e. material between 30S and 50S including neosome and ribosome. Data from Fig. 2.

below the total curve by an amount approximately equal to the quantity of eosome.

On the other hand, analyses of the pulse labelled total RNA (Yčas & Vincent, 1960; Astrachan & Fisher, 1961) and the purified 14S fraction (Midgley, 1962) show an apparent base composition intermediate between that of ribosomal RNA and the bacterial DNA. Consequently, depending on the type of observations made, the rapidly labelled fraction has been described as mostly ribosome precursor (McCarthy *et al.*, 1962) or mostly "messenger" (Gros *et al.*, 1961) or informational RNA postulated to be necessary for the genetically directed synthesis of specific proteins on ribosomes (Jacob & Monod, 1961). Kitazume, Yčas and Vincent (1962) have attempted to resolve this paradox by concluding that, in yeast, the DNA-like RNA fraction is an obligatory precursor in the formation of ribosomal RNA.

Correlation of kinetic and composition measurements therefore seemed necessary to elucidate the relative amounts of the supposed two components. The term DNA-like RNA or D-RNA is used to describe the RNA fraction whose composition is observed to be close to that of the DNA. The base composition of the rapidly labelled 14S peak of RNA was measured in five species of bacteria of widely different DNA base compositions (Midgley, 1962). Exponentially growing cultures of bacteria were labelled with P^{32} for periods of 2 or 3 per cent of the generation time, i.e. 2 to 4 min depending on the cells employed. The labelled 14S RNA was then isolated by sucrose gradient centrifugation or chromatography on DEAE cellulose (Fig. 1). The RNA was collected, TCA precipitated and its composition determined. The results are recorded in Table 1 together with the measured compositions of the bacterial ribosomal RNA (Midgley, 1962) and the DNA (Belozersky & Spirin, 1960).

In each case the composition of the 14S RNA falls between those for

TABLE 1
COMPOSITION OF 14S RAPIDLY LABELLED RNA

	Composition Mole %				
					G+C
	C	A	G	U(T)	A+U(T)
P. vulgaris					
14S RNA	21.9	27.0	27.6	23.5	0.98
DNA*	19	31	19	31	0.61
Ribosomal RNA†	21.7	26.2	31.4	20.7	1.13
B. subtilis					
14S RNA	22.5	25.3	28.0	24.2	1.02
DNA	21	29	21	29	0.72
Ribosomal RNA	22.3	25.9	31.0	20.8	1.15
E. coli					
14S RNA	22.7	25.1	29.1	23.1	1.07
DNA	26	24	26	24	1.08
Ribosomal RNA	21.9	25.1	32.6	20.4	1.20
A. aerogenes					
14S RNA	24.1	24.5	30.2	21.2	1.19
DNA	28	22	28	22	1.28
Ribosomal RNA	21.9	25.5	31.5	21.1	1.15
Ps. aeruginosa					
14S RNA	25.6	20.8	31.7	21.9	1.31
DNA	32	18	32	18	1.78
Ribosomal RNA	21.7	25.7	31.6	21.0	1.14

*Values for DNA taken from Belozersky and Spirin (1960).
†Values for ribosomal RNA taken from Midgley (1962).

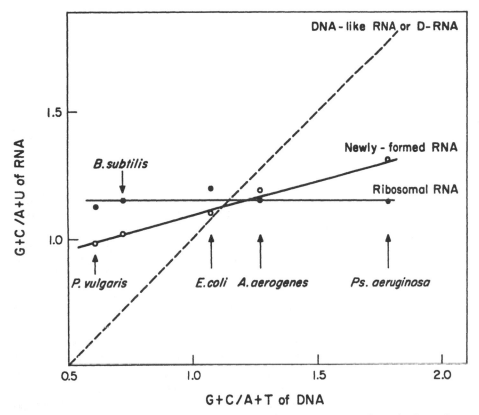

FIG. 5. Comparison of G+C/A+U ratios of ribosomal RNA and newly formed or rapidly labelled RNA with the G+C/A+T ratios for the corresponding DNA. ● ribosomal RNA. ○ newly formed RNA.

ribosomal RNA and DNA (or D-RNA) suggesting a mixture of two types of molecules. The results can be expressed in graphical form by plotting the G + C / A + U ratio for the DNA (Fig. 5). In such a plot a pure D-RNA fraction should give a slope of 1. Since the composition of ribosomal RNA is almost constant and shows no correlation with the DNA, the slope of the line through the numbers for the rapidly labelled RNA gives a rough measure of the proportion of the two types of molecule which could be present in the fraction. A reasonable fit to the data would be made by a mixture of about one-third D-RNA and two-thirds ribosomal RNA. This experiment does not establish the existence of such a mixture but does indicate that the rapidly labelled fraction of RNA cannot consist solely of D-RNA or messenger RNA.

III. SEPARATION AND PURIFICATION OF D-RNA

(a). Fractionation of newly synthesized RNA. The early labelled RNA can be separated into two fractions of different composition by differential

TABLE 2

FRACTIONATION OF P^{32} PULSE LABELLED RNA IN *E. coli*

Expt. no.	Exposure to P^{32} (min.)		Base Composition Mole %				$\dfrac{G+C}{A+U}$
			C	A	G	U	
1	1.5	Pellet*	21.2	25.0	33.1	20.8	1.18
		SN	25.5	24.4	27.2	22.9	1.11
2	2.0	Pellet	22.5	24.7	32.5	20.3	1.22
		SN	24.7	24.7	27.1	23.5	1.07
3	3.0	Pellet	21.5	25.3	32.7	20.5	1.18
		SN	25.2	24.3	26.7	23.8	1.08
4	3.0	Pellet	22.0	24.9	32.0	21.1	1.17
		SN	25.4	24.0	26.8	23.7	1.09
	Average	Pellet	21.8	25.0	32.6	20.6	1.19
		SN	25.2	24.4	26.9	23.5	1.09
		Ribosomal RNA	21.9	25.1	32.6	20.4	1.20
		DNA	26	24	26	24	1.08

*Pellet refers to that RNA remaining with the ribosomes after water treatment and consequent reduction of the ionic strength and magnesium concentration (Midgley 1962) and SN to the RNA dissociated.

dissociation from ribosomes at a Mg^{++} concentration of about 3×10^{-4} M (Midgley & McCarthy, 1962).

Table 2 contains the results of the base analyses of the various fractions together with the fraction of the labelled macromolecules recovered. The separation technique is best applied to *E. coli* material, although it has been applied with limited success to three other bacterial species (Midgley & McCarthy, 1962). Very little of the pulse labelled RNA was degraded during the procedure and the fractions obtained had base compositions very close to those of pure ribosomal RNA and of *E. coli* DNA. Distortions of the real nucleotide composition by a combination of unequal labelling of pool nucleotides (Yčas & Vincent, 1960) and nonrandomness in DNA sequences (Burton, 1960; Josse, Kaiser & Kornberg, 1961) are not apparent in the measured composition of the D-RNA. Apparently the "water shock" treatment causes the DNA-like fraction to become disassociated from the ribosomes leaving behind the labelled RNA which resembles ribosomal RNA.

(*b*). Purification of D-RNA with a DNA column. The principle of using immobilized DNA to select D-RNA molecules by complementary base pair formation developed by Bautz and Hall (1962) for T4 specific RNA has been generalized by Bolton and McCarthy (1962a) so as to be applicable to the nucleic acid of any organism. Immobilization of DNA in an agar gel preparation leads to a method for the separation of D-RNA and ribosomal RNA. The hybridization reaction is a very specific one and no reaction occurs between unrelated DNA and RNA molecules. Fig. 6 shows the specificity of the reaction of P^{32} pulse labelled RNA from *Proteus vulgaris* cells. This RNA hybridizes with the homologous DNA agar but not with an agar preparation containing T2 bacteriophage DNA of approximately the

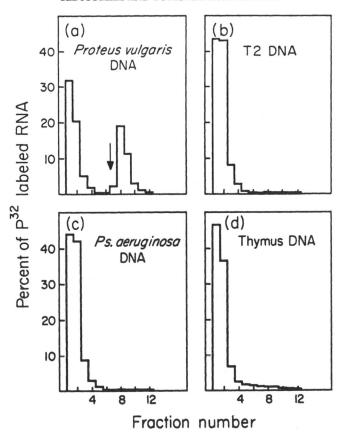

FIG. 6. The specificity of the adsorption of RNA from *P. vulgaris* labelled with P32 for 1 min to columns of DNA-agar gel. Conditions as for Fig. 2. (*a*) Agar containing *P. vulgaris* DNA, (*b*) T2 DNA, (*c*) *Ps. aeruginosa* DNA, (*d*) calf thymus DNA.

same average base composition as *P. vulgaris* DNA. Similarly there is no reaction with the gels prepared with the DNA of *Pseudomonas aeruginosa* or calf thymus.

RNA prepared from *P. vulgaris* cells exposed to P32 for one minute reacts with *P. vulgaris* DNA agar until approximately one-third of the P32 labelled RNA is hybridized after some eight hours. No further reaction takes place on longer incubation (Bolton & McCarthy, 1962a). The two components of RNA (Fig. 6a) prove to have very different base compositions (Table 3). The adsorbed material has a composition closely resembling that of the DNA and the unadsorbed RNA is apparently ribosomal. Since all the P32 is present in the rapidly labelled or 14S RNA at this time, this experiment establishes that there are indeed two types of RNA present in this component. Moreover it is in agreement with the interpretation that approximately one-third of this RNA is D-RNA and the remainder ribosomal RNA.

TABLE 3

BASE COMPOSITION OF P³² LABELLED RNA SEPARATED BY DNA-AGAR

	Mole Fraction				
	C	A	G	U(T)	%GC
Pulse labelled *P. vulgaris* RNA:					
Unadsorbed RNA 65%	22.5	23.3	32.1	22.1	55
Adsorbed RNA 35%	19.8	30.1	20.9	29.2	41
Purified 14S RNA fraction of *P. vulgaris* labelled for 5 min with P³²*	22.7	26.7	27.6	23.0	49
P. vulgaris ribosomal RNA†	21.7	26.2	31.4	20.7	53
P. vulgaris DNA‡	19	31	19	31	38

*Data from Midgley and McCarthy (1962).
†Data from Midgley (1962).
‡Data from Belozersky and Spirin (1960).

IV. RATE OF SYNTHESIS AND TURNOVER OF D-RNA

The experiments recorded above establish the amount of D-RNA present in the cell and its rate of synthesis relative to ribosomal RNA. Thus the rapidly labelled 14S fraction of RNA is roughly 3 per cent of the total cellular RNA (McCarthy *et al.*, 1962) and is about one-third D-RNA. This would fix the quantity of D-RNA at about 1 per cent. The fact that the base composition of the 14S fraction is the same after different periods of exposure to P³² (Midgley & McCarthy, 1962) suggests that the composition is a measure of the relative rates of synthesis of the two types of molecule. The flow of material into D-RNA is thus approximately half that into ribosomal RNA. These facts together with the studies of the change in base composition with the time of exposure to P³² show that the D-RNA molecules are unstable. The rapid labelling of the ribosomal portion of the 14S RNA is a consequence of the large flow of material into ribosomes and that of the D-RNA is due to degradation to low molecular weight compounds.

The constant composition of the newly formed RNA mixture indicates that the time constant for approach to constant specific radioactivity is the same for the two classes of rapidly labelled RNA. Since the time constant of the over-all fraction has already been measured (Fig. 4) at 2 to 3 min, this would seem to be an adequate estimate of the average lifetime of these molecules. It is, in fact, possible to measure this directly and also to study the reutilization of the nucleotide material provided by the degradation by the methods of analysis to be described below.

The separation of pulse labelled bacterial RNA into two components by the DNA-agar technique makes it possible to study the rate of synthesis of the D-RNA directly. Cells of *P. vulgaris* were grown in C medium containing P³² for three generations. C¹⁴-uracil was then added and samples taken for the isolation of RNA after 1, 2, 3, 5, 7 and 10 min. The fractionation of the one-minute sample is shown in Fig. 7. It is evident that about

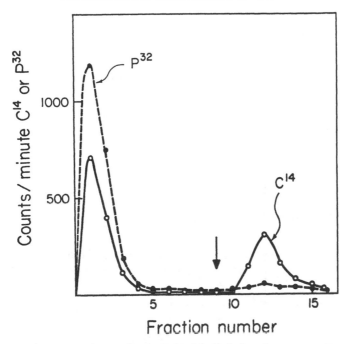

FIG. 7. The adsorption of *P. vulgaris* RNA labelled for three generations with P[32] and for 1 min with C[14]-uracil to a column of DNA agar gel. Incubation 15 hr at 60 C. Elution with eight 5 ml portions of 2 × SSC followed by eight 5 ml portions of 0.01 × SSC.

one-third of the C[14]-labelled RNA is in the hybrid peak and is accompanied by only a small fraction of the total RNA as represented by the P[32] label. The C[14] and P[32] radioactivity in the front and back peaks were computed for each time point. After normalization to the same size sample of RNA by means of the total P[32] eluted, the C[14] radioactivity in the total RNA and in the adsorbed peak were plotted (Fig. 8). A small correction was applied to the latter series of numbers to account for the small amount of ribosomal RNA appearing in the back peak. This may be owing to specific hybridization between ribosomal RNA and DNA (Yankofsky & Spiegelman, 1962; Bolton & McCarthy, 1962b). The correction can be easily estimated from a knowledge of the total RNA adsorbed in the hybrid peak as measured by the P[32] radioactivity.

The rate of entry of C[14]-uracil into total RNA produces a straight line through the origin as in *E. coli* (see Fig. 4). Apparently the initial rate of entry of label into the D-RNA accounts for about one-third of this flow. The entry of C[14]-uracil into D-RNA soon levels off indicating an average lifetime of these molecules of about two minutes. Estimation of the quantity of D-RNA from these kinetics is made somewhat inaccurate by the large correction at late times, but the curve suggests an amount corresponding to the RNA synthesized during one minute; i.e., approximately 1 per cent of the total RNA content.

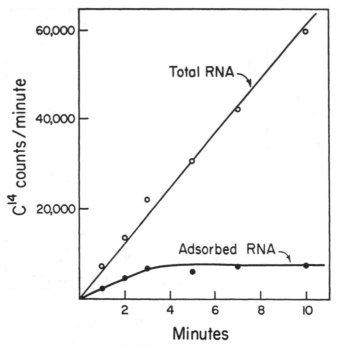

FIG. 8. The rate of synthesis of RNA adsorbable by a DNA agar gel column. Six samples of RNA from *P. vulgaris* cells grown for three generations in P[32] with a generation time of 72 min were taken after exposures of 1, 2, 3, 5, 7 and 10 min to C[14]-uracil. Each was incubated with an agar gel containing *P. vulgaris* DNA 30 μg RNA/0.5 mg DNA (see Fig. 4). The C[14] cpm in the total RNA and the adsorbable material was normalized for the amount of RNA employed by means of the P[32] cpm and plotted against time. Data from Fig. 4 and five additional analyses.

CONCLUSION

The information obtained from the various experimental approaches has been combined to give the diagram of Fig. 9. This summarizes the flow of material into the various nucleic acid components. The dashed lines indicate a convenient separation into parts analysable by different techniques. The areas of the boxes correspond to the relative quantity of each component present in growing *E. coli* cells. There are a multitude of complex reactions and interconversions symbolized by the box of low molecular weight compounds. This part of the diagram will not be discussed here further except to point out the evidence that a major fraction of the exogenously added bases can be rapidly incorporated into RNA, bypassing these relatively large nucleoside phosphate pools (McCarthy & Britten, 1962; Buchwald & Britten, 1963). The labelled compounds entering these pools do ultimately find their way into RNA.

The second region of Fig. 9 concerns the steps in ribosome biosynthesis up to the assembly of the 30S and 50S ribosomes. The 14S RNA or eosome is shown as two distinct objects or classes of objects having different roles.

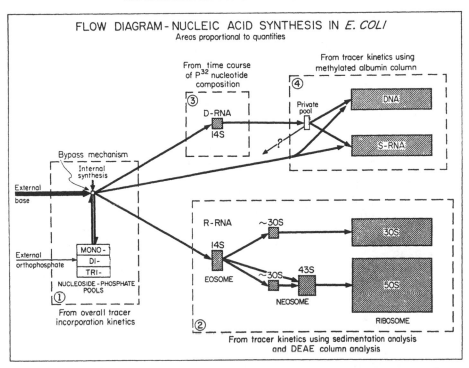

FIG. 9. Flow diagram for nucleic acid synthesis in *E. coli*. The areas of the boxes represent the relative quantities of the different elements present in exponentially growing cells. Open boxes represent low molecular weight (acid soluble) compounds and the cross-hatched boxes represent macromolecular fractions. The dashed lines show how the pattern has been separated into analysable parts and the titles indicate the classes of evidence used.

One is the first in a sequence of precursors to 30S and 50S ribosomes, and the other is a group of molecules of only transitory existence which may act as template or messenger RNA (Jacob & Monod, 1961). This RNA is degraded after an average lifetime of about two minutes and the nucleotide material reutilized for S-RNA and DNA synthesis and possibly for ribosomal RNA synthesis (Midgley & McCarthy, 1962). Evidence for this latter process is difficult to obtain and likewise the "private pool" for the degradation products is hypothetical, although it is certainly separate from the main nucleoside phosphate pool. There must however be alternative sources of material for S-RNA and DNA since the composition of the former differs from that of D-RNA and both are labelled in the presence of chloramphenicol where D-RNA is apparently not degraded so rapidly (Midgley & McCarthy, 1962).

At the moment, then, this diagram would seem to summarize satisfactorily our knowledge of the flow of material into nucleic acids in *E. coli* cells, although it is certainly subject to the addition of further features. It should be remembered also that this type of description applies to the bulk components as they are present in the cell extract, and that very little is known of their spatial distribution within the living cell. Our understanding of nucleic acid biosynthesis and function would be greatly amplified if there were available cytological evidence with which to correlate these observations.

REFERENCES

Astrachan, L., and T. M. Fisher. 1961.   Resemblance of bacterial RNA and DNA. Fed. Proc. *20*: 35a.

Bautz, E. K. F., and B. D. Hall. 1962.   The isolation of the specific RNA on a DNA cellulose column. Proc. Ntal. Acad. Sci. U.S. *48*: 400.

Belozersky, A. N., and A. S. Spirin. 1960.   *In* Nucleic acids, vol. III, ed. Chargaff and Davidson, p. 146. Academic Press.

Bolton, E. T., and B. J. McCarthy. 1962a. A general method for the isolation of RNA complementary to DNA. Proc. Natl. Acad. Sci. U.S. *48*: 1390.

Bolton, E. T., and B. J. McCarthy. 1962b.   Unpublished results.

Britten, R. J., and B. J. McCarthy. 1962.   The synthesis of ribosomes in *E. coli.* II. Analysis of the kinetics of tracer incorporation in growing cells. Biophys. J. *2*: 49.

Britten, R. J., B. J. McCarthy and R. B. Roberts. 1962.   The synthesis of ribosomes in *E. coli.* IV. The synthesis of ribosomal protein and the assembly of ribosomes. Biophys. J. *2*: 83.

Burton, K. 1960.   Frequencies of nucleotide sequences in deoxyribonucleic acids. Biochem. J. 77: 547.

Buchwald, M., and R. J. Britten. 1963.   Incorporation of RNA bases into the metabolic pool and RNA of *E. coli.* Biophys. J. *3*: 155.

Gros. F., W. Gilbert, H. H. Hiatt, G. Attardi, P. E. Spahr and J. D. Watson. 1961. Cold Spring Harbor Symp. Quant. Biol. *26*: 111.

Jacob, F., and J. Monod. 1961.   Genetic regulatory mechanisms in the synthesis of proteins. J. Mol. Biol. *3*: 318.

Josse, J., A. D. Kaiser and A. Kornberg. 1961.   Enzymatic synthesis of DNA. VIII. Frequencies of nearest neighbor base sequences in DNA. J. Biol. Chem. *236*: 864.

Kitazume, Y., M. Yčas, and W. S. Vincent. 1962.   Metabolic properties of a RNA fraction in yeast. Proc. Natl. Acad. Sci. U.S. *48*: 265.

McCarthy, B. J., and R. J. Britten. 1962.   The synthesis of ribosomes in *E. coli.* I. The incorporation of C^{14} uracil into the metabolic pool and RNA. Biophys. J. *2*: 35.

McCarthy, B. J., R. J. Britten and R. B. Roberts. 1962.   The synthesis of ribosomes in *E. coli.* III. Synthesis of ribosomal RNA. Biophys. J. *2*: 57.

Midgley, J. E. M. 1962.   The nucleotide base composition of RNA from several microbial species. Biophys. et Biochim. Acta. *61*: 513.

Midgley, J. E. M., and B. J. McCarthy. 1962.   The synthesis and kinetic behaviour of DNA-like RNA in bacteria. Biophys. et Biochim. Acta. *61*: 696.

Yčas, M., and W. S. Vincent. 1960.   A RNA fraction from yeast related in composition to DNA. Proc. Natl. Acad. Sci. U.S. *46*: 804.

Yankofsky, S. A., and S. Spiegelman. 1962.   The identification of the ribosomal RNA cistron by sequence complementarity. Proc. Natl. Acad. Sci. U.S. *48*: 1069, 1466.

THE USE OF DNA-RNA HYBRIDIZATION AS AN ANALYTICAL TOOL[*]

S. SPIEGELMAN

University of Illinois
Urbana, Illinois, U.S.A.

MARMUR AND DOTY (1961) demonstrated the specific re-formation of double stranded DNA when heat denatured DNA is subjected to a slow cool from elevated temperatures. Such reconstitution of the native duplex structure occurs only between DNA strands originating from the same or closely related organisms (Schildkraut, Marmur & Doty, 1961). The degree of biological relatedness required is about the same as that demanded by the possibility of genetic recombination. It is difficult to avoid the conclusion that such rigid specificity requirements must reflect the need for a perfect or near perfect complementarity of base sequences.

We have here, then, a method of detecting the existence of sequence complementarity between two strands of polynucleotide. The formation of a double stranded structure when mixtures of the single stranded materials are subjected to a slow cool can be accepted as evidence for the existence of complementarity.

Hall and Spiegelman (1961) sought to extend this device as a tool for analysing relations between RNA and DNA. It was known from the pioneering model experiments with synthetic homopolymers (Rich, 1960; Schildkraut *et al.*, 1961a) that hybrid duplexes composed of ribose and deoxyribose polynucleotides can be formed. It seemed likely that similar complexes might be attainable with naturally occurring polynucleotides.

However, several technical improvements had to be devised before this procedure could be usefully exploited. Previous work on duplex reconstitution used the optical methods of the analytical ultracentrifuge to detect renatured material in equilibrium density gradients of cesium chloride. It was evident from the outset that optical evidence alone would be neither certain nor sensitive enough for the purposes that we had in mind. Recourse was, therefore, had to radioactive labelling and the swinging bucket rotor of the Spinco Model L for equilibrium centrifugation which permitted the performance of definitively interpretable experiments. The principal advantage of these procedures is that they allow the actual isolation and analysis of the pertinent fractions and thus provide ready and certain identification of any hybrids formed. Further, as will be seen below, the

[*]This investigation was aided by grants in aid from the U. S. Public Health Service and the National Science Foundation.

method can be pushed to levels adequate to detect complementary sequences corresponding to as little as .01 per cent of the genome of *E. coli*. The sensitivity attainable permits the realization of experiments which can illuminate a variety of interesting biological problems.

It is the primary purpose of the present paper to illustrate the use and versatility of these methods by describing experiments which provide information relevant to the following issues: (1) the nature of the RNA synthesized in a bacterial cell infected with a virulent DNA virus; (2) the existence and selective synthesis of DNA-like RNA in normal cells subjected to a "step-down" transition from fast to slow growth; (3) the origin of ribosomal RNA; (4) the origin and biological individuality of the amino acid transfer RNA's which serve as the cellular genetic dictionary; (5) the question of homology between the nucleic acid of an RNA virus and the DNA in its host cell.

THE RNA SYNTHESIZED IN E. COLI INFECTED WITH T2 BACTERIOPHAGE

Data accumulated over the past two decades have suggested that infection of bacterial cells with virulent DNA viruses is followed by a virtually complete repression of macromolecular synthesis indigenous to the normal cells. Infected cells behave as if they can no longer follow their own genetic instructions and have become completely subservient to those transmitted to them from the genome of the viral agent.

The first suggestion that this might indeed be the case was provided by the experiments of Volkin and Astrachan (1956) who examined the nature of the RNA synthesized in the T2 *E. coli* complex by means of P^{32} pulse labelling. They concluded that a new type of RNA was synthesized distinguished by possessing a base composition homologous to the viral DNA.

The existence of an RNA peculiar to virus infected cells is inferred from the data of Volkin and Astrachan (1956) primarily from the distribution of P^{32} amongst the four nucleotides derived from an alkaline hydrolysate of total RNA. Unequal precursor labelling or non-randomness of base distribution in the polymer could have been, and were invoked, to question the validity of the inference. Nevertheless, the potential significance of these observations was clear, since unequivocal proof of the existence of an RNA specific for T2-infected cells would immediately generate a host of new experimental possibilities.

As a first step in this direction, Nomura, Hall and Spiegelman (1960) undertook to see whether a direct demonstration of the existence of T2-specific RNA was experimentally obtainable. The methods employed involved zone electrophoresis through starch columns and centrifugation in linear sucrose gradients developed by Britten and Roberts (1960). These experimental devices succeeded in establishing the existence of a T2-specific RNA as a physically distinct entity. It was found that the RNA synthesized subsequent to T2 infection could be distinguished from the principal RNA of the components by two physical differences. One was an apparent higher mobility in zone electrophoresis. The other was a greater heterogeneity in size as exhibited in the profiles observed during centrifugation in linear sucrose gradients.

The procedures employed led to the selective separation of T2-specific RNA and opened up the possibility for the next stage of the investigation of its nature. The fact that T2-RNA possessed a base ratio analogous to that of T2-DNA is of interest principally because it suggests that the similarity may go further and extend to a detailed correspondence of base sequence. The central issue of the significance and meaning of T2-RNA was indeed whether or not this was, in fact, the case. To decide whether sequence complementarity existed, Hall and Spiegelman (1961) undertook to determine whether specific hybrid structures could be formed between the RNA synthesized after T2 infection and single stranded DNA from T2. A hybrid structure involving RNA and DNA would have a lower density than free uncombined RNA and a somewhat heavier density than single stranded DNA. Separation and detection should, therefore, be attainable by equilibrium centrifugation in cesium chloride gradients. To ensure a sensitive and unambiguous detection of the hybrid, should it occur, double labelling was employed. The T2-RNA was marked with P^{32} and the T2-DNA with H^3.

The general outlines of such experiments may be briefly described. Mixtures of purified P^{32}-labelled RNA synthesized after T2 infection and tritium-labelled single stranded T2-DNA are subjected to a slow cool. The products are then separated in CsCl gradients. Fig. 1 shows the results obtained with three preparations cooled from different starting temperatures. Comparison of the profiles of H^3 and P^{32} show that in all cases a peak of P^{32} appears close to the band of tritium (denatured DNA). This new P^{32}-containing band must contain DNA-RNA hybrid having a density somewhat greater than that corresponding to denatured T2-DNA.

It was shown in the same investigation that exposure to the slow cooling process and the presence of denatured DNA are both necessary for hybrid formation. Most important, the ability of the T2-RNA to hybridize was found to be specific for T2-DNA. Of further interest is the fact that little if any hybrid structure was formed with *E. coli* DNA. This would suggest that the injection of the T2-DNA results in an inhibition of the synthesis of RNA which is complementary to the DNA of the host cell. A virulent virus can apparently prevent the formation of new genetic messages from the host genome.

In summary, the data obtained in the course of this investigation showed that the RNA molecules synthesized after infection have the ability to form a well-defined complex only with denatured DNA of the virus. The fact that such specific requirements must be met is taken to reflect a complementary correspondence in sequence between the RNA and DNA in the sense of Watson and Crick (1953).

The fact that evidence can be provided for sequence complementarity

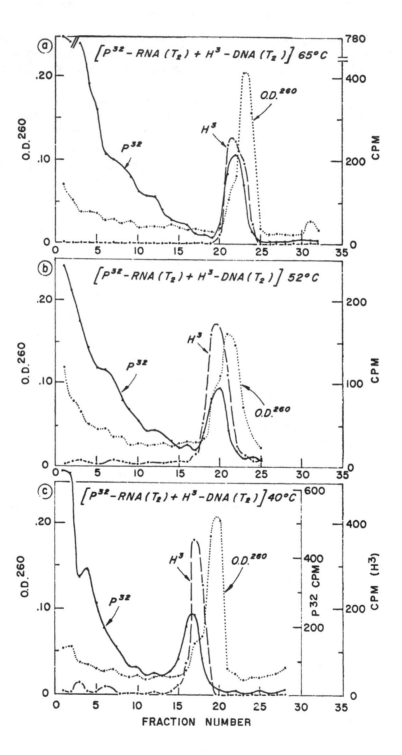

lends obvious support for the supposition that the normal process of transferring information from DNA to the protein synthesizing machine involves a mechanism whereby DNA serves as a template for the polymerization of a complementary polyribonucleotide. Complementarity was subsequently shown by a similar hybridization test with the RNA synthesized by purified RNA polymerase (Geiduschek *et al.*, 1961).

SELECTIVE SYNTHESIS OF COMPLEMENTARY* RNA IN BACTERIA

The detection of the properties of the informational RNA formed in T2-infected cells was greatly facilitated by the fact that the synthesis of the normal stable RNA components (ribosomal and transfer RNA) is suppressed. This advantage is not, however, generally present in uninfected cells and complicates, therefore, the search for normal informational or complementary RNA. However, several investigations have suggested that such a search might indeed be feasible. Thus, Yčas and Vincent (1960) infer the existence in yeast of a metabolically unstable and homologous RNA from P^{32} experiments. Further, short pulses with radioactive precursors reveal (Nomura *et al.*, 1960; Gros *et al.*, 1961) the existence of RNA in the size ranges which characterized the T2 informational RNA.

To provide definitive evidence for the existence of complementary RNA it was clearly desirable to find or devise a situation in normal cells which would be analogous to that which obtains in T2-infected cells. Essentially what was sought is a condition which suppresses ribosomal and transfer RNA synthesis while permitting prolonged formation of the informational or complementary variety. The possibility that this might, in fact, be realizable was suggested by recent studies (Kjeldgaard *et al.*, 1950; Neidhardt & Magasanik, 1960) on RNA and protein synthesis during passage from fast to slow growth.

It has been known for some time that the RNA and, therefore, the ribosome content of a cell is positively correlated with its growth rate. Consider then the situation when one subjects a culture to a "step-down" transition by transferring cells from a rich to a synthetic medium. At the moment they

*We use in the present discussion the terms "informational" or "complementary" to designate a population of RNA molecules operationally defined by the following two properties: (1) an over-all base composition analogous to homologous DNA; (2) the ability to hybridize specifically with homologous DNA. Within this class will presumably be found the "messenger" RNA postulated by Jacob and Monod (1961) to constitute the unstable programs of protein synthesis.

FIG. 1. Formation of DNA–RNA hybrid at various temperatures. CsCl-gradient centrifugation analysis. P^{32}–RNA (T2) (14 μg) and H^3–DNA (T2) (6.5 μg) were mixed in 0.6 ml 0.3 M NaCl and 0.03 M Na citrate (pH 7.8); then the solution was immediately placed in slow-cooling bath. Three identical solutions were made: (a) was placed in the bath at 65 C, (b) at 52 C, and (c) at 40 C. When bath temperature reached 26 C, CsCl and 25 μg T2–DNA were added to each solution; then they were centrifuged for 5 days at 33,000 rev/min. The last O.D. peak identifies the carrier unlabelled double stranded T2–DNA. (Hall & Spiegelman, 1961.)

are introduced into a synthetic medium, and for some time thereafter, the cells have more ribosomes than they can usefully employ. From the viewpoint of selective advantage it is perhaps not surprising to find that such "step-down" transitions are accompanied by a dramatic cessation of net RNA synthesis. Nevertheless, there is a residue of RNA formation remaining. It seemed possible that this residue might be restricted to the variety immediately required for the fabrication of new protein molecules, that is to say, to the normal informational RNA for which we were searching.

Experiments undertaken by Hayashi and Spiegelman (1961) confirmed these predictions. It was shown that the RNA synthesized during such a "step-down" transition possessed all the characteristics which had been found for the T2-specific RNA. These included base compositional homology to the DNA, metabolic instability, and polydispersity of size.

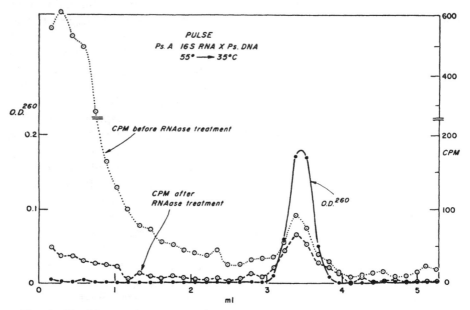

Fig. 2. Equilibrium density centrifugation (33 K 60 hr) in CsCl. A mixture of H^3-RNA (16S) from a *Ps. aeruginosa* step-down culture slow-cooled with single stranded DNA from *Ps. aeruginosa*. No marker was added. Open circles (dashed line) gives effects on the counts per minute of treatment of indicated fractions with ribonuclease prior to precipitation and counting. (Hayashi & Spiegelman, 1961.)

To complete the identification it was necessary to test for sequence complementarity as had been done in the case with T2-DNA. Fig. 2 shows a typical CsCl gradient profile of a hybridization test between *Ps. aeruginosa* informational RNA and homologous DNA. We note excellent hybrid formation as demonstrated by the peak of tritium in the DNA density region. This same figure illustrates a feature which is extremely useful in attempts at distinguishing true hybrids from non-specific aggregations. It will be noted that most of the counts corresponding to free RNA are almost completely removed by RNAase. However, the counts in the region of the hybrid are obviously much more resistant. This resistance is a characteristic feature of DNA-RNA hybrids and, as will be noted later, can be profitably used in certain types of experiments.

Specificity tests with normal informational RNA synthesized in a variety of organisms were as clear-cut and as satisfactory as had been observed in the case of the T2-specific RNA. Hybrid structures were readily formed only when the mixture contained RNA and DNA of genetic and homologous origins. It would appear, therefore, that the mechanism of information transfer from DNA genomes to the protein synthesizing mechanism is essentially a universal one and involves a complementary polyribonucleotide strand as the informed intermediary between the DNA and the protein synthesizing machines.

THE ORIGIN OF RIBOSOMAL RNA

Ribosomes are the protein synthesizing machines. The 16S and 23S RNA components, universally found in them, constitute the bulk (85 per cent) of the cellular RNA. The mode of origin of ribosomal RNA is of obvious interest. While clearly not exhaustive, two alternatives can be entertained. One would assume a DNA-dependent reaction and the other would invoke a synthetic mechanism of RNA formation which is independent of the DNA. The fact that the base composition of ribosomal RNA shows no tendency to correlate with homologous DNA (Woese, 1961; Spiegelman, 1961) is irrelevant to a choice between the two hypotheses. The presumed DNA segment involved might be so small as to constitute a statistically inadequate sample of the over-all base composition.

Posing the problem in the form of these two alternatives suggests the following question pertinent to a decision and amenable to experimental resolution. "Does DNA contain a sequence homologous to ribosomal RNA"? It is clear that, in principle, an answer to this question can be obtained by the use of DNA-RNA hybridization.

There are obvious technical difficulties inherent in using hybridization to answer the question posed (Spiegelman, 1961). The major complications stem from the numerology of the situation. For example, the 23S RNA component of the ribosomes is 1×10^6 in molecular weight so that even if a specific complex were formed it might involve only .02 per cent of the DNA available in the genome of *E. coli*. It is for this reason that hybrid structures between ribosomal RNA and homologous DNA are not observable in the usual hybridization procedures, were they to occur. One is faced with the problem of designing experiments which will detect hybridizations at very low levels. This can theoretically be accomplished by raising the specific radioactivity of the RNA used to suitable levels. Indeed, in principle, the test can be made definititive in both a positive and a negative sense. However, magnification of the sensitivity of hybrid detection by such means

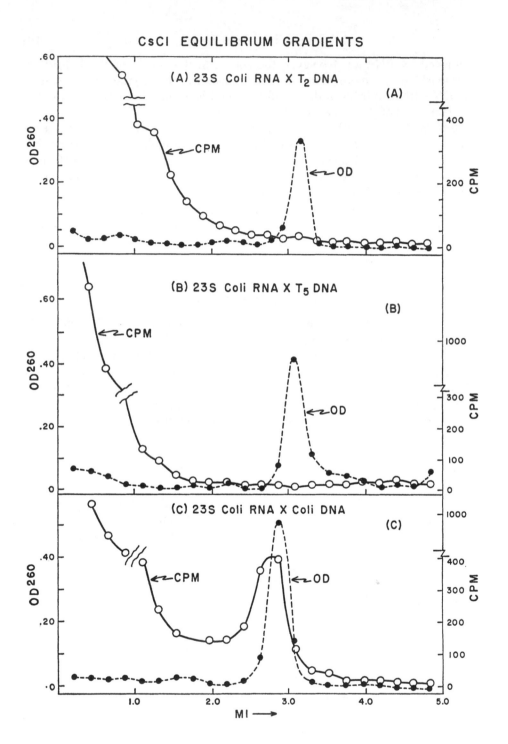

CsCl EQUILIBRIUM GRADIENTS

(A) 23S Coli RNA X T₂ DNA

(B) 23S Coli RNA X T₅ DNA

(C) 23S Coli RNA X Coli DNA

carries with it the attendant dangers that complexes will be observed which are irrelevant to the question being examined. Apparent hybrids might represent any one of the following: (a) complexes between DNA and small amounts of informational RNA contaminating the ribosomal preparations; (b) mechanical trapping of small amounts of ribosomal RNA in the strands of DNA; (c) partial hybridization resulting from accidental coincidences of complementarity over short regions.

In view of these possible difficulties, apparent hybrids with ribosomal RNA must be interpreted with caution. Observations of RNA accompanying the DNA in a density gradient must be supplemented with independent information which establishes that the RNA, so complexed, is ribosomal and that it is specifically hybridized to the DNA. Experimental procedures which provide the requisite information were devised by Yankofsky and Spiegelman (1962, I, II).

Proof that the RNA complexed in such experiments is indeed ribosomal was provided by analysis of the hybridized material which showed that the base composition was characteristically ribosomal. The fact that mechanical trapping is not an important consideration is demonstrated by Fig. 3. Here, tritium-labelled 23S RNA of *E. coli* was incubated with heat denatured DNA from T2, T5, and *E. coli* and centrifuged in cesium chloride gradients. It is clear that no complex is observable with either of the two viral DNA molecules. However, an excellent hybrid is formed in the DNA region of the homologous mixture.

The third possibility of partial hybridization due to accidental coincidences in short regions did pose a problem since it was found that false hybrids could be observed when genetically complex heterologous DNA (e.g., calf thymus DNA) is used in the test. However, it has already been noted that such false hybrids can be readily distinguished by their sensitivity to nucleolytic degradation, a feature illustrated in Fig. 4. We compare here the behavior of homologous (coli DNA $\times$ coli 23S RNA) and heterologous (calf thymus DNA $\times$ coli 23S RNA) "complexes." In the case of the homologous hybridization (Fig. 4c) there is a loss of counts in the first five minutes but the residue is virtually completely resistant to RNAase. On the other hand, in the case of the heterologous complex of thymus DNA by coli ribosomal RNA (Fig. 4f), it is impossible to distinguish the sensitivity of the apparent hybrid (H^3) from that of the internal P^{32}-RNA control.

It is apparent that the nuclease sensitivity test permits a ready distinction between the specific hybridization involving long sequences and the partial

---

FIG. 3. CsCl density gradient profiles. (a): 76 μg/ml T2 heat-denatured DNA + 3.4 μg/ml *E. coli* 23S–H^3–RNA (4.8×10^4 counts/min μg) in TMS; 0.22–ml fractions collected. (b): 76 μg/ml T5 heat-denatured DNA + 3.4 μg/ml *E. coli* 23S–H^3–RNA (4.8×10^4 counts/min μg) in TMS; 0.21–ml fractions collected. (c): 84 μg/ml *E. coli* heat-denatured DNA + 3.4 μg/ml 23S–H^3–RNA (4.8×10^4 counts/min μg) in TMS; 0.22–ml fractions collected. All 3 reaction mixtures were held at 40 C for 36 hr. Centrifugation was at 33,000 rev/min and 25 C for 72 hr. (Yankofsky & Spiegelman, 1962a.)

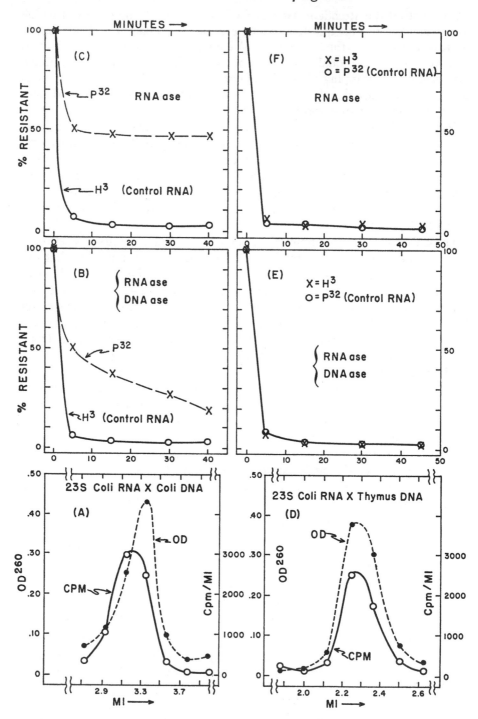

pairing of short segments which can occur by chance when the DNA is of considerable genetic complexity.

These results are consistent, then, with the conclusion that there exists a specific sequence in DNA which is complementary to homologous ribosomal RNA. Further evidence can be provided. The specific pairing of ribosomal RNA with a complementary sequence in DNA leads to the following two predictions: (1) the ratio of RNA to DNA in the specific complex should approach a maximum value at levels indicating the involvement of a minor fraction of the DNA; (2) non-ribosomal RNA should not compete for the same site.

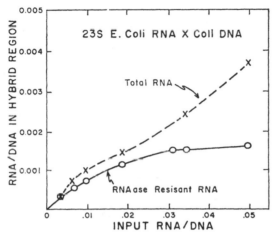

FIG. 5. Saturation curves of total and ribonuclease-resistant counts in DNA region of CsCl equilibrium gradients.

The detection of the saturation plateau requires the performance of experiments involving the following steps: (1) mixtures containing fixed amounts of heat denatured DNA and varying amounts of labelled ribosomal RNA are exposed to a slow cool from 55 C; (2) the resulting products are then subjected to equilibrium centrifugation in cesium chloride solutions to separate free RNA from that which is complexed to DNA. Again, we use nucleolytic sensitivity to distinguish between specific pairing and "noise." Fig. 5 shows the outcome of a series of such experiments. We have here a comparison of the total RNA found in the DNA density region with that

FIG. 4 (a): Apparent hybrid in DNA region after CsCl density gradient centrifugation. 114 μg/ml E. coli heat-denatured DNA + 3.1 μg/ml E. coli 23S-P^{32}-RNA (1.2 × 10^5 counts/min μg) in TMS slow-cooled from 55 C to 35 C. Centrifugation was at 33,000 rev/min and 25 C for 72 hr. (b): Resistance of apparent hybrid (a) to digestion with ribonuclease and deoxyribonuclease. (c): Ribonuclease resistance of apparent hybrid shown in (a). (d): Apparent hybrid in DNA region after CsCl density gradient centrifugation. 100 μg/ml calf thymus heat-denatured DNA + 2.72 μg/ml E. coli 23S-H^3-RNA (4.8 × 10^4 counts/min μg) in TMS, slow-cooled from 55 C to 35 C. Centrifugation was at 33,000 rev/min and 25 C for 97 hr. (e): Resistance of apparent hybrid shown in D to digestion with both ribonuclease and deoxyribonuclease. (f): Resistance of apparent hybrid shown in (d) to ribonuclease digestion. (Yankofsky and Spiegelman, 1962a).

which resists degradation by RNAase. The behavior of these two is, as might be expected, strikingly different. The total RNA shows no signs of saturation whereas the resistant residue clearly approaches a plateau corresponding approximately to an RNA–DNA ratio of .0018. The existence of this maximal level is consistent with the view that the DNA contains a restricted region capable of specifically complexing with ribosomal RNA.

To further examine the specificity of the interaction between the ribosomal RNA and its locus, competition experiments can be employed. These can be realized by using two identifying isotopic labels on different RNA preparations. If the two RNA molecules are competing for the same site,

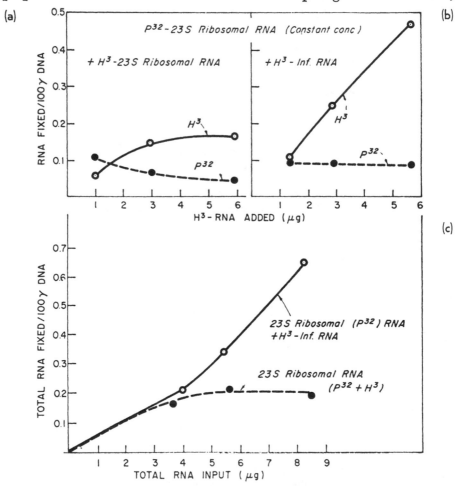

FIG. 6. Tests for competitive interactions in mixtures of ribosomal and informational RNA molecules. (a): All mixtures contained 63 μg/ml of heat denatured *E. coli* DNA and 2.66 μg/ml of *E. coli* P^{32}-23S ribosomal RNA. H^3-23S ribosomal RNA of *E. coli* varied as shown. (b): DNA and P^{32}-RNA same as (a) except that H^3-informational RNA was added in amounts indicated. (c): Same preparations as (a) and (b). Plot here is total (P^{32} + H^3) ribonuclease-stable counts/100 μg of DNA as a function of total input of RNA.

and the total concentration is at or near the saturation level, one label will displace the other as its proportion is increased in the reaction mixture. If they do not compete for the same site, fixation to the DNA of one will be essentially indifferent to the presence of the other.

To examine questions of this nature the following types of experiments were performed with *E. coli* RNA and DNA. Mixtures containing fixed levels of P^{32}-23S RNA, heat denatured DNA, and varying amounts of H^3-23S RNA were incubated and then centrifuged in cesium chloride. The amounts of P^{32} and tritium-labelled RNA fixed in the DNA and resistant to enzyme were then determined. For purposes of comparison similar experiments were carried out with H^3-complementary RNA replacing the H^3-23S RNA in the mixture. The "complementary" variety was chosen since it was known to complex well with the DNA and thus provides a test for the specificity of the ribosomal combination with DNA. Fig. 6 summarizes the outcome of such experiments. There is clear evidence (Fig. 6a) of displacement of the P^{32}-labelled ribosomal RNA as more tritium-labelled RNA of the same kind is incorporated into the complex. Further, a saturation plateau in the amount of tritium RNA complex is observed within the concentration range tested. On the other hand, when the tritium label is on the "informational" RNA its hybridization with the DNA has no effect on the ability of the DNA to combine with the P^{32}-labelled ribosomal material. In addition, no evidence of saturation is observed with the "informational" variety in the concentration range tested, indicating that this type of RNA has many more sites to which it can complex than the ribosomal RNA. This difference in saturation behavior is clearly illustrated in Fig. 6c and provides an experimental way of distinguishing between "informational" and ribosomal RNA even though both are complementary to some segments in homologous DNA at 0.2 per cent.

The hybridization experiments provide proof that specific complexes can indeed be formed between ribosomal RNA and homologous DNA. They further show that the particular region of the DNA involved corresponds to between 0.1 and 0.2 per cent of the total genome.

ON THE ORIGIN AND BIOLOGIC INDIVIDUALITY OF THE AMINO ACID TRANSFER RNA

There are excellent reasons for identifying the soluble RNA with the genetic dictionary which permits translation from the four unit language of the polynucleotides to the twenty element parlance of the proteins. It is of obvious interest to determine the relation between these RNA molecules and the genome. Again, in particular, we should like to know whether sequences exist in homologous DNA which are complementary to those which occur in the s-RNA molecules. Clearly information on this question would illuminate a number of central issues including problems of origin, uniqueness of sequences, and estimations of coding degeneracy. Giacomoni and Spiegelman (1962) showed that such complementarity does indeed exist.

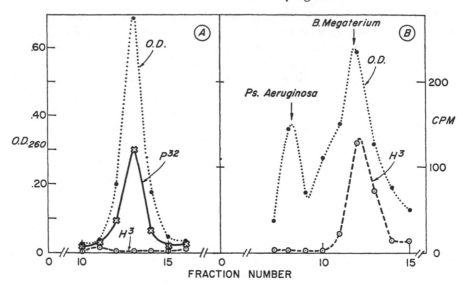

FIG. 7. Specificity of hybridization. (a) Two different s-RNA types plus one DNA; 55γ of heat denatured DNA from *E. coli* were incubated in TMS (2 hours, 72 C) with a mixture of .06 γ P^{32}-s-RNA (50,000 cpm/γ) from *E. coli* and .06 γ H^3-s-RNA (100,000 cpm/γ) from *B. megaterium*. After equilibrium density gradient centrifugation, 0.2 ml fractions were collected and diluted up to 1.2 ml. The $O.D.^{260}$ and RNAase resistant acid precipitable radioactivity were determined by counting in a Packard liquid scintillation spectrometer which permits simultaneous counting of P^{32} and H^3. Only the hybrid region is shown. The O.D. profile identifies the DNA and radio-activity, the hybrid structure.

(b) Two different DNA's plus one s-RNA. Heat denatured DNA from *B. megaterium* and *Ps. aeruginosa*, 30 γ each, were incubated in TMS with 0.06 γ of H^3-s-RNA from *B. megaterium* at 72 C for two hours (total volume was .7 ml). The hybrid region after RNAase treatment is shown. The peaks in the optical density profile identify the positions of the two DNA preparations included in the reaction mixture. (Giacomoni & Spiegelman, 1962.)

Here, as in the case of the ribosomal RNA, we were faced with a numerical difficulty of searching for sequence complementarity in a relatively restricted region of the genome. Again, it was necessary to provide auxiliary evidence to support the contention that what was being observed were hybrid structures between the DNA and the s-RNA. This took the form of demonstrating that the RNA observed in the complex was indeed s-RNA by analysis of the base composition on the hybridized material and a demonstration that the RNA in the DNA density region was much more resistant to degradation by RNAase than a free RNA control.

Convincing tests for specificity of complex formation, containing internal controls in the hybridizing process, can be readily designed (Giacomoni & Spiegelman, 1962). In the first, s-RNA preparations of two different biological origins are incubated with DNA homologous to one of them. For ease of identification each s-RNA is labelled with a different radioactive isotope. If specificity is complete, the homologous s-RNA will hybridize and the heterologous one will be excluded. In the other type of test, two

DNA preparations distinguishable by their positions in the density gradient are incubated in the presence of a labelled s-RNA homologous to one of them. If specificity exists, the isotope will be found associated only with the peak corresponding to the homologous DNA. The results of both types of tests are summarized in Fig. 7. In Fig. 7a the incubation mixture contained denatured *E. coli* DNA, P^{32}-labelled s-RNA of *E. coli* and tritium-labelled s-RNA of *B. megaterium*. We note the complete exclusion of the tritiated heterologous s-RNA from the hybrid region and excellent hybrid formation with the homologous s-RNA marked with P^{32}.

Because they have very different densities, the alternative specificity test was carried out with DNA of *Pseudomonas aeruginosa* and DNA of *B. megaterium*. A mixture of heat denatured preparations of these two DNA's was incubated with H^3-s-RNA of *B. megaterium*. The resulting profiles obtained are described in Fig. 7b. There are virtually no counts associated with the *Pseudomonas aeruginosa* DNA whereas an excellent hybrid structure is seen in the density region of the homologous *B. megaterium* DNA.

The question of the level at which saturation of the DNA occurs with s-RNA is of immediate interest to the problem of coding degeneracy. Here, the usual type of experiment is carried out where a fixed amount of DNA is incubated with various concentrations of tritiated s-RNA and the resulting complexes are separated in cesium chloride gradients. The total and the RNAase resistant counts in the DNA density regions are then determined. The results of such experiments are summarized in Fig. 8. The picture

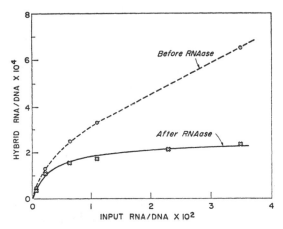

FIG. 8. Saturation curve of s-RNA *E. coli* × DNA *E. coli*. Mixtures containing 45–50 γ of heat denatured DNA plus various amounts of H^3-s-RNA (100,000 cpm/γ) in 0.85 ml TMS were incubated at 72 C for 2 hr. Following separation in the density gradient, fractions in the DNA density region were collected and divided into two aliquots. In one, the total acid insoluble radioactivity was determined. The second aliquots were further diluted to give a molarity of CsCl less than .2 and 10 γ/ml of RNAase added. They were then incubated at 25 C for 10 min. and the residual acid precipitable radioactivity was determined. In the plateau region, the whole hybrid region was pooled and the RNAase resistant residue examined by the kinetic procedure. (Giacomoni & Spiegelman, 1962.)

obtained is very similar to that observed (see Fig. 5) in the saturation experiments with ribosomal RNA. Prior to RNAase treatment no sharp plateau is observed owing to the formation of irrelevant complexes at the high RNA to DNA ratios. However, the RNAase resistant counts show abrupt evidence of saturation and a plateau is attained which suggests that .023 per cent of the DNA possesses sequences complementary to homologous s-RNA.

These experiments offer convincing evidence that specific hybrids between s-RNA and homologous DNA can indeed be detected under the proper conditions. One obvious implication of these findings is similar to that which was drawn in the case of the ribosomal RNA study. The existence of complementarity makes it likely that s-RNA originates on a DNA template. Invoking a DNA independent pathway is clearly now unnecessary.

The fact that the hybridization curve of s-RNA saturates the DNA between .02 and .03 per cent is of interest since it is consistent with what would be expected if the genetic code were degenerate. The expected saturation level can be estimated from the molecular weight equivalent to the genome of *E. coli* and the number of different kinds of s-RNA molecules each of which has a molecular weight of 2.5×10^4. If the genetic code is not degenerate, each amino acid is coded by only one triplet which implies that there are only twenty different s-RNA molecules. If the code is degenerate, more than twenty will be needed in the dictionary. The plateau predicted by the non-degenerate case is .01 per cent. The fact that it is more than twice as high suggests that some amino acids are identified with more than one s-RNA molecule. This possibility is consistent with the accumulating evidence for degeneracy which has emerged from triplet identification going on in the laboratories of Nirenberg (1962) and Ochoa (1961). It also agrees with the recently found multiplicity of s-RNA's for individual amino acids (Doctor *et al.*, 1961; Sueoka & Yamane, 1962). A direct demonstration that this multiplicity is the physical basis for degeneracy has been recently provided by Weisblum, Benzer, and Holley (1962).

The data available suggest that the genetic dictionary is universal or nearly so. However, it seems likely that the coding triplets occupy only a small proportion of the s-RNA strands. The function of the non-coding stretches of approximately 70 nucleotides is as yet unknown. They do, however, provide the opportunity for the development of biological individuality by sequence variation without disturbing the functioning of the universal triplet language. The specificity of complex formation exhibited shows that this opportunity was not neglected by biological evolution. Thus, although the s-RNA of *E. coli* can translate the genetic message of a rabbit into haemoglobin (von Ehrenstein & Lipmann, 1961), the s-RNA can be uniquely identified with the genome of its origin. The same combination of generality in use and biological uniqueness appears to obtain with the ribosomal RNA. Ribosomes are comparatively indifferent (Martin *et al.*, 1962; Speyer *et al.*, 1962; Berg & Lagerkvist, 1962) to the origin of the genetic messages to which they respond. However, their sequences are unique as demonstrated by the fact that they hybridize readily only to homologous DNA.

THE PROBLEM OF HOMOLOGY BETWEEN THE NUCLEIC ACID OF AN RNA VIRUS AND THE DNA IN ITS HOST CELL

It is obvious that a definitive decision on the existence or non-existence of homology between viral RNA and the host DNA could aid in the resolution of a number of central questions concerning the RNA viruses, including their origin, the probable mechanism involved in the replication of and transcription from an RNA genome. Consequently, Doi and Spiegelman (1962) undertook to answer the following question: "Does the DNA in the host cell contain, either before or after infection, a sequence complementary to the nucleic acid of an RNA virus?" The system used involved the RNA bacteriophage discovered by Loeb and Zinder (1961) and its host *E. coli*.

The detection of hybrids with the viral RNA involved no greater complications than had already been resolved by the experiments with ribosomal RNA. An element of assurance can be introduced into the search for complementarity with viral RNA in the form of an internal control. Ribosomal RNA (23S) and viral RNA are comparable in molecular weights, base composition, and behavior with respect to thermal disruption of their secondary structures. Consequently, in addition to serving as a test for the sensitivity level of hybrid detection, ribosomal RNA can also be employed as an internal monitor of the adequacy of the hybridization test. Thus, under conditions which yield hybrids with ribosomal RNA, the absence of such complexes with viral RNA can be accepted with confidence as a negative answer to the question of homology between viral RNA and cellular RNA.

In these experiments P^{32}-labelled phage RNA and tritium 23S-RNA were used. Results of a number of experiments are exemplified by the curves in Fig. 9. Fig. 9a shows the usual hybrid structure observed when ribosomal RNA is incubated with homologous single stranded DNA. Fig. 9b describes the completely negative outcome obtained when viral RNA is substituted for ribosomal RNA in the reaction mixture. Since the two RNA molecules are labelled with different isotopes it was possible to carry out a direct check on the significance of the negative results with the viral RNA. The two could be included in the same reaction mixture and the extent of hybridization of the DNA with either RNA examined in the presence of the other. Fig. 9c describes the result of such an experiment. Here, one sees that the tritiated ribosomal RNA formed a hybrid structure and the P^{32}-labelled viral RNA did not. A large number of experiments were carried out under a variety of other conditions with DNA from both infected and non-infected cells with identically negative results.

It is evident that neither prior to nor subsequent to infection can one find

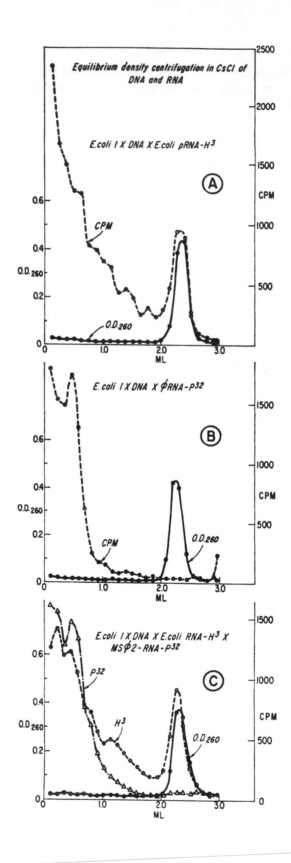

Equilibrium density centrifugation in CsCl of DNA and RNA

A. E.coli I X DNA X E.coli pRNA-H³

B. E.coli I X DNA X φRNA-p³²

C. E.coli I X DNA X E.coli RNA-H³ X MSφ2-RNA-p³²

sequences in the DNA which are complementary to the viral RNA. This outcome has a number of interesting implications which we may briefly note. They obviously lend no support to the rather attractive speculation that the RNA viruses might represent escaped genetic messages of the host. They further imply that the RNA viruses have evolved a mechanism of transcription and replication at the level of RNA and do not involve DNA in any part of the process directly. We would then predict the existence of an enzymatic mechanism involving an RNA-dependent polymerase. It seems highly unlikely that an enzyme of this sort pre-exists in the cell. All recognized nucleic acid components including informational, ribosomal and amino acid transfer RNA have been shown to be complementary to some sequence in homologous DNA. One is, therefore, led to the conclusion that the incoming viral RNA contains the structural program for this polymerase. Since this enzyme must be synthesized before replication one would further predict that the viral RNA must be conserved during its translation into protein.

SUMMARY

Experiments are described which illustrate the use of DNA-RNA hybridization as an analytical tool in the search for biologic homology. The combined use of isotopic labelling and equilibrium density centrifugation increases the sensitivity of detection to a level which permits identification of individual complementary sequences corresponding to 0.01 per cent of the total genome of *E. coli*. This has permitted the resolution of a number of interesting questions including the nature of the RNA synthesized after infection with a DNA virus, the origin of ribosomal and transfer RNA, and the problem of homology between the nucleic acid of an RNA virus and the DNA in the host cell. The potential usefulness of these procedures is far from exhausted.

FIG. 9. Equilibrium density gradient centrifugation of incubated mixtures of RNA and DNA. In all cases the peak in O.D. identifies the position of DNA in the density gradient which decreases from left to right. In addition to 50 μg of heat denatured DNA of *E. coli*, the annealing mixtures contained the following: (a) 2 μg of tritium (H^3)-labelled ribosomal RNA (40,000 cpm per μg); (b) 2 μg of P^{32}-labelled viral RNA (85,000 cpm per μg); (c) a mixture of (a) and (b). The incubation solution was 0.3 M in NaCl, and .05 M in phosphate at pH 6–8 and possessed a total volume of 0.5 ml. The mixtures were slow cooled from 55 C to 30 C over a period of approximately 17 hr. The density was then adjusted to 1.720 with CsCl and the final volume adjusted to 3.0 ml. The resulting samples were centrifuged for 72 hr at 33,000 rpm at 25 C in the SW39 rotor of the Spinco Model L ultracentrifuge. At the end, fractions of 0.12 ml were collected from the bottom of the tubes, diluted, and analysed for optical density at 260 mμ and radioactivity. Acid insoluble radioactivity was assayed on aliquots washed and dried on millipore membranes in the Packard liquid scintillation spectrometer which permits the simultaneous measurement of H^3 and P^{32}. It should be noted that although the O.D. 260 was measured on the whole sample the radioactivity was assayed on a fraction. The cpm given must be multiplied by 5.6 to convert to the total sample. (Doi & Spiegelman, 1962.)

REFERENCES

Berg, P., and V. Lagerkvist. 1962. Acides ribonucleiques et polyphosphates. C.N.R.S., Paris.

Britten, R. J., and R. B. Roberts. 1960. High resolution density gradient sedimentation analysis. Science *131*: 32–33.

Doctor, B. P., J. Agper and R. W. Holley. 1961. Fractionation of yeast amino acid acceptor ribonucleic acids by countercurrent distribution. J. Biol. Chem. *236*: 1117–1120.

Doi, R.H., and S. Spiegelman. 1962. Homology test between the nucleic acid of an RNA virus and the DNA in the host cell. Science *138*: 1270.

Geiduschek, E. P., T. Nakamoto and S. B. Weiss. 1961. Complementary interaction with deoxyribonucleic acid. Proc. Natl. Acad. Sci. U.S. *47*: 1405–1415.

Giacomoni, D., and S. Spiegelman. 1962. Origin and biologic individuality of the genetic dictionary. Science *138*: 1328.

Gros, F., H. Hiatt, W. Gilbert, C. G. Kurland, R. W. Risebrough and J. D. Watson. 1961. Unstable ribonucleic acid revealed by pulse labelling of *Escherichia coli.* Nature *190*: 581–585.

Hall, B. D., and S. Spiegelman. 1961. Sequence complementarity of T$_2$-deoxyribonucleic acid and T$_2$-specific ribonucleic acid. Proc. Natl. Acad. Sci. U.S. *47*: 137–146.

Hayashi, M., and S. Spiegelman. 1961. The selective synthesis of informational RNA in bacteria. Proc. Natl. Acad. Sci. U.S. *47*: 1564–1580.

Jacob, F., and J. Monod. 1961. Genetic regulatory mechanisms in the synthesis of proteins. J. Mol. Biol. *3*: 318–356.

Kjeldgaard, N. O., O. Maaløe and M. Schaechter. 1958. The transition between different physiological states during balanced growth of *Salmonella typhimurium.* J. Gen. Microbiol. *19*: 607–616.

Loeb, T., and N. D. Zinder. 1961. A bacteriophage containing RNA. Proc. Natl. Acad. Sci. U.S. *47*: 282–289.

Marmur, J., and P. Doty. 1961. Thermal renaturation of deoxyribonucleic acids. J. Mol. Biol. *3*: 585.

Martin, R. G., J. H. Matthaei, O. W. Jones, and M. W. Nirenberg. 1962. Ribonucleotide composition of the genetic code. Biochem. Biophys. Res. Comm. *6*: 410–414.

Neidhardt, F. C., and B. Magasanik. 1960. Studies on the role of ribonucleic acid in the growth of bacteria. Biochim. et Biophys. Acta *42*: 99–116.

Nirenberg, M. W., J. H. Matthaei and O. W. Jones. 1962. An intermediate in the biosynthesis of polyphenylalanine directed by synthetic template RNA. Proc. Natl. Acad. Sci. U.S. *48*: 104–109.

Nomura, M., B. D. Hall and S. Spiegelman. 1960. Characterization of RNA synthesized in *Escherichia coli* after bacteriophage T2 infection. J. Mol. Biol. *2*: 306–326.

Ochoa, S., D. P. Burma, H. Kroger, and J. D. Weill. 1961. Deoxyribonucleic acid-dependent incorporation of nucleotides from nucleotide triphosphates into ribonucleic acid. Proc. Natl. Acad. Sci. U.S. *47*: 670–679.

Rich, A. 1960. A hybrid helix containing both deoxyribose and ribose polynucleotides and its relation to the transfer of information between the nucleic acids. Proc. Natl. Acad. Sci. U.S. *46*: 1044.

Schildkraut, C. L., J. Marmur, R. Fresco, P. Doty. 1961a. Formation and properties of polyribonucleotide-polydeoxyribonucleotide helical complexes. J. Biol. Chem. *236*: PC 2–4.

Schildkraut, C. L., J. Marmur, and P. Doty. 1961. The formation of hybrid

DNA molecules and their use in studies of DNA homologies. J. Mol. Biol. 3: 595.

Spiegelman, S. 1961. The relation of informational RNA to DNA. Cold Spring Harbor Symposia on Quantitative Biology 26: 75.

Speyer, J. R., P. Lengyel, C. Basilio, and S. Ochoa. 1962. Synthetic polynucleotides and the amino acid code. IV. Proc. Natl. Acad. Sci. U.S. 48: 441–448.

Sueoka, N., and T. Yamane. 1962. Fractionation of amino acylacceptor RNA on a methylated albumin column. Proc. Natl. Acad. Sci. U.S. 48: 1454.

Volkin, E., and L. Astrachan. 1956. Phosphorus incorporation of Escherichia coli ribonucleic acid after infection with bacteriophage T_2. Virology 2: 149–161.

Watson, J. D., and F. H. C. Crick. 1953. Genetic implications of the structure of deoxyribonucleic acid. Nature 171: 964–967.

Woese, C. R. 1961. Composition of various ribonucleic acid fractions from micro-organisms of different deoxyribonucleic acid composition. Nature 189: 920–921.

von Ehrenstein, G., and F. Lipmann. 1961. Experiments on hemoglobin biosynthesis. Proc. Natl. Acad. Sci. U.S. 47: 941–950.

Weisblum, B., S. Benzer and R. H. Holley. 1962. A physical basis for degeneracy in the amino acid code. Proc. Natl. Acad. Sci. U.S. 48: 1449.

Yankofsky, S. A., and S. Spiegelman. 1962a. The identification of the ribosomal RNA cistron by sequence complementarity. I, Specificity of complex formation. II, Saturation of and competitive interaction at the RNA cistron. Proc. Natl. Acad. Sci. U.S. 48: 1069–1077, 1466–1472.

Yčas, M., and W. S. Vincent. 1960. An RNA fraction from yeast related in composition to DNA. Proc. Natl. Acad. Sci. U.S. 46: 804–811.

ON THE BIOSYNTHESIS OF HEMOGLOBIN IN RETICULOCYTE RIBOSOMES *

GUNTER VON EHRENSTEIN

Department of Biophysics, School of Medicine
The Johns Hopkins University
Baltimore, Maryland, U.S.A.

IN SPITE OF the great stimulation the field of protein biosynthesis has received by the finding (Nirenberg & Matthaei, 1961; Lengyel *et al.*, 1961; Martin *et al.*, 1962; Matthaei *et al.*, 1962; Speyer *et al.*, 1962; Lengyel *et al.*, 1962; Basilio *et al.*, 1962) that artificial polynucleotides could be utilized by ribosomes as templates for the synthesis of polypeptide chains, the study of the biosynthesis of a real protein can still be useful.

THE RETICULOCYTE SYSTEM

Reticulocytes are immature red cells which have lost their cell nucleus before entering the peripheral circulation. In spite of the loss of the nucleus they continue to synthesize protein and 80 to 90 per cent of the newly synthesized protein is hemoglobin.

Hemoglobin consists of four polypeptide chains, two α- and two β-chains containing 141 and 146 amino acids respectively. Each chain carries one molecule of heme as a prosthetic group. The complete amino acid sequence of both chains of human hemoglobin is known (Braunitzer *et al.*, 1961; Guidotti *et al.*, 1962). The amino acid composition of the tryptic and chymotryptic peptides of hemoglobins from different species is very similar (Braunitzer & Matsuda, 1961; Diamond & Braunitzer, 1962; Naughton & Dintzis, 1962).

A cell-free system prepared from rabbit reticulocytes (Schweet *et al.*, 1958) synthesizes hemoglobin at about 1 per cent of the rate in the intact cells. For studying hemoglobin synthesis in a cell-free system the components of Fig. 1 are required (Schweet *et al.*, 1958; Bishop *et al.*, 1961; von Ehrenstein & Lipmann, 1961). C^{14}-aminoacyl-sRNA can be substituted for the bracketed components as amino acid donor, thus eliminating variables associated with amino acid activation and amino acid-sRNA synthesis (von Ehrenstein and Lipmann, 1961; Bishop *et al.*, 1961; Nathans *et al.*, 1962).

*This work was supported by research grants from the National Institutes of Health, U.S. Public Health Service and the National Science Foundation. It was begun while the author was a Fellow of the Helen Hay Whitney Foundation.

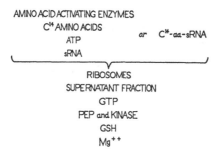

FIG. 1. Components of the reticulocyte ribosomal system.

In contrast to the synthesis of hemoglobin in the intact cell, the cell-free system is only capable of completing unfinished polypeptide chains present on the ribosomes (Bishop *et al.*, 1960; Knopf, 1962). Therefore, it is necessary to follow the incorporation of radioactive amino acids.

The hemoglobin chains grow on the template sequentially from the free amino end toward the free carboxyl end (Bishop *et al.*, 1960; Dintzis, 1961; Naughton & Dintzis, 1962; Knopf, 1962).

By mixing ribosomes of one species with supernatant from another species it has been shown that the ribosomes carry the information for the type of hemoglobin synthesized (Bishop *et al.*, 1961; Arnstein *et al.*, 1962). Contradictory results (Lamfrom, 1961; Kruh *et al.*, 1961) are most likely to be explained by hybridization of nascent single hemoglobin chains on the ribosomes with the "wrong" hemoglobin present in large excess in the supernatant (von Ehrenstein, unpubl. exp.).

HEMOGLOBIN TEMPLATE RNA

During the past years, several studies on protein synthesis in cell-free preparations of microbial origin have implicated DNA-dependent RNA synthesis in this process (Tissières *et al.*, 1960; Tissières & Hopkins, 1961; Matthaei & Nirenberg, 1961; Wood & Berg, 1962; Eisenstadt *et al.*, 1962; Kameyama & Novelli, 1962). In conjunction with the occurrence in normally growing micro-organisms (Yčas & Vincent, 1960; Gros *et al.*, 1961; Hayashi & Spiegelman, 1961) and phage-infected bacteria (Volkin & Astrachan, 1956; Nomura *et al.*, 1960; Volkin, 1960; Brenner *et al.*, 1961) of a transient informational or "messenger" RNA molecule to serve as template for the synthesis of only one or very few protein molecules (Jacob & Monod, 1961), this RNA should have a rate of turnover comparable to the rate of protein synthesis.

It was particularly interesting to test this notion in reticulocytes since these cells very actively synthesize hemoglobin in the absence of any detectable DNA. Also, it was realized that a radioactive label would be very

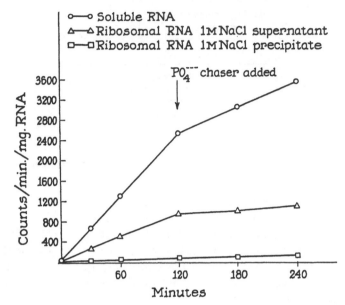

FIG. 2. Incorporation of P³²-orthophosphate into soluble and ribosomal RNA by intact rabbit reticulocytes. Conditions as in Table 1.

TABLE 1

INCORPORATION OF P³²-ORTHOPHOSPHATE INTO RNA FRACTIONS AND C¹⁴ AMINO ACIDS INTO HEMOGLOBIN BY RABBIT RETICULOCYTES *in vitro*

Incorporation	μμmole per 10 ml of packed cells per minute
Amino acids into hemoglobin	990,000
Phosphate into s-RNA	52
Ribosomal RNA	
1 M NaCl precipitate	4.7
1 M NaCl supernatant	4.5
Debris RNA	
1 M NaCl precipitate	27
1 M NaCl supernatant	30

30 ml of packed reticulocytes were made up in 100 ml of a reaction mixture described by Bishop *et al.* (1960). To half of this reaction mixture, 1 mc carrier-free P³²-othophosphate and to the other half 4 μmoles of C¹⁴ leucine (1 × 10⁷ cpm) were added. Both flasks were incubated at 37 C. Aliquots were removed at various intervals, and the cells were fractionated into ribosomes, 100,000 × g supernatant and "debris" (10,000 × g pellet) as described by Schweet *et al.* (1958). RNA was prepared from these fractions by an extraction procedure involving sodium dodecylsulfate and phenol. The RNA fractions were precipitated with 1 M sodium chloride solution after ethanol precipitation and dialyzed. Hemoglobin was prepared from the 100,000 × g supernatant by ammonium sulfate precipitation between 45 and 90 per cent saturation.

useful during the isolation of the hemoglobin template RNA. Incorporation of various precursors into different RNA fractions was studied under conditions of maximal hemoglobin synthesis. Fig. 2 shows the incorporation of P^{32}-orthophosphate into RNA fractions of intact reticulocytes. Essentially the same results were obtained using C^{14}-uracil, C^{14}-adenosine, and C^{14}-guanosine as RNA precursors. There was no indication of a rapidly labelled RNA fraction in the ribosomes even after exposure of the cells to the various labelled precursors for as short a time as 10 seconds. It should be emphasized that great care must be taken to avoid contamination of the reticulocytes with white blood cells and nucleated erythroblasts. The higher incorporation of radioactivity (Table 1) into the RNA of a "debris"-fraction which mainly contains the reticulocyte ghosts is presumably due to contamination of this fraction with white cells and nucleated red cells.

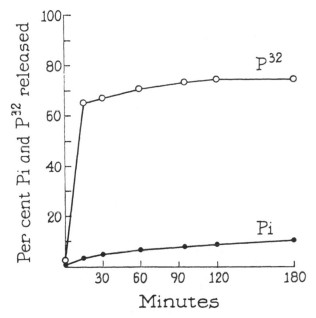

FIG. 3. Release of inorganic phosphate Pi and P^{32} after digestion of the soluble RNA with crude snake venom. Conditions and analysis as described by Weiss (1960).

In order to localize the incorporated P^{32} in the polynucleotide chains, the labelled RNA fractions were digested with crude snake venom and the release of P^{32} and inorganic phosphate was determined at various intervals. Most of the label in the s-RNA (Fig. 3) and in the high molecular weight ribosomal RNA (Fig. 4) is localized near the 3'-end of the chains, thus indicating mainly end group addition, whereas the high molecular weight RNA isolated from the "debris" fraction is almost uniformly labelled (Fig. 5) indicating *de novo* synthesis of RNA chains.

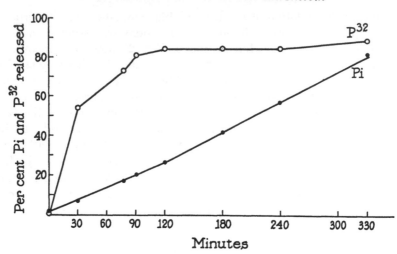

FIG. 4. Release of inorganic phosphate Pi and P[32] after digestion of the high molecular weight ribosomal RNA with crude snake venom. Conditions as in Fig. 3.

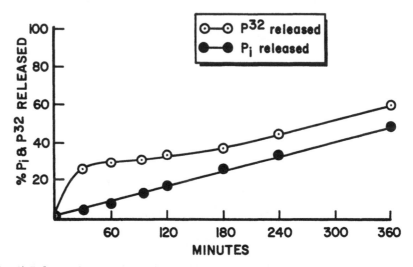

FIG. 5. Release of inorganic phosphate Pi and P[32] after digestion of the high molecular weight RNA of the "debris" fraction with crude snake venom. Conditions as in Fig. 3.

When the rate of amino acid incorporation into hemoglobin was compared with the rate of P[32]-orthophosphate, C[14]-uracil or C[14]-guanosine incorporation into RNA, the rate of amino acid incorporation was several orders of magnitude greater than the rate of incorporation of the RNA precursors (Table 1). Although further proof is needed assuming that the specific activity of the pool of nucleoside-triphosphates—in the case of P[32] the specific activity of their ester phosphate—accurately represents the specific activity of the RNA precursor pool, this result would indicate a rather stable template, the renewal of which is several orders of magnitude below the rate of amino acid incorporation (Nathans *et al.*, 1962). Similar results have recently also been obtained by Holt *et al.* (1962) and Marks (personal communication).

The possibility that the reticulocytes are endowed with a large supply of template RNA, which subsequently is broken down during hemoglobin synthesis, is unlikely, in view of the fact that some thousand hemoglobin chains are synthesized per ribosome before the reticulocyte matures into a red cell.

Since it was demonstrated that certain RNA fractions will serve as templates in the *E. coli* ribosomal system (Nirenberg & Matthaei, 1961; Ofengand & Haselkorn, 1961), we tried to develop an assay system for the hemoglobin template RNA using the *E. coli* ribosomal system.

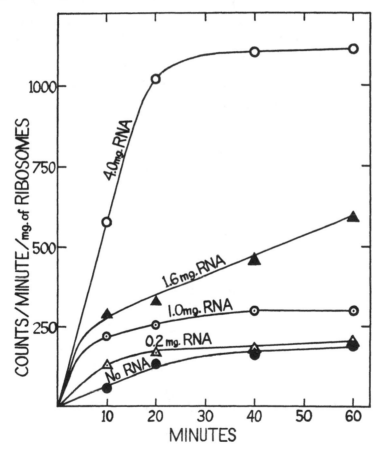

FIG. 6. Kinetics of C^{14}-leucine incorporation in the *E. coli* ribosomal system with different concentrations of reticulocyte ribosomal RNA. The incubation conditions were as described by Nirenberg and Matthaei (1961). Each point represents the hot trichloracetic acid (TCA) insoluble counts of 0.5 ml reaction mixture.

Different RNA fractions were isolated from reticulocytes and tested for stimulation of amino acid incorporation in the *E. coli* system. RNA prepared from washed ribosomes was found to be most effective in stimulating amino acid incorporation. A time curve with four RNA concentrations is shown in Fig. 6. In an experiment using C^{14}-lysine and C^{14}-arginine, 60 per cent of the incorporated radioactivity was released from the ribosomes and after addition of carrier hemoglobin 30 per cent moved with the hemoglobin band in starch gel electrophoresis. However, counting the tryptic peptides after isolation on paper by the method of Dintzis (1961) it was found that only some 10 of the 36 hemoglobin peptides contained radioactivity and that there were many radioactive spots which did not correspond to any of the hemoglobin peptides.

These preliminary results suggest either that there might be RNA templates for other proteins than hemoglobin in the reticulocyte ribosomes, or that the structural RNA of the ribosomes can serve as a template in the *E. coli* system leading to the synthesis of "junk" polypeptide chains. Similar discouraging results have also been obtained by Tsugita *et al.* (1962) who found that, at most, only about 10 per cent of the protein synthesized by the *E. coli* system under the influence of TMV–RNA is similar but not identical with TMV-protein.

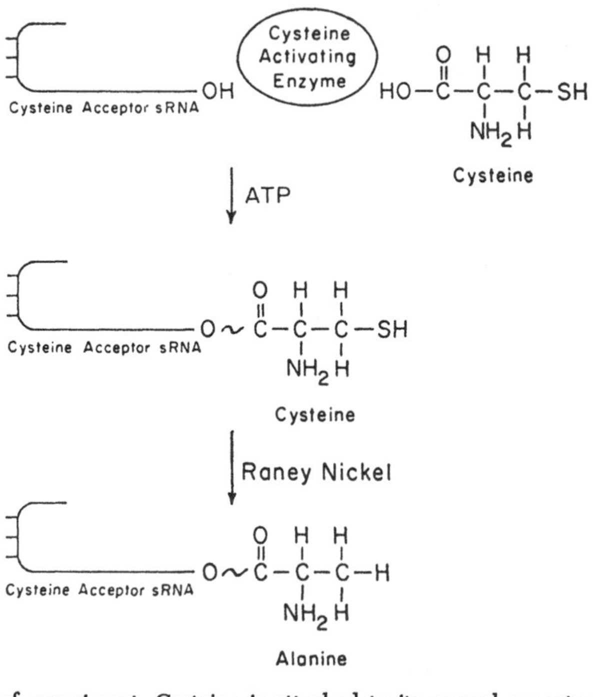

FIG. 7. Plan of experiment. Cysteine is attached to its normal accepter s-RNA by the cysteine activating enzyme. Raney Nickel converts the cysteine, while still attached, to alanine, producing the hybrid Ala-s-RNA^{CySH} (Chapeville *et al.*, 1962). The coding properties of the hybrid molecule are then investigated.

The possibility that abnormal proteins are formed because of a different amino acid code in *E. coli* and rabbit seems to be excluded on the basis of results which will be discussed below.

ADAPTOR FUNCTION OF S-RNA

According to the "adaptor" hypothesis of Crick (1958) and Hoagland (1959) the position of a particular amino acid in a polypeptide chain would be determined not by the amino acid itself, but by hydrogen bonding between the RNA template and a complementary nucleotide sequence in the s-RNA carrying the amino acid.

This hypothesis was tested by attaching cysteine to its normal acceptor s-RNA, and converting it, while still attached to its s-RNA, to alanine, by reduction with Raney Nickel, producing the hybrid Ala-sRNA^{CySH} (Chapeville *et al.*, 1962). Fig. 7 illustrates this procedure. The coding properties

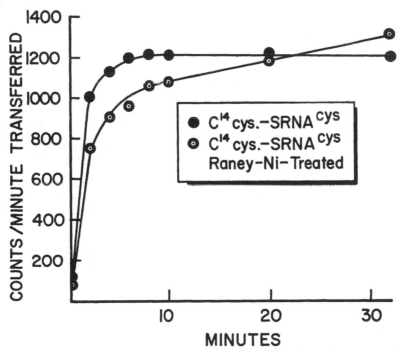

Fig. 8. Kinetics of transfer with untreated C14-CySH-s-RNA^{CySH} (●) and with Raney Nickel treated C14-CySH-s-RNA^{CySH} (○) containing 60 per cent of the radioactivity as alanine and 40 per cent as cysteine. Conditions as described by von Ehrenstein and Lipmann (1961). 100 mg of reticulocyte ribosomes were incubated in a final volume of 10 ml with: (1) 20 mg (63,250 cpm) of untreated *E. coli* s-RNA charged with C14-cysteine and a complete mixture of non-radioactive amino acids minus cysteine, and (2) 20 mg (59,500 cpm) of Raney Nickel–treated *E. coli* s-RNA charged with C14-cysteine only and in addition 20 mg of untreated *E. coli* s-RNA charged with a complete mixture of non-radioactive amino acids minus cysteine. Aliquots of 0.1 ml were precipitated, washed with hot TCA and counted. The counts per minute transferred refer to the total reaction mixture.

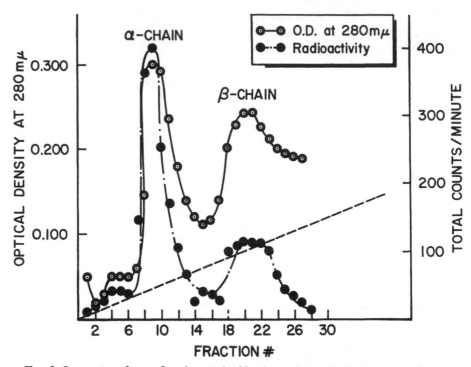

FIG. 9. Separation of α- and β-chains of rabbit hemoglobin labelled in the reticulocyte ribosomal system by transfer of C14-Ala-sRNA^Ala. Incubation conditions as described by von Ehrenstein and Lipmann (1961), except that 32 mg of ribosomes were incubated in a final volume of 3.5 ml with 20 mg (1.35 × 10^5 cpm) of *E. coli* s-RNA charged with C14-alanine and a complete mixture of non-radioactive amino acids minus alanine. Separation on a carboxymethylcellulose (CMC) column using a linear gradient of buffer between 0.2 M formic acid–0.02 M pyridine and 2 M formic acid–0.2 M pyridine (Dintzis, 1961). The total volume of each fraction was 7 ml. Aliquots of 1 ml were dried on planchettes and counted.

of the hybrid were examined by the use of poly U G which stimulates incorporation into polypeptide of cysteine but not alanine. Alanine attached to the cysteine acceptor is incorporated, indicating that the adaptor hypothesis is correct in this case (Chapeville *et al.*, 1962). It remained to be shown, however, that the result obtained with the artificial U G polymer carries over to the synthesis of a natural protein. This was tested in the reticulocyte system, in collaboration with B. Weisblum and S. Benzer. A full account of these experiments will be published shortly (von Ehrenstein, Weisblum, Benzer, 1962).

It has been shown (von Ehrenstein & Lipmann, 1961) that hemoglobin is formed by direct transfer from aminoacyl-s-RNA in a system containing reticulocyte ribosomes and *E. coli* s-RNA charged with amino acids. The experimental plan was therefore to perform three transfer experiments with reticulocyte ribosomes and *E. coli* s-RNA charged with (1) C14-CySH-sRNA^{CySH}, (2) C^{14}-Ala-sRNA^{Ala}, (3) Raney Nickel–treated C^{14}-CySH-sRNA^{Cys}; and to analyse the hemoglobin formed.

The Raney Nickel treatment of the CySH-sRNA^{CySH} had converted 60 per cent of the radioactivity into Ala-sRNA^{CySH}. The extent of reduction of cysteine into alanine was determined by paper electrophoresis at pH 1.9 as described previously (Chapeville *et al.* 1962). The time curve of the transfer with the treated preparation was comparable to that obtained with the nonreduced preparation (Fig. 8), as had already been shown in the *E. coli* ribosome–poly U G system (Chapeville *et al.*, 1962). At the end of the incubation, 20 mg of carrier hemoglobin were added to each reaction mixture and the ribosomes were removed by centrifugation. Ribonuclease (3μg/ml) was added to the supernatant to break down the s-RNA and globin was prepared by the acid acetone method. The globin was separated into α- and β-chains on a column of carboxymethyl cellulose as described by Dintzis (1961). Alanine is transferred from authentic C^{14}-Ala-sRNA^{Ala} into both α and β chain (Fig. 9) whereas for unknown reasons cysteine from the unreduced C^{14} CySH-sRNA^{CySH} is transferred only into the α-chain (Fig. 10). As expected, the Raney Nickel–treated C^{14}-CySH-sRNA^{CySH} containing 60 per cent of the hybrid C^{14}-Ala-sRNA^{CySH} behaves like the unreduced C^{14}-CySH-sRNA^{CySH} transferring only into the α-chain (Fig. 11).

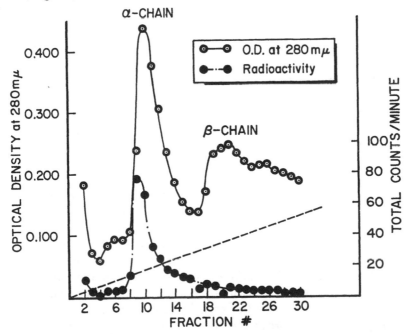

FIG. 10. Separation of α- and β-chains of rabbit hemoglobin labelled in the reticulocyte ribosomal system by transfer of C^{14}-CySH-sRNA^{CySH}. Incubation conditions as in Fig. 8. Separation on a CMC column as in Fig. 9. Aliquots of 2 ml were dried and counted.

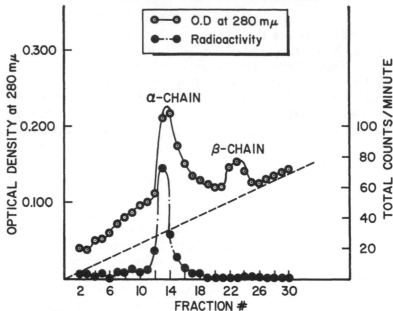

Fig. 11. Separation of α- and β-chains of rabbit hemoglobin labelled in the reticulocyte ribosomal system by transfer of Raney Nickel–treated C14-CySH-s-RNACySH containing 60 per cent of the radioactivity as alanine and 40 per cent as cysteine. Incubation conditions as in Fig. 8. Separation on a CMC column as in Fig. 9. Aliquots of 0.5 ml were dried and counted.

For further analysis we therefore concentrated on the peptides of the α-chain. The peptides were separated after trypsin digestion by electrophoresis and chromatography on paper (Dintzis, 1961), with the modification that mercaptoethanol was present during the entire procedure to keep the cysteine in the SH-form. The peptides were eluted and counted in an end window counter with a background of 1.5 counts per minute. The samples and the background were counted alternately for a time long enough to reduce the standard deviation of the corrected counts to less than ±10 per cent.

There is only one cysteine in the α-chain of rabbit hemoglobin (Diamond & Braunitzer, 1962; Naughton and Dintzis, 1962) and the cysteine containing peptide remains in the trypsin-resistant core. While these experiments were in progress Diamond and Braunitzer (1962) showed that this peptide is liberated by digestion of the α-chain core with chymotrypsin. They furthermore showed that the cysteine containing chymotryptic peptide did not contain alanine. Two more peptides containing alanine but no cysteine were liberated from the core by chymotrypsin.

The trypsin resistant cores were eluted from the paper and after digestion with chymotrypsin in the presence of mercaptoethanol, the peptides were separated by paper electrophoresis at pH 4.5 and chromatography (Dintzis, 1961), eluted and counted.

TABLE 2

ANALYSIS OF ALANINE AND CYSTEINE CONTAINING PEPTIDES OF
RABBIT HEMOGLOBIN

Peptide No.	Number of alanine residues	Number of cysteine residues	Total (cpm)	Incorporated	
				Alanine (cpm)	Cysteic acid (cpm)
A—After transfer of C^{14}-Ala-sRNA^{Ala}					
1	1	0	0	0	0
4	2	0	0	0	0
9	1	0	1.3	0.9	0
8+9	1	0	2.9	1.3	0
10	3	0	9.1	4.7	0
13	0	1	0	0	0
14	1	0	4.0	2.2	0
15	3	0	15.3	7.6	0
B—After transfer of C^{14}-CySH-sRNA^{CySH}					
13	0	1	13.1	0	5.4
All others	—	0	0	0	0
C—After transfer of Raney Nickel–treated C^{14}-CySH-sRNA^{CySH}					
13	0	1	10.2	3.1	1.6
All others	—	0	0	0	0

Isolation and counting of the peptides is described in the text. The peptides are numbered according to Diamond and Braunitzer (1962) corresponding to their sequence in the polypeptide chain from the free amino end to the free carboxyl end. Peptides 1–10 were identified by their position on the paper after electrophorsis and chromatography at right angles using the data of Naughton and Dintzis (1962). Peptides 13–15 were identified by their amino acid composition as determined by the semiquantitative paper electrophoresis method described by Naughton and Hagopian (1962). 0— indicates ±0.17 counts per minute.

The tryptic and chymotryptic peptides were oxidized with performic acid, hydrolyzed in 6 N HCl for 36 hr at 105 C. The HCl was evaporated and after addition of alanine and cysteic acid as carriers the amino acids were separated by paper electrophoresis at pH 1.9. The alanine and the cysteic acid spots were cut out, eluted and counted.

No C^{14}-alanine was found in the cysteine containing peptide after transfer of either authentic C^{14}-Ala-sRNA^{Ala} (Table 2A), or unreduced C^{14}-CySH-sRNA^{CySH} (Table 2B). With the Raney Nickel-treated preparation containing 60 per cent C^{14}-Ala-sRNA^{CySH}, two-thirds of the counts appear in the alanine spot after hydrolysis of the cysteine containing peptide (Table 2C). In addition no C^{14}-alanine was detected in the alanine containing peptides after transfer of the treated preparation (Table 2C).

The alanine containing peptides #1 and #4 near the free amino end of the α-chain do not contain C^{14}-alanine after transfer of C^{14}-Ala-sRNA^{Ala} (Table 2A). This is explained by the fact that the cell-free system is unable to start new chains on the ribosomes (Bishop et al., 1960; Knopf, 1962) and that the chains grow from the free amino end toward the free carboxyl end (Bishop et al., 1960; Dintzis, 1961; Naughton & Dintzis, 1962; Knopf, 1962). The increase of the specific activity of the alanine residues in the peptides going from the amino end toward the carboxyl end of the chain (Table 2) is also due to this peculiarity of the cell-free system.

We conclude then, that the adaptor hypothesis is correct in the synthesis of a natural protein.

This proof of the adaptor function of the *E. coli* s-RNA in the reticulocyte ribosomal system corroborates our earlier conclusions (von Ehrenstein & Lipmann, 1961) that the *E. coli* s-RNA can recognize directly the nucleotide sequences on the RNA template for hemoglobin proving the identity of the amino acid code of these two organisms.

ACKNOWLEDGEMENT

I wish to express my gratitude to Dr. Fritz Lipmann for his advice and encouragement during my stay in his Laboratory at the Rockefeller Institute.

REFERENCES

Arnstein, H. R. V., R. A. Cox and J. A. Hunt. 1962. Function of polyuridylic acid and ribonucleic acid in protein biosynthesis by ribosomes from mammalian reticulocytes. Nature *194*: 1042–1044.
Basilio, C., A. J. Wahba, P. Lengyel, J. F. Speyer and S. Ochoa. 1962. Synthetic polynucleotides and the amino acid code. V. Proc. Natl. Acad. Sci. U.S. *48*: 613–616.
Bishop, J., G. Favelukes, R. Schweet and E. Russell. 1961. Control of specificity in haemoglobin synthesis. Nature *191*: 1365–1368.
Bishop, J., J. Leahy and R. Schweet. 1960. Formation of the peptide chain of hemoglobin. Proc. Natl. Acad. Sci. U.S. *46*: 1030–1038.
Braunitzer, G., R. Gehring-Müller, N. Hilschmann, K. Hilse, G. Hobom, V. Rudloff und B. Wittmann-Liebold. 1961. Die Konstitution des normalen adulten Humanhämoglobins. Z. Physiol. Chem. *325*: 283–286.
Braunitzer, G., und G. Matsuda. 1961. Die Analyse der tryptischen Peptide des Pferdehämoglobins. Z. Physiol. Chem. *325*: 91–93.
Brenner, S., F. Jacob and M. Meselson. 1961. An unstable intermediate carrying information from genes to ribosomes for protein synthesis. Nature *190*: 576–581.
Chapeville, F., F. Lipmann, G. von Ehrenstein, B. Weisblum, W. J. Ray, Jr. and S. Benzer. 1962. On the role of soluble ribonucleic acid in coding for amino acids. Proc. Natl. Acad. Sci. U.S. *48*: 1086–1092.
Crick, F. H. C. 1958. On protein synthesis. Symp. Soc. Exp. Biol. *12*: 138–163.
Diamond, J. M., and G. Braunitzer. 1962. Alpha-chain of rabbit hemoglobin. Nature *194*: 1287–1288.
Dintzis, H. M. 1961. Assembly of the peptide chains of hemoglobin. Proc. Natl. Acad. Sci. U.S. *47*: 248–261.
Eisenstadt, J. M., T. Kameyama and G. D. Novelli. 1962. A requirement for gene-specific deoxyribonucleic acid for the cell-free synthesis of β-galactosidase. Proc. Natl. Acad. Sci. U.S. *48*: 652–659.
Giudotti, G., R. J. Hill and W. Konigsberg. 1962. The structure of human hemoglobin. II. The separation and amino acid composition of the tryptic peptides from the α and β chains. J. Biol. Chem. *237*: 2184–2195.
Gros, F., H. Hiatt, W. Gilbert, C. G. Kurland, R. W. Risebrough, and J. D. Watson. 1961. Unstable ribonucleic acid revealed by pulse labelling of *Escherichia coli*. Nature *190*: 581–585.

Hayashi, M., and S. Spiegelman. 1961. The selective synthesis of informational RNA in bacteria. Proc. Natl. Acad. Sci. U.S. *47*: 1564–1580.

Hoagland, M. B. 1959. The present status of the adaptor hypothesis. *In* Structure and function of genetic elements. Brookhaven Symposia in Biology No. *12*: 40–45.

Holt, C. E., E. Herbert and P. B. Joel. 1962. RNA metabolism of intact rabbit reticulocytes. Fed. Proc. *21*: 381.

Jacob, F., and J. Monod. 1961. Genetic regulatory mechanisms in the synthesis of proteins. J. Mol. Biol. *3*: 318–356.

Kameyama, T., and G. D. Novelli. 1962. The synthesis of β-galactosidase by a cell-free preparation from *Escherichia coli*. Proc. Natl. Acad. Sci. U.S. *48*: 659–666.

Knopf, P. M. 1962. Hemoglobin synthesis in a cell-free system. Thesis, Mass. Inst. Technology.

Kruh, J., J. Rosa, J. C. Dreyfus et C. Schapira. 1961. Synthèse d'hémoglobines par des systèmes acellulaires de réticulocytes. Biochim. et Biophys. Acta. *49*: 509–519.

Lamfrom, H. 1961. Factors determining the specificity of hemoglobin synthesized in a cell-free system. J. Mol. Biol. *3*: 241–252.

Lengyel, P., J. F. Speyer and S. Ochoa. 1961. Synthetic polynucleotides and the amino acid code. Proc. Natl. Acad. Sci. U.S. *47*: 1936–1942.

Lengyel, P., J. F. Speyer, C. Basilio and S. Ochoa. 1962. Synthetic polynucleotides and the amino acid code. III. Proc. Natl. Acad. Sci. U.S. *48*: 282–287.

Martin, R. G., J. H. Matthaei, O. W. Jones and M. W. Nirenberg. 1962. Ribonucleotide composition of the genetic code. Biochem. Biophys. Res. Comm. *6*: 410–414.

Matthaei, J. H., and M. W. Nirenberg. 1961. Characteristics and stabilization of DNAase-sensitive protein synthesis in *Escherichia coli* extracts. Proc. Natl. Acad. Sci. U.S. *47*: 1580–1588.

Matthaei, J. H., O. W. Jones, R. G. Martin and M. W. Nirenberg. 1962. Characteristics and composition of RNA coding units. Proc. Natl. Acad. Sci. U.S. *48*: 666–677.

Nathans, D., G. von Ehrenstein, R. Monro and F. Lipmann. 1962. Protein synthesis from aminoacyl-soluble ribonucleic acid. Fed. Proc. *21*: 127–133.

Naughton, M. A., and H. M. Dintzis. 1962. Sequential biosynthesis of the peptide chains of hemoglobin. Proc. Natl. Acad. Sci. U.S. *48*: 1822–1830.

Naughton, M. A., and H. Hagopian. 1962. Some applications of two-dimensional ionophoresis. Anal. Biochem. *3*: 276–284.

Nirenberg, M. W., and J. H. Matthaei. 1961. The dependence of cell-free protein synthesis in *Escherichia coli* upon naturally occurring or synthetic polyribonucleotides. Proc. Natl. Acad. Sci. U.S. *47*: 1588–1602.

Nomura, M., B. D. Hall and S. Spiegelman. 1960. Characterization of RNA synthesized in *Escherichia coli* after bacteriophage T2 infection. J. Mol. Biol. *2*: 306–326.

Ofengand, J., and R. Haselkorn. 1962. Viral RNA-dependent incorporation of amino acids into protein by cell-free extracts of *E. coli*. Biochem. Biophys. Res. Comm. *6*: 469–474.

Schweet, R., H. Lamfrom and E. Allen. 1958. The synthesis of hemoglobin in a cell-free system. Proc. Natl. Acad. Sci. U.S. *44*: 1029–1035.

Speyer, J. F., P. Lengyel, C. Basilio and S. Ochoa. 1962. Synthetic polynucleotides and the amino acid code. IV. Proc. Natl. Acad. Sci. U.S. *48*: 441–448.

Speyer, J. F., P. Lengyel, C. Basilio and S. Ochoa. 1962. Synthetic polynucleotides and the amino acid code. II. Proc. Natl. Acad. Sci. U.S. *48*: 63–68.

Tissières, A., D. Schlessinger and F. Gros. 1960. Amino acid incorporation into proteins by *Escherichia coli* ribosomes. Proc. Natl. Acad. Sci. U.S. *46*: 1450–1463.

Tissières, A., and J. W. Hopkins. 1961. Factors affecting amino acid incorporation into proteins by *Escherichia coli* ribosomes. Proc. Natl. Acad. Sci. U.S. *47*: 2015–2023.

Tsugita, A., H. Fraenkel-Conrat, M. W. Nirenberg, and J. H. Matthaei. 1962. Demonstration of the messenger role of viral RNA. Proc. Natl. Acad. Sci. U.S. *48*: 846–853.

Volkin, E. 1960. The function of RNA in T2-infected bacteria. Proc. Natl. Acad. Sci. U.S. *46*: 1336–1349.

Volkin, E., and L. Astrachan. 1956. Phosphorus incorporation of *Escherichia coli* ribonucleic acid after infection with bacteriophage T2. Virology *2*: 149–161.

Von Ehrenstein, G., and F. Lipmann. 1961. Experiments on hemoglobin biosynthesis. Proc. Natl. Acad. Sci. U.S. *47*: 941–950.

Von Ehrenstein, G., B. Weisblum and S. Benzer. 1963. Proc. Natl. Acad. Sci. U.S. *49*: in press.

Weiss, S. B. 1960. Enzymatic incorporation of ribonucleoside triphosphates into the interpolynucleotide linkages of ribonucleic acid. Proc. Natl. Acad. Sci. U.S. *46*: 1020–1030.

Wood, W. B., and P. Berg. 1962. The effect of enzymatically synthesized ribonucleic acid on amino acid incorporation by a soluble protein-ribosome system from *Escherichia coli*. Proc. Natl. Acad. Sci. U.S. *48*: 94–104.

Yčas, M., and W. S. Vincent. 1960. An RNA fraction from yeast related in composition to DNA. Proc. Natl. Acad. Sci. U.S. *46*: 804–811.

SYMPOSIUM III

INSECT MICROBIOLOGY

Chairman: L. BAILEY

A. KRIEG

Crystalliferous Bacteria

D. M. MacLEOD AND T. C. LOUGHHEED

Entomogenous Fungi

ANTON KOCH

The Symbionts in Wood-Destroying Insects

C. VAGO

La Pathogénèse des viroses d'insectes

JOHN PAUL KRAMER

The Entomophilic Microsporidians

CHAIRMAN'S REMARKS

L. BAILEY

Rothamsted Experimental Station
Harpenden, England

INSECT MICROBIOLOGY has become an important part of agricultural and forestry entomology in the past twenty years, partly because of some remarkable advances in fundamental knowledge—particularly of the virus infections that cause the polyhedroses and of the crystalliferous bacilli—but mostly because of the clear demonstrations that microbes, especially those I mention together with some species of fungi, sometimes control insect pests remarkably well. With this promise of economic gain further fundamental studies are being increasingly urged, notably by E. A. Steinhaus at Berkeley. Already such work is actively pursued in many parts of the world, especially in Canada whence some of the most important results have come.

In the past, insect microbiology played a significant part in the origins of microbiology itself in the celebrated works of Agostino Bassi and of Louis Pasteur. They worked with the silkworm; and the pathogenic microbes of this insect, together with those of the honey bee, subsequently provided much of the material for insect microbiology, at least until recent times. It is noteworthy that the subject was originally studied, as it is today, because it had to do with practical problems associated with insects of economic importance: it has lacked academic appeal because it has no apparent intrinsic uniformity. Perhaps, as Steinhaus suggests, insect microbiology will play a leading part in a general study of the immense and poorly known field of invertebrate microbiology and pathology, but at present it has developed very unevenly; few workers have studied it for its own sake and those aspects of obvious practical significance have had most attention.

However, the current practical theme of insect microbiology in agriculture—the microbial control of insect pests—has been well discussed in the past few years so it was decided that this symposium should be concerned with wider aspects of the subject and should take as comprehensive a view of insect microbes as possible. Furthermore, it seemed appropriate for this Congress that emphasis should be laid more on microbiological than on entomological aspects. Accordingly, the speakers in this Symposium were asked to consider the nature and ecology of the variety of entomogenous micro-organisms with which they are concerned. I trust this request has allowed sufficient scope to enable them to give of their best.

CRYSTALLIFEROUS BACTERIA

A. KRIEG

Biologische Bundesanstalt
Institut für biologische Schädlingsbekämpfung
Darmstadt, Germany

Bacillus thuringiensis and related bacilli are facultative pathogens which can be cultivated on simple media such as nutrient broth. During sporulation of these bacilli a spore and one or two parasporal bodies ("Restkörper") are formed within each cell (Berliner, 1915; Mattes, 1927; Hannay & Fitz-James, 1955). The parasporal inclusions are of regular, bipyramidal form, and therefore are called "crystals."

According to their appearance and cultural characteristics, all crystalliferous bacteria of the *B. thuringiensis* group are closely related to *Bacillus cereus*. In fact, Toumanoff and Le Corroller (1959) proposed placing the crystal-producing bacteria in this species, as they do not agree with Heimpel and Angus (1958) that the formation of parasporal crystals is sufficient reason to justify species status. For example Toumanoff *et al.* (1955), De Barjac and Bonnefoi (1962), and Lysenko (1960) reported spontaneous loss of ability to form crystals in some strains of crystalliferous bacteria (*B. thuringiensis* var. *alesti*, var *sotto*, and var. *thuringiensis*). Fitz-James and Young (1959) caused loss of crystals by formalin treatment of *B. thuringiensis*. The inverse process, spontaneous production of crystals by simple straits of *B. cereus* and by strains of *B. thuringiensis*, which had become a-crystalliferous, was observed by Toumanoff *et al.* (1955) and by his collaborator Le Corroller (1958) after passage of these bacilli through larvae of the wax moth (*Galleria mellonella* (L.)). However, as wax moth larvae are often latently infected with *B. thuringiensis* (see below) it may be possible that Toumanoff and Le Corroller did not isolate the inoculated strains but rather another one (comp. Heimpel & Angus, 1960).

Serological analyses of *B. thuringiensis* strains have been made by several workers. Using agglutination tests Shvecova (1959) observed highly specific antigen patterns in different strains of *B. thuringiensis*. The spore antisera of distinct strains react not only with the homologous spore antigen, but also with the antigen of homologous vegetative cells. This reaction was reciprocal. Lamanna and Jones (1961) tested agglutinogenic relationships between the spores of the crystalliferous bacteria and the spores of other bacilli. They also found strain-specific and, therefore, very complex antigenic patterns. It was surprising that they could demonstrate serological cross reactions not only between spores of *B. thuringiensis* and *B. cereus*, but also between the spores of these bacilli and *Bacillus anthracis*. Norris (1961) observed a common spore-precipitogen present in all strains of crystalliferous bacteria and of *B. cereus* studied. De Barjac and Bonnefoi (1962) studied 24 different strains of crystalliferous bacilli by flagellar agglutination reaction and found 6 groups, each with a different H-antigen. No serological relationship, however, was found between these strains and the a-crystalliferous *B. cereus* strain (A 30) which according to Toumanoff can be converted to a crystalliferous one (see above).

As shown by several authors (Heimpel & Angus, 1958; Toumanoff & Le Corroller, 1959; Krieg, 1961; De Barjac & Bonnefoi, 1962) the study of biochemical properties may be important for solving taxonomic problems of *B. thuringiensis*. About 10 different metabolic characters make it possible to classify the known crystalliferous bacilli into 6 biochemical groups which correspond to the 6 serological groups of H-antigens (De Barjac and Bonnefoi). The biochemical and serological groups are represented by the following types: *B. thuringiensis* var. *thuringiensis*; var. *alesti* (or *euxoae*); var. *sotto* (or *dendrolimus*); var. *galleriae*; var. *entomocidus* (or *subtoxicus*); and *Bacillus finitimus*.

According to Angus (1956), the parasporal crystals of *B. thuringiensis* are composed of 17 amino acids, and contain no nucleic acids or carbohydrates. Monro (1961a, b) found that normal sporulation with formation of crystals takes place not only during incubation in optimal media, but also under suitable conditions in a nutrient-free medium. He showed further that crystal protein antigens are absent from vegetative cells and that water-soluble, antigenically related precursors are not present even in sporulating cells during the period of crystal formation. Therefore, it is suggested that the crystal protein is derived from material already present in the vegetative cells but that the precursors are antigenically unrelated. Krywienczyk and Angus (1960) indicate that only the toxic component in the crystals of different varieties of *B. thuringiensis* is the same since the other antigentic material of the crystals is serologically different.

INSECT PATHOLOGY

It is well known that *B. thuringiensis* is pathogenic to lepidopterous larvae when ingested whereas *B. finitimus* and *B. cereus* are not. The parasporal crystals are highly toxic and cause a gut paralysis in caterpillars (Hannay, 1953; Angus, 1953, and others).

Heimpel and Angus (1959) observed that different species of Lepidoptera react differently after contamination with a pathogenic crystalliferous bacillus. These authors compared the type of pathogenic reaction and the solubility of crystals in alkali with the pH in the gut of the host and found three groups. The first is represented by silkworms (e.g., *Bombyx mori* L.) and hornworms (e.g., *Protoparce sexta* (Johan)) which exhibit a general paralysis some hours after being fed either with sporulated cultures of *B. thuringiensis* or with the toxin of crystals alone. The pH in the gut of these larvae is very high (about 9.5 to 10.5) and Heimpel and Angus suggested that a rapid dissolution of the toxic crystals takes place in the gut even though the spores cannot germinate. The toxin damages the gut-wall, and permeation of alkali from the gut into the body cavity leads to an increase of the pH of the haemolymph and causes general paralysis.

The second group, to which the majority of Lepidoptera belong, does not show general paralysis, but only a paralysis of the gut. Thus, feeding is stopped a short time after they have ingested the spore-crystal-complex and they die after several days. In Pieridae the pH of the gut is about 7.5 to 9.5, i.e. lower than in the first group. Therefore, germination and multiplication of bacilli is possible and the increase in the pH of the haemolymph after paralysis of the gut is not very striking. Tanada (1953) reported that ingestion of *B. thuringiensis* by the imported cabbage worm (*Pieris rapae* (L.)) was followed by an invasion of the bacilli into the body cavity causing death of the larvae by septicaemia.

A third group is represented by the larvae of the Mediterranean flour moth (*Anagaster kühniella* (Zell.)) in which the reaction in the gut is nearly neutral. The toxin alone gives no effect, but it is suggested that here it plays a role of pace-maker of the general infection, because a synergism between the effect of spores and crystals is reported by Heimpel and Angus (1959) and by Burgerjon and Yamvrias (1959). The caterpillars of *A. kühniella* die after invasion of bacilli into their hemocoel (Berliner, 1915; Mattes, 1927).

To these three groups Martouret (1962) adds a fourth that contains the larvae of Lepidoptera which are resistant to the spore-crystal-complex. In larvae of some Noctuidae, for example, no toxic effect occurs although the pH of the gut reaches a high value (9.5 to 10.2). Martouret believes that the effectiveness of crystalliferous bacteria depends as much on the action of proteinases as on the pH of the gut. He noted three types. In the first one, to which belong all sensitive species of Lepidoptera (e.g., *Pieris brassicae* (L.)) the crystals are broken down rapidly to highly toxic fragments. In the second type, represented by some Agrotiidae (e.g., *Agrotis segetum* (Schiff.) and *Agrotis ypsilon* (Huf.)), enzymatic digestion produces only non-toxic fragments. In the third type no digestion of parasporal crystals takes place (e.g., *Barathra brassicae* (L.), *Rhyacia saucia* Hbn. ab margaritosa Haw.). The larvae of both the second and the third types are resistant to crystalliferous bacteria.

The results of Martouret suggest that the parasporal crystal is only the precursor, but not the toxic principle itself. In sensitive hosts the dissolved crystals may have a destructive effect on the gut-wall. Tanada (1953) and Heimpel and Angus (1959) observed that the texture of the epithelial layers in the mid-gut was destroyed in susceptible hosts a short time after ingestion of a crystal-containing spore preparation and cells were liberated into the lumen. To explain the mode of action, further observations are necessary.

Though most authors described only the effects on Lepidoptera of sporulated cultures (i.e., spores and crystals), Toumanoff and Vago (1953), Vaňková (1957), and Krieg (unpubl.) also observed infections when vegetative cells had been applied perorally. In these cases, it seems that substances other than the toxic crystals may be pace-makers of an infection.

Toumanoff and Vago (1953) reported that phospholipase C, produced by several crystalliferous bacilli, may be harmful to caterpillars. Large amounts of phospholipase are produced by *B. thuringiensis* var. *sotto*, var. *alesti*, and by many strains of *B. cereus*, but no phospholipase is found in cultures of *B. thuringiensis* var. *entomocidus* (Heimpel & Angus, 1958; Krieg, 1961; De Barjac & Bonnefoi, 1962).

McConnell and Richards (1959) found an insecticidal agent in filtrates of *B. thuringiensis* cultures applied parenterally. Similarly a peroral insecticidal effect of filtrates of cultures fed over a long time (4 to 10 days) in high doses has been reported (Burgerjon & De Barjac, 1960; Krieg & Herfs, 1963). In contrast to the crystal toxin and phospholipase C the filtrable agent is dialysable and heat-stable. It induces intoxication without stopping feeding and is more effective by injection into the body cavity.

Large amounts of the filtrable heat-stable agent are formed by vegetative cells of most strains of *B. thuringiensis* var. *thuringiensis*; some varieties produce it in smaller amounts whereas *B. thuringiensis* var. *sotto* produces none. The production of the filtrable heat-stable agent and of phospholipase, however, is not limited to crystalliferous bacteria. It is also found in cultures of many *B. cereus* strains. The chemical composition of the filtrable agent and its mode of action are unknown as yet.

The prolonged peroral application of high doses of the filtrable agent kills not only Lepidoptera but also Diptera, Hymenoptera, and Coleoptera. Therefore, the over-all effects of *B. thuringiensis* as reported in the literature may be the result not only of the toxic parasporal crystals but also of heat-stable toxic substances secreted into the culture medium.

The effectiveness of insect pathogens depends on the nature of the host, its species, strain, instar, physiological stage. Different races of one species may show some differences. Krieg (unpubl.) compared the susceptibility to *B. thuringiensis* of a Canadian inbred strain of *Bombyx mori* with a "wild strain" from Germany under comparable conditions. The German silkworms showed a significantly higher resistance than the Canadian ones. It is a question whether such demonstrable differences in the reaction of races or strains of hosts are genetically fixed or not. Yamvrias (1961) subjected larvae of *Anagasta kühniella* to sublethal doses of *B. thuringiensis* but noticed no enhancement of resistance after seven generations.

Mortality curves indicate that the susceptibility of larvae decreases with their age. According to the study of Wiegand (1960) on *Hyponomeuta malinellus* Zell., however, the sensitivity of caterpillars is generally constant if measured in terms of dose per unit volume rather than in terms of dose per insect. The physiological status of insects is related to individual disposition and may be changed by stressors (see below).

Epizootics caused by *B. thuringiensis* have been reported by several authors in mass-rearings of *Bombyx mori, Anagasta kühniella,* and *Galleria mellonella* but the conditions which cause these epizootics in populations of Lepidoptera are relatively unknown. To explain the epizootic waves in *B. mori* populations Toumanoff (1960) suggested a vertical transmission of bacilli from one generation to the next.

Norris (1961) found latency of crystalliferous bacilli in *G. mellonella* colonies and repeatedly isolated such bacilli from the faeces of reared caterpillars which showed no signs of any disease. Latently infected larvae were also recorded by Krieg (unpubl.) in laboratory colonies of *A. kühniella*. Two to 8 per cent of the eggs of this strain were found to be contaminated externally when cultured on nutrient agar plates.

Schütte (unpubl.) observed that, in such latently infected colonies of *A. kühniella,* an epizootic arose as a result of crowding. When a population density of 20,000 eggs per kilogram of wheat flour was used no outbreak occurred, but when the density was increased to 30,000 eggs per kilogram, an epizootic destroyed the colony. This suggests that epizootics arise in latently infected populations when stressors (such as starvation) appear and that a high population density supports horizontal spreading.

Epizootics are reported in many other Lepidoptera (comp. Krieg, 1961), and spontaneous infections in the Homopteron, *Cicada plebeia* (Scop.) (Vago, 1951), and in the Hymenopteron, *Pristiphora erichsonii* (Htg.) (Smirnoff & Heimpel, 1961).

Since the detection of crystalliferous bacteria as insect pathogens by Berliner fifty years ago, their utilization in biological control has been investigated. These studies have been intensified in the last few years since commercial preparations of the spore-crystal-complex became available in North America and Europe. Russian formulations are prepared by governmental agencies.

A detailed account of the many successful field trials cannot be given here, but one field experiment may be of special interest. Talalaev (1958) induced an artificial epizootic against the Siberian moth (*Dendrolimus sibiricus* Tschetv.) by means of *B. thuringiensis* var. *dendrolimus.* He observed some spread of the infection in the field, but in the larvae of advanced instars, which were relatively resistant to the disease, the infection remained latent for several months. Only after hibernation of the caterpillars did the disease become manifest and the dead pupae became reservoirs of the crystalliferous bacilli.

The larvae of more than 100 other lepidopterous species are sensitive to preparations of the spore-crystal-complex, so that crystalliferous bacilli are a useful specific weapon against many harmful caterpillars (comp. Heimpel & Angus, 1960; Krieg, 1961).

REFERENCES

Angus, T. A. 1953. Studies of *Bacillus* spp. pathogenic for silkworm. Can. Dept. Agr. Bi.-Mo. Rept. 9: 1–2.

Angus, T. A. 1956. Extraction, purification, and properties of *Bacillus sotto* toxin. Can. J. Microbiol. 2: 416–426.

De Barjac, H., and A. Bonnefoi. 1962. Essai de classification biochimique de 24 souches de *Bacillus* du type *B. thuringiensis*. Entomophaga 7: 5–31.

Berliner, E. 1915. Ueber die Schlaffsucht der Mehlmottenraupe (*Ephestia kühniella* Zell.) und ihren Erreger *Bacillus thuringiensis* n.sp. Z. angew. Entomol. 2: 29–56.

Burgerjon, A., and H. De Barjac. 1960. Nouvelles données sur le rôle de la toxine soluble thermostable produite par *Bacillus thuringiensis* Berliner. Compt. rend. Acad. Sci., Paris 251: 911–912.

Burgerjon, A., and C. Yamvrias. 1959. Titrage biologique des préparations à base de *Bacillus thuringiensis* Berliner vis-à-vis de *Anagasta* (*Ephestia*) *kühniella* Zell. Compt. rend. Acad. Sci., Paris 249: 2871–2872.

Le Corroller, Y. 1958. A propos de la transformation de souches banales de *B. cereus* Frank. et Frank. en souches cristallophores pathogènes pour les insectes. Ann. Inst. Pasteur 94: 670–673.

Fitz-James, P. C., and I. E. Young. 1959. Comparison of species and varieties of the genus *Bacillus*. Structure and nucleic acid content of spores. J. Bacteriol. 78: 743–754.

Grison, P. 1961. L'utilisation d'une bactérie *Bacillus thuringiensis* dans la lutte biologique contre les insectes nuisibles. *In* La Lutte biologique contre les insectes ravageurs. Université de Paris, Palais de la Découverte, A 277: 3–25.

Hannay, C. L. 1953. Crystalline inclusions in aerobic spore-forming bacteria. Nature 172: 1004.

Hannay, C. L., and P. C. Fitz-James. 1955. The protein crystals of *Bac. thuringiensis* Berliner. Can. J. Microbiol. 1: 694–710.

Heimpel, A. M., and T. A. Angus. 1958. The taxonomy of insect pathogens related to *Bacillus cereus* Frankland and Frankland. Can. J. Microbiol. 4: 531–541.

Heimpel, A. M., and T. A. Angus. 1959. The site of action of crystalliferous bacteria in Lepidoptera larvae. J. Insect Pathol. 1: 152–170.

Heimpel, A. M., and T. A. Angus. 1960. Bacterial insecticides. Bacteriol. Rev. 24: 266–288.

Krieg, A. 1961. *Bacillus thuringiensis* Berliner. Ueber seine Biologie, Pathogenie und Anwendung in der biologischen Schädlingsbekämpfung (In memoriam Dr. Ernst Berliner (1880–1957)). Mitt. Biol. Bundesanstalt, Berlin-Dahlem, Heft Nr. 103, 79 pp.

Krieg. A., and W. Herfs. 1963. Empfindlichkeit verschiedener Insektenarten gegenüber den "Exotoxinen" von *Bacillus thuringiensis* Berliner. In press.

Krywienczyk, J., and T. A. Angus. 1960. A serological comparison of the para-sporal bodies of three insect pathogens. J. Insect Pathol. 2: 411–417.

Lamanna, C., and L. Jones. 1961. Antigenic relationship of the endospores of *Bacillus cereus*–like insect pathogens to *Bacillus cereus* and *Bacillus anthracis*. J. Bacteriol. *81*: 622–625.

Lysenko, O. 1960. Cited after Heimpel, A. M. and T. A. Angus. 1960.

Martouret, D. 1962. Les toxines de *Bacillus thuringiensis* et leur processus d'action chez les larves de Lépidoptères. Meded. Landbouwhoogesch., Opzoek. stat., Gent, *26*: 1116–1126.

Mattes, O. 1927. Parasitäre Krankheiten der Mehlmotten-Larven und Versuche über ihre Verwendbarkeit als biologische Bekämpfungsmittel (Zugleich ein Beitrag zur Zytologie der Bakterien). Sitzungsber. Ges. Beförderung ges. Naturwiss., Marburg, *62*: 381–417.

McConnell, E., and H. G. Richards. 1959. The production by *Bacillus thuringiensis* Berliner of a heat-stable substance toxic for insects. Can. J. Microbiol. *5*: 161–168.

Monro, R. E. 1961a. Protein turnover and the formation of protein inclusions during sporulation of *Bacillus thuringiensis*. Biochem. J. *81*: 225–232.

Monro, R. E. 1961b. Serological studies on the formation of protein parasporal inclusions in *Bacillus thuringiensis*. J. Biophys. Biochem. Cytol. *11*: 321–331.

Norris, J. R. 1961. Bacteriophages of *Bacillus cereus* and crystal-forming insect pathogens related to *B. cereus*. J. Gen. Microbiol. *26*: 167–173.

Smirnoff, W., and A. M. Heimpel. 1961. A strain of *Bacillus thuringiensis* var. *thuringiensis* Berliner isolated from the larch sawfly, *Pristiphora erichsonii* (Hartig). J. Insect Pathol. *3*: 347–351.

Shvecova, O. I. 1959. Biologische Besonderheiten verschiedener entomopathogener Sporenbildner in Verbindung mit der Ausbildung ihrer Einschlüsse. *In* Biologičeskij Metod Bor'by s Vrediteljami Rastenij (edit.: Telenga, N. A., Ščerbinovskij, N. S. & Djadečko, N. P.). Izdatel'stvo Akademii Nauk Ukrainskoi SSR, Kiev, 192–201. (Orig. Russian).

Talalaev, E. V. 1958. Künstliche Induktion einer septikämischen Epizootie in Larven von *Dendrolimus sibiricus* (Tschetv.) (Lep. Lasiocampidae). Ent. Obozr. (Rev. Ent. USSR) *37*: 641–652. (Orig. Russian).

Tanada, Y. 1953. Susceptibility of the imported cabbageworm to *Bacillus thuringiensis* Berliner. Proc. Hawaii. Ent. Soc. *15*: 159–166.

Toumanoff, C. 1960. Observations sur la transmission héréditaire de la flacherie des vers à soie (*Bombyx mori* L.). Ann. Inst. Pasteur *98*: 367–372.

Toumanoff, C., and Y. Le Corroller. 1959. Contribution à l'étude de *Bacillus cereus* Frank. et Frank. cristallophores et pathogènes pour les larves de lépidoptères. Ann. Inst. Pasteur, Paris: *96*: 680–688.

Toumanoff, C., M. Lapied, and L. Malmanche. 1955. Au sujet de souches cristallophores entomophytes de *cereus*. Observations sur leurs inclusions cristallines. Ann. Inst. Pasteur *89*: 644–653.

Toumanoff, C., and C. Vago. 1953. Recherches sur l'effet toxique de *Bacillus cereus* var. alesti vis-à-vis des vers à soie. Ann. Inst. Pasteur *84*: 623–628.

Vago, C. 1951. Bactérémie de la Cigale: *Cicada plebeia*. Bull. Soc. zool. France *76*: 383–386.

Vaňková, J. 1957. (Studien der Wirkung von *Bacillus thuringiensis* im Versuchsbetriebsmasstab.) Csl. biologie *6*: 114–120.

Wiegand, H. 1960. Der Wirkungsbereich von *Bacillus thuringiensis* Berliner. Tagungsber. Nr. 29, Dtsch. Akad. Landwiss., Berlin (Wiss. Sitzung der DAL, Berlin, 16.12.59).

Yamvrias, C. Cited after Grison, P., 1961.

ENTOMOGENOUS FUNGI

D. M. MacLEOD* and T. C. LOUGHHEED

Insect Pathology Research Institute
Department of Forestry
Sault Ste. Marie, Ontario, Canada

ENTOMOGENOUS FUNGI offer a wide variety of challenging problems that merit the attention of microbiologists other than those interested mainly in biological control. The application of some of the newer techniques developed in other fields would almost certainly lead to a new understanding of these organisms, and no doubt eventually add to the success that has already been obtained with them under natural field conditions.

In this paper, therefore, it is our aim to examine this topic in a general way and, at the same time, to treat in more detail certain aspects considered to be of special interest.

We acknowledge our debt to the authors of the original publications, of several reviews, and especially to Dr. M. F. Madelin for allowing us to see a manuscript copy of his contribution to the forthcoming book "Insect Pathology, an Advanced Treatise" to be published by Academic Press Inc.

IN VITRO CULTIVATION

Nutrition

Investigations concerning *in vitro* cultivation of entomogenous fungi are not extensive and have been reviewed in recent publications (MacLeod, 1959; Müller-Kögler, 1959). The majority of attempts to cultivate the various fungal pathogens *in vitro* have made use of various kinds of complex natural media, especially those rich in protein. Schweizer (1947) has shown that the housefly parasite *Entomophthora muscae* (Cohn) Fres. grows well on cold-sterilized meat extract-gelatin with added blood or serum and glucosamine. Growth was stimulated by including fats extracted from flies. An egg-yolk medium developed by Müller-Kögler (1959) is also of interest in that it supports the growth of a number of *Entomophthora* species. However, not all members of this group require a complicated medium. Wolf (1951) demonstrated that *Entomophthora apiculata* Thaxter and *Entomophthora coronata* (Cost.) Kevorkian can be grown upon a dextrose-asparagine-salts synthetic medium. Both species are apparently autotrophic with respect to vitamins and other growth factors. Smith (1954) later reported that *E.*

*Dr. MacLeod presented this paper on invitation of the Congress Committee. Contribution No. 38, Insect Pathology Research Institute.

coronata also grows well in a medium containing only mineral salts, arginine hydrochloride, dextrose, and distilled water.

Benham and Miranda (1953) found that some *Beauveria* strains require thiamine for optimal growth. MacLeod (1960) found that a variety of chemicals stimulated the growth of *Hirsutella gigantea* Petch but none, either singly or in combination, equalled the effect obtained with yeast extract, acid casein hydrolyzate, or Bacto-casitone. The enhanced growth associated with the casein products suggests that the active factor may be a peptide. Working with the same organism, Loughheed (1961) showed that some substance in liver fraction L stimulates the formation of synnemata, the stalk-like outgrowths upon which spores are eventually produced.

The nutritional studies, though limited, nevertheless serve as a basis for the development of chemically defined media capable of supporting full growth of the various insect fungal parasites. A more detailed knowledge of the nutritional requirements of these organisms may be of value in elucidating their physiological activities connected with sporulation, the development of a yeast-like stage, and the problem of host specificity. The growth factors in the natural products at present used may prove to be familiar substances but it is possible that some may be new compounds or at least of hitherto unrecognized importance.

Sporulation

Reproduction in many of the entomogenous fungi is mainly or conclusively by the formation of asexual spores (conidia) but practically nothing is known of the controlling mechanisms. In many cases when a pathogen is established in pure culture on artificial media, sporulation does not occur (Benham & Miranda, 1953; MacLeod, 1954, 1959; Loughheed, 1961). With fungi generally, it is fairly well established that the processes involved in sporulation are quite different from those associated with vegetative growth. According to Morton, England, and Towler (1958) sporulation is often favoured by those conditions which are adverse to mycelial growth, such as falling or low food supply, but this is not always the case. Various apparently unrelated factors have been recorded as inducing or stimulating sporulation in different species. In a given species the occurrence of sporulation is likely to depend on a complex of factors which act together to stimulate the requisite metabolic processes.

Recently there have been a number of publications concerned with sporulation in some non-entomogenous fungi which open up new fields of work. Behal and Eakin (1959) have developed the technique of using inhibitors of single developmental stages to elucidate the sporulation process. Cantino and co-workers have probably gone further than anyone in explaining sporulation at the enzyme level (for a review see Cantino and Turian, 1959). Hadley and Harrold (1958,a,b) and Hunt (1957) have shown that fungi may produce certain substances which trigger off the sporulation phase. Application of these various techniques to entomogenous fungi would certainly yield valuable information.

Metabolism

Biochemists have found that fungi are ideal organisms for much of their work; for example, in sorting out metabolic pathways, for the isolation of pure enzymes, for the study of radiation effects, for producing new antibiotics, etc. As a result, there is a large body of knowledge relating to procedures and techniques for use with fungi. Apparently no entomogenous fungi have been used for this type of work, but if these techniques were applied it should not take long to acquire many interesting data. It would be especially valuable to know what metabolic changes accompany the morphological differentiations which occur during the life cycles of these fungi.

Some publications dealing with the isolation of metabolic products have appeared in recent years. Vining, Kelleher, and Schwarting (1962) have found that the red pigment formed by *Beauveria bassiana* (Bals.) Vuill. is oosporein, an antibiotic of widespread occurrence in fungi. Kodaira (1961) has isolated a yellow powder, also from *B. bassiana*, which has strong antibiotic properties. Loughheed and MacLeod (1958) reported the production of a number of extracellular polysaccharides by *H. gigantea*. In addition there are a number of accounts of toxins produced by entomogenous fungi, but these will be considered in a later section.

HOST-PARASITE RELATIONSHIPS

Infection Chains

Gäumann (1950) has suggested the term "infection chain" to describe the process by which an infectious disease can maintain itself by continual reinfection. Continuous infection chains invariably lead without a break directly from one host to another and if these are interrupted the disease dies out. In the temperate zone, however, an intermittent infection chain is more common, since the winter season, during which host insects are unavailable, interrupts this serial transmission. In such cases the gap must be bridged by an overwintering stage of the pathogen.

Some members of the Fungi Imperfecti, for example *Beauveria, Metarrhizium, Isaria,* and *Hirsutella,* persist as a compact mass of interwoven vegetative hyphae. The following spring various types of spore-bearing cells may arise from this pseudosclerotium.

It is generally believed that *Entomophthora* and *Massospora* species overwinter by means of resting spores, which are formed in abundance by many species toward the end of the infection phase. These thick-walled spores are generally formed within the body of the insect and may be either sexual (zygospores) or asexual (azygospores).

The circumstances that give rise to the development of resting spores are imperfectly understood but may be one or more of the following: low temperature, low humidity (Dustan, 1924, 1927), exhaustion of nutrients (Schweizer, 1947), high carbon dioxide concentration (Emerson, 1950), host resistance, and hormonal or endogenous chemical activity of the host

(Cochrane, 1958). Hepden and Folkes (1960) have made the interesting observation that zygospore formation in *Rhizopus sexualis* (Smith) Callen is accompanied by a change in the RNA/DNA ratio.

It has been found that it is difficult to induce germination in resting spores (MacLeod, 1963). It is possible that a "maturation period" is essential. Hall and Halfhill (1959) found that heat treatment up to 93 C for 10 minutes stimulated germination of spores of *Entomophthora virulenta* Hall and Dunn. However, the relation of this treatment to germination under natural conditions has not been explained. If germination could be brought about at will, these spores would be an ideal biological control agent since their extreme hardiness would be of great advantage in field operations.

In many cases insects killed by fungi gradually disintegrate and fall to the ground. The soil thus becomes an important reservoir of infectious agents whose subsequent development is not yet clear. It is known that many of the Fungi Imperfecti including *Beauveria, Isaria,* and *Metarrhizium* species are frequently associated with mycotic diseases of insects that hibernate in the soil (MacLeod, 1954; Donaubauer, 1959; Balfour-Browne, 1960). On the other hand, the entomophthorous species generally attack free feeding larvae or adults or both (MacLeod & Heimpel, 1955). Where the latter have been found in cocoons it is believed that infection had taken place before the insect had left the host plant. These observations suggest that members of the Fungi Imperfecti can enter a saprophytic phase and temporarily maintain life in the mycelial stage in the soil, whereas the entomophthorous species must exist in a passive state. In the latter case, germination must be stimulated by the host, either through contact in the soil or with airborne spores. The resting spores may either give rise directly to a penetration tube or produce so-called "spring conidia"; subsequent infections are spread by asexual propagative spores throughout the growing season or until unfavourable conditions once again cause the formation of the resting stage.

The soil conditions most favourable for the growth of the pathogenic Fungi Imperfecti are not known. There can, however, be no doubt that pH, moisture, and temperature are important factors among those influencing their growth, and thus their effectiveness as pathogens. Their efficacy may be limited in part by competitive action of rapidly growing saprophytic Actinomycetes or other soil micro-organisms (Donaubauer, 1959; Wartenberg & Freund, 1961).

Insects may be readily infected but for a disease to expand to epizootic proportions a number of conditions must occur simultaneously: a large population of susceptible insects, a high infective capacity in the pathogen, and optimal environmental conditions for its development (Gäumann, 1950). It is not often that all the factors affecting these conditions are synchronized, which helps to explain the rather infrequent occurrence of fungal epizootics. It may also account for the fact that while there are many pathogenic fungi only a few ever give rise to epizootics.

It is apparent from the limited knowledge available that considerably more information is needed on the epidemiology and ecology of these infectious agents, before they can be utilized to the best advantage.

Pathogenesis

Entomogenous fungi, once they infect a susceptible host, develop quite rapidly and death usually occurs within a period of 2 to 14 days. The course of the disease may be divided into three stages: penetration, growth and development before the death of the host, and growth and development after the death of the host. These will be considered in turn.

Entrance of the pathogen into a host may be gained by direct penetration of the integument (MacLeod, 1963); or through natural openings, such as the digestive tract (Gabriel, 1959), the spiracles (Lepesme, 1938), and by growing inward through secreted honeydew (Harris, 1948); or through wounds (Müller-Kögler & Huger, 1960). Of these, the more usual portal of entry is believed to be directly through the outer integument into the body cavity.

It is known that spore germination followed by hyphal extension occurs on the surface of the insect prior to direct penetration. In the few publications dealing with the penetration process there is no mention of any organized external structure similar to the appressorium formed by many plant pathogens. However, this does not exclude the possibility that mechanical pressure has some role in this process.

It is generally accepted that penetration by hyphae is preceded by local enzymic degradation of the integument. Unfortunately, many authors have considered only the chitin portion of the integument and have ignored the other components of this complex structure and, therefore, have not provided a complete explanation. There is also evidence that certain chemical compounds in the integument of some insects may act as inhibitors (Koidsumi, 1957) or stimulants (Notini & Mathlein, 1944; Schweizer, 1947) of fungal development.

Once the pathogen has penetrated to the haemocoele, the hyphae fragment and multiply as free-floating unicellular yeast-like forms (de Bary, 1867, 1869; Thaxter, 1888; Speare, 1920, Gäumann & Dodge, 1928). These cells reproduce by a process of division and budding and are carried in the haemolymph throughout the body of the insect. They may attack the haemocytes, but their main effect is to block the blood circulation (Smith, 1961) which in turn leads to a general disintegration of tissue. In some cases the muscles are directly attacked resulting in typical lethargic symptoms (Lepesme, 1938) or cessation of feeding.

The production of toxins during this phase is one factor that has not received the attention that it deserves. In some cases toxins themselves may be the cause of death, in other cases their principal role may be as one of several debilitating factors. Both Burnside (1930) and Toumanoff (1931) were convinced that a toxin was involved in the death of honey bees infected by *Aspergillus flavus* Link. Toumanoff extracted a toxic compound from the mycelium of both *A. flavus* and *B. bassiana*. Dresner (1950) also concluded that germinating spores of *B. bassiana* produced a toxin but did not try to isolate the substance. Recently Kodaira (1961) showed that nine fungi, which cause various muscardine diseases in silkworms, all produce toxic culture filtrates. He also showed that a toxin was present in the blood of infected, dying silkworms. Moreover, working mainly with *Metarrhizium anisopliae* (Metsch.) Sorokin and *Aspergillus ochraceus* Wilm., he isolated four pure crystalline toxins from the culture filtrates. Kodaira identified two as cyclic dipeptides which he regards as products resulting from the breakdown of the medium rather than true fungal toxins. However, the other two compounds, Destruxins A and B, can also be isolated from the mycelium. A number of their properties have been determined although their chemical structure is not yet clear.

At about the time of the host's death most of the pathogens revert to the mycelial form before attacking the remaining tissues. The stimulus for this reversion has never been explained. The fat bodies are among the first of the softer tissues to disappear; the muscles, nerve fibres, malpighian tubes, and hypodermal tissues are attacked in turn until only fragments of the tracheae can be observed. Invariably the gradual depletion of the host nutriments is accompanied by some striking changes in the morphology of the pathogen. *Beauveria* species and other Fungi Imperfecti produce conidiophores and conidia; *Entomophthora* species may form either conidiophores and conidia or resting spores or both, while other fungi including *Sorosporella* species may develop chlamydospores. The application of the highly sensitive staining techniques (Zimmerman, 1957; Kelly, Morgan, & Saini, 1962) recently developed especially for fungi will no doubt reveal other aspects of these changes. It may be mentioned that the reversible transformation of some fungi from the mycelium to the yeast-like form has been investigated in some detail, but no similar work on entomogenous fungi has been published. The recent progress in insect cell culturing (Vago, 1959) may make it possible to use this technique to learn more about this morphological transition.

Ainsworth (1955) has commented on the growing appreciation of the view that fungi are normally saprophytes and only incidentally are they parasites of men and animals. Some entomogenous fungi may be similar (Boyce & Fawcett, 1947; Sussman, 1951; Müller-Kögler & Huger, 1960) but others (e.g., *Beauveria* and *Isaria*) must be regarded primarily as parasites and only incidentally as saprophytes. Still others, like some *Entomophthora* and *Massospora*, do not grow saprophytically but only as obligate parasites. The *Laboulbeniales*, which attack but do not destroy their host, are the culminating form of this group of parasites.

EXPERIMENTAL TAXONOMY

Investigations on the morphology and taxonomy of species of the many genera of entomogenous fungi are still an important part of the study of the biological control of insects. There has been a tendency in the past, and indeed to some extent even now, to assume that parasitic forms found on new hosts should be assigned new specific names even when few, if any, morphological differences exist. This has been particularly so in the genus *Entomophthora* where a recent review listed 104 specific names (MacLeod, 1963). There is little doubt that some of these are synonyms and that the taxonomy of this group should be studied in detail in order to eliminate the present confusion. Within the past twenty-five years the papers on the genus *Beauveria* by Benham and Miranda (1953) and by MacLeod (1954) are the only ones of any significance in which the experimental taxonomic approach had been used. Their conclusions were based upon the morphological variability of single spore cultures grown under controlled conditions. The great variability of form and behaviour so characteristic of fungi is now generally recognized and should always be kept in mind, particularly when dealing with the taxonomy of new isolates.

Within the last year there have been two reports of misidentifications involving entomogenous fungi (Molitoris, 1962; Vining *et al.*, 1962). This should remind us once again that insect pathologists must know the correct names and synonymy of the fungi with which they are working; otherwise results cannot be correctly evaluated by others and may lead to serious misunderstanding.

No paper on the cytology of insect fungal pathogens has been published since the contribution by Schweizer in 1947 in which he summarized his painstaking study of the cytology of *E. muscae* throughout its life history. With the aid of a new staining technique Schweizer (1942, cited by Cutter, 1951) obtained some excellent nuclear preparations. The large size and chromaticity displayed by nuclei of this organism led Cutter (1951) to conclude that large nuclear volume may be a common characteristic of obligate fungal parasites of both plants and animals.

Finally, for the student of comparative cytology in the fungi, there are still some unsolved problems. Should the various entomophthorous species be treated as one genus, or do they belong in two or more distinct genera? A cytological study, along with single spore culturing, may confirm that the perfect stages described by Schaerffenberg (1955, 1957, 1959) are, as stated, the sexual stages of the form-genera *Beauveria* and *Metarrhizium* respectively.

CONCLUSION

Entomogenous fungi, because of their mode of life, their varied character, and their economic importance, should be of interest to the mycologist and the microbiologist alike. Unquestionably they offer some exciting possibilities for fundamental laboratory study; in many cases the methods have already been developed with other fungi. We have tried to point out in this paper some of the specific problems that remain unsolved.

Published data indicate that fungi can be an effective natural control factor but the results obtained with artificial dissemination have been inconsistent and not always up to expectations. It is suggested that the acquisition of additional fundamental knowledge of these pathogens will enable us to develop new approaches for increasing the effectiveness of fungi as biological control agents.

References

Ainsworth, G. C. 1955. Pathogenicity of fungi in man and animals. *In* Mechanisms of microbial pathogenicity, ed. J. W. Howie and A. J. O'Hea, pp. 242–262. Cambridge University Press, Cambridge, England, 333p.

Balfour-Browne, F. L. 1960. The green muscardine disease of insects, with special reference to an epidemic in a swarm of locusts in Eritrea. Proc. Roy. Entomol. Soc. (London), A *35*: 65–74.

Bary, A. de. 1867. Zur Kenntniss insektentödtender Pilze. Botan. Ztg. *25*: 1–7; 9–13; 17–21.

Bary, A. de. 1869. Zur Kenntniss insektentödtender Pilze. Botan. Ztg. *27*: 586–593; 601–606.

Behal, F. J., and R. E. Eakin. 1959. Metabolic changes accompanying the inhibition of spore formation in *Aspergillus niger*. Arch. Biochem. Biophys. *82*: 448–454.

Benham, R. W., and J. L. Miranda. 1953. The genus *Beauveria*, morphological and taxonomical studies of several species and two strains isolated from wharf-piling borers. Mycologia *45*: 727–746.

Boyce, A. M., and H. S. Fawcett. 1947. A parasitic *Aspergillus* on mealybugs. J. Econ. Entomol. *40*: 702–705.

Burnside, C. E. 1930. Fungous diseases of the honeybee. U.S. Dept. Agr. Tech. Bull. *149*, 43 p.

Cantino, E. C., and G. F. Turian. 1959. Physiology and development of lower fungi (PHYCOMYCETES). Ann. Rev. Microbiol. *13*: 97–124.

Cochrane, V. W. 1958. Physiology of fungi. John Wiley and Sons, Inc., New York. 524p.

Cutter, V. M. 1951. The cytology of the fungi. Ann. Rev. Microbiol. *5*: 17–34.

Donaubauer, E. 1959. Ueber eine Mykose der Latenzlarve von *Cephaleia abietis* L. Sydowia. Ann. Mycol. Ser. 2, *13*: 183–222.

Dresner, E. 1950. The toxic effect of *Beauveria bassiana* (Bals.) Vuill. on insects. J. New York Entomol. Soc. *63*: 269–278.

Dustan, A. G. 1924. Studies on a new species of *Empusa* parasitic on the green apple bug (*Lygus communis* var. *novascotiensis* Knight) in the Annapolis Valley. Proc. Acad. Entomol. Soc. *9*: 14–36.

Dustan, A. G. 1927. The artificial culture and dissemination of *Entomophthora sphaerosperma* Fres., a fungus parasite for the control of the European apple sucker (*Psyllia mali* Schmidb.). J. Econ. Entomol. *20*: 68–75.

Emerson, R. 1950. Current trends of experimental research on the aquatic PHYCOMYCETES. Ann. Rev. Microbiol. *4*: 169–200.

Gabriel, B. P. 1959. Fungus infection of insects via the alimentary tract. J. Insect Pathol. *1*: 319–330.

Gäumann, E. A. 1950. Principles of plant infection. (English edition by W. B. Brierly.) Hafner Publishing Co., New York. 543 p.

Gäumann, E. A., and C. W. Dodge. 1928. Comparative morphology of fungi. McGraw-Hill, New York. 701 p.

Hadley, G., and C. E. Harrold. 1958a. The sporulation of *Penicillium notatum* Westling in submerged liquid culture. I. The effect of calcium and nutrients on sporulation intensity. J. Exptl. Botany 9: 408–417.

Hadley, G., and C. E. Harrold. 1958b. The sporulation of *Penicillium notatum* Westling in submerged liquid culture. II. The initial sporulation phase. J. Exptl. Botany 9: 418–425.

Hall, I. M., and J. C. Halfhill. 1959. The germination of resting spores of *Entomophthora virulenta* Hall and Dunn. J. Econ. Entomol. 52: 30–35.

Harris, M. R. 1948. A phycomycete parasitic on aphids. Phytopathology 38: 118–122.

Hepden, P. M., and B. F. Folkes. 1960. A possible relationship between nucleic acid metabolism and the initiation of zygospores of *Rhizopus sexualis*. Nature 185: 254–255.

Hunt, P. 1957. Physiological aspects of the formation of sclerotia by *Rhizoctonia solani* and some other fungi. Ph.D. thesis, Univ. of Bristol. 154 p.

Kelly, J. W., P. N. Morgan and N. Saini. 1962. Detection of tissue fungi by sulfation and metachromatic staining. Arch. Pathol. 73: 70–73.

Kodaira, Y. 1961. Biochemical studies on the muscardine fungi in the silkworms, *Bombyx mori*. J. Fac. Textile Sci. Technol. No. 25, Ser. E, Agr. Sericult. No. 5: 1–68.

Koidsumi, K. 1957. Antifungal action of cuticular lipids in insects. J. Insect Physiol. 1: 40–51.

Lepesme, P. 1938. Recherches sur une Aspergillose des Acridiens. Bull. Soc. d'Hist. nat. de l'Afrique du Nord 29: 372–384.

Loughheed, T. C., and D. M. MacLeod. 1958. Extracellular metabolic products of a *Hirsutella* species. Nature 182: 114–115.

Loughheed, T. C. 1961. The effect of nutrition on synnemata formation in *Hirsutella gigantea* Petch. Can. J. Botany 39: 865–873.

MacLeod, D. M. 1954. Investigations on the genera *Beauveria* Vuill. and *Tritirachium* Limber. Can. J. Botany 32: 818–890.

MacLeod, D. M. 1959. Nutritional studies on the genus *Hirsutella*. I. Growth response in an enriched liquid medium. Can. J. Microbiol. 37: 695–714.

MacLeod, D. M. 1960. Nutritional studies on the genus *Hirsutella*. III. Acid-hydrolyzed casein and amino acid combinations as sources of nitrogen. J. Insect Pathol. 2: 139–146.

MacLeod, D. M. 1963. Entomophthorales infections. In Insect pathology, an advanced treatise, vol. II, ed. E. A. Steinhaus. Academic Press Inc., New York. 689 pp.

MacLeod, D. M., and A. M. Heimpel. 1955. Fungal and bacterial pathogens of the larch sawfly. Can. Entomol. 87: 128–131.

Molitoris, P. 1962. Identification of purported *Agaricus campestris* strains (NRRL 2334, 2335, 2336) as *Beauveria tenella* (Delacroix Siem.). Nature 194: 316.

Morton, A. G., D. J. F. England and D. A. Towler. 1958. The physiology of sporulation in *Penicillium griseofulvum* Dierckx. Trans. Brit. Mycol. Soc. 41: 39–51.

Müller-Kögler, E. 1959. Zur Isolierung und Kultur insektenpathogener Entomophthoraceen. Entomophaga 4: 261–274.

Müller-Kögler, E. and A. Huger. 1960. Wundinfektionen bei Raupen von *Malacosoma neustria* (L.) durch *Penicillium brevi-compactum* Dierckx. Z. angew. Entomol. 45: 421–429.

Notini, G., and R. Mathlein. 1944. Grönmykos fororsakad av *Metarrhizium anisopliae* (Metsch.) Sorok. I. Grönmykosen som biologiskt insektbekämpningsmedel. Stat. Väx. Medd. 43: 1–58.

Schaerffenberg, B. 1955. Die Hauptfruchtform (ascus-form) von *Beauveria bassiana* (Vuill.) Link und *B. densa* (Vuill.) Link. Z. Pflanzenkrh. 62: 544–549.

Schaerffenberg, B.   1957.   Infektions- und Entwicklungsverlauf des insektentötenden Pilzes *Beauveria bassiana* (Vuill.) Link. Z. angew. Entomol. *41*: 395–402.

Schaerffenberg, B. Von.   1959.   Zur Biologie und Oekologie des insektentötenden Pilzes *Metarrhizium anisopliae* (Metsch.) Sorok. Z. angew. Entomol. *44*: 262–271.

Schweizer, G.   1942.   Pflanzen und Tier. Gustav Fischer, Jena. 224 p. Cited by Cutter, 1951.

Schweizer, G.   1947.   Ueber die Kultur von *Empusa muscae* Cohn und anderen Entomophthoracean auf kalt sterilisierten Nährböden. Planta, *35*: 132–176.

Smith, M. C. W.   1954.   The nutrition and physiology of *Entomophthora coronata* (Cost.) Kevorkian. Dissertation Abstr. *13*: 648–649.

Smith, O. E.   1961.   Control of the European corn borer with the fungi, *Metarrhizium anisopliae* and *Beauveria bassiana*. Dissertation Abstr. *22*: 686.

Speare, A. T.   1920.   Further studies of *Sorosporella uvella*, a fungous parasite of noctuid larvae. J. Agr. Research *18*: 399–439.

Sussman, A. S.   1951.   Studies of an insect mycosis. I. Etiology of the disease. Mycologia *43*: 338–350.

Thaxter, R.   1888.   The Entomophthoraceae of the United States. Memoirs Boston Soc. Nat. Hist. *4*: 133–201.

Toumanoff, C.   1931.   Action des champignons entomophytes sur les abeilles. Ann. Parasitol. *9*: 462–482.

Vago, C.   1959.   Recherches sur la culture de tissus en virologie des insectes. Entomophaga *4*: 23–36.

Vining, L. C., W. J. Kelleher and A. E. Schwarting.   1962.   Oosporein production by a strain of *Beauveria bassiana* originally identified as *Amanita muscaria*. Can. J. Microbiol. *8*: 931–933.

Wartenberg, H., und K. Freund.   1961.   Der Konservierungseffekt antibiotischer Mikroorganissen an Konidien von *Beauveria bassiana* (Bals.) Vuill. Zentr. Bakteriol. Parasitenk. *114*: 718–724.

Wolf, F. T.   1951.   The cultivation of two species of *Entomophthora* on synthetic media. Bull. Torrey Botan. Club 78: 211–220.

Zimmerman, L. E.   1957.   Some contributions of the histopathological method to the study of fungus diseases. Trans. New York Acad. Sci. Ser. 2, *19*: 358–371.

ON THE ROLE OF THE SYMBIONTS IN WOOD-DESTROYING INSECTS

ANTON KOCH

Paul Buchner Institut für Experimentelle Symbioseforschung
Regensburg, Germany

OF THE WONDERS of symbioses between animals and vegetal micro-organisms, which have been made manifest chiefly by Paul Buchner and his school, comparatively little seems to be known abroad. The reason for this may be that his comprehensive book *Endosymbiose der Tiere mit pflanzlichen Mikroorganismen* (1953) and his numerous other papers on the subject were published in German and are therefore less readily available to many Anglo-American readers. Therefore I am especially happy to have the opportunity of giving you a small view of this most interesting subject by reporting on the role of the symbionts in xylophagous insects.

Endosymbiosis is observed in well-defined categories of animals, mainly in connection with their nutritional physiology. It is found in all blood-sucking animals (so far as they feed on vertebrate blood throughout their life), and in almost all insects living on plant juices. Many wood-destroyers, too, have enrolled the services of symbionts. This fact, pointed out by Buchner (1928), has led to the discovery of further instances of symbiosis.

Today I will confine myself to the symbiosis of wood-destroying insects. Time is limited, so that I can discuss only a small selection. I hope to show in an ascending scale the ever closer amalgamation of the vital spheres of insects and micro-organisms.

At the lowest rung are the Ambrosia-growers. These insects grow the fungi outside of their bodies, either in special "fungus gardens" (leaf-cutting ants and termites) or in the walls of the tunnels they bore in the wood. Examples are found amongst beetles in most Ipidae, the Platypodidae and Lymexylonidae; amongst Hymenoptera, in the Siricidae (Buchner, 1930).

It had long been known that the wood-dwelling Ipidae and Platypodidae live in association with various strains of Ambrosia fungi, each strain being specific for each kind of insect. But little was known of the mode of transfer of the fungi (Neger, 1911; Schneider-Orelli, 1913; Strohmeyer, 1918) until the careful investigations of Francke-Grosmann (1956 a, b; 1960) shed light on this problem.

In the females of Xylodendron species the fungi hibernate in the pre-thoracic oil glands: in *Xylosandrus* and *Anisandrus* it is in saccular extensions of the intersegmental skin between pre- and mesonotum; in *Xyleborus saxeseni* a fungal depot is provided by a depression surrounded by protective hairs at the anterior border of the elytra. In *Platypus cylindrus* vernal reinfection of the wood is achieved by greasy masses of Ambrosia fungi carried in the deeply indented posterior portion of the mesonotum. Many similar examples could be given.

In all these cases explantation of the fungi is a passive process occurring when the female, in quest of fresh breeding places, burrows into the wood. The work of gnawing aids the disposal of cutaneous secretions and thereby the growth of the fungi. So long as the influence of the beetle's secretion persists, the fungi can maintain themselves in the burrow walls. In these cases there can be no question of a true "cultivation" of the fungi.

The availability of the fungi needed for the nurture of the young brood is most securely achieved in those cases where the fungi are brought into direct contact with the egg. A good example of this is afforded by the Lymexylonidae. Their larvae burrow in the wood of beech, oak, birch, fir and pine. The tunnels made by *Hylecoetus dermestoides*, for example, are lined with a creamy layer of fungal mycelia on which the larvae feed. The septate mycelia produce at their free ends spherical, thick-walled appendages particularly rich in glycogen (Buchner, 1928, 1930). In the cold season the fungal growth recedes, but in spring a luxuriant growth of the fungi develops afresh; the bottle-shaped sporangia are found in the pupal cradles and near the outlet of the tunnels. The same spores as were present in these asci were found by Buchner in two spacious pouches of the laying apparatus in the *Hylecoetus* female; the pouches are in direct communication with the vagina, their mucous secretion provides for adhesion of the fungal spores to the chorion, and thus for their transfer to previously uninfected wood.

This is the first step in the evolution of more highly organized symbioses. The wood wasp uses a similar mode of transfer. Here we find two pear-shaped ejaculatory organs opening on either side of the genital aperture. They contain one to three cells of oidia of a basidiomycete embedded in the mucous secretion of a large gland (Buchner, 1928). Thus when the egg is laid, the secretion laden with oidia will adhere to its anterior and posterior poles. How the organs are filled is not yet known. Francke-Grosmann (1939) found no fungi in old pupae of *Paururus juvencus*, but older imagines, which had not yet emerged from the wood, had become infected. Probably the apparatus for coating the egg is filled in the pupal cradle. In the early stages only hyphae are found; the characteristic oidia do not appear until the egg is deposited. In order to complete the picture of symbiosis in the Siricidae the observations of Parkin (1941, 1942) may be mentioned: In *Sirex gigas* and *Sirex cyaneus* larvae of different ages, a narrowly circumscribed area of the hypopleural fold of the first abdominal segment was found to be filled with fungi. Here also the fungal carpet grown on the walls of the tunnels serves as larval food.

A far closer relationship with the symbionts has been established for the Anobiidae which live in the dead wood of deciduous trees and conifers.

Among them only *Sitodrepa* and *Lasioderma*, which are pests of our provisions (cereals, tobacco), have altered their mode of life. The others have taken a further step by providing within their body a habitat for their symbionts. The portal of entry for such symbionts, all belonging to the Saccharomycetes, is undoubtedly the mouth. Four voluminous diverticula of the anterior mid-gut harbour the yeasts in their greatly hypertrophied cells, each species having a different strain of yeast. The infected intestinal cells have lost their brush border, their plasma is almost entirely replaced by the symbionts, their nuclei are deeply indented. (Buchner, 1921; Breit-sprecher, 1928; Grinbergs, 1961).

During metamorphosis some of the symbionts are transferred to much more slender diverticula of the imago's mid-gut; the remainder of the symbionts pass into the intestinal lumen and almost all are voided, together with the decomposing intestinal epithelium, at the first defaecation of the newly hatched imago. If one compares the symbiont-bearing areas of the intestine in different Anobiidae, a rising level of development is noted. It begins in *Dorcatoma* with simple bulges in the gut, still full of faecal material; it ends in *Ptilinus* with diverticula almost entirely separated from the gut and communicating with the intestinal lumen only by two long narrow channels (Gräbner, 1954). Thus true homes for the symbionts seem to have developed from such simple intestinal diverticula.

In this type of symbiosis continuity of infection is maintained, for, when the egg is deposited, the symbionts are transferred to its surface by a smearing apparatus. This consists of paired intersegmental ducts of varying length, some of which are provided with glandular cells and retentive hairs. Already in the newly hatched imago these ducts are filled with symbiotic yeasts which have wandered up from the end-gut via the anus into the sheath of the ovipositor. The yeasts find a suitable nutrient medium in the glandular secretion in which they multiply actively. Besides this mechanism there is a second pair of symbiont reservoirs formed by two vaginal pouches, which assure the transfer. These may grow into voluminous sacs as in *Anobium striatum*; in *Hylecoetus* they are in open communication with the lowest part of the vagina. This twofold mechanism guarantees security of transfer. As soon as the larva emerges, symbionts attached to particles of the egg-shell find their way into the previously sterile diverticulum cells and provide the origin for the more extensive colonization of the symbiotic organs. Thus the cycle is completed, except for a brief interruption during embryogenesis (Buchner, 1928).

At this stage a discussion of the symbiotic mechanism in the Cerambycidae follows naturally. It closely resembles that of the Anobiidae, but differs in the following respect. After completion of larval development all the symbionts completely disappear from the intestine, except in females which retain in their intersegmental sacs a small residue of symbionts, which infect the egg surface. Here, too, as in the larval diverticula each species of Cerambycidae has its own specific symbiont; all are species of *Candida*

(Heitz, 1927; Ekblom, 1931, 1932; W. Müller, 1934; Schanderl, 1942; Gräbner, 1954; Jurzitza, 1959; Jurzitza, Kühlwein and Kreger-van Rij, 1960). In a detailed study Schomann (1937) found that symbionts are carried only by those cerambycid larvae which burrow in the wood of conifers and dead deciduous trees. But he also found that even in species of Cerambycidae carrying no symbionts, the females possess small intersegmental sacs; these evidently form a normal part of the beetle's organism. Recently Grinbergs (1961) investigated several species belonging to different groups of Cerambycidae in Chile (Prioninae, Cerambycinae, and some undetermined forms); he found no symbiotic arrangements, but yeasts were present in their intestinal content and were determined to be *Candida*.

Time forbids me to discuss the very interesting group of the Curculionidae, but I would like to report on the Lyctidae which I have studied personally (Koch, 1936; Gambetta, 1927). They present quite a different type of symbiosis which finds its counterpart in the related family of the Bostrychidae (Buchner, 1954). Lyctidae and Bostrychidae surpass all previously described insects by the closeness of their adaptation and commensalism. Lyctus harbours two different pleomorphic strains of bacteria which are housed in separate zones of two oval, slightly lobate mycetomata. These organs are found in the posterior third of the larval body, embedded in adipose tissue between the gut and the gonads. The main mass of the mycetoma consists of enormous syncytia which enclose the one symbiont, a spherical to sausage-shaped organism that stains rather poorly. The cortical zone of the mycetoma consists of smaller syncytia which enclose the second, better staining symbiont. The whole organ is covered by a delicate layer of epithelium.

This new method of harbouring the symbionts in the space between gut and hypodermis requires a very different method to assure their transfer from the maternal body to the egg cells. The proximity of the mycetomata to the ovarioles favours their direct passage through the follicular epithelium. As soon as the first eggs from the fourteen ovarioles have completed the formation of yolk, special forms of the symbionts, serving only for the transfer, emigrate from both zones of the mycetomata. Through temporary gaps in the surface of the follicular epithelium they penetrate into the germinal blastema, whereupon the gaps close and the chorion starts to form.

The fate of the symbionts during embryogenesis need not be discussed. It suffices to state that at an early stage the original mixture of the two kinds of symbionts undergoes an orderly rearrangement and each type finds its proper domicile in the embryonal mycetoma.

In *Lyctus*, therefore, the symbiotic cycle is completely closed, whereas in the Anobiidae there remains a gap during the period of embryogenesis. This temporary sterility in the Anobiidae is of great help to the research worker in his endeavour to separate the two symbiotic partners, which is essential when studying the true meaning of symbiosis. This leads us to the cardinal problem in research on symbiosis: What part does the symbiont play in the life of its host? From all that I have said so far the idea must emerge that—in contrast to parasitic systems—the host makes the utmost endeavour to preserve the symbiotic bond once it has been knit. He cares for the accommodation of his symbionts and for their maintenance from one generation to another!

Obviously in many cases, if not in all, nutritional problems represent the essential link between the two partners. One need but think of the far more competent chemical activity of the micro-organisms and of the fact that symbiosis is found in animals with a particularly one-sided mode of feeding, as with the wood-eaters. A guide to the solution of the problem is afforded by insects and other animals that suck the blood of vertebrates: symbionts are found exclusively in those which feed on blood all their life, for example lice, bedbugs, Triatomidae, Pupiparae, ticks, and the leech, *Hirudo medicinalis*. Temporary blood-suckers, like the mosquitoes, *Phlebotomus*, fleas, *Stomoxys*, have no symbionts, since during their early life they have lived on different food containing bacteria and are therefore able to do without symbionts (Buchner, 1930).

The wood-eating insects also guide us to the solution of our problem. Wood is rich in carbohydrate and the small amount of protein present occurs only in the outermost layers of the tree trunk: that is why the larvae of *Hylotrupes bajulus*, devoid of symbionts, rarely penetrate into the heart-wood: they cannot survive in pure cellulose (Becker, 1942a,b).

In contrast the larvae of *Anobium punctatum* are completely independent of the protein content of the wood. Becker (1942c) was able to keep them alive in pure bleached cellulose for many months and they even grew a little. This is explained by the fact that in the genus Anobium symbiosis has attained its acme (Breitsprecher, 1928). Other Anobiidae, as well as the Lyctidae, restrict themselves to the more nourishing areas of the sap-wood (*Ernobius mollis, Lyctus linearis*) or prefer, like *Dendrobium pertinax*, to burrow in mouldy wood (Becker, 1942c, 1951). In experiments with artificial feeding of xylophagous insects their development was shown to be speeded up by the addition of protein or even of peptone and certain amino acids (Becker, 1942c, 1943, 1949). Likewise *Xestobium rufovillosum* develops faster in mouldy than in healthy wood.

Confirmatory evidence is furnished by Schomann's (1937) observation that all those Ceramycidae which burrow in fresh deciduous trees have no symbionts. The imagines of symbiont-bearing Ceramycidae which feed on the sugar-rich juices of plants do not need the symbionts any longer; they throw them overboard at the terminal stage of their development, a sign that the symbionts are required only during the period of growth.

Further pathways of research give a clearer insight into the physiological role of the symbionts. During the last three decades various methods have been elaborated for obtaining insects free of symbionts, and for *in vitro* cultivation of the symbionts themselves. This allows the research worker to study host and symbiont separately and to investigate the physiological competence of each partner. There is not time for a detailed discussion of the numerous relevant experiments (Koch, 1960, 1962); only the most important results will be summarized.

Loss of the symbionts is always followed by severe deficiency signs in the host. Lice deprived of their symbionts present symptoms of excessive hunger, are weak and listless, and show marked changes in their ovaries (Aschner and Ries, 1931; Aschner, 1934): Sterile larvae of *Sitodrepa* (*Stegophilus*) are unable to develop and die at the first shedding of their skin (Koch, 1933). Grave disturbance of growth and difficulty in shedding their skin are a characteristic consequence of loss of the symbionts in phytophagous and blood-sucking bugs (Brecher and Wigglesworth, 1944; Bewig and Schwartz, 1956; H. J. Müller, 1956; Schorr, 1957). The vital need for the symbiont is confirmed by similar signs of arrested development in aposymbiontic Blattidae (Frank, 1955; Brooks and Richards, 1955; Richards and Brooks, 1958; Selmair, 1962). It has thus been proved that the symbionts supply non-specific foodstuffs which supplement the extremely one-sided diet of their hosts. At the time when these facts were discovered in the louse (Aschner and Ries, 1931; Aschner, 1934) and *Sitodrepa* (Koch, 1933) vitamin research was still in its infancy. Today we know that the food-supplements needed by such insects are vitamins of the B-group (thiamine, riboflavin, pyridoxine, nicotinic acid, pantothenic acid, folic acid, beta-biotin), choline chloride, a sterol (ergosterol or cholesterol), and the biogenic amine carnitine (Fröbrich, 1939, 1952, 1953a, b; Fraenkel, 1952; Fraenkel and Blewett, 1943; Blewett and Fraenkel, 1944; Offhaus, 1939, 1952, 1958; Fröbrich and Offhaus, 1952; Schwarz and Koch, 1954; Pant and Fraenkel, 1954; Puchta, 1955). And we know that these vitamins are produced wholly or in part by the symbionts.

This fact has been proved wherever cultivation of the symbiont was successful. It is fairly easy to grow the fungi from the tunnels bored by *Hylecoetus*, the Ipidae, and *Sirex* (Grosmann, 1930; W. Müller, 1934; Francke-Grosmann, 1939, 1952) and it is not difficult to cultivate the symbiotic yeasts of the Cerambycidae and Anobiidae (Heitz, 1927; Ekblom, 1931, 1932; W. Müller, 1934; Schanderl, 1942; Pant and Fraenkel, 1954; Gräbner, 1954; Jurzitza, Kühlwein, and Kreger-van Rij, 1960; Kühlwein and Jurzitza, 1961).

With the Tribolium test, developed by my collaborators and myself, we were able to determine the content in vitamins and their synthesis by *in vitro* cultures of symbionts and Ambrosia fungi; with this method we were able to test even the vitamin content of the insects' normal habitat. The results of these tests afford unmistakable proof of the important part played by the symbionts in the life of their hosts. All the micro-organisms we investigated were excellent sources of the essential B-vitamins, as well as carnitine which is vital for the metamorphosis of the insect *Tribolium confusum* (Koch, 1956). In their vitamin content they are hardly inferior to beer wort or *Torulopsis utilis*. Therefore it is evident why loss of the symbionts is readily compensated by addition of brewers' yeast.

When it is considered that each individual micro-organism is species-specific, i.e., adapted to its particular host, it can be anticipated that both qualitative and quantitative differences occur in their vitamin content. Such differences are even found in the fungi of *Hylecoetus* and *Xyleborus* with their particularly rich yield of vitamins (Koch, 1956; Francke-Grosmann, 1956b). The *Sitodrepa* symbionts are less efficient vitamin producers than those of *Lasioderma*; they produce less biotin than those of *Ernobius*. This was shown by Pant and Fraenkel (1954) by exchanging the symbionts in the two bettle species: on a diet free from thiamine, *Lasioderma* larvae infected with *Sitodrepa* symbionts fail to grow; but in the same medium *Sitodrepa* larvae, infected with *Lasioderma* symbionts, develop. This was confirmed by recent work of Kühlwein and Jurzitza (1961). They investigated the synthesizing ability of the symbionts of *Sitodrepa* larvae grown in Hansen's solution (KH_2PO_4 0.3%, $MgSO_4$ 0.3%, glucose 5%, peptone from Merck's casein 1%) as well as a purely synthetic medium in which the peptone was replaced by $(NH_4)_2SO_4$ 1%. In neither of these media could they detect any vitamin production by these symbionts. This does not agree, however, with earlier work of Gräbner (1954) who used ammonium sulphate agar in diffusion cultures (Kanz, 1958); when he tested this medium before and after inoculation with *Sitodrepa* symbionts, he definitely observed production of folic acid, biotin B_1, B_2, B_6, and pantothenic acid. He found that *Sitodrepa* larvae, deprived of their symbionts, fail to grow on diets devoid of thiamine, riboflavin, pyridoxine, nicotinic and pantothenic acids; all these substances—with the exception of nicotinic acid—are passed into the agar by the symbionts (Blewett & Fraenkel, 1944; Pant & Fraenkel, 1954; Gräbner, 1954). These discrepancies may perhaps be attributed to differences in the technique employed by the two groups of workers.

Jurzitza (1959) also studied the metabolism of some symbionts of Ceramycidae (*Leptura rubra, Harpium mordax, Harpium inquisitor*) and obtained remarkable results with them. With the exception of *Candida rhagii*, the symbiont of *Harpium (Rhagium) inquisitor*, and the symbionts of *Gaurotes virginea*, all the symbiont strains proved to be vitamin-heterotrophic, i.e., unable to produce all the vitamins needed for their host's nutrition. The yeast from *Leptura rubra* can synthesize thiazole but not pyrimidine, the other component of thiamine; hence it must be considered as thiamine-heterotrophic. On the other hand, the symbionts of *Harpium* are only heterotrophic for biotin. Even between the two closely related *Candida* strains of *Harpium mordax* and *Harpium inquisitor* there are very marked differences in their synthesizing capacity. A further point of interest is that, with the exception of *Leptura rubra* yeasts, all the Cerambycidae symbionts can utilize urea. Thus they may also take an active part in the nitrogen metabolism of their hosts; this has, in fact, been proved to be the case with the symbionts of *Pseudococcus citri* (Fink, 1952).

As was to be expected, the examination of different kinds of wood revealed a marked vitamin deficiency. Apart from choline chloride and the occasional occurrence of pyridoxine and folic acid none of the other vitamins was detected. Therefore the vitamins of the symbionts of xylophagus insects provide an ideal supplement to the vitamin-deficient food of their hosts and open up to them a sphere of life otherwise inaccessible. The symbionts therefore have a multiple task. They provide or supplement the necessary vitamins and protein and they participate in their host's nitrogen metabolism by using the host's metabolic by-products. Their utilization of atmospheric nitrogen, reported by Schanderl (1942), has not been confirmed (Stapp, 1951; Jurzitza, 1959).

REFERENCES

Aschner, M. 1934.   Studies on the symbiosis of the body-louse. I. Elimination of the symbionts by centrifugation of the eggs. Parasitology *26*: 309–314.

Aschner, M., and E. Ries. 1931.   Das Verhalten der Kleiderlaus bei Ausschaltung ihrer Symbionten. Z. Morph. u. Oekol. d. Tiere *26*: 529–590.

Becker, G. 1942a.   Untersuchungen über die Ernährungsphysiologie der Hausbockkäferlarven. Z. vergl. Physiol. *29*: 315–388.

Becker, G. 1942b.   Beobachtungen und experimentelle Untersuchungen zur Kenntnis des Mulmbockkäfers (*Ergates faber* L.). Z. angew. Entomol. *29*: 1–30.

Becker, G. 1942c.   Oekologische und physiologische Untersuchungen über die holzzerstörenden Larven von *Anobium punctatum* de Geer. Z. Morph. u. Oekol. d. Tiere *39*: 98–152.

Becker, G. 1943.   Zur Oekologie und Physiologie holzzerstörender Käfer. Z. angew. Entomol. *30*: 304–218.

Becker, G. 1949.   Beiträge zur Oekologie der Hausbockkäfer-Larven. Z. angew. Entomol. *31*: 135–174.

Becker, G. 1951.   Ueber einige Ergebnisse und Probleme der angewandten Entomologie auf dem Holzschutzgebiet. Verh. Dt. Ges. angew. Entomol. e. v. 1949: 47–70.

Bewig, F. E. and W. Schwartz. 1956.   Untersuchungen über die Symbiose von Tieren mit Pilzen und Bakterien. VII. Ueber die Physiologie der Symbiose bei einigen blutsaugenden Insekten. Arch. Mikrobiol. *24*: 174–208.

Blewett, M. and G. Fraenkel. 1944.   Intracellular symbiosis and vitamin requirements of two insects, *Lasioderma serricorne* and *Sitodrepa panicea*. Proc. Roy. Soc. London (B) *132*: 212–221.

Brecher, G., and V. B. Wigglesworth. 1944.   The transmission of *Actinomyces rhodnii* Erikson in *Rhodnius prolixus* Stål (Hemiptera) and its influence on the growth on the host. Parasitology, *35*: 220–227.

Brooks, M., and G. A. Richards. 1955.   Intracellular symbiosis in cockroaches. I. Production of aposymbiotic cockroaches. Biol. Bull. *109*: 22–39.

Breitsprecher, E. 1928.   Beiträge zur Kenntnis der Anobiidensymbiose. Z. Morph. u. Oekol. d. Tiere *11*: 495–538.

Buchner, P. 1921. Studien an intrazellularen Symbionten. III. Die Symbiose der Anobiiden mit Hefepilzen. Arch. Protistkde. *42*: 320–336.

Buchner, P. 1928. Holznahrung und Symbiose. Springer Verlag, Berlin.

Buchner, P. 1930. Tier und Pflanze in intrazellularer Symbiose. Verlag Gebrüder Bornträger, Berlin.

Buchner, P. 1953. Endosymbiose der Tiere mit pflanzlichen Mikroorganismen. Verlag Birkhäuser, Basel/Stuttgart.

Ekblom, T. 1931. Cytological and biochemical researches into the intracellular symbiosis in the intestinal cells of *Rhagium inquisitor* L. (I). Skand. Arch. Physiol. *61*: 35–48.

Ekblom, T. 1932. Cytological and biochemical researches into the intracellular symbiosis in the intestinal cells of *Rhagium inquisitor* L. (II). Skand. Arch. Physiol. *64*: 279–298.

Fink, R. 1952. Morphologische und Physiologische Untersuchungen an den intrazellulären Symbionten von *Pseudococcus citri* Risso. Z. Morph. u. Oekol. d. Tiere *41*: 78–146.

Fraenkel, G. 1952. The role of symbionts as sources of vitamins and growth factors for their insect hosts. Tijdschr. Entomol. *95*: 183–196.

Fraenkel, G., and M. Blewett. 1943. The vitamin-B-complex requirements of several insects. Biochem. J. *37*: 686–695.

Francke-Grosmann, H. 1939. Ueber das Zusammenleben von Holzwespen mit Pilzen. Z. angew. Entomol. *25*: 647–680.

Francke-Grosmann, H. 1956a. Zur Uebertragung der Nährpilze bei Ambrosiakäfern. Naturwiss. *43*: 286–287.

Francke-Grosmann, H. 1956b. Hautdrüsen als Träger der Pilzsymbiose bei Ambrosiakäfern. Z. Morph. u. Oekol. d. Tiere *45*: 275–308.

Francke-Grosmann, H. 1960. Ein orales Uebertragungsorgan der Nährpilze bei *Xyleborus mascarensis* Eichh. (Scolytidae). Naturwiss. *47*: 405.

Frank, W. 1955. Einwirkung verschiedener Antibiotica auf die Symbionten der Küchenschabe *Blatta orientalis* L. und die dadurch bedingten Veränderungen am Wirtstier. Verh. Dt. Zool. Ges. Tübingen 1954: 381–388.

Fröbrich, G. 1939. Untersuchungen über Vitaminbedarf und Wachstumsfaktoren bei Insekten. Z. vergl. Physiol. *27*: 335–383.

Fröbrich, G. 1953a. Darstellung von Konzentraten des "Tribolium-Imago-Faktors" (TIF) und seine vermutliche chemische Natur. Naturwiss. *40*: 344–345.

Fröbrich, G. 1953b. Der "Tribolium-Imago-Faktor" (TIF) durch Carnitin ersetzbar. Naturwiss. *40*: 556.

Fröbrich, G., and K. Offhaus. 1952. Ein neuer Nahrungsfaktor, der die Metamorphose von *Tribolium confusum* Duv. (Tenebrionidae, Coleoptera) ermöglicht. Naturwiss. *39*: 575.

Gambetta, L. 197. Ricerche sulla simbiosi ereditaria di alcuni coleotteri silofagi. Ric. Morf. e Biol. Animale *1*: 3–17.

Gräbner, K. E. 1954. Vergleichende morphologische und physiologische Studien an Anobiiden- und Cerambycidensymbionten. Z. Morph. u. Oekol. d. Tiere *41*: 471–528.

Grinbergs, J. 1961. Untersuchungen über Vorkommen und Funktion symbiontischer Mikroorganismen bei holzfressenden Insekten Chiles. Arch. Mikrobiol. *41*: 51–78.

Grosmann, H. 1930. Beiträge zur Kenntnis der Lebensgemeinschaft zwischen Borkenkäfern und Pilzen. Z. Parasitkde. *3*: 56–102.

Heitz, E. 1927. Ueber intrazelluläre Symbiose bei holzfressenden Käferlarven (I). Z. Morphol. u. Oekol. d. Tiere *7*: 279–305.

Jurzitza, G. 1959. Physiologische Untersuchungen an Cerambycidensymbionten. Arch. Mikrobiol. *33*: 305–332.

Jurzitza, G., H. Kühlwein, and N. J. W. Kreger-van Rij. 1960. Zur Systematik einiger Cerambycidensymbionten. Arch. Mikrobiol. *36*: 229–243.

Kanz, E. 1958. Bakterienkultivierung im Symbioseverfahren durch eine neue Form der Ammenplatte. Arch. f. Hygiene u. Bakt. *142*: 288–320.

Koch, A. 1933. Ueber das Verhalten symbiontenfreier Sitodrepalarven. Biol. Zentr. *53*: 199–203.

Koch, A. 1936. Symbiosestudien. I. Die Symbiose des Splintkäfers, *Lyctus linearis* Goeze. Z. Morph. u. Oekol. d. Tiere *32*: 92–136.

Koch, A. 1956. The experimental elimination of symbionts and its consequences. Exptl. Parasitol. *5*: 481–518.

Koch, A. 1960. Intracellular symbiosis in insects. Ann. Rev. Microbiol. *14*: 121–140.

Koch, A. 1962. Grundlagen und Probleme der Symbioseforschung. Med. Grundl. Forsch. *4*: 64–156.

Kühlwein, H., and G. Jurzitza. 1961. Studien an der Symbiose der Anobiiden. I. Mitteilung: Die Kultur der Symbionten von *Sitodrepa panicea* L. Arch. Mikrobiol. *40*: 247–260.

Müller, H. J. 1956. Experimentelle Studien an der Symbiose von *Coptosoma scutellatum* Geoffr. Z. Morph. u. Oekol. d. Tiere *44*: 459–482.

Müller, W. 1934. Untersuchungen über die Symbiose von Tieren mit Pilzen und Bakterien. III. Mitteilung: Ueber die Pilzsymbiose holzfressender Insektenlarven. Arch. Mikrobiol. *5*: 84–147.

Neger, F. W. 1911. Zur Uebertragung des Ambrosiapilzes von *Xyleborus dispar*. Naturw. Z. Land- u. Forstwiss. *9*: 223–225.

Offhaus, K. 1939. Der Einfluss von wachstumsfördernden Faktoren auf die Insektenentwicklung unter besonderer Berücksichtigung der Phytohormone. Z. vergl. Physiol. *27*: 384–428.

Offhaus, K. 1952. Der Vitaminbedarf des Reismehlkäfers *Tribolium confusum* Duval. I. Mitteilung: Ueber den für *Tribolium confusum* lebensnotwendigen wasserunlöslichen Hefeanteil. Z. Vitamin-, Hormon- u. Fermentforsch. *4*: 555–563.

Offhaus, K. 1958. Der Vitaminbedarf des Reismehlkäfers *Tribolium confusum* Duval. II. Mitteilung: Weitere Ergebnisse über den für *Tribolium confusum* lebensnotwendigen, wasserunlöslichen Hefeanteil (TIF=Tribolium-Imago-Faktor). Z. Vitamin-, Hormon- und Fermentforsch. *9*: 196.

Pant, N. C., and G. Fraenkel. 1954. Studies on the symbiotic yeasts of two insect species, *Lasioderma serricorne* F. and *Stegobium paniceum* L. Biol. Bull. *107*: 420–432.

Parkin, E. A. 1941. Symbiosis in larval *Siricidae*. Nature *147*: 329.

Parkin, E. A. 1942. Symbiosis and siricid woodwasps. Ann. Appl. Biol. *29*: 268–274.

Puchta, O. 1955. Experimentelle Untersuchungen über die Symbiose der Kleiderlaus *Pediculus vestimenti* Burm. Z. Parasitkde. *17*: 1–40.

Richards, A. G., and M. Brooks. 1958. Internal symbiosis in insects. Ann. Rev. Entomol. *3*: 37–56.

Schanderl, H. 1942. Ueber die Assimilation des elementaren Stickstoffs der Luft durch die Hefesymbionten von *Rhagium inquisitor* L. Z. Morph. u. Oekol. d. Tiere *38*: 526–533.

Schneider-Orelli, O. 1913. Untersuchungen über den pilzzüchtenden Obstbaumborkenkäfer *Xyleborus* (*Anisandrus*) *dispar* und seinen Nährpilz. Zbl. Bakt. II, Abt. *38*: 25–110.

Schomann, H.   Die Symbiose der Bockkäfer.   Z. Morph. u. Oekol. d. Tiere *32*: 542–612.

Schorr, H. 1957.   Zur Verhaltensbiologie und Symbiose von *Brachypelta aterima* Först. (Cynidae, Heteroptera). Z. Morph. u. Oekol. d. Tiere *45*: 561–602.

Schwartz, W. 1935.   Untersuchungen über die Symbiose von Tieren mit Pilzen und Bakterien. IV. Mitteilung: Der Stand unserer Kenntnisse von den physiologischen Grundlagen der Symbiosen von Tieren mit Pilzen und Bakterien. Arch. Mikrobiol. 6: 369–460.

Schwarz, I., and A. Koch. 1954.   Vergleichende Analyse der wichtigsten Wachstumsvitamine der Blütenpollen nebst einer Bemerkung über die Verteilung der Vitamine in Buchensämlingen. Wiss. Z. d. M. Luther-Univ. Halle-Wittenberg *4*: 7–20.

Selmair, E. 1962.   Beiträge zur Wirkung wachstumsfördernder Stoffe auf die Entwicklung der Blattiden (*Blattella germanica* L.). Z. Parasitkde. *21*: 321–362.

Stapp, C. 1951.   Zur Frage der Bindung atmosphärischen Stickstoffs durch hautbildende Hefen. Arch. Mikrobiol. *16*: 48–52.

Strohmeyer, H. 1918.   Die Morphologie des Chitinskelettes der Platypodiden. Arch. Naturgesch. A *84*: 1–25.

LA PATHOGÉNÈSE DES VIROSES D'INSECTES

C. VAGO

Laboratoire de Cytopathologie
Saint Christol-les-Ales, France

LES MALADIES À VIRUS des insectes présentent depuis longtemps un intérêt agronomique, car elles peuvent contribuer à la diminution naturelle des pullulations de défoliateurs, être la cause de pertes dans les élevages d'insectes utiles, et être employées en lutte biologique contre les ennemis des cultures.

Toutefois, un autre aspect s'est dessiné depuis une cinquantaine d'années : l'approfondissement des processus intratissulaires. Celui-ci était d'abord lié à l'agriculture devant la nécessité d'expliquer des phénomènes écologiques, mais on s'est aperçu des facilités qu'offre le travail sur insectes pour l'étude des problèmes de virologie générale. Ainsi, récemment les recherches sur la multiplication des virus, la formation des corps d'inclusion et la transmission intraovulaire sont devenues nombreuses. Elles représentent un ensemble hétérogène que nous traiterons en choisissant les points de gravité autour desquels les problèmes d'actualité convergent : la pathogénèse aigüe, la présence de virus sans manifestation de maladie, et la pathogénèse « in vitro ».

I. PATHOGÉNÈSE DES VIROSES AIGÜES

Les viroses d'insectes qu'elles soient à corps d'inclusion, (polyèdries nucléaires, cytoplasmiques, nucléaires intestinales, granuloses) ou dépourvues de ces corps (sacbrood, virose de *Pseudaletia*, maladie irisante de *Tipula*, peut-être hydropisie des Scarabéides) n'ont été étudiées que sur quelques cas. L'infection, le passage à travers les tissus, et la multiplication intracellulaire sont plus ou moins approfondies, selon les difficultés techniques propres à chaque phase.

A. *Ingestion*

Pour les virus libres, l'existence de ce stade est admise *a priori*.

Chez les polyèdries ou granuloses, l'ingestion a une signification particulière : la libération des virus à partir des corps d'inclusion. Vago et Croissant (1959) et Vago (1962) ont filmé, en contraste de phase, le comportement des polyèdres de *Bombyx mori* L. dans le suc intestinal et ont montré la formation de fentes, l'éclatement en « peau d'orange », et la dissolution des fragments. Au microscope électronique sur coupes ultrafines on voit, au cœur des polyèdres, des vacuoles entourant les virus, lesquels s'échappent en masse au niveau des fentes.

Le sort des virus libérés dans la lumière intestinale est mal connu. Il est probable qu'ils subissent des dommages sous l'action du suc intestinal dont la réaction alcaline et probablement aussi un composant (Kitajima, 1932; Masera, 1954) récemment isolé (Suzuki, 1937; Aizawa, 1962) les inactivent. Il faut cependant supposer que les virus possédent une résistance, car certains arrivent malgré tout à infecter les cellules sensibles.

B. *Passage jusqu'aux cellules sensibles*

On suppose *a priori* que les virus ayant une affinité vis à vis des cellules intestinales peuvent y pénétrer directement après leur ingestion ou leur libération. Pour ceux affectant les tissus de la cavité générale, la traversée de plusieurs tissus serait nécessaire. Mais nos connaissances sur la phase comprise entre la libération des virus et leur réapparition dans les noyaux des cellules, sont réduites. Peut-être les virus pénétrent-ils au niveau des glandes, ou des tubes de Malpighi. Nous ignorons également sous quelle forme les virus traversent l'hémolymphe.

C. *Pathogénèse intracellulaire*

La pénétration des virus dans les cellules fait partie de la phase inconnue de la pathogénèse. Chez les viroses nucléaires, s'ajoute aussi leur passage à travers le cytoplasme pour accéder au noyau. Nous avons quelques données sur l'éclipse des virus, consistant en la disparition d'éléments infectieux, pendant un certain temps après l'inoculation. Ce phénomène observé chez plusieurs virus de vertébrés ou chez les bactériophages, a été signalé pour la polyédrie de *B. mori* par Yamafuji et coll. (1954), par Aizawa (1959) et par Krieg (1958). L'absence du pouvoir infectieux de l'hémolymphe a été constatée par Heitor et Vago (1963) chez *Galleria mellonella* L., peu après l'infection buccale.

La grande majorité des travaux concernent la « phase à lésions » de la pathogénèse. Parmi les virus libres, un rangement très régulier dans le cytoplasme a été noté dans la maladie irisante de *Tipula* (Smith, 1955b).

Pour les polyédries nucléaires, rappelons que déjà Conte et Levrat (1906) et Paillot (1933) ont vu chez *B. mori* une agglomération de taches chromatophiles. Chez une polyédrie nucléaire intestinale, Benz (1960) a observé pour ces masses de chromatine, des changements lors de la réaction du Feulgen de négatif en positif. De même, Wittig (1960) et Huger (1960) ont remarqué des trainées dans le noyau de cellules adipeuses atteintes de granulose.

En microscopie électronique, on observe des batonnets dans ces agglomérats, lesquels sont appelés par certains auteurs « virogenic stroma » (Xeros, 1956) et correspondent probablement au « viroplasme » souvent décrit chez les vertébrés. Dans le cas des granuloses, ce lieu de formation de virus serait près de la membrane nucléaire (Huger et Krieg, 1961) et entouré d'ergastoplasme. Pour les polyédries cytoplasmiques, des corps élémentaires cocciformes (Smith, 1956; Xeros, 1956) ont été vus dispersés ou en « stroma », dans le cytoplasme des cellules intestinales.

La formation d'une membrane autour des virus nucléaires est admise. Bergold (1950) distingue à l'intérieur des membranes, des stades de développement du virus; formes courtes, recourbées et droites. Sur coupes ultrafines, ces stades sont difficiles à suivre, et Bird (1959) envisage la sortie des bâtonnets des membranes, après des cycles de développement.

A la formation des membranes se rattache le groupement des virus en faisceaux. Il semble que celui-ci serait lié aux souches de virus : ceux de *G. mellonella* (Vago et coll., 1962), d'*Antheraea pernyi* Guer. (Vago, Sisman, 1959) de *Pterolocera amplicornis* Walk. (Day et coll., 1958) ou de *Lymantria dispar* L. (Morgan et coll., 1955) se groupent en faisceaux de 3 à 25 bâtonnets alors que ceux de *B. mori* ou de *Plusia gamma* L. (Lepine et coll., 1953) sont dispersés individuellement. Vago, Croissant et Lepine (1962) pensent que ce n'est qu'une substance entourant les virus qui les réunit.

La phase la plus caractéristique de la pathogénèse des polyèdries et des granuloses, est la formation des corps d'inclusion. Celle-ci serait un épi-phénomène (Vago, Croissant, 1960) et malgré les données sur la composition des polyèdres (Bergold, 1958) nous n'avons aucune conception précise sur son mécanisme. Il est généralement admis que ces corps sont les résultats de l'activité des virus sur le métabolisme cellulaire et qu'ils ont plus de parenté avec les protéines cellulaires qu'avec celles du virus. L'histologie en microscopie électronique a montré une structure de rangement macromoléculaire (Morgan et coll., 1955, Day et coll., 1958, Vago et Croissant, 1960) ainsi que l'inclusion des virus par cristallisation progressive de la masse de protéine (Day et coll., 1958; Bird, 1959; Vago et Croissant, 1960). Toutefois, Vago, Croissant et Lepine (1955) signalent une accumulation des virus à l'endroit de la formation des polyèdres de *B. mori*; ainsi que Smith (1955a) chez *T. paludosa*.

Chez une granulose, Hughes (1952) montre différents degrés de déposition des protéines autour des bâtonnets, jusqu'à la formation des granules. Par contre, Huger et Krieg (1961) sur coupes ultrafines remarquent le détachement des granules d'une masse hémogène.

Pour les virus cytoplasmiques, les images électroniques reflètent un processus d'incorporation des virus ronds dans les polyèdres intestinaux (Smith, 1956).

Sur le dernier stade de pathogénèse les observations signalent chez toutes les viroses à corps d'inclusion, un appauvrissement en virus et une accumulation des corps d'inclusion.

II. ACTION DE VIRUS SANS MALADIE AIGÜE

On a remarqué depuis longtemps, les signes de présence de virus dans les insectes sans pouvoir reconnaître des altérations pathologiques. Il s'agit d'observations hétérogènes, dont certaines sont liées à la pathogénèse aigüe et concernent une phase latente, d'autres révèlent par des traitements particuliers la présence de virus normalement restés sans action, enfin d'autres sont relatives aux virus étrangers transmis dans les tissus d'insectes.

A. *Latence des virus d'insectes*

On a l'habitude de traiter sous cette dénomination un ensemble de phénomènes remarqués dès la fin du siècle dernier, chez les Lépidoptères normalement sujets aux polyèdries nucléaires. Il s'agit de l'apparition, souvent massive, de cette maladie après action d'un facteur abiotique, sans que l'on ait à supposer une infection virale externe. Rappelons que ces phénomènes ont été attribués soit à l'alternance de phases chroniques et aigües des viroses dans les populations de *Lymantria monacha* L. ou *L. dispar* (Wahl, 1909, 1910, 1911, 1912; Roegner-Aust, 1947), soit simplement à une forme d'infection faible (Paillot, 1930), soit enfin à la production endogène de virus (Acqua, 1930) et notamment par transformation de nucléoprotéines normales en protéine de virus (Yamafuji, 1952).

Vago (1951) a étudié ce phénomène dans le cadre de la pathologie comparée, et l'a rapproché de la « latence » en admettant la présence, dans certains Lépidoptères « d'éléments portant la potentialité d'un virus » et a pensé qu'il serait illusoire d'envisager des spéculations sur sa nature exacte. Depuis, la plupart des auteurs acceptent plutôt la « latence » que la « production endogène » pour interpréter leurs observations. Smith (1952) estime que la vie en élevage déclenche les viroses chez les Lépidoptères. Les chocs de chaleur (Wellenstein, 1942; Yamafuji & Kosa, 1944; Vago, 1951; Ishimori & Osawa, 1952) et de froid (Ooba, 1956; Aruga & Arai, 1959) semblent pouvoir faire apparaître des polyèdries et des granuloses. De même, les rayons solaires, ultraviolets ou X (Vago, 1951; Krieg, 1956; Karpov, 1959; Smirnoff, 1961) ont montré un effet dans certains cas. Enfin, l'action de substances chimiques absorbées à faibles doses : nitrites, hydroxylamine, fluorure de sodium (Yamafuji, 1952; Veneroso, 1934; Vago, 1953; Aruga, 1958) a été particulièrement suivie.

Si l'on compare ces observations avec les phénomènes semblables signalés comme « infections inapparentes » en pathologie médicale, ou végétale, on doit penser aux virus provoquant des infections chroniques et à ceux existant sous forme « latente » et qui ne sont décelables que sous l'action de certaines influences. A première vue, l'apparition des viroses d'insectes sous l'effet de facteurs abiotiques ferait penser sans hésitation à la deuxième catégorie et au rôle d'un virus incomplet. Toutefois, les réponses sérologiques étant mal connues et peut-être aussi, réduites chez les insectes, on peut imaginer à la suite d'un trouble métabolique, aussi bien une reprise d'activité des virus normaux, que la recombinaison à partir d'éléments incomplets. La pathologie comparée fournit des exemples pour les deux cas : le virus de Theiler, la choriomeningite lymphocytaire ou certains virus végétaux pour le premier, la lysogénie des bactériophages pour le second. D'ailleurs, même en virologie générale, les hésitations sont nombreuses et il est probable que différents mécanismes existent. C'est pour cette raison que nous avons différents mécanismes existent. C'est pour cette raison que nous avons employé il y a dix ans la définition d' « éléments portant la potentialité d'un virus » et même aujourd'hui, il semble difficile de donner plus de précisions.

En effet, les phénomènes observés, sont très variables. Les viroses peuvent être provoquées dans un lot d'insectes et non dans un autre, et les doses actives de substances chimiques ne sont pas toujours les mêmes (Steinhaus & Dineen, 1960; Bird, 1961, etc . . .). Nous pensons que l'inconstance des résultats serait due au manque de précisions concernant les conditions physiologiques et avant tout au fait de ne pas avoir exclu tout apport externe de virus, comme l'ont fait Vago, Fosset et Meynadier (1961) avec l'élevage aseptique et individuel de Lépidoptères phytophages et de G. *mellonella* alimenté sur milieu de composition connue. Ce moyen pourrait apporter des éclaircissements sur la transmission des virus des polyèdries ou des granuloses par les oeufs de Lépidoptères, indispensables pour la définition de la forme de la latence. C'est également par cette technique et par celle des cultures de tissus que nous voyons un rapprochement des formes incomplètes de virus.

B. *Anomalies héréditaires et transmissibles*

Un aspect génétique de la pathogénèse virale a été remarqué dans quelques cas. En dehors de l'étude de l'absence héréditaire et transmissible de certains "seta sensoriels" à peine abordée chez les acariens *Tetranychus* (Boudreaux, 1959), l'exemple le plus suivi concerne le Diptère *Drosophila melanogaster* Meig. dont certains adultes meurent après anesthésie au gaz carbonique alors que la majorité reprend sa vie normale (L'Heritier, 1954). Cette sensibilité s'étant révélée transmissible par inoculation d'hémolymphe (L'Heritier & Hugon de Scoeux, 1947) les éléments infectieux ont été rapprochés des virus. En effet, ils se multiplient avec conservation d'un titre élévé pendant toute la vie de l'insecte (Plus, 1954). Il est particulièrement intéressant que les particules infectieuses transmises par la femelle peuvent créer deux situations dans la descendance : soit la multiplication de particules infectieuses amenant un état de sensibilité au gaz carbonique, soit l'état «stabilisé» dans lequel le virus a une concentration moins forte mais se transmet indéfiniment à toute la descendance, par les femelles et dans certaines mesures par les mâles. Cette situation se complique par des modalités appelées ρ et ultra- ρ, pour le moment sommairement définis.

Ces données permettent d'établir certaines comparaisons avec la latence des bactériophages (Jacob, 1954). En effet, la continuité génétique et le déclenchement d'une action freinante vis-à-vis des éléments surinfectants, observés chez les prophages se retrouvent chez le σ. Il est cependant vraisemblable que le virus de la Drosophile ne soit pas particulièrement lié aux chromosomes, ce qui semble être le cas pour les prophages (L'Heritier, 1962). Bien qu'il ne soit pas exclu que le prophage ait aussi une relation extra-chromosome avec la bactérie lysogène.

Peu de rapprochements peuvent être établis avec d'autres virus d'insectes. Le virus de la Drosophile n'a pas été isolé à l'état pur, sa forme n'a pu être définie au microscope électronique. On ignore l'organe dans lequel les éléments infectieux sont localisés, et celui qui subit les modifications permettant l'action mortelle du gaz carbonique. Il paraît souhaitable d'étudier les éventuelles lésions cellulaires décelables par l'histochimie, par la microscopie électronique et par la culture de tissus. En effet, nous ne pouvons considérer le virus de la Drosophile comme entièrement « non pathogène ». Malgré l'absence de mortalité, la sensibilité au gaz carbonique paraît obligatoirement liée à une modification cytopathologie encore inconnue et sans conséquence sur la mouche dans les conditions naturelles où la concentration en gaz carbonique est insuffisante pour que joue la déficience due au virus.

C. *Comportement des virus transmis par les insectes*

Des exemples toujours plus nombreux montrent que certains virus d'animaux et de végétaux absorbés par les insectes vecteurs pénètrent dans les tissus du vecteur et y accomplissent même certaines activités.

Pour les virus de végétaux Storey (1932) a révélé que dans certaines lignées de *Cicadulina mbila* Naude les virus des stries du maïs passent dans l'hémolymphe et Fukushi (1933, 1940) a pensé à une multiplication en voyant le maintien du pouvoir infectieux des cicadelles *Nephotettix apicalis* Horsc. pendant six générations. Black (1941) a montré par la suite que la concentration du virus de la jaunisse de l'aster dans le corps de la cicadelle vectrice augmente au moins cent fois. Maramorosch (1952) a réalisé à partir d'une cicadelle nourrie sur plante malade, 10 inoculations d'insecte à insecte avec dilution de 10.000 fois, entre chaque passage, sans que les cicadelles aient perdu de leur pouvoir infectieux. Des preuves semblables ont été apportées, par Day (1955), Heinze (1959) et surtout par Stegwee et Ponsen (1958), concernant le virus de l'enroulement de la pomme de terre et son hôte l'aphide *Myzus persicae* (Sulz.)

La multiplication des virus d'animaux dans les tissus des tiques ou les moustiques, a également été observée. Le titre du virus de la fièvre jaune augmente dans le corps de *Aedes aegypti* (Whitman, 1937). Pour le virus de la dengue, l'évidence de la multiplication n'a pas été établie, mais la persistance de l'infectiosité pendant au moins 174 jours chez *A. aegypti* la fait supposer (Lavier, 1958).

Les signes cytologiques de la multiplication ont été recherchés. Chez les végétaux, Dobroscky (1929), Blattny (1931), Hartzell (1937), Sukhov (1940) n'ont pu déceler que des altérations incertaines, mais Littau et Maramorosch (1956, 1960) ont observé une déformation du noyau des cellules adipeuses de la cicadelle *Macrosteles fascifrons* Stal. vectrice de la jaunisse de la reine-marguerite. Vago (1958) note des altérations nucléaires chez l'aphide *M. persicae* ayant absorbé du virus de l'enroulement de la pomme de terre. Il examine ces altérations aussi au microscope électronique.

La reconnaissance de virus serait une tâche extrêmement difficile, leur forme et leur localisation n'étant pas connues et leur concentration étant probablement faible.

Nous ignorons à l'heure actuelle la nature de l'action des virus sur le vecteur. La vie des cicadelles porteuses du virus de la jaunisse de la reine marguerite est dans certains cas prolongée et dans d'autres inchangée (Severin, 1945, 1947). Le virus du « dwarf » de l'oranger réduit le métabolisme du vecteur (Yoshii & Kiso, 1957). Jensen (1958) note une mortalité précoce des cicadelles porteuses du virus de la maladie X de l'Ouest. La signification de ces données serait à vérifier, car on ne sait pas si les effets bénéfiques ou nocifs ne seraient pas d'ordre écologique ou éthologique.

Chez les virus de vertébrés, l'absence d'effet pathogène cliniquement visible est de régle. La vie des *A. aegypti* porteurs du virus de méningo-encéphalomyélite n'est pas raccourcie et l'on ne décèle aucune lésion (Goret & Joubert, 1958). Les mêmes auteurs estiment qu'il s'agit de septicémie chez *A. aegypti*, pour la méningoencéphalite équine. L'examen systématique des tissus s'imposerait.

Une interférence entre virus semble se produire dans les cellules de certains vecteurs. L'infection de *Macrosteles* avec une souche de virus de la jaunisse de la reine marguerite empêche la transmission d'une autre souche (Kunkel, 1955). D'autres facteurs, tel que la « dominance » d'un virus compliquent ce phénomène (Maramorosch, 1957, 1958, Jensen, 1959).

Enfin, l'affinité du virus vis-à-vis du vecteur, semble être une partie instable du cycle viral. Si l'on entretient certains virus transmis par les cicadelles ou par les aphides, uniquement par passages sur plantes, l'infection ne se produit plus par le circuit à travers le corps du vecteur (Black, 1935; Hollings, 1955; Swenson, 1957; Watson, 1958).

III. PATHOGÉNÈSE IN VITRO

Des éclaircissements sur la pathogénèse virale ayant été obtenus sur cultures de cellules de vertébrés, des études semblables ont été envisagées pour les virus d'Insectes. Les premières tentatives de cultiver un tissu d'insecte remontent au début du siècle. mais les résultats obtenus sont pendant longtemps, restés dans les limites d'une survie dans l'hémolymphe (Goldschmidt, 1915; Paillot, 1924a,b; Frew, 1928; etc . . .), d'extraits d'insectes (Lewis & Robertson, 1916) ou de solutions salines empiriques. Les cultures ont été améliorées par l'emploi de milieux (Glaser, 1917; Trager, 1935), se rapprochant de l'hémolymphe des insectes (Wyatt, 1956; Shaw, 1956; Vago & Chastang, 1958, 1960a,b; Grace, 1958a). Enfin, l'obtention des couches monocellulaires par digestion enzymatique des tissus (Aizawa & Vago, 1959a) a ouvert de plus larges possibilités d'études virologiques.

L'infection virale en culture a été progressivement réalisée. Glaser (1917) n'obtient pas de résultats probants, tandis que Trager (1935) observe, dans la culture de fibroblastes de *B. mori*, la formation de polyèdres de Borrelinavirus. Aizawa et Vago (1959b) réalisent *in vitro* la pathogénèse de Borrelinavirus bombycis avec les virus de l'hémolymphe, ceux libérés de corps d'inclusion, et par mise en culture d'ovaires faiblement virosés. Cette infection a été obtenue aussi en culture d'hémocytes de Lépidoptères (Vago, 1959; Martignoni & Scallion, 1961). Certaines différences dans l'apparition des polyèdres dans les fibroblastes, selon les milieux ont été attribuées à la latence des virus (Grace, 1958b).

Les cultures cellulaires à durée contrôlée sont particulièrement propices à l'étude détaillée de la pathogénèse cellulaire. En microscopie électronique cependant, le seul travail réalisé à l'heure actuelle, est celui de Vago (1960, 1962) concernant des coupes ultrafines de cellules de Lépidoptères infectés en culture, montrant les stades successifs de la multiplication des virus, leur dispersion et leur inclusion dans les polyèdres.

La culture de tissus de Lépidoptères a servi également à tester l'absorption des virus des polyèdries sur les cellules (Aizawa, 1959).

Le problème si discuté de l'infection virale interspécifique a également été étudié *in vitro*. Vago (1959, 1962) a obtenu l'infection de gonades femelles de *B. mori* par des explants virosés de *G. mellonella* cultivés ensemble.

Le rapport de la multiplication des virus avec l'intensité du métabolisme cellulaire a été étudié à l'aide de fibroblastes de Lépidoptères (Vago, 1959; Vago & Chastang, 1960) en définissant la période de survie pendant laquelle l'infection et la formation des polyèdres sont possibles.

Le comportement des virus étrangers dans les cellules d'insectes, a été également suivi en cultures. Trager (1938) conserve le virus de l'encéphalite équine dans des tissus de *A. aegypti* en survie, (Rehacek & Pesek, 1960), le virus d'encéphalite dans ceux des tiques et Maramorosch (1956) le virus de la jaunisse de la reine marguerite dans les cellules d'une cicadelle.

CONCLUSIONS

Nous avons tenu à présenter, sous la dénomination «pathogénèse virale» non pas les détails de déroulement de maladies aigües, comme cela est habituellement fait, mais des phénomènes apparemment hétérogènes. Nous avons ainsi attiré l'attention sur les liens étroits entre les problèmes relatifs aux viroses aigües (dont une phase peut se relier à une période latente) aux virus appelés « non pathogènes » (lesquels causent malgré tout certaines anomalies) et aux virus transmis par les vecteurs (avec phases pathogènes dans d'autres organismes). En effet, il ne nous semble pas possible de comprendre le mécanisme du rapport cellule-virus, sans intensifier, dans l'avenir, les recherches comparatives sur les relations entre le type pathogène, le type transmis, et les formes dites « intégrées » des virus, malgré la très grande diversité d'extériorisation de leurs effets.

BIBLIOGRAPHIE

Acqua, C. 1930. Il bombice del gelso. G. Cesari, Ascoli Piceno, 373.

Aizawa, K. 1959. Mode of multiplication of silkworm nuclear polyhedrosis virus. J. Insect Pathol. *1*: 67–74.

Aizawa, K. 1962. Antiviral substance in the gut-juice of the silkworm *Bombyx mori* (Linnaeus). J. Insect Pathol. *4*: 72–76.

Aizawa, K., et C. Vago. 1959a. Culture "in vitro" de cellules séparées de tissu d'Insectes. Compt. rend. Acad. Sci., Paris *249*: 928–930.

Aizawa, K., et C. Vago. 1959b. Sur l'infection à Borrelinavirus en culture de tissu d'insectes. Ann. Inst. Pasteur *96*: 455–460.

Aruga, H. 1958. Mechanism of resistance to virus diseases in the silkworm *Bombyx mori* L. (IV) (V) (VI). J. Sericult. Sci., Japan *27*, 5–9.

Aruga, H., et N. Arai. 1959. Studies on the induction of polyhedroses by the low temperature treatment in the silkworm, *Bombyx mori*. J. Sericult. Sci., Japan *28*: 362–368.

Benz, G. 1960. Histopathological changes and histochemical studies on the nucleic acid metabolism in the polyhedrosis-infected gut of *Diprion hercyniae* Hartig. J. Insect Pathol. *2*: 259–273.

Bergold, G. H. 1950. The multiplication of insect viruses as organisms. Can. J. Res. *28*: 5–11.

Bergold, G. H. 1958. Viruses of insects. Handbuch Virusforsch. *4*: 60–142.

Bird, F. T. 1959. Polyhedrosis and granulosis viruses causing single and double infections in the spruce budworm *Choristoneura fumiferana* Clemens. J. Insect Pathol. *1*: 406–430.

Bird, F. T. 1961. Transmission of some insect viruses with particular reference to ovarial transmission and its importance in the development of epizootics. J. Insect Pathol. *3*: 352–380.

Black, L. M. 1941. Further evidence for multiplication of the aster-yellows virus in the aster leafhopper. Phytopathology *31*: 120–135.

Black, L. M. 1953. Loss of vector transmissibility by viruses normally insect transmitted. Phytopathology *43*: 466.

Blattny, C. 1931. Is it possible to detect the presence of the virus causing some diseases of potatoes in their carriers, the aphids? S. B. Böhm, Ges. Wiss. 7.

Boudreaux, H. B. 1959. A virus like transovarian factor affecting morphology in spider mites. J. Insect Pathol. *1*: 270–280.

Conte, A., et D. Levrat. 1906. Les maladies du ver à soie. La grasserie. Laboratoire d'Etudes de la Soie, Lyon *13*: 41–60.

Day, M. F. 1955. The mechanism of the transmission of potato leaf roll virus by aphids. Austral. J. Biol. Sci. *8*: 498–513.

Day, M. F., J. L. Farrant et C. Potter. 1958. The structure and development of a polyhedral virus affecting the moth larva, *Pterolocera amplicornis*. J. Ultrastruct. Res. *2*: 227–238.

Dobroscky, J. D. 1929. Is the aster-yellows virus detectable in its insect vector? Phytopathology *19*: 1009.

Frew, J. G. H. 1928. A technique for the cultivation of insect tissues. J. Exptl. Biol. *6*: 1–11.

Fukushi, T. 1933. Transmission of the virus through the eggs of an insect vector. Proc. Imp. Acad., Japon *9*: 457–460.

Fukushi, T. 1940. Further studies on the dwarf disease of rice plant. J. Fac. Agr. Hokkaido Univ. *45*: 83–154.

Glaser, R. W. 1917. The growth of insect blood cells in vitro. Psyche *24*: 1–7.

Goldsmidt, R. 1915. Some experiments on spermatogenesis in vitro. Proc. Natl. Acad. Sci. U.S. *1*: 220–22.

Goret, P., et L. Joubert. 1958. Destinée des ultravirus des maladies animales chez les arthopodes vecteurs. Rev. Pathol. Gén. Physiol. Clin. *58*: 1849–1872.

Grace, T. D. C. 1958a. Effects of various substances on growth of silkworm tissues in vitro. Austral. J. Biol. Sci. *11*: 407–417.

Grace, T. D. C. 1958b. Induction of polyhedral bodies in ovarian tissues of the tussock moth "in vitro". Science *128*: 249–250.

Hartzell, A. 1937. Movement of intracellular bodies associated with peach yellow. Contr. Boyce Thompson Inst. *8*: 375.

Heinze, K. 1959. Phytopathogene Viren und ihre Ueberträger. Duncker et Humbolt, Berlin.

Heitor, F., et C. Vago. 1963. Evolution des virus de la polyèdrie après infection orale de *Galleria mellonella* L. (sous presse).

Hollings, M. 1955. Investigation of Chrysanthemum viruses. I. Asperny flower distortion. Ann. Appl. Biol. *43*: 86–102.

Huger, A. 1960. Ueber die Natur des Fadenwerkes bei der Granulose von *Choristoneura murinana* (HBN) (Lepidoptera, Tortricidae). Naturwiss. *15*: 1–3.

Huger, A., et A. Krieg. 1961. Electron microscope investigations on the virogenesis of the granulosis of *Choristoneura murinana* (HBN.) J. Insect Pathol. *3*: 183–196.

Hugues, K. M. 1952. Development of the inclusion bodies of granulosis virus. J. Bacteriol. *64*: 375–380.

Ishimori, N., et M. Osawa. 1952. Provocation of polyhedral disease in silkworm by injection of hydrogen peroxide. I. A single use of hydrogen peroxide. Med. and Biol. *22*: 172–176.

Jacob, F. 1954. Recherches sur la lysogénie. Thèse, Paris. Inst. Pasteur, Masson.

Jensen, D. D. 1958. Reduction in longevity of leafhoppers carrying peach yellow leaf roll virus. Phytopathology *48*: 394.

Jensen, D. D. 1959. A plant virus lethal to its insect vector. Virology *8*: 164–175.

Karpov, A. E. 1959. On polyhedral disease in the silkworm induced by rays. Compt. Rend. Acad. Sci. Ukraine SSR. *9*: 1015–1018.

Kitajima, E. 1932. Studies on the polyhedral disease of the silkworm. Bull. Kagoshima Imp. Coll. Agr. *10*: 163–190 (en japonais).

Krieg, A. 1956. "Endogene Virusentstehung" und Latenzproblem bei Insektenviren. Arch. ges. Virusforsch. *6*: 472–481.

Krieg, A. 1958. Verlauf des Infektionstiters bei stäbchenförmigen Insekten-Viren. Z. f. Naturforsch. *13*: 27–29.

Kunkel, L. O. 1955. Cross protection between strains of yellows type viruses. Adv. Virus Research *3*: 251–273.

Lavier, G. 1958. Le sort chez le vecteur, des virus de la fièvre jaune, de la dengue et de la fièvre de trois jours. Rev. Pathol. Gén. Phys. Clin. *58*: 1873–1885.

Lepine, P., C. Vago et O. Croissant. 1953. Mise en évidence au microscope électronique du virus de la polyèdrie de *Plusia gamma* L. (Lepidoptera). Ann. Inst. Pasteur *85*: 170–173.

Lewis, M. R., et W. R. Roberts. 1916. Référence. Biol. Bull. *30*: 99.

L'Heritier, Ph. 1954. Le virus héréditaire de la Drosophile. *Dans* Problèmes actuels de virologie. Masson, Paris.

L'Heritier, Ph. 1962. Les relations du virus héréditaire de la Drosophile avec son hôte. Ann. Inst. Pasteur. *102*: 511–526.

L'Heritier, Ph., et F. Hugon de Scoeux. 1947. Transmission par greffe et injection de la sensibilité héréditaire au gaz carbonique chez la Drosophile. Bull. Biol. Fr. et Belg. *81*: 70–81.

Littau, V. C., et K. Maramorosch. 1956. Cytological effects of aster-yellows virus on its insect vector. Virology *2*: 128–130.

Littau, V. C., et K. Maramorosch. 1960. A study of the cytological effects of aster yellows virus on its insect vector. Virology *10*: 483–500.

Maramorosch, K. 1952. Direct evidence for the multiplication of aster-yellows virus in its insect vector. Phytopathology *42*: 59–64.

Maramorosch, K. 1956. Multiplication of aster-yellows virus in "in vitro" preparations of insect tissues. Virology *2*: 369–376.

Maramorosch, K. 1957. Cross-protection studies of two types of corn stunt virus. Phytopathology *47*: 23.

Maramorosch, K. 1958. Cross-protection between two strains of corn stunt virus in an insect vector. Virology *6*: 448–459.

Martignoni, M. E., et R. J. Scallion. 1961. Preparation and uses of insect hemocyte monolayers in vitro. Biol. Bull. *121*: 507–520.

Masera, E. 1954. Sul contenuto microbico intestinale del baco da seta e sull'etiologia della flaccidezza. Agr. Venezia *8*: 714–735.

Morgan, C., G. H. Bergold, D. H. Moore, et H. M. Rose. 1955. The macro-molecular paracrystalline lattice of insect viral polyhedral bodies demon-strated in ultrathin sections examined in the electron microscope. J. Biophys. Biochem. Cytol. *1*: 187–190.

Ooba, H. 1956. The nature of artificially induced grasserie and flacherie in larvae of the silkworm *Bombyx mori*. J. Sericult. Sci., Japan *25*: 211.

Paillot, A. 1924a. Sur les altérations cytoplasmiques et nucléaires au cours de l'évolution de la grasserie des vers à soie. Compt. rend. Acad. Sci. *179*.

Paillot, A. 1924b. Sur une nouvelle maladie des chenilles de *Pieris brassicae* et sur les maladies du noyau chez les Insectes. Compt. rend. Acad. Sci. *179*: 1353.

Paillot, A. 1930. Traité des maladies du ver à soie. Doin, Paris.

Paillot, A. 1933. L'infection chez les insectes. G. Patissier, Trevoux (Ain), France.

Plus, N. 1954. Etude de la multiplication du virus de la sensibilité au gaz carbonique chez la Drosophile. Bull. Biol. Fr. et Belg. *88*: 248–293.

Rehacek et Pesek. 1960. Propagation of Eastern Equine Encephalomyelitis (EEE) virus in surviving tick tissues. Acta Virol. *4*: 241–245.

Roegner-Aust, 1947. Der Infektionsweg bei der Polyederkrankheit der Nonne. Naturwiss. *34*: 158.

Severin, H. H. P. 1945. Evidence of nonspecific transmission of California aster-yellows virus by leafhoppers. Hilgardia *17*: 21–59.

Severin, H. H. P. 1947. Longevity of noninfective and infective leafhoppers on a plant nonsusceptible to a virus. Hilgardia *17*: 541–543.

Shaw, E. J. 1956. A glutamic acid-glycine medium for prolonged maintenance of high mitotic activity in grasshopper neuroblasts. Exptl. Cell Research *11*: 580–86.

Smirnoff, W. A. 1961. A virus disease of *Neodiprion swainei* Middleton. J. Insect Pathol. *3*: 29–46.

Smith, K. M. 1952. Latency in viruses and the production of new virus diseases. Biol. Rev. *27*: 347–357.

Smith, K. M. 1955a. Intranuclear changes in the polyhedrosis of *Tipula paludosa* (Meig). Parasitology *45*: 482–487.

Smith, K. M. 1955b. Morphology and development of insect viruses. Adv. Virus Research *3*: 199–220.

Smith, K. M. 1956. The structure of insect virus particles. J. Biophys. Biochem. 2: 301–306.

Stegwee, D., et M. B. Ponsen. 1958. Multiplication of potato leaf roll virus in the Aphid *Myzus persicae* (Sulz). Entomol. Exp. Appl. *1*: 291–300.

Steinhaus, E. A., et J. P. Dineen. 1960. Observations on the role of stress in a granulosis of the variegated Cutworm. J. Insect Pathol. *2*: 55–65.

Storey, H. H. 1932. The inheritance by an insect vector of the ability to transmit a plant virus. Proc. Roy. Soc. London (B) *125*: 455–477.

Sukhov, K. S. 1940. X-bodies in salivary glands of *Delphax striatella* Fallen the carrier of Zakukhvanie. Compt. rend. Acad. Sci., U.R.S.S. *27*: 377.

Suzuki, T. 1937. Studies on the silkworm nuclear polyhedrosis. Bull. Imp. Kyoto Sericult. Coll. *1*: 225–338 (en japonais).

Swenson, K. G. 1957. Transmission of bean yellow mosaic virus by aphids. J. Econ. Entomol. *50*: 727–731.

Trager, W. 1935. Cultivation of the virus of grasserie in silkworm tissue cultures. J. Exptl. Med. *61*: 501–513.

Trager, W. 1938. Multiplication of the virus of equine encephalomyelitis in surviving mosquito tissues. Am. J. Trop. Med. *18*: 387–393.

Vago, C. 1951. Phénomène de "Latentia" dans une maladie à ultravirus des Insectes. Rev. Can. Biol. *10*: 299–308.

Vago, C. 1953. Facteurs alimentaires et activation des viroses latentes chez les Insectes. Compt. rend. 6ème Congr. Intern. Microbiol. *5*: 556–564.

Vago, C. 1958. Les signes cytologiques du passage des virus végétaux dans l'organisme de leurs Insectes vecteurs. Rev. Pathol. Gén. Physiol. Clin. *703*: 1837–1847.

Vago, C. 1959. Recherches sur la culture de tissus en virologie des Insectes. Entomophaga *4*: 23–36.

Vago, C. 1960. Les virus d'invertébrés et leur mode d'action. Conf. Inst. Bota. Univ. Montpellier.

Vago, C. 1962. Etude au microscope électronique de la libération des virus, à partir des polyèdres dans le suc intestinal des Lépidoptères (sous presse).

Vago, C., et S. Chastang. 1958. Culture "in vitro" d'un tissu nymphal de Lépidoptère. Expérientia *14*: 426–429.

Vago, C., et S. Chastang. 1960a. Culture de tissus d'huîtres. Compt. rend. Acad. Sci. *250*: 2751–2753.

Vago, C., et S. Chastang. 1960b. Culture de Borrelinavirus dans les organes d'Insectes en survie. Compt. rend. Acad. Sci. *251*: 903–905.

Vago, C., et O. Croissant. 1959. Recherches sur la pathogénèse des viroses d'Insectes. La libération des virus dans le tube digestif de l'Insecte à partir des corps d'inclusion ingérés. Ann. Epiphy. *1*: 5–18.

Vago, C., et O. Croissant. 1960. Etude au microscope électronique de la pathogénèse virale intranucléaire de la "Grasserie". Arch. ges. Virusforsch. *10*: 126–138.

Vago, C., O. Croissant, et P. Lepine. 1955. Démonstration au microscope électronique du développement intranucléaire du virus de la grasserie. Ann. Inst. Pasteur *89*: 364–366.

Vago, C., O. Croissant et P. Lepine. 1962. Intérêt de la méthode histologique dans la caractérisation au microscope électronique des virus d'Insectes. Ann. Inst. Pasteur *102*: 749–753.

Vago, C., J. Fosset et G. Meynadier. 1961. Elevage aseptique d'Insectes phytophages. Rev. Path. Veg. Ent. Agr. France *40*: 111–129.

Vago, C., et J. Sisman. 1959. Mise en évidence du virus de la polyédrie d'*Antheraea pernyi* (Lepidoptera). Arch. Ges. Virusforsch. *9*: 267–271.

Veneroso, A. 1934. La malattia della poliedria nel *Bombyx mori* L. provocata da foglia intossicata da fluori. Boll. R. Staz. Sper. Gels. Bach., Ascoli Piceno, *13*: 1.

Wahl, B. 1909, 1910, 1911, 1912. Ueber die Polyederkrankheit der Nonne (*Lymantria monacha* L.). Zentr. Ges. Forstw. *35*: 164–172, 212–215; *36*: 193–212; *37*: 247–268; *38*: 355–378.

Watson, M. A. 1958. The specificity of transmission of some nonpersistent viruses. Proc. 10th Intern. Congr. Ent., Montreal, August 1956, *3*: 215–219.

Wellenstein, G. 1942. Die Nonne in Ostpreusen. Paul Parey, Berlin.

Whitman, L. 1937. The multiplication of the virus of yellow fever in *Aedes aegypti*. J. Exptl. Med. *66*: 133–143.

Wittig, G. 1960. Untersuchungen am Blut gesunder und granulosekranker Raupen von *Choristoneura murinana* (HBN.) (Lepidoptera, Tortricidae). Z. angew. Entomol. *46*: 385–400.

Wyatt, S. S. 1956. Culture in vitro of tissue from the silkworm *Bombyx mori*. L. J. Gen. Physiol. *39*: 841–852.

Xeros, N. 1956. The virogenic stroma in nuclear and cytoplasmic polyhedroses. Nature *178*: 412–413.

Yamafuji, K. 1952. Mechanism of artificial virus formation in silkworm tissues. Enzymologia *15*: 223.

Yamafuji, K., et Y. Kosa. 1944. Zum Chemismus der Entstehung des Virus. Biochem. Z. *317*: 81–85.

Yamafuji, K., F. Yoshihara, et M. Sato. 1954. Eclipse period of polyhedral disease. Enzymologia *17*: 152–154.

Yoshii, H., et A. Kiso. 1957. Studies on the nature of insect transmission in plant viruses. II. Some researches on the unhealthy metabolism in the viruliferous plant hopper *Geisha distintissima* WAL.; which is the insect vector of the dwarf disease of Satsuma orange. Virus *7*: 315–320.

THE ENTOMOPHILIC MICROSPORIDIANS

JOHN PAUL KRAMER

Illinois Natural History Survey
Urbana, Illinois, U.S.A.

PERHAPS THE MOST APPROPRIATE WAY to introduce my subject is to describe briefly those micro-organisms known as the microsporidians. Taxonomically, they belong to the order Microsporidia of the class Sporozoa of the phylum Protozoa. Morphologically, they possess a highly refractive univalved spore which typically contains a single amoeboid sporoplasm and a remarkable coiled organelle called the polar filament. Ecologically, they are obligate cytozoic parasites which attack other protozoans, invertebrate metazoans, and poikilothermic vertebrates. Entomologically, they are the most important group of protozoans that fatally parasitize insects.

Nearly 200 species of entomophilic microsporidians have been described. About 25 per cent of these species have been reported from Lepidoptera, and another 25 per cent have been described from Diptera, particularly from those flies with aquatic larvae. The remaining 50 per cent of the known species parasitize Thysanura, Ephemeroptera, Odonata, Orthoptera, Isoptera, Plecoptera, Anoplura, Hemiptera, Homoptera, Coleoptera, Trichoptera, and Siphonaptera. Most of these species have been treated in a recent monograph by Weiser (1961).

The habitats of these microsporidians include one or more of the following: epithelium of the gut, fat bodies, muscles, Malpighian tubes, silk glands, tracheal matrix, subcutaneous connective tissues, leucocytes, oenocytes, nerve fiber, and gonads. It is important to note here that certain species are host and tissue specific while others attack a variety of hosts and tissues.

For this symposium I shall briefly discuss some of the more obvious characteristics of the entomophilic microsporidians and their biology. The discussion will be arbitrarily limited to five topics: morphology, life history, transmission, spore longevity, and effects on the host.

MORPHOLOGY

An appreciation of the diversity found among the microsporidians and an understanding of their biology require some knowledge of their form and structure. I shall not attempt to catalogue all of the available information on this subject. Instead, I shall briefly discuss the major features of the spore with some reference to the developmental stages found in schizogony and sporogony.

The spore is the most characteristic form of the microsporidian. In most species it is ovoidal to pyriform; in others it may be bacilliform, reniform, or spherical with intermediate forms. The spores of most species are 3 to 7 microns in length and about 1.50 to 2.50 microns in breadth. A few are more than 20 microns long and 3 microns wide. Several species are as small as 1.25 microns by 1 micron. Indeed, the microsporidian spore is one of the smallest animal cells known.

The spore membrane or shell is generally smooth and structureless. As has been noted, the spore usually contains one sporoplasm and one coiled

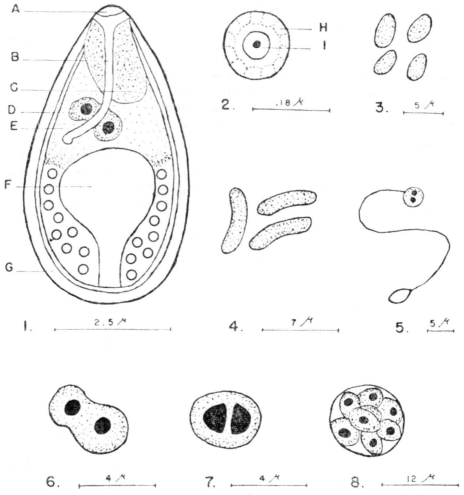

Figs. 1–8. Microsporidia. 1: Longitudinal section of spore; A, polar cap; B, polar filament; C, polaroplast; D, nuclei of sporoplasm; E, sporoplasm; F, vacuole; G, spore membrane. 2: Cross section of polar filament; H, wall; I, central axial structure. 3: *Nosema whitei* spores. 4: *Octosporea muscaedomesticae* spores. 5: Germinated spore of *N. whitei*. 6: A microsporidian schizont. 7: A microsporidian diplokaryon. 8: A microsporidian pansporoblast with eight spores. (All figures redrawn and modified from various authors, see text.)

polar filament. The arrangement of these structures within the spores of different species is variable. However, the general organization of a plistophoran spore described by Lom and Vávra (1961) is probably representative of the order as a whole. The shell of the spore of this microsporidian is about .10 of a micron in thickness except at the frontal pole where its thickness is reduced to .02 of a micron. The anterior one-third of the spore is nearly filled with a delicate structure called the polaroplast. Under the thin membrane at the front end of the spore is a polar cap. The polar filament attached to this cap runs along the polaroplast to the rear of the spore where it is wound in a spiral. The unattached end of the filament rests within the spore cavity. The filament, which is about .15 of a micron in diameter, is a hollow tube composed of elongate vertically-arranged fibrils. Within the lumen of the filament is another thin tube which contains a thin axial fiber. A vacuole, filled with a liquid of low viscosity, occupies the posterior part of the spore. The remainder of the space within the spore is filled by the binucleate sporoplasm.

The sporoplasm or amoebula which has emerged from the spore is a rounded body, generally .5 to 2 microns in diameter, with compact cytoplasm and two nuclei. In some species the sporoplasm apparently multiplies extracellularly, giving rise to planonts which are uninucleate; in other respects they resemble sporoplasms. Sporoplasms and/or planonts enter host cells where they produce schizonts which are rounded bodies of various dimensions with 1 to 16 nuclei. The schizonts produce more schizonts. Schizogony terminates with the formation of diplokarya in which the nuclei undergo a kind of sexual reproduction (see Weiser, 1961). The diplokarya produce sporonts which are generally oval in form. A sporont may develop into a single sporoblast which produces a single spore. The sporont may also grow, and its nuclei divide into 2, 4, 8, 16 or more daughter nuclei. Each of these daughter nuclei becomes the nucleus of a sporoblast. In this manner comparatively large bodies are formed which contain 2, 4, 8, 16 or more sporoblasts. These large bodies are the pansporoblasts. Each sporont within a pansporoblast develops into a single spore. It should be noted here that the classification of the Microsporidia is based upon the shape and size of spores, the number of spores present in the pansporoblasts, and upon host as well as tissue specificity (see Codreanu, 1961; Weiser, 1961).

LIFE HISTORY

The spore is the stage of the microsporidian that is usually transmitted from one insect to another. It enters the host by the oral route as a contaminant in food or drink. In the lumen of the cardia, or the anterior midgut, the spore germinates. The germination of the microsporidian spore is truly a remarkable process by which the delicate sporoplasm gains entry to the gut epithelium while avoiding the rigors of the gut environment with its ever-churning mixture of food, bacteria, and digestive juices. Several workers have observed various stages of germination *in vitro* (Gibbs, 1956; Kramer, 1960; Lom and Vávra, 1961; West, 1960). From a synthesis of their reports, the chain of events seems to begin with an expansion or displacement of the polaroplast which in turn exerts pressure on the polar filament. Next the end of the polar filament attached to the frontal pole of the spore begins to turn inside out. Within a fraction of a second, the entire filament is everted and the sporoplasm is forced through the filament and is injected into the gut epithelium of the host.

Sporoplasms, lodged in the wall of the gut, soon enter the coelomic cavity where they are circulated in the hemolymph. Probably within 48 hours, the sporoplasms enter the cells of certain tissues of the host. For example, the sporoplasms of *Nosema* (=*Perezia*) *pyraustae* (Paillot) invade the silk glands and Malpighian tubes of the larval European corn borer (*Ostrinia nubilalis*) while those of *Nosema whitei* Weiser invade the fat body cells of the larval red flour beetle (*Tribolium castaneum*).

The microsporidian now situated in a favorable medium, represented by the cell cytoplasm, undergoes schizogony. The schizonts produced move into other cells; eventually entire organs are invaded. Within seven to eight days, tremendous numbers of spores are formed. When tissues of the enteron or its appendages are heavily parasitized, host cells burst and release the spores which are then passed in the feces. The liberation of spores formed in other tissues involves other phenomena which will be discussed in the next section.

TRANSMISSION

As was mentioned, the microsporidian generally enters the host by the oral route. However, it may also be transmitted within the egg of the host, and in a few instances it is transmitted by a hymenopterous vector. For convenience these three modes of transmission will be treated separately although it is important to realize that some microsporidians are transmitted in more than one way.

Transmission Per Os. The sources of spores for oral transmission are often the by-products of the diseased insect. The most important of these is the feces. For example, the spore-laden feces of blow flies infected with *Octosporea muscaedomesticae* Flu are deposited on carrion where they are ingested by other susceptible larval and adult hosts (Kramer, unpublished data). Another important by-product is the secretion of infected accessory glands. In this instance the eggs from an infected female are joined or covered with an adhesive substance containing spores. As the larval insect emerges from the egg, it chews and ingests a portion of the chorion or shell including the contaminated adhesive. This phenomenon has been observed in several microsporidian infections of Lepidoptera including a nosematosis of the European corn borer caused by *Nosema pyraustae* (see Kramer, 1959a). Other by-products which may directly contaminate the food of susceptible hosts include vomitus, exuviae, and silk.

The tissues of the diseased insect are a second source of spores. Direct transmission of spores from these tissues to susceptible hosts occurs among cannibalistic forms such as the larva of the corn earworm (*Heliothis zea*) with its parasite *Nosema heliothidis* Lutz and Splendor (Kramer, unpublished data). Transmission of spores from infected tissues may involve a mechanical vector such as a predatory insect or bird. For example, the spores of *Thelohania hyphantriae* Weiser ingested with the diseased caterpillar (*Hyphantria cunea*) pass through the alimentary tract of a silphid beetle (*Xylodrepa quadripunctata*) without injury and contaminate the food of other caterpillars (Weiser, 1957).

A third source of spores is the body of the insect killed by the microsporidian. Physical factors such as wind, rain, and water currents break up the spore-laden carcass and disperse its contents over large areas. In this way spores contaminate the general environment of the insect.

Transovarial Transmission. Transmission of a microsporidian to progeny by invasion of the ovary and infection of the egg involves vegetative stages of the parasite as well as spores. Histological studies of infected ovaries have shown that nurse cells, the germarium, follicular epithelium, and other tissues harbor singly or in combination schizonts, spores, and intermediate stages (see Zimmack and Brindley, 1957; Thomson, 1958; Weiser, 1958). In the yolk of freshly laid eggs of *N. pyraustae*—infected moths, I have found vegetative stages and spores (Kramer, 1959a). As the development of the embryonic borer progresses, the deutoplasm or yolk becomes more or less transparent. In infected eggs it is therefore quite easy to observe the spores through the chorion. Just before the fully developed borer chews its way out of the egg, it swallows the mixture of liquids remaining within the shell, including the spores (Kramer, unpublished data). The parasite may also be absorbed into the developing embryo from the contaminated deutoplasm as has been reported in the case of *Nosema otiorrhynchi* Weiser which attacks the weevil *Otiorrhynchus ligustici* (Weiser, 1958).

That spores are transmitted by the male parent to its offspring has been demonstrated in at least one instance. Thomson (1958) observed this phenomenon in *Glugea* (*=Perezia*) *fumiferanae* (Thomson), the microsporidian parasite of the spruce budworm (*Choristoneura fumiferana*). Apparently spores are passed to the female in the spermatophores and stored in the spermatheca; they then enter the micropile of the egg with the sperm.

Transmission by a Vector. A few species of Microsporidia are injected into their lepidopterous hosts by hymenopterous parasites. In such cases the ovipositor of the wasp or its eggs are contaminated with spores. A larval wasp living within an infected caterpillar eventually acquires the microsporidian by ingesting the tissues of its host. Adult wasps developing from infected larvae retain the microsporidian within their alimentary tracts and reproductive organs. In this way a new generation of infected vectors is produced (see Payne, 1933; Allen, 1954; Blunk, 1954).

From an ecological viewpoint, the prime attribute of the microsporidian spore is its ability to withstand unfavorable external conditions when separated from the tissues of its host. How long these dormant spores, scattered throughout the general environment of the insect, remain viable depends primarily upon the water content of their immediate surroundings. In most cases spores resting on a damp surface, in water, or within the moist carcass of the host remain infective for two to six months at temperatures of 15 to 20 C. At temperatures of 5 to 10 C, such spores retain their infectivity for at least a year. In one case it has been shown that spores of *Nosema apis* Zander stored in sterile distilled water at about 5 C were infective for nearly seven years (Revell, 1960). Generally, excessive bacterial contamination in the environment of the microsporidian spore adversely affects its longevity. Most free spores subjected to drying at 15 to 25 C or to freezing are probably killed within a month (Weiser, 1961). However, spores of *Nosema whitei* dried at room temperatures remain viable for at least three months (Kramer, unpublished data), while frozen spores of *Glugea fumiferanae* remain viable for about four months (Thomson, 1958).

EFFECTS ON THE HOST

What a microsporidian does to an insect depends upon the site of infection. Those species attacking vital tissues such as the mid-gut epithelium may rather quickly and severely disrupt the physiology of the host. In contrast, microsporidians attacking only fat bodies slowly deplete the energy reserves of the host and thereby adversely influence its metamorphosis, especially at the time of pupation. The numbers of spores entering the host is an important factor in some instances. When excessive numbers of spores are ingested by the host, its gut-wall is often severely damaged by the polar filaments of the germinating spores. Bacteria enter the coelomic cavity through the perforated gut wall, a septicemia develops, and the insect dies within three to five days (see Weiser and Lysenko, 1956). In such cases the microsporidian has no opportunity to establish itself. Generally a microsporidian alone does not kill the host in less than seven days. As we will see, certain abiotic agents may interact with the microsporidian infection to the detriment of the host.

Our knowledge of the effects of microsporidian parasites on insects is based primarily upon the results of studies on diseased populations. Some conclusions drawn from these studies are briefly summarized below.

Mortality is high. In the European corn borer, for example, less than 15 per cent of congenitally infected larvae generally reach adulthood while at least 75 per cent of disease-free borers attain maturity under optimal conditions (see Kramer 1959a).

Development is often abnormal. Infected insects are generally undersized and slow to mature. Adults may have underdeveloped genitalia (see Finlayson and Walters, 1957). In a few cases, fatally infected larvae are unusually large; this suggests that the parasite may upset the hormone balance within the insect (Fisher and Sanborn, 1962).

Reproductive potential is reduced. The heavily infected female may produce no eggs or comparatively few eggs (see Zimmack and Brindley, 1957).

Mobility is impaired. The infected insect is typically sluggish and is easily caught by predators. It is often unable to undertake migratory flights (see Canning, 1962).

Sensitivity to DDT is increased. Parasitosis of certain beetles and lepidopterous larvae accelerates the lethal effect of this insecticide when it is applied topically. (Rosicky, 1951; Morgan, 1960).

Sensitivity to temperature is increased. During periods of abnormally hot or cold weather, the mortality rate among N. *pyraustae*—infected larval corn borers is greater than the mortality rate among healthy borers (see Kramer, 1959b).

Finally, it is important to realize that microsporidians are often "good" parasites; that is, they consume only enough of the substance of the host to maintain their kind.

REFERENCES

Allen, H. W. 1954. Nosema disease of *Gnorimoschema operculella* (Zeller) and *Macrocentrus ancylivorus* Rohwer. Ann. Entomol. Soc. Am. 47: 407–424.

Blunk, H. 1954. Mikrosporidien bei *Pieris brassicae* L., ihren Parasiten und Hyperparasiten. Z. angew. Entomol. 36: 316–333.

Canning, E. U. 1962. The pathogenicity of *Nosema locustae* Canning. J. Insect Pathol. 4: 248–256.

Codreanu, R. 1961. Sur la structure bicellulaire des spores de *Telomyxa* cf. *glugeiformis* Leger et Hesse, 1910, parasite des nymphes d'*Ephemera* (France, Roumanie) et les nouveaux sous-ordres des Microsporidies, Monocytosporea nov. et Polycytosporea nov. Compt. rend. Acad. Sci. 253: 1613–1615.

Finlayson, L. H., and V. A. Walters. 1957. Abnormal metamorphosis in saturniid moths infected by a microsporidian. Nature 180: 713–714.

Fisher, A. F., Jr., and R. C. Sanborn. 1962. Production of insect juvenile hormone by the microsporidian parasite *Nosema*. Nature 194: 1193.

Gibbs, A. J. 1956. *Perezia* sp. (Fam. Nosematidae) parasitic in the fat-body of *Gonocephalum arenarium* (Coleoptera, Tenebrionidae). Parasitology 46: 48–53.

Kramer, J. P. 1959a. Some relationships between *Perezia pyraustae* Paillot (Sporozoa, Nosematidae) and *Pyrausta nubilalis* (Hübner) (Lepidoptera, Pyralidae). J. Insect Pathol. 1: 25–33.

Kramer, J. P. 1959b. Observations on the seasonal incidence of microsporidiosis in European corn borer populations in Illinois. Entomophaga 4: 37–42.

Kramer, J. P. 1960. Observations on the emergence of the microsporidian sporoplasm. J. Insect. Pathol. 2: 433–439.

Lom, J., and J. Vávra. 1961. Niektóre wyniki badán nad ultrastrukturą spor pasożyta ryb *Plistophora hyphessobryconis* (Microsporidia). Wiadomošci Parazytol. 7: 828–832.

Morgan, C. A.   1960.   The susceptibility of microsporidian-infected larvae of the European corn borer, *Pyrausta nubilalis* (Hübner) to DDT intoxication. M.S. Thesis, Univ. of Illinois, Urbana. 26 pp.

Payne, N. M.   1933.   A parasitic hymenopteron as a vector of an insect disease. Entomol. News *44*: 22.

Revell, I. L.   1960.   Longevity of refrigerated nosema spores—*Nosema apis*, a parasite of honey bees. J. Econ. Entomol. *53*: 1132–1133.

Rosicky, B.   1951.   Nosematosis of *Otiorrhynchus ligustici*. II. The influence of the parasitation by *Nosema otiorrhynchi* Weiser 1951 on the susceptibility of the beetles to insecticides. Věstník Českoslov. zool. spol. *15*: 219–234.

Thomson, H. M.   1958.   Some aspects of the epidemiology of a microsporidian parasite of the spruce budworm, *Choristoneura fumiferana* (Clem.). Can. J. Zool. *36*: 309–316.

Weiser, J.   1957.   Mikrosporidiemi působená onemocnění bekyně velkohlavé a zlatořitné. Věstník Českoslov. zool. spol. *21*: 65–82.

Weiser, J.   1958.   Transovariale Uebertragung der *Nosema otiorrhynchi* W. 1958. Věstník Českoslov. zool. spol. *22*: 10–12.

Weiser, J.   1961.   Die Mikrosporidien als Parasiten der Insekten. Monograph. angew. Entomol. (Beih. Z. angew. Entomol.) No. 17. 149 pp.

Weiser, J., and O. Lysenko.   1956.   Septikemie bource morušového. Českoslov. mikrobiol. *1*: 216–222.

West, A. F., Jr.   1960.   The biology of a species of *Nosema* (Sporozoa: Microsporidia) parasitic in the flour bettle *Tribolium confusum*. J. Parasitol. *46*: 747–754.

Zimmack, H. L., and T. A. Brindley.   1957.   The effect of the protozoan parasite *Perezia pyraustae* Paillot on the European corn borer. J. Econ. Entomol. *50*: 637–640.

SYMPOSIUM IV

PSYCHROPHILIC MICRO-ORGANISMS

Chairman: M. INGRAM

J. L. STOKES

General Biology and Nomenclature of Psychrophilic Micro-organisms

A. H. ROSE

Biochemistry of the Psychrophilic Habit:
Studies on the Low Maximum Temperature

J. L. INGRAHAM

Factors Affecting the Lower Limits of Temperature for Growth

CHAIRMAN'S REMARKS

M. INGRAM

Low Temperature Research Station
Cambridge, England

MICROBIOLOGISTS who investigate habitats other than the bodies of warm-blooded animals have to deal with micro-organisms possessing temperature relations different from those of the mesophilic bacteria of classical medical and veterinary bacteriology. Because there are now many such microbiologists, working on micro-organisms, for example, in soil, or in the sea, or in water or foods, this is a subject of wide general interest, eminently suitable for a symposium at this Congress.

The general characteristic of these organisms of "natural" habitats is their ability to grow promptly and rapidly at lower temperatures than the mesophiles, and accordingly the name psychrophile has been commonly applied to them. It is unfortunate that literal interpretation of the word psychrophile, "cold-loving," implies that these organisms prefer cold conditions, because this is not true of most of the organisms to which the name psychrophile is commonly applied. These, like other organisms, accelerate in growth with increase of temperature over most of the tolerable range, roughly up to 25 C in this case. The misnomer seems especially unfortunate as it now becomes plain that micro-organisms exist which cannot tolerate temperatures above about 15 C, i.e. which really are "cold-loving" and might truly be called psychrophiles. One school of thought believes that this symposium on psychrophilic micro-organisms should have dealt exclusively with organisms of the latter kind; a view which, though justified linguistically, seems premature as little is yet known about them.

To avoid such misconceptions, the term psychrotroph (i.e., cold-growing) has recently been proposed for all organisms able to grow at temperatures near 0 C. This term has the advantage of focussing attention on the important general characteristic to which the organisms in question owe their dominance in nature and hence their importance in our discussions. Dr. Stokes will take up this question of nomenclature in terms of temperature relations, and the argument as to which measure of "growth" is best chosen to express the relation with temperature.

An organism of this kind is usually regarded as having maximum, optimum, and minimum temperatures for growth which are lower than those of the mesophiles. This, however, is not always the case: one need only recall the existence of faecal streptococci capable of growing over the range 44 to 0 C, though they are never regarded as psychrophiles because their optimum temperature is near the upper limit. Dr. Rose will be speaking particularly about the upper temperature limit, and Dr. Ingraham about the lower. It seems important to realize, from the outset, that there may be no relation between the several temperature characteristics.

GENERAL BIOLOGY AND NOMENCLATURE OF PSYCHROPHILIC MICRO-ORGANISMS

J. L. STOKES

Department of Bacteriology and Public Health
Washington State University
Pullman, Washington, U.S.A.

THE VERY FACT that the present symposium is being held indicates a considerable general interest in psychrophilic micro-organisms. This is not a new but rather a renewed interest. Psychrophiles have been known and investigated for seventy-five years, ever since psychrophilic bacteria were isolated and described by Forster (1887).

The reasons for this renewed interest are both basic and applied. Most microbiological research in the past and also now concerns mesophilic organisms which grow in the range of approximately 10 to 50 C. To a much lesser but yet considerable extent thermophilic organisms which grow at temperatures as high as 70 to 80 C also have been investigated. Perhaps it was time therefore for concentrated attention to be applied to micro-organisms at the opposite end of the biological temperature scale, to the psychrophiles which can grow at 0 C and even lower temperatures and which had been somewhat neglected by microbiologists. It is apparent that psychrophiles present intriguing problems of taxonomy, morphology, nutrition, physiology and biochemistry. Moreover it is clear that psychrophiles must be of paramount importance in the various cycles of matter in the cold regions of the earth—the oceans and the polar regions and also in temperate zones during the winter season. Also, the modern trend towards the production of frozen foods, and the storage of foods at low temperatures for relatively long periods of time, accentuates the importance of psychrophiles as spoilage organisms. These are the major factors which are responsible for the current marked interest in psychrophiles.

TERMINOLOGY

Much controversy has centered on the matter of terminology. This has been valuable in that it has forced microbiologists to think critically about the properties of psychrophiles especially those properties which differentiate psychrophiles from other types of micro-organisms. The term "psychrophile" was used first by Schmidt-Nielsen (1902) for micro-organisms which grow at 0 C. Almost immediately other investigators objected to the term because it implied, incorrectly, that the low temperature micro-organisms preferred the cold whereas actually they grew better at higher temperatures, 20 C and above. As a result other more appropriate names were proposed such as psychrocartericus or cold-conquering by Rubentschik (1925), psychrotolerant or cold-tolerant by Horowitz-Wlassowa and Grinberg (1933) and psychrotrophic or cold-thriving by Eddy (1960). All of the definitions proposed are based on one or more of the cardinal temperatures, the minimum, optimum and maximum temperatures for growth. Before we become too deeply involved in the matter of terminology perhaps we should examine the cardinal temperatures of representative low temperature bacteria.

Minimum temperature. The minimum growth temperatures of various psychrophilic bacteria are listed in Table 1. Growth occurs down to about −10 C. At these low temperatures the organisms must be incubated for

TABLE 1
MINIMUM AND OPTIMUM GROWTH TEMPERATURES
OF PSYCHROPHILIC BACTERIA*

Investigator	Organisms	Minimum °C	Optimum °C
Bedford	Marine	−7.5	20–30
Haines	Achromobacter	−3	—
Ingraham	Pseudomonads	—	20–37
Müller	Bacterium A	—	25–30
Smart	Various	−9	—
Straka and Stokes	Antarctic	−7	20–35
Sulzbacher	Pseudomonas	−8	—
Upadhyay and Stokes	Facultative anaerobes	—	20–30
Zobell and Conn	Marine	—	18–37

*Ingram & Stokes (1959); Straka & Stokes (1960); Upadhyay & Stokes (1962).

many weeks or months before appreciable growth occurs. Possibly growth can take place below −10 C if the culture medium can be prevented from freezing. Enzymatic activity can be detected at considerably lower temperatures and there have been a few reports of microbial growth, especially molds, below −10 C. In general, however, such low temperatures prevent growth perhaps by damaging cell membranes, by causing dehydration of the cells and culture medium, by promoting the accumulation of high salt concentration in the medium owing to desiccation and by slowing down enzymatic activity to a critical level.

The minimum growth temperature of −10 C for psychrophiles is far below the +10 C for mesophilic micro-organisms. It is useful for characterizing psychrophiles but is of limited value for identifying them partly because of the slowness of multiplication. Growth at the considerably higher temperature of 0 C, however, was proposed originally by Forster (1887) as the unique property of low temperature bacteria. In his paper on luminous bacteria published in 1887 Forster stated: ". . . our bacteria exhibit at certain temperatures a very special property which to my knowledge, at least with pure cultures, has not been previously observed. . . . they grow almost as well in the ice box as at the usual room temperature and even when tubes of streaked nutrient gelatin are placed in a container packed with finely crushed ice in the ice box, that is, at 0 C."

In my opinion, the development of easily visible growth within about one week at 0 C is still the best way of distinguishing and identifying low temperature micro-organisms. If incubation is continued for many months even typical mesophiles may grow somewhat at 0 C. Perhaps a higher growth temperature such as 5 C could be used and still separate psychrophiles from mesophiles. But it must be recognized that the higher the temperature adopted for differentiation, the greater is the possibility of including border-line organisms and mesophiles. Dairy microbiologists prefer a distinguishing temperature of about 8 C because it is common in commercial holding and distribution channels of dairy products. This relatively high temperature, however, will permit the growth of some frankly mesophilic organisms.

Optimum temperature. This is defined, usually, as the temperature at which growth is most rapid. Optimum growth temperatures for a number of psychrophilic bacteria are shown in Table 1. The optimum for most of them is 30 C or lower, although some grow best at 37 C. This is in sharp contrast to the frequently encountered definition of psychrophiles in text-books as organisms which grow best below 20 C. Recent evidence, however, indicates unequivocally that psychrophiles with an optimum temperature below 20 C exist in nature. They appear to be mainly yeasts. Several strains of *Candida* isolated by Lawrence *et al.* (1959) from grape juice stored at low temperatures grew optimally at 11 C and failed to grow at 21 C. Likewise, strains of *Candida scottii* isolated from Antarctic soil by Margaret di Menna (1960) grew best in the range of 4 to 15 C and many of them failed to grow at 15 to 20 C. Dr. Eimhjellen of the Technical University of Norway at Trondheim, has isolated a gram-negative, rod-shaped bacterium from sea-water which develops best at about 15 C and does not grow at 20 C (personal communication).

Perhaps such micro-organisms, which might be called strict or obligate psychrophiles, are more common in nature than is now apparent. If these organisms cannot grow at the usual room temperature of 20 to 25 C, they may die rapidly when brought into the laboratory. Success in isolation may require therefore rigorous maintenance of low temperatures throughout the isolation procedure.

It has been suggested by some investigators that the optimum growth temperature be defined as that which gives the largest cell crop rather than the most rapid growth. In general, the largest cell crops are produced at temperatures considerably below those at which growth is most rapid. For example, as shown in Table 2, Hess (1934) found that *Pseudomonas fluorescens* multiplied most rapidly at 20 C but produced the largest number of cells at 5 C. We have obtained similar results with a facultatively anaerobic psychrophilic bacterium (Upadhyay & Stokes, 1962).

No explanation has been offered for this curious phenomenon of greater total growth at lower temperatures. During the past year, Sinclair and

TABLE 2

GROWTH OF *Pseudomonas fluorescens* IN BUFFERED
NUTRIENT BROTH AT VARIOUS TEMPERATURES*

Growth	Temperature			
	20° C	5° C	0° C	−3° C
Generation time, minutes	85	401	1813	3408
Maximum cell count per ml × 10⁻⁶	995	1850	1590	1200+
Days required to reach maximum	3	29	46	60

*Hess (1934).

Stokes (1963) investigated this phenomenon and found a relatively simple explanation for it. The investigators who have observed the striking effect of temperature on cell crop used stationary cultures of aerobic organisms. In stationary cultures the initial dissolved oxygen in the medium is rapidly consumed by the multiplying cells and is not replaced rapidly enough from the atmosphere because of its low rate of diffusion and limited solubility. As a result, O_2 exhaustion limits growth in stationary cultures. When the incubation temperature is lowered, however, the solubility of O_2 increases and more O_2 becomes available for growth. Therefore, growth continues for a longer period of time, although slowly, at the lower temperatures and this leads eventually to larger final cell crops. The correctness of this explanation is indicated by the data in Table 3. Under stationary conditions and therefore O_2 limitation *Pseudomonas fluorescens* produces approximately twice as many cells at 10 C as at 30 C. However, when the cultures are aerated vigorously by shaking so that O_2 is not limiting, the maximal cell crop is the same at both temperatures.

TABLE 3

EFFECT OF TEMPERATURE AND AERATION ON THE
GROWTH OF *Pseudomonas fluorescens**

	Stationary		Aerated	
	30° C	10° C	30° C	10° C
Maximum viable count per ml × 10⁻⁹	8	14	18	17
Hours to reach maximum crop	27	94	30	72

*In trypticase soy broth.

It would be impractical to use crop yield as a measure of optimum growth temperature because of the long incubation periods required at the low temperatures. Moreover, our results indicate that crop yield is meaningless with respect to the effect of temperature on microbial growth since it is controlled by the availability of oxygen and not by temperature.

Maximum temperature. Perhaps surprisingly, the maximum growth temperatures of many psychrophilic micro-organisms can be quite high. Bedford (1933) found that although 37 of 60 strains could not grow above 30 C (5 not above 25 C), 13 had a maximum growth temperature of 37 C, 5 of 40 C, 2 of 42.5 C and 3 of 45 C. This is probably representative of psychrophilic bacteria.

Maximum growth temperatures have been used to subdivide psychrophiles. According to Hucker (1954), strict psychrophiles cannot grow at 32 C whereas facultative psychrophiles can grow at that temperature. Similarly, Rose (1962) sets the maximum growth temperature for strict or obligate psychrophiles at 25 C and for facultative psychrophiles at 30 C.

Because of the wide range of maximum growth temperatures, it would seem preferable to base the subdivision on optimum rather than maximum temperatures. On this basis, psychrophiles which grow most rapidly below 20 C would be classified as strict or obligate whereas those which develop most rapidly at 20 C or above would be facultative.

Conclusions. There are differences of opinion concerning the nomenclature and even the properties of micro-organisms which grow at low temperatures. These differences, however, are neither large nor critical. My own inclination is to retain the term psychrophile because of its long and wide usage; to define psychrophiles as micro-organisms which grow rapidly enough at 0 C to become macroscopically visible in about a week, in order to exclude mesophiles; to subdivide psychrophiles into strict or obligate and facultative depending on whether they grow most rapidly below 20 C or at and above 20 C. I do not expect that these views will receive universal acceptance.

ECOLOGY AND TYPES

Psychrophilic micro-organisms are very widely distributed in nature. They have been isolated in appreciable and frequently large numbers from air, water, soil, plants, animals and a great variety of foods. They are present in the temperate and polar regions of the earth and in the oceans. Their ability to grow at both low and moderate temperatures confers upon them an ecological and competitive advantage over mesophiles and this may be responsible, in part, for their wide distribution.

There are psychrophilic bacteria, yeasts, molds and actinomycetes. Recent investigations have been concerned mainly with psychrophilic bacteria in foods of plant and animal origin. The types isolated are predominantly gram-negative rods of the genus *Pseudomonas* and to a much lesser extent of *Achromobacter, Flavobacterium* and *Alcaligenes.* Occasionally, species of *Serratia, Proteus, Corynebacterium, Micrococcus* and other genera have been isolated. This limited range in bacterial types may be more apparent than real. Most isolations have been made from foods and with a limited variety of culture media and environmental conditions. It is quite possible that many additional bacterial types will be isolated when other habitats and cultural conditions are employed. Suggestive supporting evidence is our finding that of 30 strains of unidentified psychrophiles from Antarctica only 23 per cent were gram-negative rods. The preponderant group included gram-positive and gram-negative cocci and gram-negative cocco-bacilli (Straka & Stokes, 1960). Likewise elective cultures of soil, water and various foods at 0 C and strictly anaerobic conditions led to the isolation of 83 strains of facultatively anaerobic psychrophiles only 47 per cent of which were gram-negative rods. The majority consisted of 41 per cent gram-positive non-sporeforming rods and 12 per cent gram-negative cocci (Upadhyay & Stokes, 1962). Strictly anaerobic psychrophilic bacteria have not yet been isolated although they probably exist in nature.

It is noteworthy that psychrophilic yeasts can be readily isolated from Antarctic soils (di Menna, 1960). Recently 113 identified species of molds which grow at 5 C and below were isolated from frozen food products (Gunderson, 1961). They included species of *Mucor, Rhizopus, Penicillium, Alternaria, Cladosporium* and other genera. Psychrophilic strains of actinomycetes have been isolated but this group of micro-organisms has not been investigated extensively.

The polar regions and the oceans undoubtedly will be prolific sources of diverse morphological and physiological psychrophilic micro-organisms. These sources merit extensive and intensive investigation.

REFERENCES

Bedford, H. 1933. Marine bacteria of the northern Pacific Ocean. The temperature range for growth. Contrib. Can. Biol. and Fisheries 7: 431–438.
di Menna, Margaret E. 1960. Yeasts from Antarctica. J. Gen. Microbiol. 23: 295–300.
Eddy, B. P. 1960. The use and meaning of the term "psychrophilic." J. Appl. Bacteriol. 23: 189–190.
Forster, J. 1887. Ueber einige Eigenschaften leuchtender Bakterien. Centr. Bakteriol. Parasitenk. 2: 337–340.
Gunderson, M. F. 1961. Mold problem in frozen foods. Proc. Low Temperature Microbiol. Symp., Campbell Soup Co., Camden, New Jersey: 299–310.
Hess, E. 1934. Effects of low temperatures on the growth of marine bacteria. Contrib. Can. Biol. and Fisheries, Ser. C, 8: 491–505.
Horowitz-Wlassowa, L. M., and L. D. Grinberg. 1933. Zur Frage über psychrophile Mikroben. Zentr. Bakteriol. Parasitenk., Abt. II, 89: 54–62.
Hucker, G. J. 1954. Low temperature organisms in frozen vegetables. Food Technol. 8: 79–82.
Ingraham, J. L., and J. L. Stokes. 1959. Psychrophilic bacteria. Bacteriol. Rev. 23: 97–108.
Lawrence, N. L., Wilson, D. C. and C. S. Pederson. 1959. The growth of yeasts in grape juice stored at low temperatures. II. Appl. Microbiol. 7: 7–11.
Rose, A. H. 1962. Temperature relationships among micro-organisms. Wallerstein Lab. Comm. 25: 5–18.
Rubentschik, L. 1925. Ueber die Lebenstätigkeit der Urobakterien bei einer Temperatur unter 0°. Centr. Bakteriol. Parasitenk., Abt. II, 64: 166–174.
Schmidt-Nielsen, S. 1902. Ueber einige psychrophile Mikroorganismen und ihr Vorkommen. Centr. Bakteriol. Parasitenk., Abt. II, 9: 145–147.
Sinclair, N. A., and J. L. Stokes. 1963. Role of oxygen in the high cell yields of psychrophiles and mesophiles at low temperatures. J. Bacteriol. 85: 164–167.
Straka, R. P., and J. L. Stokes. 1960. Psychrophilic bacteria from Antarctica. J. Bacteriol. 80: 622–625.
Upadhyay, J., and J. L. Stokes. 1962. Anaerobic growth of psychrophilic bacteria. J. Bacteriol. 83: 270–275.

BIOCHEMISTRY OF THE PSYCHROPHILIC HABIT: STUDIES ON THE LOW MAXIMUM TEMPERATURE

A. H. ROSE

Department of Bacteriology, King's College,
University of Durham, Newcastle upon Tyne, England

THE DISTINCTIVE PROPERTY of psychrophilic micro-organisms which distinguishes them from mesophiles is the ability to grow well at temperatures just above 0 C. In what is probably a minority of psychrophiles, this low minimum temperature is accompanied by a low maximum temperature, as shown by the inability of the organism to grow at temperatures above about 30 C. This has led some workers in the field to recognize two distinct classes of psychrophiles—obligate and facultative (Rose, 1962). Examples of each of these classes have been known for well over fifty years. Until recently, however, microbiologists have paid little attention to the biochemical bases of these relatively low maximum and minimum temperatures. The recent upsurge of interest in the subject is a result not only of an increasing awareness of the economic importance of psychrophilic micro-organisms, but also of a realization that thermal energy can be an important factor in the control of cell metabolism.

Since low maximum and low minimum temperatures are not always found together, it is probably fair to assume that they have different biochemical bases. The low maximum temperatures of obligate psychrophiles are in a range in which many mesophiles grow optimally and are well inside the extremes of the biokinetic zone, and this strongly suggests that the biochemical basis of this property is associated with certain abnormally heat-sensitive cell constituents. Enzymes have long been recognized as, on the whole, the most heat-sensitive group of cell constituents, and so it is to an examination of the enzymes in obligate psychrophiles that biochemists have turned in their quest for a biochemical explanation of the low maximum temperature. It is well to remember, however, that other cell constituents, such as DNA and possibly RNA, may also show some degree of abnormal heat sensitivity and might therefore have some effect on the maximum temperature for growth of an organism.

But if we assume for the present that the biochemical basis of the low maximum temperature is to be found in the behaviour, and hence structure, of one or more enzymes in psychrophilic micro-organisms, then the problem is one of discovering which of the hundreds of enzymes in any one organism show abnormal heat sensitivity. Moreover, once the biochemist has located one of these enzymes, he has to decide whether it is in any way responsible for the low maximum temperature of the organism.

In my own laboratory, we have been studying the biochemical basis of the low maximum temperature in an obligately psychrophilic species of *Cryptococcus*, an encapsulated yeast. This organism was isolated by my former colleague, Dr. Walter J. Nickerson, from decomposing *Laminaria* collected during an expedition to Labrador. It has been described (Hagen & Rose, 1961) and would appear to be a previously unreported species of *Cryptococcus* although it closely resembles *C. terricolus*, a species recently isolated from Norwegian soils (Pedersen, 1958).

Preliminary experiments showed the obligately psychrophilic nature of this yeast and this was confirmed following more definitive studies on the effect of temperature on growth of the organism. Using a simple glucose-salts-vitamins medium (pH 4.5), the final cell crop was greatest in cultures incubated at 21 C although the yeast grew equally rapidly at 25 C. At 3 C, growth was also rapid after a lag period lasting approximately five days. But, at temperatures of 30 C and above, no growth of the yeast was observed.

Then, quite by accident, we found that, although this yeast would not grow in freshly inoculated cultures at 30 C, it could be induced to do so for a period on being transferred from 16 to 30 C, after which growth ceased. The rate and extent of growth at 30 C depended upon the duration of the

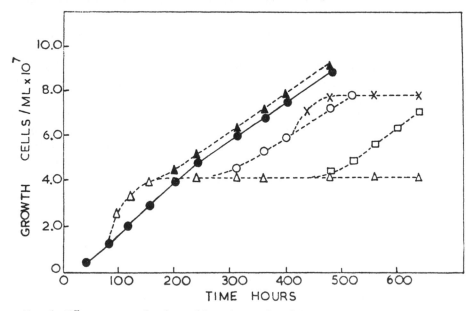

Fig. 1. Effect on growth of an obligately psychrophilic cryptococcus of transferring cultures from 16 C (●) to 30 C after 80 hr (△) and later transferring back to 16 C after 152 hr (▲), 200 hr (○), and 320 hr (□); growth of cultures following a second transfer from 16 C to 30 C after 417 hr is also shown (×).

incubation period at 16 C. Closely similar results were obtained when cultures were transferred from 25 C to 30 C. When cultures that had stopped growing at 30 C after being transferred from 16 C were returned to 16 C, growth resumed after a lag period which was proportional to the duration of the incubation period at 30 C (Fig. 1). No growth was observed, however, when cultures that had been incubated at 37 C after inoculation were transferred to 16 C.

Certain other psychrophilic yeasts, mainly *Candida* species, have been found to behave similarly on being transferred from 16 C to 30 C although with no organism is the stimulation of growth at 30 C following transfer from 16 C as great as with the psychrophilic cryptococcus. Several other psychrophilic yeasts which have been examined fail to grow on being transferred from 16 C to 30 C although they remain viable at the higher temperature.

The discovery of this transferring phenomenon appeared to provide a new and more rigorous method for studying the biochemical basis of the low maximum temperature in obligate psychrophiles for, by comparing the biochemical activities of organisms in cultures that had been transferred from 16 C to 30 C with that of organisms that had been maintained at 16 C, it might be possible to discover differences that would indicate a basis for the low maximum temperature.

Preliminary experiments along these lines did not reveal any marked

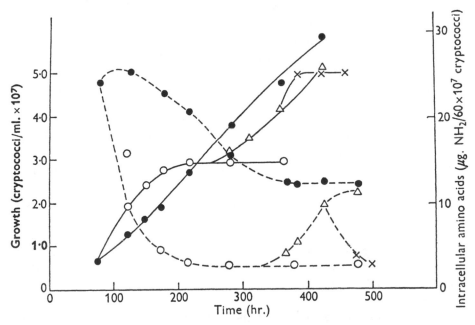

FIG. 2. Growth of an obligately psychrophilic crytococcus (–), and size of the intracellular amino acid pool (---) following the transfer of cultures from 16 C (●) to 30 C (○) after 72 hr, followed by a return to 16 C (△) after a further 144 hr. The effect of a second transfer from 16 to 30 C is also shown (×).

differences in the contents of DNA, RNA, acid-soluble ultraviolet-absorbing substances or total protein in cryptococci grown at 16 C compared with organisms from cultures of the same age which had been transferred to 30 C after 120 hr at 16 C. But, when the sizes of the intracellular amino acid pools in cryptococci grown under each of these conditions were compared, it was found that the pool was rapidly depleted when the incubation temperature was raised, but was replenished when the culture was returned to 16 C (Fig. 2). This decrease in the size of the intracellular amino acid pool was shown not to be the result of excretion of amino acids. Moreover, provision of exogenous amino acids in the form of bacteriological peptone did not enable the yeast to continue growing at 30 C.

One reason, therefore, for the failure of the cryptococcus to continue multiplying at 30 C after being transferred from 16 C was because it lacked the ability to synthesize some or all amino acids and to accumulate these from the medium. So our attention was directed to the biosynthetic precursors of amino acids in the cryptococcus.

To begin with, a study was made of the effect of a change in incubation temperature on the total keto acid content of the cryptococcus since certain key amino acids are known to be synthesized from α-keto acids. It was shown that, although the total keto acid content of the cryptococcus increased slightly during incubation at 16 C, there was, after an initial slight increase, a steady decline in the amounts of these acids in cryptococci from cultures that had been transferred from 16 C to 30 C. This decrease corresponded to the decline in the size of the intracellular amino acid pool. But the difference was that the depleted keto acid pool could be replenished by adding certain tricarboxylic acid cycle intermediates to the culture, and this enabled the yeast to continue to grow at 30 C. Transfer from 16 C to 30 C therefore creates an additional nutritional demand by the cryptococcus. However, freshly inoculated cultures of the organism in media supplemented with α-ketoglutarate fail to grow at 30 C and the cultures need to be incubated for about 96 hr at 16 C before addition of the keto acid brings about maximum stimulation of growth at 30 C (Fig. 3).

We are still some way from being able to explain fully the biochemical basis of the low maximum temperature in this organism. But the results so far obtained have shown the value of the transferring technique in localizing the area of metabolism containing the heat-sensitive reactions, thereby obviating the indiscriminate search for abnormally heat-sensitive enzymes. Work is now in progress on the next stages of the problem, and we already have preliminary evidence showing that, in cell-free extracts, certain tricarboxylic acid cycle enzymes in the cryptococcus are denatured at around 30 C.

We have also started looking at the biochemical bases of the low maximum temperatures in other obligately psychrophilic yeasts. None of these studies has yet progressed to the stage we have reached with the psychrophilic cryptococcus. But already it appears that we were fortunate in first

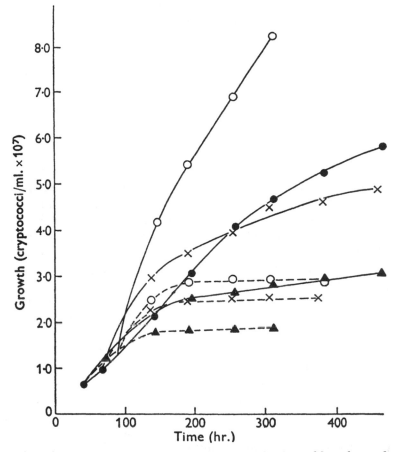

FIG. 3. Effect of addition of α-ketoglutarate on growth of an obligately psychrophilic cryptococcus in cultures transferred from 16 to 30 C after 48 hr (▲—▲), 72 hr (×—×) and 96 hr (○—○). At the time of transfer, each of the triplicate cultures received 0.5 ml of a sterile 12 per cent (w/v) solution (pH 4.5) of potassium α-ketoglutarate. Growth of control cultures which did not receive α-ketoglutarate on being transferred to 30 C is shown with dotted lines. Growth of cultures maintained throughout at 16 C is also shown (●—●).

tackling the problem using the cryptococcus. This organism is able to grow well at 30 C after being transferred from 16 C but this is not true of several of the other organisms so far examined. Clearly, the behaviour at 30 C following an incubation at 16 C will depend upon the type of enzyme or enzymes showing abnormal heat-sensitivity. It is conceivable that these enzymes may be concerned with the cell division process with the result that the organism is completely incapable of multiplying at 30 C. Also, in the psychrophilic cryptococcus, the biochemical changes brought about by a transfer from 16 C to 30 C, a depletion of the intracellular amino acid pool, were comparatively easy to study.

The above account is in the nature of a progress report of what could well be a fairly protracted investigation. But it is worth considering the significance of the results obtained and their bearing on theories relating to the maximum temperature in obligate psychrophiles.

Several theories have been put forward to explain the biochemical basis of the low maximum temperature in obligate psychrophiles but, in the context of modern biochemistry, only two of these merit detailed consideration.

The theory which has received by far the greatest measure of support postulates that obligate psychrophiles have certain exceptionally thermolabile enzymes inactivation of which leads directly to a cessation of growth. To date, no such enzyme from an obligately psychrophilic organism has been isolated and studied in detail although, as already mentioned, preliminary results with the psychrophilic cryptococcus have indicated that certain tricarboxylic acid cycle enzymes fall into this category. Interesting studies have, however, been made with mutant strains of mesophilic microorganisms which, unlike the wild types, are unable to grow in simple basal media at temperatures above about 30 C, and so resemble obligate psychrophiles in having abnormally low maximum temperatures. One of the first of these was reported by Maas and Davis (1952). A mutant strain of *Escherichia coli*, which required pantothenate at all temperatures, gave rise to occasional mutants requiring pantothenate only above 30 C. Extracts of the heat-sensitive mutant contained an enzyme capable of synthesizing pantothenate from pantoate and β-alanine, but which, unlike the corresponding enzyme from the wild type, lost 90 per cent of its activity during 25 min at 35 C. One particularly interesting result of this study was that the thermolabile enzyme was also abnormally unstable to treatment with urea, a well-known protein denaturing reagent. Closely similar results were obtained by Horowitz and Fling (1953) with a thermolabile tyrosinase from a mutant strain of *Neurospora crassa*, and several other examples of low maximum temperature mutants have since been reported. Also of interest in this connexion is the report by Lichstein and Begue (1960) who found a strain of *Saccharomyces cerevisiae* which would grow at 38 C only in media containing pantothenate although, at 30 C and below, it is capable of abundant growth in pantothenate-free media. There is clearly a need for further work on the biochemical basis of the maximum temperature of mesophilic micro-organisms and this should be of benefit to studies on the low maximum temperature in obligate psychrophiles.

A second theory which has been put forward attempts to explain the inability of obligate psychrophiles to grow at temperatures greater than about 30 C by postulating that, at these temperatures, these organisms synthesize or accumulate a metabolic poison. The two theories are not mutually exclusive for it would seem possible for an enzyme to be inactivated at higher temperatures and, although it does not lead directly to a cessation of growth, to cause the accumulation of an intermediate that inhibits the activity of other enzymes. Lichstein and Begue (1960) suggested that their observations on S. *cerevisiae* may be explained on this basis. This type of explanation is much more plausible than the suggestion that obligate psychrophiles, presumably with the aid of enzymes having relatively high minimum temperatures, synthesize a metabolically foreign substance at the higher temperatures. It is worth noting, in connexion with this theory, the recent work of Horiuchi, Horiuchi and Novick (1961) on a mutant strain of E. *coli* in which the regulatory system controlling the synthesis of β-galactosidase has become thermolabile. The presence of a similar type of thermolabile repression mechanism could form the basis of the low maximum temperature in obligate psychrophiles.

Use of the transferring technique might be expected to give information on the possible accumulation of an inhibitor by analysis of organisms transferred from a lower temperature to one above the maximum temperature for growth. Also if the inability of an organism to grow at the higher temperature is caused by an accumulation of a metabolic intermediate, then one might expect a period of detoxification before growth resumes on returning the culture to the lower temperature. In addition tests for production of an inhibitor can be made by examining the effect on growth at lower temperatures of extracts prepared from organisms transferred to a temperature above the maximum for growth.

Studies on the biochemical basis of the low maximum temperature in obligately psychrophilic micro-organisms, although so far few in number, will undoubtedly further our understanding of the effects of thermal energy on enzymes. They should, I believe, be carried out alongside studies on the maximum temperature in mesophiles and also thermophiles, for only in this way can we begin to formulate an over-all picture of the effect of thermal energy on biological systems.

ACKNOWLEDGMENT

Figs. 2 and 3 are reproduced by kind permission of the editors of the *Journal of General Microbiology*.

REFERENCES

Hagen, P-O., and Rose, A. H. 1961. A psychrophilic cryptococcus. Canad. J. Microbiol. 7: 287–294.

Hagen, P-O., and Rose, A. H. 1962. Studies on the biochemical basis of the low maximum temperature in a psychrophilic cryptococcus. J. Gen. Microbiol. 27: 89–99.

Horiuchi, T., Horiuchi, S., and Novick, A. 1961. A temperature-sensitive regulatory system. J. Mol. Biol. 3: 703–704.

Horowitz, N. H., and Fling, M. 1956. Studies of tyrosinase production by a heterocaryon of *Neurospora crassa*. Proc. Natl. Acad. Sci. U.S. 42: 498–501.

Lichstein, H. C., and Begue, W. J. 1960. Increased nutritional requirements of

Saccharomyces cerevisiae as a result of incubation at 38° C. Proc. Soc. Exptl. Biol. Med. *105*: 500–503.

Maas, W. K., and Davis, B. D.   1952.   Production of an altered pantothenate-synthesizing enzyme by a temperature-sensitive mutant of *Escherichia coli*. Proc. Natl. Acad. Sci. U.S. *38*: 785–797.

Pedersen, T. A.   1958.   *Cryptococcus terricolus* nov. sp., a new yeast isolated from Norwegian soils. Compt. rend. Lab. Carlsberg *31*: 93–103.

Rose, A. H.   1962.   Temperature relationships among micro-organisms. Wallerstein Lab. Comm. *25*: 5–18.

FACTORS AFFECTING THE LOWER
LIMITS OF TEMPERATURE FOR GROWTH

J. L. INGRAHAM

University of California
Davis, California, U.S.A.

PSYCHROPHILES are characterized by having a lower minimal temperature for growth than other bacteria. In this discussion I should like to consider some possible reasons for this difference, and also consider the more general question of the factors that make any bacterium stop growing at low temperature.

Ingraham (1958) compared the growth rate of a psychrophile and a mesophile as a function of temperature (Fig. 1) and obtained two curves of similar shape with that of the psychrophile being displaced about 8 to 10

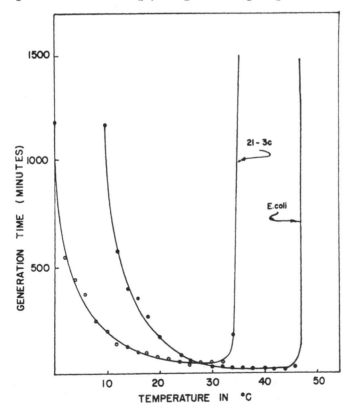

FIG. 1. Effect of temperature on the generation time of a typical mesophile (*E. coli*) and a psychrophile (21–3c). Cultures were grown aerobically in complex media. (Ingraham, 1958)

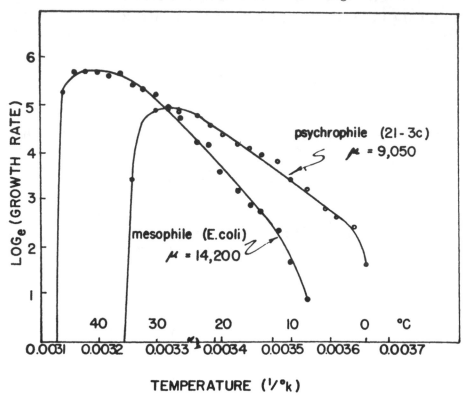

FIG. 2. Arrhenius plot of the data shown in Fig. 1. (Ingraham, 1958)

degrees lower. However, when the same data were presented in the form of an Arrhenius plot (Fig. 2) another interesting difference became apparent. This was that the slope of the linear portion of the curve is less for the psychrophile than for the mesophile.

In an isolated chemical system, the slope of the Arrhenius plot is a measure of the activation energy of the reaction. In complex biological processes, the corresponding quantity is without precise physical meaning and is termed the "temperature characteristic" (μ).

The difference in temperature characteristic between psychophile and mesophile seemed to offer an explanation for the difference in minimal growth temperature. We reasoned that certain enzymes of psychrophiles might catalyze reactions at a lower activation energy than would the corresponding enzyme from mesophiles. Accordingly, the activation energies of three pairs of enzymes from a psychrophile and a mesophile were measured (Ingraham & Bailey, 1959). No significant differences were found. A comparison of isocitric acid dehydrogenase from *E. coli* and from a psychrophilic pseudomonad is shown in Fig. 3. The slopes are identical. Respiration experiments were also unsuccessful in explaining the differences in temperature characteristics of growth.

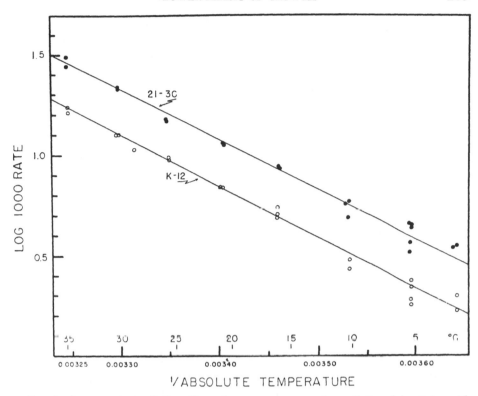

FIG. 3. A comparison of the effect of temperature on the activity of isocitric acid dehydrogenase from a psychrophile and a mesophile. 21–3c, a sonic extract from a psychrophilic pseudomonad. K-12, a sonic extract from *E. coli*. (Ingraham and Bailey, 1959)

More recently we have considered the problem which we feel is an essential prerequisite to understanding the differences between psychrophiles and mesophiles: why do bacteria have a minimum temperature for growth? Otto Rahn put the question quite clearly a number of years ago when he wrote, "Since growth and fermentation are chemical reactions, they should continue, though at a greatly reduced rate of speed until the medium freezes solid. This is certainly not always the case with bacteria; most cease to grow at temperatures 5, 10, or more degrees above freezing."

The question of why bacteria have a minimal temperature for growth can also be stated in a slightly different way: why does the temperature characteristic for growth rate increase dramatically at low temperature (Fig. 2) and eventually become infinite? In this form, the question of minimal temperature of growth becomes a part of a more general biological question, because the phenomenon of increased temperature characteristics at low temperature is very common in the biological world. During the 1920's it was verified in such diverse processes as the chirping rate of crickets and the activities of the human brain.

A number of hypotheses have been proposed to explain the phenomenon. Blackman (1905) proposed that the rate of a biological process is set by the rate of a certain "master reaction." As temperature is decreased, reactions with progressively greater activation energies would become rate-limiting causing the temperature characteristic of the over-all process to increase. Recently severe objections to the Blackman hypothesis have been raised (Senez, 1962).

Kistiakowsky and Lumry (1949) approached this problem by analyzing the effect of temperature on the rate of hydrolysis of urea by urease. In the presence of 0.034 M sodium sulphite, the temperature characteristic of the reaction increases sharply below 20 C, but in the absence of the inhibitor the temperature characteristic is linear to 0 C. They assumed that a rapid equilibrium reaction exists between active enzyme and sulphite-yielding inactive enzyme. If the Δ H of this reaction is negative, the equilibrium constant will increase at low temperature so that a decreasing amount of the enzyme will be in the active form, and, consequently, the temperature characteristic of the over-all process will increase. These authors suggest that this sort of explanation may well account for the common observation of increased temperature characteristics in biological systems at low temperature.

Marr and Ingraham developed another model to account for the phenomenon (unpublished data). They considered a branched system (Fig. 4) in which A yields B which in turn yields C and D. They assumed that the reaction B to C is productive of cell growth and B to D is non-productive, and that A to B and B to C have a high activation energy while B to D has a low activation energy. They further assumed that the order of the reaction B to D is considerably lower than with B to C. From these assumptions a plot of the log of the rate of C formation against the reciprocal of absolute temperature mimics the Arrhenius plot of bacterial growth rate (Fig. 5).

The foregoing hypotheses all assume that the curvalinearity of the Arrhenius plot is a direct result of complex chemical kinetics. They predict an immediate change in growth rate with a change in temperature.

A second type of explanation is that growth at low temperature changes

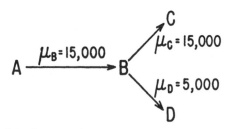

FIG. 4. Proposed model which results in an increased temperature characteristic at low temperature.

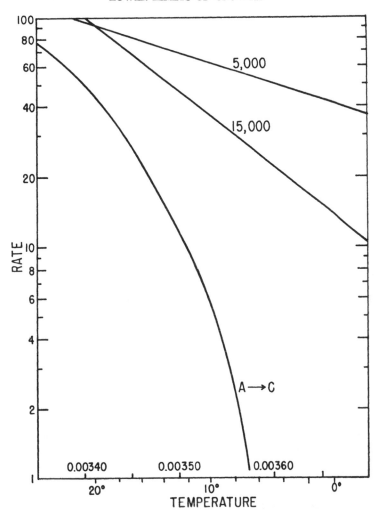

FIG. 5. Arrhenius plot of the rate of the reaction A to C shown in Fig. 4 as compared with reaction A to B (15,000) and B to D (5,000).

the composition of cells in such a way that they grow less rapidly than would be expected from kinetic considerations alone.

To distinguish between these two types of explanations, Ng, Ingraham, and Marr (1962) did a series of experiments in which exponentially growing cultures of *E. coli* ML30 were subjected to abrupt changes in temperature. They found that the Arrhenius plot of growth rate of *E. coli* ML30 growing in glucose-minimal medium is essentially linear down to 20 C, and that below that temperature the temperature characteristic increases sharply (Fig. 6). Temperature shifts, up or down, within the range of constant temperature characteristic were found to be followed by continued exponential growth at a rate characteristic of the new temperature. However,

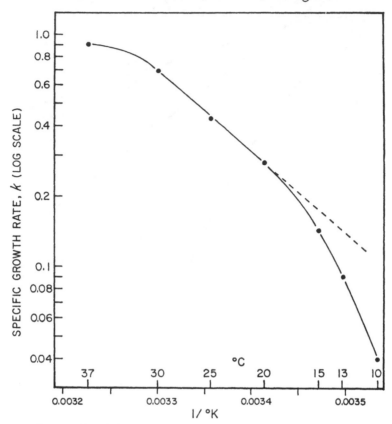

Fɪɢ. 6. Arrhenius plot of the specific growth rate of *E. coli* ML30 growing aerobically in basal-glucose medium. The ordinate is the specific growth rate (log scale), and the numbers below the abscissa are reciprocals of the absolute temperature. (Ng, Ingraham and Marr, 1962)

if the shift was made from a temperature below 20 C to one greater than 20 C transient growth rates were observed. Immediately after the increase in temperature, the culture increased exponentially at a rate intermediate to those normal for the initial and the final temperature. The growth rate immediately following the increase in temperature was found to be a function of the lower temperature, but in all cases the transition from the intermediate to normal rate for the high temperature occurred after about 2.3 doublings (Fig. 7).

If the temperature shift was made from a temperature above 20 C to one below 20 C transient growth rates were also observed (Fig. 8). Immediately after the temperature was decreased, the cultures stopped growing for a period of several hours after which time the culture grew more rapidly than the rate at which they normally grow at low temperature for approximately one doubling. Then the normal rate of growth for the low temperature was assumed.

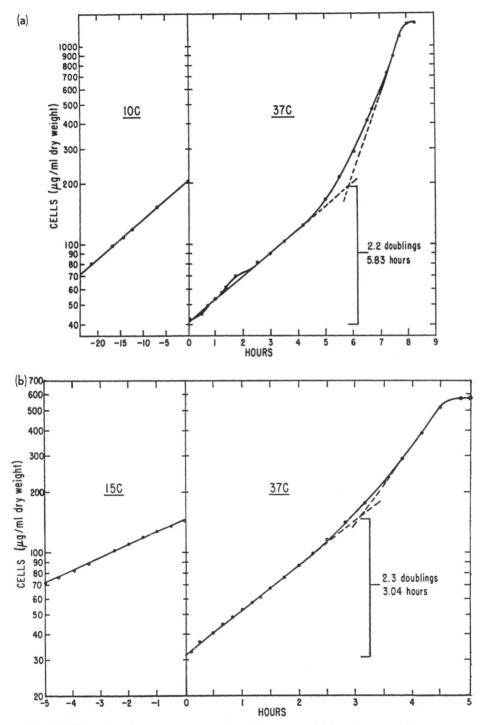

Fig. 7. Effect of an increase in temperature from 10 C (7a) and 15 C (7b) to 37 C on the growth of *E. coli* ML30. Culture was grown in basal-glucose medium to a density of about 280 µg dry weight/ml; the change in temperature was effected by rapidly transferring 60 ml of culture to 240 ml of the same medium previously equilibrated and saturated with oxygen at the indicated temperature. (Ng, Ingraham and Marr, 1962).

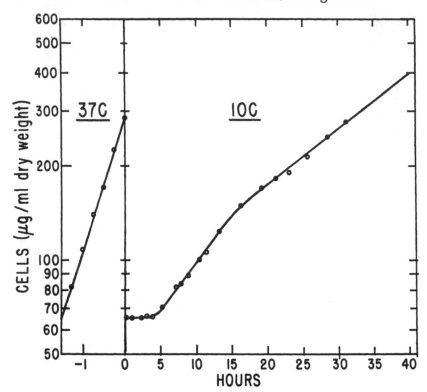

FIG. 8. Effect of a decrease in temperature from 37 C to 10 C on the growth of *E. coli* ML30. Techniques of transfer are the same as those indicated in the legend of Fig. 7. (Ng, Ingraham and Marr, 1962)

These "step-up" and "step-down" experiments were followed by turbidity measurements. However, selected experiments were done by counting viable cells to establish that death of cells did not account for the observed results.

These results indicate that growth of *E. coli* below 20 C results in metabolic damage which depresses the growth rate beyond that which would be expected from kinetic considerations alone.

A likely form of damage which might result from growth at low temperature is damage to the regulatory system of the cell. Accordingly, Ng, Ingraham and Marr (1962) studied the effect of temperature on the formation of certain inducible enzymes.

Catabolite repression of β-galactosidase, i.e. the inhibition of β-galactosidase induction by the presence of certain readily oxidizable substrates such as glucose, was considered first. It was found that catabolite repression of β-galactosidase induction, i.e. the glucose effect, disappears below about 20 C (Fig. 9). Since Neidhardt and Magasanik (1956) have shown that catabolite repression results from the accumulation of certain intermediates within the cell it seemed possible that the observed release from the glucose

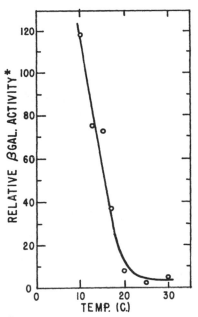

*Activity with glucose as a carbon source/activity with succinate as a carbon source X100 in presence of 5×10^{-4} M TMG.

Fig. 9. Relative specific activity of β-galactosidase as a function of growth temperature. Cells were grown in basal-glucose and basal-succinate media containing 5×10^{-4} M thiomethyl-β-D-galactoside. Relative activity is the quotient times 100 of the specific activity of cells grown on glucose and succinate. (Ng, Ingraham and Marr, 1962)

effect at low temperature may merely reflect a selective slowing of glucose catabolism with respect to growth at low temperature. However, by comparing cell yield and glucose disappearance from cultures growing exponentially at 30 and 13 C (Fig. 10) no evidence of a slower relative rate of glucose catabolism was found at the low temperature. In fact, the yield constant was slightly lower at 13 C than at 30 C. Also no differences in the amount of lactic acid or volatile acids could be detected in the medium between the cultures growing at 13 and 30 C. Hence, low temperature exerts its effect at a more fundamental level of cellular control.

The effect of growth temperature on the inducible enzyme, tryptophanase, was selected for investigation, since this enzyme is also under control of catabolite repression. It was found that tryptophanase is not relieved from catabolite repression; further, tryptophanase cannot be induced at low temperature (13 C) even in media which do not cause catabolite repression at high temperature. As a result, *E. coli* ML30 does not grow at 13 C in a medium in which tryptophan is present as the only source of carbon. On prolonged incubation of *E. coli* ML30 at 13 C in this medium, however, growth was found to occur. Examination of the resulting culture revealed that mutants were present (Ng & Gartner, 1962). The mutants are consti-

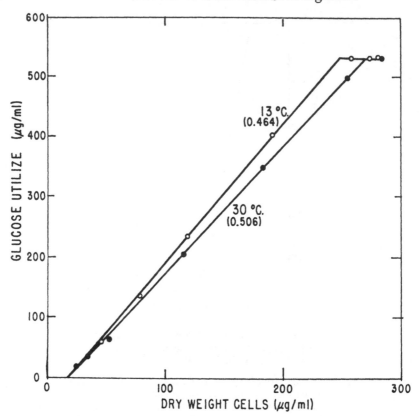

FIG. 10. Yields of *E. coli* ML30 as a function of glucose disappearing from basal-glucose medium during exponential growth at 13 C and 30 C. Numbers in parentheses indicate μg of bacterial cells (dry weight)/μg glucose utilized before exhaustion of glucose from the medium. (Ng, Ingraham and Marr, 1962)

tutive for tryptophanase at 30 C and are inducible at 13 C as compared with the wild type which is inducible at 30 C and cannot be induced at 13 C.

In summary, we feel that the marked increase in the temperature characteristic for growth rate of *E. coli* at low temperature which results in the existence of a minimal temperature for growth is a consequence of metabolic damage. Growth at low temperature (below 20 C) is a prerequisite to the expression of this damage, and subsequent growth at a higher temperature (above 20 C) is required to correct it. Since we have found major changes in the control of enzyme synthesis below 20 C it seems likely that these changes may indeed be a part of the damage in question. Possibly these observations may serve as a basis for understanding why psychrophiles are capable of growth at lower temperatures than mesophiles.

A commonly cited theory of minimal temperature for growth is the lipid theory. This theory, expressed by Gaughran (1947) and others, is based on the general observation that organisms grown at low temperature have a greater proportion of unsaturated fatty acids or of more highly unsaturated fatty acid in their lipids than if they are grown at higher temperatures.

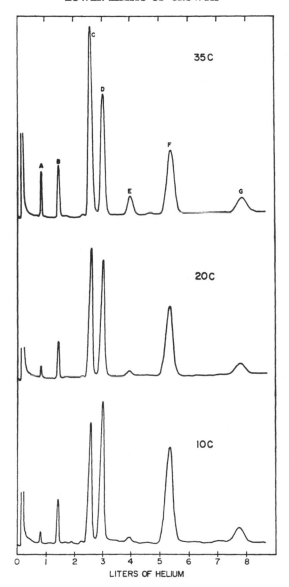

FIG. 11. Tracings of gas-liquid chromatograms of the methyl ester of fatty acids from *E. coli* harvested during exponential growth in glucose-minimal medium at 35 C, 20 C, and 10 C. A—laurate (saturated); B—myristate (saturated); C—palmitate (saturated); D—hexadecenoate (unsaturated); E—methylene hecadecanoate (cyclopropane fatty acid); F—octadecenoate (unsaturated); G—β-hyroxymyristate. (Marr and Ingraham, 1962)

Such observations have been made with plants (Howell & Collins, 1957), insects (Fraenkel & Hopf, 1940), and micro-organisms (Terroine, Hatterer & Roehrig, 1930; Gaughran, 1947). Even homiothermic organisms (Dean & Hilditch, 1933) undergo similar changes in surface lipids in response to environmental temperature. The "lipid theory" holds that the temperature at which lipids become so highly unsaturated that they no longer fulfill their essential structural role in the cell is the minimal temperature for growth of that cell.

Recently, Marr and Ingraham (1962) examined the effect of the temperature of growth on the fatty acid content of *E. coli* using the technique of gas chromatography. All previous studies of this type with micro-organisms have been done by determining iodine numbers.

Tracings of gas-liquid phase chromatograms of the fatty acids of *E. coli* grown at 10 C, 20 C, and 35 C in glucose-minimal medium are shown in Fig. 11. It can be seen that the relative proportions of unsaturated fatty acids increase dramatically as the temperature of growth is decreased.

If the glucose-minimal medium is supplemented with yeast extract or with casamino acids, the proportions of unsaturated fatty acids also increase at low temperatures of growth. However, at all temperatures the proportions of unsaturated fatty acids are higher in cells grown in minimal medium. This difference persists at 10 C which is near the minimum for *E. coli* in both these media. These results clearly establish that fatty acid composition does not set the minimum temperature for growth of *E. coli*.

REFERENCES

Blackman, F. F. 1905. Optimal and limiting factors. Ann. Bot. *19*: 281–295.
Dean, H. K., and T. P. Hilditch. 1933. The body fats of the pig. III. The influence of body temperature on the composition of depot fats. Biochem. J. *27*: 1950–1956.
Fraenkel, G., and H. S. Hopf. 1940. Temperature adaptation and degree of saturation of phosphatides. Biochem. J. *34*: 1085–1092.
Gaughran, E. R. L. 1947. The saturation of bacterial lipids as a function of temperature. J. Bacteriol. *53*: 506.
Howell, R., and F. I. Collins. 1957. Factors affecting linolenic and linoleic acid content of soybean oil. Agron. J. *49*: 593–597.
Ingraham, J. L. 1958. Growth of psychrophilic bacteria. J. Bacteriol. *76*: 75–80.
Ingraham, J. L., and G. F. Bailey. 1959. Comparative study of effect of temperature on metabolism of psychrophilic and mesophilic bacteria. J. Bacteriol. *77*: 609–613.
Kistiakowsky, G. H., and R. Lumry. 1949. Anomalous temperature effects in the hydrolysis of urea by urease. J. Am. Chem. Soc. *71*: 2006–2013.
Marr, A. G., and J. L. Ingraham. 1962. Effect of temperature on the composition of fatty acids in *Escherichia coli*. J. Bacteriol. *84*: 1260–1267.
Neidhardt, F. C., and B. Magasanik. 1956. The effect of glucose on the induced biosynthesis of bacterial enzymes in the presence and absence of inducing agents. Biochem. et Biophys. Acta *21*: 324–334.
Ng, H., and T. K. Gartner. 1963. Selection of mutants of *Escherichia coli* constitutive for tryptophanase. J. Bacteriol. *85*: 245–246.
Ng, H., J. L. Ingraham and A. G. Marr. 1962. Damage and derepression in *Escherichia coli* resulting from growth at low temperatures. J. Bacteriol. *84*: 331–339.
Senez, J. C. 1962. Some considerations on the energetics of bacterial growth. Bacteriol. Revs. *26*:95–107.
Terroine, E. F., C. Hatterer and P. Roehrig. 1930. Les acides gras des phosphatides chez animaux poikilothermes, les végétaux supérieurs et les microorganismes. Bull. Soc. Chem. Biol., Paris *12*: 682–702.

SYMPOSIUM V

ENZYMES IN SOILS

Chairman: G. H. PETERSON

E. HOFMANN

The Origin and Importance of Enzymes in Soil

A. D. McLAREN

Enzyme Activity in Soils Sterilized by Ionizing Radiation
and Some Comments on Micro-Environments in Nature

G. HOFFMANN

Synthetic Effects of Soil Enzymes

C. G. DOBBS

Factors in Soil Mycostasis

CHAIRMAN'S REMARKS

G. H. PETERSON

Purdue University
Lafayette, Indiana, U.S.A.

IN RECENT YEARS increasing attention has been given to the detection of specific enzymes and metabolic pathways in soil. An objective inherent in these studies has been to obtain information on the intensity of certain biological events taking place in soil that cannot be provided by the enumeration of the micro-organisms involved in the transformations.

For example, the urease activity may be estimated by determining the rate at which added urea is hydrolysed by a sample of soil previously treated with a sterilizing agent to prevent the enrichment of urea-decomposing micro-organisms. To correlate urease activity of the soil with the number of urea-decomposing micro-organisms present would not be an easy task since many diverse forms can affect the decomposition.

Furthermore, since the enzyme content of the individual cells as they are found in the soil cannot be measured, and both the enzymes present in non-viable cells and those liberated from lysed cells may be active, a poor correlation may exist between the number of micro-organisms capable of carrying out a specific transformation and the actual intensity of the transformation.

Thus, as suggested by J. H. Quastel, "it is . . . essential, for an understanding of the metabolic processes taking place in a complex system such as soil, to turn to the study of the biochemistry of the soil itself, this being treated as far as possible as a biological unit."

THE ORIGIN AND IMPORTANCE OF ENZYMES IN SOIL

E. HOFMANN

Institut für Agrikulturchemie
Technische Hochschule, München
Weihenstephan, Germany

THERE IS NO DOUBT that the majority of soil phenomena have a biological origin, or at least have biological factors implicated. Micro-organisms, therefore, condition a soil and in large part govern its fertility level (Norman, 1955; Pochon & De Barjac, 1958). We are in agreement about the importance of micro-organisms although our studies on the activity of enzymes in soil have frequently been considered contradictory to the classical microbiological methods.

One has to admit that studies on the species and numbers of micro-organisms do contribute a great deal to our knowledge of the microbial life of soils. Such studies are necessary, but one must not forget the disadvantages and errors involved in enumeration.

The evolution of carbon dioxide has frequently been used to determine the total respiratory activity of micro-organisms in soil. The results obtained by this method have considerable value but the technique again has inherent disadvantages.

It is because of the disadvantages of the classical methods of determining microbiological activity in soil that we have turned to the study of soil enzymes. All biochemical reactions are catalysed by enzymes, each of which is specific for a single reaction. We are convinced that the activity and metabolism of soils are not due to numbers of micro-organisms alone but to a combination of numbers and the activity of enzymes. It is obvious that the micro-organisms are responsible for the production of these enzymes. We have shown that soils containing a large number of micro-organisms also exhibit high enzyme activity. At the same time we have demonstrated that the enzyme activity found in various horizons parallels the findings of microbiologists.

It is not our intention to diminish the value of the data obtained in the field of soil microbiology. Such studies have given us a deep insight into microbial life in soil and the activity therein. This type of analysis has three main weaknesses which detract from its significance: (1) Enumeration techniques yield values that are too low. (2) The numbers of organisms in soil are not constant but vary considerably under the influence of temperature, humidity, manuring and other factors. As a result, repeated estimations are necessary to determine an average value. (3) The numbers thus determined are not related to activity. Activity is dependent upon enzyme production which does not necessarily involve all of the soil flora.

In our studies on the determination of biological activity through enzyme activity we have been concerned primarily with the decomposition and transformations of organic substances. The initial step in their breakdown generally involves a hydrolysis.

$$2 \times \text{Glucose} = \text{Maltose} + \text{H}_2\text{O}$$
$$\text{Maltose} + \text{H}_2\text{O} + \text{Maltase} = 2 \text{ Glucose}$$

For example, a molecule of sucrose is broken by the intercession of a molecule of water and by the action of saccharase to form molecules of glucose and fructose. The large molecules of starch, cellulose, pectin and albumin can be broken down in a similar manner. In our studies we have been concerned with saccharase (Hofmann & Seegerer, 1951; Hofmann *et al.*, 1953), urease, amylase, β-glucosidase and phosphatase activity in soils (Hofmann & Hoffmann, 1954, 1955).

Studies of microbiologists have shown that the numbers of micro-organisms in soil decrease with depth. Since enzymes are products of micro organisms we have investigated the relationship between numbers and the quantity and activity of enzymes at different horizons in two soil profiles. These data are presented in Table 1. It is evident from this table that both numbers and activity decrease with depth.

TABLE 1

NUMBER OF BACTERIA IN RELATION TO SACCHARASE ACTIVITY

Profile	Depth cm.	Bacterial numbers $\times 10^6$	Saccharase activity*
A	0–10	7.3	6.6
	10–20	7.1	6.2
	20–40	4.1	4.2
B	0–10	7.6	6.4
	10–20	6.2	6.2
	20–40	3.2	3.8

*ml of 0.1 N sodium thiosulphate to titrate monosaccharides liberated from 2 gm soil during 24 hr incubation at 37 C (Lehmann-Maquenne method).

Microbiologists have also stated that the numbers of micro-organisms depend on the soil pH. Generally neutral soils contain a high number of organisms, especially bacteria. In acid soils bacterial numbers decrease while fungi increase. In this respect it is of interest that bacterial enzymes have a pH optima of 6–7 while those of fungi have a lower range at pH 4–5. Table 2 shows the effect of acid and neutral soils on the activity of saccharase. Greatest activity in the neutral soil was found at a pH of around 6 while in the acid soil the range for optimum activity was quite large

TABLE 2
SACCHARASE ACTIVITY IN RELATION TO SOIL pH

| | Saccharase activity in | |
pH	acid soil	neutral soil
4.1	7.4	6.6
4.7	8.8	7.8
5.0	8.7	9.0
5.6	8.5	9.6
6.1	8.7	9.6
6.7	6.5	7.4
7.0	5.9	7.0

TABLE 3
ENZYME ACTIVITY AT DIFFERENT HORIZONS IN A PROFILE

| Depth cm. | Saccharase* | | β-glucosidase† | | Urease‡ | |
	field	meadow	field	meadow	field	meadow
0–10	8.5	14.8	2.0	4.0	7.9	16.8
10–20	9.4	7.3	1.6	1.8	7.0	11.0
20–40	5.0	3.0	1.0	0.8	3.2	8.1
40–60	3.3	2.6	1.0	0.4	1.2	2.3
60–80	2.3	0.6	0.3	0.3	0.9	1.0
80–100	2.3	0.5	0.2	0.3	0.0	0.7
150–170	—	0.1	—	—	—	—

*As in Table 1.
†As in Table 1 except incubation time 96 hr.
‡ml of 0.1 N NaOH required to neutralize ammonia liberated from 10 gm soil
during 48 hr incubation at 37 C. For details of methods see Bergmeyer, 1962,
and Herrmann *et al.*, 1955.

(pH 4.7–6.1) probably owing to the enzymes of fungi. It is likely that in
the neutral soil the fungal enzymes played only a small part.

We have known for a long time that the microbial flora of meadow soils
(under permanent vegetation) is at or near the surface. Table 3 presents
data showing the effect of depth of sampling on enzyme activity in a field
and meadow soil. In the field soil maximum activity was found at a depth
of 5–10 cm.

Enzyme activity varies with the soil type. For example, the saccharase
activity increased from a low value in sand (0.9), through moderate values
in a calcareous base peat (6.1), and neutral clay (6.5) to high values in
calcareous clay soil from a field (9.8) and a meadow (14.6).

The life of a soil is closely allied to its fertility so we also determined
the effect of artificial fertilizers on enzymatic activity (Table 4). It will be
noted that the long-term application of nitrogen increased the activity of
the enzymes, particularly of urease.

As shown in Table 5, both nitrogen and phosphorous increased enzyme
activity while potassium had little effect.

We have already stated that our studies were initiated with the idea
of producing a more satisfactory estimation of microbial activity than that

TABLE 4

FERTILIZER APPLICATION AND ENZYME ACTIVITY
(Trial field for 30 years)

Fertilizer and date of sampling	Saccharase	β-glucosidase	Urease
7.3.53			
PK	6.3	1.6	2.7
PK + 1 × N	6.9	1.9	3.5
PK + 2 × N	7.3	2.0	3.6
16.7.53			
PK	6.7	1.8	3.0
PK + 1 × N	7.3	2.2	3.3
PK + 2 × N	7.8	2.8	3.5

TABLE 5

FERTILIZER APPLICATION AND ENZYME ACTIVITY

Soil	Untreated	Treatment			
		PK	NK	NP	NPK
Calcareous clay	6.9	6.9	7.4	10.4	10.5
Marshy	5.0	6.8	6.4	7.5	7.5
Sand	2.4	3.1	3.0	3.3	3.9
Clay	4.8	5.3	6.5	7.6	7.6

obtained by enumeration of micro-organisms. Originally we felt that the enzyme activity determined was representative of the number of micro-organisms present at the time of sampling; however, we now realize that this conclusion was not altogether true. It is now evident that much of the enzyme activity in soil takes place in the absence of cells. Since a large part of the soil organic matter is insoluble and cannot enter into the bacterial cells, it is first broken down by extracellular enzymes. In addition, after death of the cells, autolysis occurs which liberates enzymes. These enzymes are not destroyed but remain active in soil. We are now of the opinion that extracellular enzymes and enzymes adsorbed on soil colloids are responsible for the greatest part of microbial activity at the time of sampling. In our investigations we have shown that, despite marked seasonal variations in the numbers of micro-organisms, the enzymatic activity of soil hardly varies. This would suggest that the enzymes of the living cells play only a small part in total enzyme activity. However, if soils are treated so that the numbers of micro-organisms slowly increase we find that the level of enzyme activity also increases. The reverse situation is also true.

It is for these reasons that we feel that the determination of the level of enzyme activity is of greater value in assessing the microbial activity of a soil than enumeration of the organisms present. There is no doubt that the two methods used in conjunction with one another would be the most worthwhile.

REFERENCES

Bergmeyer, H. U. 1962. Methoden der enzymatischen Analyse. Weinheim, pp. 720, 779, 854, 901.

Herrmann, R., R. Thun and E. Knickmann. 1955. Handbuch der landw. Versuchs- u. Untersuchungsmethodik (Methodenbuch). Band I. Die Untersuchung von Böden. Verlag Neumann, Radebeul und Berlin, III Auflage: 222–224.

Hofmann, E., and A. Seegerer. 1951. Ueber das Enzymsystem der Kulturböden (I). Biochem. Z. 322: 174.

Hofmann, E., W. Schmidt and I. Niggemann. 1953. Ueber das Enzymsystem der Kulturböden (II, III). Biochem. Z. 324: 125, 313.

Hofmann, E., and G. Hoffmann. 1954. Ueber das Enzymsystem der Kulturböden (V). Biochem. Z. 325: 329.

Hofmann, E., and G. Hoffmann. 1955. Ueber das Enzymsystem unserer Kulturböden. Z. Pflanzenern., Düngg. u. Bodenkunde 70: 97, 104, 114; 77: 245–251.

Norman, A. G. 1955. The place of microbiology in soil science. Adv. Agron. 7: 399.

Pochon, J., and H. De Barjac. 1958. Traité de microbiologie des sols. Paris.

ENZYME ACTIVITY IN SOILS STERILIZED BY IONIZING RADIATION AND SOME COMMENTS ON MICRO-ENVIRONMENTS IN NATURE

A. D. McLAREN

Department of Soils and Plant Nutrition
College of Agriculture, University of California
Berkeley, California, U.S.A.

SOIL IS A LIVING TISSUE and, as such, contains nearly all the enzymes which characterize the biological world. For want of precise experimental methods, however, the concept of enzyme activity in soil is not clearly developed. The soil biochemist cannot say definitely whether an enzyme acting on a suitable substrate in soil is part of a cell, is free in soil solution or is adsorbed on clays, humus, etc. The subject is of interest to the plant physiologist since organic forms of nitrogen, phosphorus and sulphur are metabolized by microbes with, eventually, a liberation of these elements as inorganic plant nutrients. Conceivably, in addition, the liberation from some organic compounds can be mediated by enzymes on root surfaces or adsorbed on soil particles in the root environment.

Let us suppose we wish to discover if glycerol phosphate (GP) added to soil, or phytin, normally in soil, are plant nutrients. Following the addition of these sustances to a soil, mineralization by micro-organisms takes place, with the liberation of inorganic phosphate (P_i). If one could sterilize soil in such a way that the soil would retain its normal chemical and physical structure, would the investigator then be able to evaluate the organic nutrition of plants? To anticipate, let me state that irradiation is just the tool we need (McLaren, Reschetko & Huber, 1957), but two unanticipated problems remain: irradiated soil contains one or more active phosphatases (McLaren, Luse, & Skujins, 1962), and so do intact sterile plant roots (Estermann & McLaren, 1961). If hydrolysis of GP occurs at a more rapid rate at the rhizoplane than the rate of utilization of P_i by plants, then the concept of uptake and utilization of GP *per se* by plants is difficult to pursue further. Kinetic studies with isotopically labelled GP and P_i might be useful in differentiating between the absorption of these two forms of phosphorus by roots. Here, however, I should like to discuss enzyme action in terms of micro-environments at interfaces within soil and the nature of soil phosphatase activity. The other aspects of the larger problem have been discussed in the references cited.

THE SOIL ENVIRONMENT

Soils contain a range of particle sizes varying from gravel to clay (less than 0.002 mm). These particles are not "pure" but are complexed with organic polymeric substances (humus) and inorganic salts and are interspersed with water and gases. On and among these particles are micro- and macro-organisms in vast numbers and of many kinds. The micro-organisms number in the billions per gram of soil in a typical field soil so that the soil may be regarded as a living tissue (Quastel, 1946; Thimann, 1955). Obviously, enzyme action and microbial activity in such a heterogenous system differ drastically from those in classical bacteriological media, not so much in *function*, perhaps, as *in form*. Because of the efflorescence of salts, the influx of rain and carbon dioxide from the atmosphere, or the growth of micro-organisms which secrete or utilize acids, soil properties, such as pH, can vary appreciably in microscopic and submicroscopic dimensions.

Kubiena (1938) points out that the pH in soil (measured with a microelectrode) varies from point to point as a result of CO_2 secretion of roots. Thus plant roots always live in a medium with a lower pH than is found in soil pastes with macro-electrode systems. We can also think of the submicroscopic domain, of the effective pH in the liquid phase within a few to a few hundred angstrom units from the surfaces of clay particles, or within gel matrices: wherever charged surfaces exist, the effective pH near the surface will be different from that of the bulk liquid phase in which a charged particle is located.

Micro-environments can be of great interest and are doubtless important determinants in the lives of micro-organisms. For example, Thimann (1955) cites an observation by Rahn that the optimum moisture film thickness for growth of *Bacillus mycoides* is 20–40 microns. The optimum is determined in part by oxygen availability. He also points out that neither in pure nor in enrichment cultures can any of the nitrifiers grow at a pH less than 6 and suggests that nitrification in acid soils is brought about by nitrifying bacteria attached to mineral particles where the local pH is higher. The opposite now seems to be the case (McLaren & Skujins, 1963).

The Concept of Surface Concentrations

By way of illustration, let us examine the concept of pH at a "point," i.e. at the surface of a soil particle, and see what consequences this may have for enzyme action. In Fig. 1 we see a negatively charged colloidal particle suspended in water and surrounded by a counterion cloud of hydrogen ions. Since the particle is negatively charged, it attracts hydrogen ions so that the effective concentration of the ions near the surface is greater than elsewhere. *At equilibrium the activities of hydrogen ion are equal everywhere, but clearly the pH is not* (pH = log $1/(H^+)$, where H^+ is the hydrogen ion concentration). We shall designate the pH at the surface

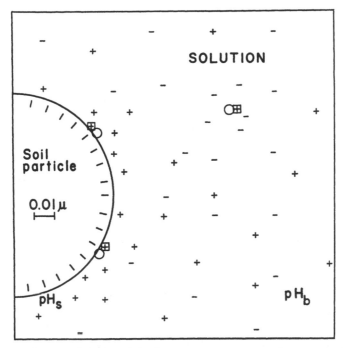

Fig. 1. Distribution of hydrated hydrogen ions, +, around a negatively charged colloidal particle. The small circles represent essentially neutral (isoionic) enzyme molecules and the squares represent positively charged substrate molecules. The hydrogen ion concentration near the surface is represented as pH_s and that in bulk solution as pH_b.

as pH_s and that in bulk solution as pH_b; they are related by the Hartley-Roe equation, namely $pH_s = pH_b + \zeta/60$ at 25°. ζ is the electro-kinetic potential of the particle. That is, a negatively charged particle will have an effective hydrogen ion concentration (not activity) near its surface which is greater than that found in bulk solution. The essence of this equation has been substantiated experimentally by Chattoraj and Bull (1959).

Referring again to Fig. 1, we see that an enzyme, for example chymotrypsin at $pH_b = 9$ whereat it is active but nearly neutral, approaching a positively charged protein substrate molecule "sees" fewer H^+ in the neighborhood of the substrate in solution than it does if it acts on the same substrate adsorbed on the surface of the particle. In solution, the pH optimum for enzyme action with this example is two pH units lower than for the action on the surface of kaolin or bentonite clay, in accord with theory (McLaren, 1960).

These elementary considerations stimulated Hattori and Furusaka (1959, 1960) to investigate the importance of $(pH_b - pH_s)$ in terms of the nutrition of *E. coli* absorbed on an anion exchange resin. Initial rates of oxidation of succinate and asparagine with free and absorbed cells were observed at various concentrations of substrate at pH 7. The rate reached a maximum at a higher concentration of succinate with absorbed than with free cells. Some effect would be anticipated on the basis of the attraction of negatively charged substrate by a positively charged resin surface, an attraction which could be expected to increase the effective nutrient supply over that in bulk solution. On this basis, the cells should be oxidizing substrate at a maximum rate at lower bulk concentrations of substrate while in the absorbed state as compared with their metabolism in the solution state. Although the shift in the maximum for the adsorbed state is not in the direction predicted by the above theory in this example, an influence of a surface on metabolism is unmistakable. With the zwitter ion asparagine, no shift was found. The approach of Hattori and Furusaka would also be of interest with cysteine as a nutrient; with cysteine we would also be dealing with variations in oxidation–reduction potentials near a charged surface.

Evidence for Enzyme Action at Solid–Liquid Interfaces

Since the classic work of Sumner and Northrop three decades ago, publications on the kinetics of purified enzymes in solution must run into many thousands of papers. Yet most enzyme reactions in nature seem to take place at solid– or gel–liquid interfaces and not in solution (McLaren, 1960). Let us review some of what is known of enzyme reactions at surfaces.

Trurnit (1953) has studied the action of chymotrypsin on bovine serum albumin adsorbed on glass slides first covered with a film of chromium and barium stearate. In this instance the digestion of the protein substrate was actually followed by a loss in thickness of the substrate layers. The Arrhenius coefficient of the reaction was 8–9 kcal/mole, which is less than corresponding reactions in solution, probably because of interfacial forces. If substrate is adsorbed on kaolin subsequent to the adsorption of chymotrypsin, the reaction rate is less than if the substrate is adsorbed first, showing an influence of surface on the surface mobility of molecules, but what is even more striking, as already mentioned, is that the pH optimum of the enzyme is shifted after adsorption (McLaren & Estermann, 1957). Both the pH shift and change in activation energy of proteolysis are convincing evidence that reaction takes place on the surface and not as a result of elution of enzyme and/or substrate back into solution. With montmorillonite the case is also clear: protein molecules absorbed between the sheets of the expanding clay lattice can be digested by proteolytic enzyme which also enters the clay particles (Estermann & McLaren, 1959). Pinck and Allison (1961), on the basis of some preliminary assays of crude urease (containing over 99 per cent protein impurity) in the presence of clays, suggested that sorbed enzyme is eluted from the surface and acts on urea only while in solution. They also questioned the scheme that any enzyme sorbed on a surface acts enzymatically. Apparently they were unaware of the earlier, definitive exploration of this field. In the exploratory work, checks were made for possible elution of the proteins during the reaction and the elution was found to be unimportant (Estermann & McLaren, 1956).

Chymotrypsin was studied below its isoelectric point and in the pH range of maximum sorption, whereas Pinck and Allison studied urease above its isoelectric point and in a pH range where it has little tendency to adsorb to a negatively charged surface. A pertinent observation is that chymotrypsin can be *chemically* reacted with and thereby firmly attached to a solid and is then still active on substrates in solution (Mitz & Summaria, 1961).

An alternate situation, probably the more prevalent one in nature, is the action of a hydrolytic enzyme in solution on an insoluble substrate, such as the action of trypsin on thiogel (Tsuk & Oster, 1961), of pepsin on insoluble ovalbumin (Mazia, 1950), of cellulase on cellulose (Thimann, 1955) and of soil enzymes on soil organic matter. The kinetics of such reactions have been discussed and the general equation for the initial velocity of the reaction is (McLaren, 1962):

$$v = \frac{k(E_o)A}{[(E_o)A_E + A_E/K_m + A - a]}$$

where A is the surface area of the substrate, a is the surface occupied by enzyme, (E_o) is the total concentration of enzyme, A_E is the area occupied per mole of adsorbed enzyme, and K_m is the equilibrium constant for the association of the substrate surface with enzyme in solution. Whenever A is small relative to (E_o), this equation is of the form of

$$v = \frac{a(E_o)}{1 + \beta(E_o)} ,$$

a and β being constants; the equation includes the empirical form found experimentally by Tsuk and Oster, namely $v = \gamma E_o^{1/n}$, γ and n being constants.

In a study of esterase activity in soil, Haig (1955) fractionated a fine sandy loam in order to find the particle size with which esterase activity in soil is most closely associated. The clay fraction had the greatest activity toward phenyl acetate although the silt fraction had considerable. The sand fractions had very little. Pure clays and autoclaved soil had none. The esterase was so firmly bound to the clay fraction (mostly montmorillonite) that it could not be extracted or eluted with phosphate, ethylammonium, pyridine or sonic oscillation. Attempts to extract soil urease and phosphatase were also unsuccessful.

ENZYME ACTION IN STERILE SOIL

An exhaustive and valuable review of soil enzymes has been published by Kiss (1958). In order to study enzyme actions in soil apart from the living micro-organisms one must be able to treat the soil to meet these requirements (Drobnik, 1961): (1) prevent assimilation of products of enzymatic reactions; (2) prevent liberation of intracellular enzymes; (3) prevent inactivation of enzymes present in soil, and of course (4) prevent further synthesis of exo-enzymes by living cells. This is a large bill, aside from the fact that we do not know if any soil enzyme is outside of dead cells.

Appreciable amounts of extracellular enzymes in natural soil probably do not exist since as proteins they would be nutrients for other microbes. Soil has a very low amount of total protein, perhaps not much more than that in microbial tissue. The use of reagents such as toluene or chloramphenicol to inhibit enzyme formation are suspect since these agents may be metabolites (Abd-el-Malek *et al.*, 1961; Drobnik, 1961). Toluene has been found to fulfil item (1) with glucose and aspartic acid and inhibits respiration with sucrose (Drobnik, 1961). Claus and Mechsner (1960) present data, obtained by the plating method, which demonstrate that multiplication of micro-organisms can take place in soil in the presence of toluene and substrate; this is not consistent with Drobnik's observations, however. Regarding the second requirement, toluene is thought to be a "plasmolyticum" which causes autolysis of bacteria and liberation of enzymes into the soil (Hofmann & Niggemann, 1953).

Perhaps the most nearly ideal "reagent" for sterilizing soil and meeting the requirements is ionizing radiation. Either an electron beam of high intensity (5–10 Mev), hard X-ray or gamma radiation will do. Since the soil can be irradiated dry there need be no autolysis and all requirements can presumably be met (McLaren *et al.*, 1957). Urease action does not increase appreciably after irradiation (McLaren *et al.*, 1957; Vela & Wyss, 1962), phosphatase decreases somewhat (McLaren, Luse & Skujins, 1962) and tryptic activity is nil in soil receiving 5 Mrep (mega roentgen equivalent physical) of the electron beam. This dose of irradiation is more than enough to kill all organisms (defined as inability to multiply by plating on soil extract agar). Any change in physical and chemical properties during irradiation seems to be small. Irradiated soil is a fine medium for microbial and plant growth. Nevertheless, there remains a very important question: is the residual enzyme activity in sterile soil both in dead cells and in or on soil particles? Urea, as a small molecule, could diffuse into dead cells and the ammonia and CO_2 could diffuse out again. Trypsin activity in soil is apparently different. Native soil shows tryptic activity, but the substrate benzoylarginine amide apparently does not diffuse into dead cells since no ammonia was released by trypsin-like action in irradiation sterilized soil (a dose of 3–5 Mrep is not enough to reduce most enzymes to a small fraction of their initial activity). Practically speaking, Hofmann and Seegerer (1951) believed that a determination of enzyme activity in soil is a more dependable measure of soil fertility than microbe counts; the enzyme content is more constant than microbe counts, indicating that enzymes are persistent in soil. The stability of soil enzymes is believed to be a function of the adsorbed state on clays, etc. Perhaps the application of classical cytological reactions to soil will reveal the site of soil enzyme activity.

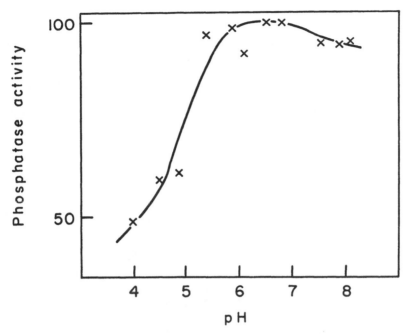

Fig. 2. Relative activity rate of phosphatase action on GP in sterile Dublin clay loam as a function of pH.

A dose of about 10^6 rep kills all fungi in soil and 2×10^6 rep kills all bacteria. The survival curves are not of the semi-log type, since we are dealing with a mixed population (McLaren *et al.*, 1962). During the delivery of these doses soil phosphatase activity declines somewhat. With sterile soil and further irradiation one can study the radiation sensitivity of soil phosphatase; the sensitivity is comparable to that of wheat phosphatase and other purified enzymes (Skujins, Braal and McLaren, 1962).

The pH activity curve for phosphatase action in radiation sterilized soil is plotted in Fig. 2. The activity has a broad pH optimum as might be expected for a mixture of acid and alkaline phosphatases. The curve is quite different from that for barley root phosphatase (Esterman & McLaren, 1961). It probably reflects both a heterogeneity of microbial origins and the molecular environments of enzyme action in soil. Clearly the presence of enzyme action in soil sterilized by this discriminating, differential method makes it most difficult to assess the possible utilization of unaltered organic nutrients by plants under natural conditions.

ACKNOWLEDGEMENT

This work was supported in part by a U.S.A.E.C. Contract AT (11–1)–34; 50 and USPH Grant (G 4236).

REFERENCES

Abd-el-Malek, Y., M. Monib and A. Hazm. 1961. Chloramphenicol, a simultaneous carbon and nitrogen source for a *Streptomyces* sp. from Egyptian soil. Nature *189*: 775–776.

Chattoraj, D. K., and H. B. Bull. 1959. Electrophoresis and surface charge. J. Am. Chem. Soc. *63*: 1809–1813.

Claus, D., and K. Mechsner. 1960. Ueber die Brauchbarkeit der von Ed. Hofmann Ausgearbeiteten. Methoden zur Bestimmung der Enzyme in Boden. Plant and Soil *12*: 195.

Drobnik, J. 1961. On the role of toluene in the measurement of the activity of soil enzymes. Plant and Soil *14*: 94–95.

Estermann, E. F., and A. D. McLaren. 1959. Stimulation of bacterial proteolysis by absorbents. J. Soil Sci. *10*: 64–78.

Estermann, E. F., and A. D. McLaren. 1961. Contribution of rhizoplane organisms to the total capacity of plants to utilize organic nutrients. Plant and Soil *15*: 243–260.

Haig, A. D. 1955. Some characteristics of esterase- and urease-like activity in soil. Ph.D. Thesis, University of California, Davis, California.

Hattori, T., and C. Furusaka. 1959. Chemical activities of *Escherichia coli* adsorbed on a resin. Biochim. et Biophys. Acta *31*: 581–582.

Hattori, T., and C. Furusaka. 1959. Chemical activities of *E. coli* adsorbed on a resin, "Dowex-1." Nature *184*: 1566–1567.

Hattori, T., and C. Furusaka. 1960. Chemical activities of *E. coli* adsorbed on a resin. J. Biochem. *48*: 831–837.

Hofmann, E., and J. Niggemann. 1953. Ueber das Enzymsystem unserer Kulturböden. Biochem. Z. *324*: 308–310.

Hofmann, E., and A. Seegerer. 1957. Die Enzyme im Boden als Faktoren seiner Fruchtbarkeit. Naturwissenschaften *6*: 141–142.

Kiss, I. 1958. Soil enzymes. *In* I. M. Csapo, *Talajtan* (Soil Science), Mezögazdasagri es Erdeszeti Allami Könyukiado (State Agro-Silvic Publisher), Bucharest, Roumania.

Kubiena, W. L. 1938. Micropedology, pp. 121, 206–207. Collegiate Press, Inc., Ames, Iowa.

McLaren, A. D. 1960. Enzyme action in structurally restricted systems. Enzymologia *21*: 356–364.

McLaren, A. D. 1962. Use of mole fractions in enzyme kinetics. Arch. Biochem. Biophys. *97*: 1–3.

McLaren, A. D., and E. F. Estermann. 1956. The absorption and reactions of enzymes and proteins on kaolinite. III. The isolation of enzyme-substrate complexes. Arch. Biochem. Biophys. *61*: 158–173.

McLaren, A. D., and E. F. Estermann. 1957. Influence of pH on the activity of chymotrypsin at a solid–liquid interface. Arch. Biochem. Biophys. *68*: 157–160.

McLaren, A. D., R. A. Luse and J. Skujins. 1962. Sterilization of soils by irradiation and some further observations on soil enzyme activity. Proc. Soil Sci. Soc. Am. *26*: 371–377.

McLaren, A. D., L. Reschetko and W. Huber. 1957. Sterilization of soil by irradiation with an electron beam, and some observations on soil enzyme activity. Soil Science *83*: 497–502.

McLaren, A. D., and J. J. Skujins. 1963. Nitrification by *Nitrobacter agilis* on surfaces and in soil with respect to hydrogen ion concentration. Can. J. Microbiol. (in press).

Mazia, D. 1950. Fiber protein structure in chromosomes and related investigations on protein fibers. Ann. N.Y. Acad. Sci. *50*: 954–967.

Mitz, M. A., and L. J. Summaria. 1961. Synthesis of biologically active cellulose derivatives of enzymes. Nature *189*: 576–577.

Pinck, L. A., and F. E. Allison. 1961. Adsorption and release of urease by and from clay minerals. Soil Sci. *91*: 183–188.

Quastel, J. H. 1946. Soil Metabolism. The Royal Institute of Chemistry of Great Britain and Ireland, London.

Skujins, J. J., L. Braal and A. D. McLaren. 1962. Characterization of phosphatase in a terrestrial soil sterilized with an electron beam. Enzymologia *25*: 125–133.

Thimann, K. V. 1955. The life of bacteria, pp. 228–260. Macmillan Co., New York.

Trurnit, H. J. 1953. Studies of enzyme systems at a solid–liquid interface. Arch. Biochem. Biophys. *47*: 251–271.

Tsuk, A. G., and G. Oster. 1961. Determination of enzyme activity by a linear measurement. Nature *190*: 721–722.

Vela, G. R., and O. Wyss. 1962. The effect of gamma radiation on nitrogen transformations in soil. Bacteriol. Proc. 62nd Annual Meeting: 24.

SYNTHETIC EFFECTS OF SOIL-ENZYMES

G. HOFFMANN

Bayerische Hauptversuchsanstalt für Landwirtschaft
Technische Hochschule, München
Weihenstephan, Germany

MANY INVESTIGATIONS have proved that enzymes of different kinds, and especially hydrolases, are present in soils. Numerous observations have shown that they are localized chiefly on the humus-coated particles of the silt and clay fractions. But so far no one has succeeded in extracting these soilborne enzymes from the colloidal particles, on which they are adsorbed strongly in an as yet unknown manner (Conrad, 1940; Hoffmann, 1958). Contrary to these findings commercial urease, added to soil and being artificially adsorbed, showed cationic properties and could be released partially by salt solutions (Pinck & Allison, 1961). This latter type of fixation may, of course, differ widely from the natural retention of enzymes by soils and naturally occurring enzymes could not be detected or their activity measured by desorption experiments. Fermi tried desorption in 1910 but was unable to extract any of the very stable enzymes, such as carbohydrases, urease, etc., present in each soil. He detected only proteolysis but we now know that the corresponding enzymes in soils are unstable and are often missing (Hoffmann & Teicher, 1957).

The only way to explore soil enzymology, then, was to determine the metabolites liberated during the contact of a specific substrate with the soil itself as enzyme-carrier. To confirm the real enzymatic nature of a breakdown, thus detected, additional experiments were necessary. Since all enzymes are proteins, heat lability, inhibition as by heavy metals, and activation by different compounds were used by us (Hofmann & Hoffmann, 1958) and others in proof of this fact. However, results of this kind are not too specific with regard to a distinct single enzyme.

We therefore looked for a more detailed proof. It has been known for a long time that synthetic steps occur during the hydrolytic decomposition of carbohydrates by enzymes. The monomers liberated are connected together to compounds different from the substrate. Some are also transferred by the hydrolysing enzyme to intact molecules of the substrate, or of the new compounds mentioned before, thus forming further products with a higher degree of polymerization than the substrate. The linkage of these new saccharides is always more resistant to the hydrolytic action of the producing enzyme than that of the substrate. Thus the new products accumulate.

Such syntheses are characteristic for certain enzymes and they often occur in solution if the enzyme is brought in contact with monomeric compounds of its specific substrate. For example, maltose and isomaltose are found in pure glucose solutions containing yeast extract (Hill, 1898) and gentiobiose if emulsin from almonds or other sources is present (Bourquelot & Herissey, 1913). Similar reactions were also detected with other specific enzymes, for example proteases (Wasteneys & Borsok, 1924). Although these facts have been well known since the end of the nineteenth century, only recent work, using chromatographic partition of the products formed, could show the real extent of the syntheses initiated by the hydrolases (Peat et al., 1952).

We assumed that, if the same syntheses could be observed in soil samples as with plant and microbial enzymes, it would be good proof of the exclusively enzymatic nature of the changes in organic compounds in soil. Our first experiments using the normal method of determining soil invertase activity (Thun et al., 1955) encouraged us to continue this field of exploration. We found on the chromatograms, along with the usual breakdown products of sucrose, a single fructose-containing compound with a smaller R_F value than that of the substrate.

From the literature it was known that a five-week incubation with fairly purified enzymes was necessary to obtain sufficient amounts of new compounds (Peat et al., 1952). But the soil is only a crude enzyme preparation and since purification of soil enzymes is impossible, we had to look for a technique which avoided too long incubation at the normal enzyme level. First we increased the natural enzyme content of a carefully selected loamy soil rich in particles able to adsorb enzymes. We mixed it with 7.5 per cent of alfalfa-meal, autoclaved to destroy its own enzymes. This mixture, moistened to 60 per cent of its water capacity, was incubated for 10 days at room temperature, during which time microbial development increased the normal enzyme activity of the sample approximately tenfold. The soil was then air dried, passed through a 2 mm sieve, and used as an enzyme preparation.

The method of incubation was similar to the normal one, except that we did not add any buffer and thus the troublesome removal of inorganic ions from the solutions to be chromatographed could be avoided.

To each 10 gm of the soil, treated with 4 ml of toluene, were added 20 ml of solutions of different substrates. Their concentration was 20 per cent w/v for sugars, 10 per cent for the glycoside arbutin (β-D-glucosidohydroquinone) and 1/15 M for amino acids and pyruvic acid respectively. The samples were incubated at 37 C for at most 40 days. They were swirled gently each day and toluene was added as needed. At intervals, 4 μl aliquots were transferred to paper.

For chromatography the circular technique described by Giri and Rao (1952) was used, with 20 spots on the circle around the centre of the sheet. Each spot could be charged with 2 μl of solution at one time without overlapping with neighbouring ones. Samples from each experiment with a sample of enzyme over the total incubation time were spotted on each half sheet. Different solvent systems were used (Reindel & Hoppe, 1953) but the Partridge mixture in a single-phase form was preferred.

In each of these experiments, a large number of synthetic compounds were found after non-enzymatic reversions had been excluded.

The results with maltose are shown in Plate I, Fig. 1. The control for maltose at the zero time is shown on the left. In the middle is the reference run with glucose at the top and maltose about half-way up. The other sectors are arranged in a time sequence from left to right (8 hr, 1, 5, 10, 15, 20, 30, 40 days). Maltose decreases continuously while glucose, the sole breakdown product, increases approximately by the same amount. After only 8 hours incubation, the first synthetic products appear in the position of the trisaccharides, and after one day are followed by tetrasaccharides. The principal fractions of each zone of the same degree of polymerization are the polymeric homologous compounds of maltose, such as maltotriose and tetraose. From the 5th day on more sugars are formed in the position of disaccharides. In the later stages of the experiment one of these becomes the principal compound. This is probably not a product of maltase (α-glucosidase) action but of β-glucosidase action.

Similar patterns were found with cellobiose and lactose as substrates, and β-glucosidase and β-galactosidase respectively as corresponding enzymes. All of the new compounds shown on Fig. 1 were reducing.

The soil invertase acts preferentially as a transfructosidase. All of the major synthetic compounds contain fructose. In contrast to the new compounds built up by aldohexoses, they are not reducing. In Fig. 2 two groups each of three wedge-shaped strips are shown, the left group from the 8th, the right one from the 20th day of incubation. The single strips are cut from three different sheets, and each sprayed with a different reagent to elucidate the composition of the spots. The strip at the far left, stained with aniline-diphenylamine-phosphate (Buchan & Savage, 1952), shows the total sugars. This reagent is less sensitive than the second, β-naphtol with sulphuric acid (Reindel & Hardt, 1955), which develops ketoses and ketose containing saccharides only and therefore more compounds, all of them containing fructose, can be seen. On the next strip appear the reducing sugars of invertase action, glucose and fructose (detected with silver-nitrate/ammonia) (Dedonder, 1952). One single weak spot of higher molarity appears, which is reducing but does not contain fructose. This demonstrates the ability of soil-invertase to perform transglucosidative linkages too. The second group of strips taken at a later term of incubation gave similar results.

The action of β-glucosidase on the phenolic glycoside arbutin during the first 9 hours of incubation is shown in Fig. 3. To detect phenolic compounds we developed a spray with dibromquinonchlorimide and sodium-dicarbonate (Hofmann & Hoffmann, 1958). When used on the upper left quadrant it revealed a number of synthetic compounds, the composition of which is

PLATE I

FIGS. 1–4. Paper chromatograms showing effect of soil enzymes. Synthetic effect of soil on maltose (1), sucrose (2) and arbutin (3). Aspartic acid amino-transferase action (4). See text for details.

still unknown. Silver nitrate, applied to the lower right quadrant, is less sensitive and does not distinguish between phenols and reducing sugars. Therefore the upper right quadrant was sprayed, with the aniline-reagent, specific for sugars, but only glucose was detected. Some days later new carbohydrates were formed, fewer in number but similar to those on the cellobiose sheet. To the lower left quadrant soil blanks which contained neither sugars nor phenols were applied. In the middle of each quadrant the reference substances hydroquinone, arbutin and glucose are visible.

To detect amino-transferase action of soils, pyruvic acid was used as an acceptor. The result with aspartic acid as the amino group donor is shown in Fig. 4. The reference compounds are located in the middle of the pattern. The section on the right side is the soil blank, which is free of detectable amino acids. After the transfer of the amino group to the acceptor compound, alanine is synthesized, and increases with time as the substrate decreases. The enzyme also reacts with leucine, valine, glutamic acid and other amino acids.

More examples could be presented, all showing similar results. Autoclaved soil fails to produce any action on organic matter but the action of natural soil and of purified enzymes is qualitatively similar; both cause the appearance of different compounds of the same or of a higher degree of polymerization than the substrate used, as well as the normal products of enzymatic breakdown. These results support our hypothesis that the changes on organic substances effected by soil samples really are of an enzymatic nature. Furthermore this suggests that the soil enzymes in their natural location should be able to bring about the same changes on organic substances derived from plant residues as they do *in vitro*.

Normally the destruction of the latter is executed by soil micro-organisms. But the cell-free soil enzymes are assumed to take over some of the microbial duties during periods unfavourable for microbial life. They form different stable organic compounds, related to some factors of soil fertility. Such a substance was recently described by Kiss (1961). We can conclude that the soil enzymes themselves are a valuable part of the soil biology. No doubt they are derived mostly from soil micro-organisms, but they are also able to act in the absence of organisms as an independent biologic factor in soil fertility.

REFERENCES

Bourquelot, E., H. Herissey and J. Coine. 1913. Synthèse biochimique d'un sucre du groupe des hexobioses, le gentiobiose. Compt. rend. Acad. Sci. Paris 157: 732–734.

Buchan, J. L., and R. I. Savage. 1952. Paper chromatography of some starch conversion products. Analyst 77: 401–406.

Conrad, J. P. 1940. Hydrolysis of urea in soils by thermolabile catalysis. Soil Sci. 49: 253–263.

Dedonder, R. 1952. Les glucides du topinambour. I. Mise en évidence d'une série de glucofructosanes dans les tubercles du topinambour. Isolement, analyse, et structure des termes les moins polymbrisés. Bull. Soc. Chim. Biol. Paris *34*: 144–156.

Fermi, C. 1910. Sur la présence des enzymes dans le sol, dans les eaux et dans la poussière. Zentr. Bakt., II Abt. *26*: 330–334.

Giri, K. V., and N. A. N. Rao. 1952. A technique for the identification of amino-acids separated by circular paper chromatography. Nature (London): *169*: 923–924.

Hill, A. C. 1898. Reversible zymohydrolysis. J. Chem. Soc. *73*: 634–658.

Hoffmann, G. 1958. Wirkungsweise, Verteilung und Herkunft einiger Enzyme im Boden. Doctor Thesis, T.H. München.

Hoffmann, G., and K. Teicher. 1957. Ueber das Enzymsystem unserer Kulturböden. VII. Proteasen (II). Z. Pflanzenern., Düngg. u. Bodenkunde 77(122): 243–251.

Hoffmann, G., and K. Teicher. 1957. Ueber das Enzymsystem unserer Kulturböden. VII. Proteasen (II). Z. Pflanzenern., Düngg. u. Bodenkunde 77(122): 97–104.

Hofmann, E., and G. Hoffmann. 1958. Eine Methode zur Erkennung phenolischer Körper auf Papierchromatogrammen. Naturwiss. *45*: 337–338.

Kiss, S. 1961. Ueber die Anwesenheit von Lävansucrase in Boden. Naturwiss. *48*: 700.

Peat, S., W. J. Whelan and K. A. Hinson. 1952. Synthetic action of almond emulsin. Nature (London), *170*: 1056–1057.

Pinck, L. A., and F. E. Allison. 1961. Adsorption and release of urease by and from clay minerals. Soil Sci. *91*: 183–188.

Reindel, F., and W. Hoppe. 1953. Verbesserung des Trennungseffektes bei der Papierchromatographie durch die Formgebung des Papierstreifens. Naturwiss. *40*: 245.

Reindel, F., and M. Hardt. 1955. Systematische Auftrennung der löslichen Kohlenhydrate und Amino-säuren einer Braugerste, ihrer Vermälzungsstadien bzw. ihrer Reifestadien am Halm mit Hilfe der Papierchromatographie. Brauwiss. *8*: 186–191.

Thun, R., R. Herrmann and E. Knickmann. 1955. Handbuch der landw. Versuchs- und Untersuchungsmethodik (Methodenbuch). Band I. Verlag Neumann, Radebeul und Berlin, III Auflage: 223.

Wasteneys, H., and H. Borsok. 1924. The enzymatic synthesis of proteins. I. The synthesizing action of pepsin. J. Biol. Chem. *62*: 15–29.

FACTORS IN SOIL MYCOSTASIS

C. G. DOBBS

University College of North Wales, Bangor, Wales

MYCOLOGISTS, especially those working with the pathogenic soil fungi, have from time to time observed that fungal spores fail to germinate when they are in contact with soil under conditions in which one would expect them to do so. At Bangor we came across this phenomenon in a context of soil fungal ecology, and after an investigation concluded that it was widespread, indeed almost universal, in surface soils, and must be attributed to the action of water-soluble inhibitors of biological origin.

Our original article in *Nature* (Dobbs & Hinson, 1953) was entitled: "A Widespread Fungistasis in Soils" but we have since been persuaded to use the word "mycostasis" and hope that other authors will concur. Since then the phenomenon has been fully and often independently confirmed by many workers, too numerous for references in this short paper; but despite considerable progress we are still not much wiser about the exact nature of the inhibition, beyond a broad confirmation of the speculation (Hinson, 1954) that it is produced by some soil bacteria and actinomycetes.

After the pioneer work of W. H. Hinson (see also Dobbs & Hinson, 1960; Dobbs, Hinson & Bywater, 1960) its continuation at Bangor was ensured by three successive two-year grants from the Forestry Commission, to whom thanks and acknowledgments are due, as well as to the three research workers who have held these grants, certain aspects of whose work I am reporting here: Joan Bywater (now Mrs. N. W. Daniels), D. Alun Griffiths, and Nancy C. Carter. This work, in so far as it has been published, has appeared under the title "Studies in Soil Mycology" in the annual Reports on Forest Research of the Forestry Commission from 1957 onwards: Dobbs & Bywater, 1957, 1959; Dobbs, Bywater & Griffiths, 1960; Dobbs & Griffiths, 1961, 1962.

MATERIAL AND METHODS

The main methods used have been the cellulose film test and the preparation of sterile filtered water-extracts of soil.

Cellulose film was adopted as our chief test material only after we had assured ourselves of the reality of the inhibition by other means: by direct burying of spores in soil, and by the use of pipe clay, sintered glass, collodion and agar. Burying and partial recovery of spores can give only a crude check; and though an artificial factor is necessarily introduced with any test material, we are satisfied that thin cellulose film introduces the least disturbance for the maximum convenience and accuracy.

The important thing seems to be to avoid test materials which themselves inhibit (such as soda-glass) or which might differentially stimulate mycostatic micro-organisms. Autoclaved agar, owing to its uncertain composition, might be suspect on both counts, though it has been useful in testing mycelial growth. Cellulose film, we are satisfied, besides being far more convenient, is not subject to either of these criticisms. It does not seem to be attacked by bacteria during the period of the test, or until the later stages of its decomposition by fungi (Tribe, 1960), but should it liberate nutrients, these could only be sugars which would tend to break down mycostasis. Such a breakdown, accompanied by bacterial proliferation, has in fact been seen when the sweet plasticizer on the film has been incompletely removed. It should be added that all test materials must provide surfaces for microbial proliferation and will hold up moisture and reduce aeration when placed on a soil, but since the soil-mass itself is a labyrinth of such surfaces, this does not seem a valid objection.

British Cellophane Ltd's non-moistureproof PT 300 film, about 20μ thick, was selected. A 2 in. square of this is boiled and then autoclaved in water, smeared or brushed with the test spores, and pressed firmly on or in the moist soil, which may be left as a lump, but for our standard assay method is contained within a 10 ml aluminium or glass cap, filled level, with the film pressed on the surface, providing margins not in contact with the soil which serve as controls. The whole is incubated 48 hours at 27° over water in a covered bowl before five replicated counts of about 100 spores are made on the soil-contact area and on the control area, the result being expressed as percentage spores germinated. The control is not accurate as it shows moisture variations, not experienced by the soil-contact area, but it serves as an assurance that the spores used are of normal viability, and reveals qualitative differences, including stimulated growth where this occurs. The two test fungi used were *Penicillium frequentans* Westling and *Mucor ramannianus* Möller, of which only the latter was used for our standard soil assay.

W. H. Hinson was the first to prepare inhibitory sterile water-extracts of normal soils by Seitz-filtration in air through filter papers, testing in sealed McCartney vials (Dobbs, Hinson & Bywater, 1960), and to show that the inhibitor is unstable in water. Griffiths later developed a method of incubating the moist soil at 30°, pressure-filtering (using a No. 6 reconstituted cellulose Membranfilter), storing and testing spore germination in the extract on washed agar against water controls, all under an atmosphere of nitrogen (Dobbs & Griffiths, 1961, 1962). This has yielded extracts giving a range of germination levels from 2 per cent up to control level, and above where sugars are present. The controls have given much trouble owing to their variability, and the use of thoroughly washed agar and of conductivity-water is essential. Recently, Carter has been able to standardize methods sufficiently to demonstrate a consistent and significant reduction in germination of under 20 per cent (see Figs. 3 and 4) from one soil collection stored long enough to achieve equilibrium. She has also shown that incubation under nitrogen, or at 30°, is not essential, as inhibitory extracts can also be obtained from moistened soil kept in air out of doors.

Methods used by Griffiths in the study of the extracts have included heating, bubbling oxygen through them, and extracting with organic solvents: diethyl ether, petroleum ether, benzene, acetone, chloroform. In each case the water fraction was removed and tested against spores by the washed agar method, while the organic solvents were evaporated away under nitrogen, and the residues taken up with water and tested against spores. Extracts were also passed through columns of washed activated charcoal and of alumina. Soil-contact germination tests were made with a range of Membranfilters graded as to pore-size down to 5 mμ.

Methods used in the study of the relation between mycostasis and soil sugars have included Wager's (1954) modification of the Shaffer-Hartman copper reagent method. Water-extracts of soils were made by bubbling oxygen-free nitrogen through a soil-and-water mixture for 20 minutes before filtration. Sugar content, as measured on a Spekker absorptiometer, was expressed as mg glucose-equivalent per gram soil. Chromatograms were later run for sugars by the butanol/pyridine/water method using extracts made both with sodium hydroxide and with water.

RESULTS

The cellulose film test has been used to demonstrate the universal production of the inhibition by moist, surface soils (unless masked by sugars), and its reduction or absence in deep sterile subsoils; its biological, in some cases bacterial, origin, its "competitive" relationship with sugars (and also citrate), its seasonal variation in forest soils, and differences between different sites and soil-layers, and the existence of more stable, or non-sugar-sensitive, types of inhibition in certain, mainly calcareous, soils, which is now under investigation.

The long suspected involvement of certain soil bacteria and actinomycetes in soil mycostasis has gradually become clearer, especially from the work of Park (1956) as regards bacteria and Stevenson (1956) and Lockwood (1959) for actinomycetes. By 1958 we had observed the association between mycostasis on cellulose films floating on water overlying soil and the accumulation of bacteria on their under surface, and also with soil bacteria travelling up from wet soil into filter paper (Dobbs, Hinson & Bywater, 1960); and in the same year Dr. Bywater obtained restoration of mycostasis in chrome-washed sterile sand both by air infection and by inoculation with live soil or sand. From the mycostatic patches in these sands only bacteria could be isolated. Out of seven strains, some isolated several times, Griffiths found three, all gram-negative rods, to produce mycostatic effects in culture on test films; the other four, all gram-positive, did not (Dobbs, Griffiths & Bywater, 1960). Of the more recent work, that relating to the sugar relation-

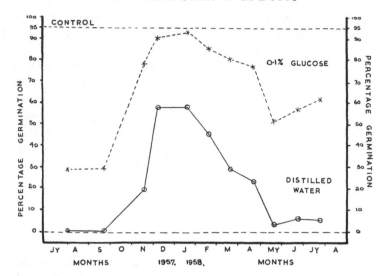

FIG. 1. Average germination, tested monthly by the cellulose film method, of spores of *Mucor ramannianus* on 12 forest soils. Full line: samples moistened with distilled water; broken line: with 0.1 per cent glucose solution.

ships of the inhibition, the properties of extracts, and spore-feeding experiments, will be briefly dealt with.

Sugar Relationships

A three-year monthly germination assay of twelve forest soils (litter, humus and mineral layers on four sites) showed an irregular seasonal variation in the inhibition, with higher germination in the winter, and significantly more in the litter than in the other layers. Over-all percentage averages were: litter 34.8, humus 9.5, mineral 8.9. A parallel assay during the first year, using 0.1 per cent glucose solution as against distilled water to moisten the soil, gave a similar curve but at about 40 per cent higher germination level (Fig. 1). This was followed up in 1959–60 by a parallel estimation of the glucose-equivalent of reducing sugars in the tested soil-samples, which again gave a similar seasonal variation (Fig. 2). The association with germination was found significant by the χ^2 test ($P < .01$).

Chromatograms run with extracts of one of these soils (humus under pine) gave spots for ribose, sorbose and galactose, with an unidentified spot of high molecular weight, presumably a polysaccharide, since it showed a decrease after hydrolysis with acid, with increase in the spots for ribose and galactose. Freezing the soil before extraction gave the same spots for sugars but somewhat larger; autoclaving much larger, with a further spot for xylose, later found in an extract from untreated soil.

This observation (Dobbs & Griffiths, 1961) of free sugars in water-extracts of forest soil is of some interest. Forsyth (1950) and Bernier (1958) have drawn attention to the presence of a polysaccharide fraction yielding a

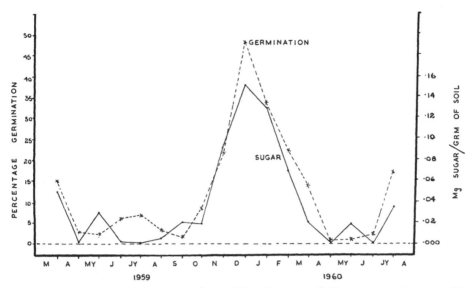

Fig. 2. Average germination, tested monthly, of spores of *Mucor ramannianus* on 12 forest soils (broken line) in relation to content of reducing sugars (full line).

range of sugars on hydrolysis, including galactose and xylose (Bernier, 1958) but the role played by the sugars themselves in the soil has had little or no attention. In fact we could find no record of them, although Nagar (1962) has since reported free monosaccharides in soil organic matter and has found glucose in four widely different soils. We have so far not found glucose in our forest soil.

Preliminary tests by Griffiths showed a surprising lack of counter-inhibitory effect on the part of these soil-sugars as compared with glucose. This did not tally with the results of Jackson (1960) who found that all of a range of sugars tested increased germination over soil, although monosaccharides did so more than disaccharides.

Recently Dr. Elizabeth H. Evans has carried out at Bangor a thoroughly replicated test of the effects of glucose, sorbose, galactose, ribose and xylose, each at three molarities 0.005, 0.01 and 0.05, on the germination of two test fungi (*M. ramannianus* and *P. frequentans*) on agar over glass and over soil. Full details cannot be given here, but the results broadly show that all the sugars stimulate germination of both fungi over soil. Glucose, however, always shows germination increasing with molarity, while all the other four somewhere showed, in one or more of the combinations of treatment, a germination reduced by increased molarity, of which the most extreme example was shown by galactose with the spores of *P. frequentans* over soil, which gave percentage germinations, with increasing molarity: 56.5; 55.4; 0.6. Such results may help to explain the occasional low or zero germination of spores on soil which has an appreciable content of reducing sugars.

Soil-Extracts

These have confirmed the presence of a soluble, very unstable inhibitor in some sterile soil-filtrates. (See also the work of Stover, 1958.) It is convenient to use the singular for brevity, but the variable properties of the extract probably indicate a complex of active substances.

Hinson (1954) found that sterile extract lost about half its activity in a sealed vial in 50 hr. Later we found that, when exposed to the air, an active extract lost activity only slightly in 12 hr, but completely in 24 hr. When oxygen was bubbled through it, the extract lost 65 per cent of activity in 5 min, 100 per cent in 7 min. Temperature relations were also somewhat variable. Most extracts tested lost activity when heated to 60°, but a few did so as low as 30°, while some survived 60°.

Of the organic solvents used, only the diethyl-ether fraction gave a rather feeble inhibition with extract of a pine humus soil. The activity of water-extracts passed through washed neutral charcoal was completely removed. Tests with graded filters showed passage of the inhibitor through the whole range, down to a pore-size of 50 A, while wet Cellophane, according to the makers, is usually quoted as having a pore-size about 20 A.

Lingappa and Lockwood (1961) made the interesting speculation that the spores themselves may act as micro-habitats in the soil, stimulating the growth of inhibitory microbes around them. Recently we have been testing this idea at Bangor by spore-feeding experiments on a mineral soil under spruce which was giving mildly, but consistently, inhibitory extracts. The results of two experiments by Dr. Carter can be seen in Figs. 3 and 4.

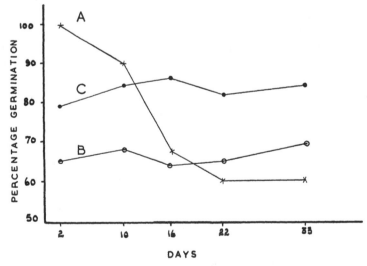

FIG. 3. A—germination of test spores in sterile extract of mineral soil under spruce "fed" with one large initial dose of unwashed spores of the test fungus (*Mucor ramannianus*). B—germination in extract of untreated sample of the same soil. C—germination in conductivity-water.

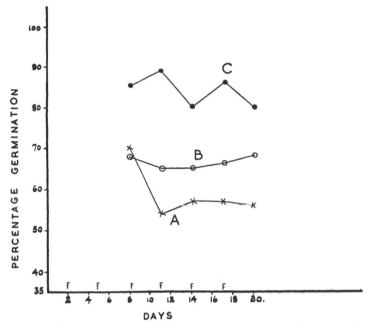

FIG. 4. A, B and C as in Fig. 3; except that in A there was no large initial dose, but washed spores were "fed" into the soil in small doses at three-day intervals on the days marked "f".

These show germination of test spores of M. *ramannianus* at intervals of days: in conductivity water (C); in successive sterile filtered extracts of the same soil sample made up each time to field capacity with conductivity water before extraction (B); and in similar extracts of another sample of the same soil-collection subjected to "feeding" with spores of the test fungus (A). The difference between B and C was significant throughout.

In the first experiment (Fig. 3) the A sample was given one massive initial dose of spores collected, without washing, from eight malt cultures. The early stimulus can be attributed to sugars thus introduced, but after 16 days germination had sunk to the level of the untreated soil extract and thereafter was reduced significantly ($P < .05$) below it. In the second experiment (Fig. 4) the spores were washed by twice centrifuging in water, and were added in very much smaller doses at three-day intervals to the soil. The reduction in germination on and after the 11th day below the level shown by the untreated soil was persistent and highly significant ($P < .01$). The total spore-dose at the end was less than one-sixth of the initial dose given in the first experiment. Even if the extra inhibition shown in Fig. 3 could be attributed in whole or in part to a mutual spore effect, this would not account for any large part of that shown in Fig. 4, which may therefore reasonably be attributed mainly to the stimulation of inhibitory organisms by the freshly added spores.

DISCUSSION

Lingappa and Lockwood (1961) have also drawn useful attention to the fact that soil mycostasis, as demonstrated by test materials such as agar and Cellophane, is due to the growth of soil microbes on their surfaces, and not to a reserve of toxic substances in the soil. This has not been in question since the microbial origin and unstable properties of this type of inhibition became clear; but as they rightly point out, the effect upon test materials may throw light on the nature of the phenomenon in the natural soil. Most of their tests were made with water agar, but they also showed that a trace of soil can render Cellophane mycostatic, which tallies also with our own observations. However, for reasons given earlier, we are satisfied that if the cellulose test-film exerts any selective effect in favour of the inhibiting organisms, this can scarcely be owing to the film, but must be attributed to the test-spores themselves, which have only a 20μ separation from the soil surface.

The question remains whether the phenomenon, as it occurs in the soil, consists mainly in the proliferation of inhibitory organisms on the actual spore surface, forming a sort of "sporosphere" surrounding each spore. The demonstration of inhibitory soil filtrates, and the examination of spores recovered from the soil, do not in general support this idea. At Bangor we have made a special study of soil-spores and both Hinson (Dobbs & Hinson, 1960) and Mrs. Anderson (unpublished) have found that they are nearly all closely covered and obscured by mineral or organic matter. It seems probable that it is this surrounding material which becomes mycostatic whenever conditions favour microbial growth, while exudates from the spore may possibly favour the mycostatic organisms. Conditions of aeration within the soil-mass would permit longer survival of the inhibitor(s) than outside it, which would be consistent with the observation that spores will germinate in minute soil fragments (e.g., in buried slide-traps) when they are separated from the mass.

There has been much discussion as to whether the inhibitors responsible for microbial soil mycostasis should be regarded as antibiotics, and they may well, of course, come under that broad label. But there is no evidence yet to show that they are toxic to fungi, or are the same substances which produce lysis in spores and hyphae, while the inhibition probably has survival value for spores in preventing germination below a nutrient level which would allow of extension and sporing. Whatever we call them they have a characteristic instability, but their most interesting property is their "competitive" relationship with sugars, and also with citrate. This suggests we are dealing with some sort of antimetabolite. It is clear that we are still on the fringes of a large field of research in biochemistry, microbiology and mycology, which cannot be ignored in any consideration of microbial ecology in the soil.

REFERENCES

Bernier, B. 1958. Characterisation of polysaccharides isolated from forest soils. Biochem. J. 70: 590–599.

Dobbs, C. G., and J. Bywater. 1957. Report on Forest Research for 1957, pp. 92–94. H.M.S.O. London.

Dobbs, C. G., and J. Bywater. 1959. Report on Forest Research for 1958, pp. 97–104. H.M.S.O. London.

Dobbs, C. G., J. Bywater and D. A. Griffiths. 1960. Report on Forest Research for 1959, pp. 94–100. H.M.S.O. London.

Dobbs, C. G., and D. A. Griffiths. 1961. Report on Forest Research for 1960, pp. 87–92. H.M.S.O. London.

Dobbs, C. G., and D. A. Griffiths. 1962. Report on Forest Research for 1961, pp. 95–100. H.M.S.O. London.

Dobbs, C. G., and W. H. Hinson. 1953. A widespread fungistasis in soils. Nature. 172: 197–199.

Dobbs, C. G., and W. H. Hinson. 1960. Some observations on fungal spores in soils. In The ecology of soil fungi, pp. 33–42. Liverpool University Press.

Dobbs, C. G., W. H. Hinson and J. Bywater. 1960. In The ecology of soil fungi, pp. 130–147. Liverpool University Press.

Forsyth, W. G. C. 1950. Studies on the more soluble complexes of soil organic matter. II. The composition of the soluble polysaccharide fraction. Biochem. J. 46: 141–146.

Hinson, W. H. 1954. A study in the biology of soil moulds. Ph.D. Thesis, University of Wales.

Jackson, R. M. 1960. Soil fungistasis and the rhizosphere. In The ecology of soil fungi, pp. 168–176. Liverpool University Press.

Lingappa, B. T., and J. L. Lockwood. 1961. The nature of the widespread soil fungistasis. J. Gen. Microbiol. 26: 473–485.

Lockwood, J. L. 1959. Streptomyces spp. as a cause of natural fungi-toxicity in soils. Phytopathology 49: 327–331.

Nagar, B. R. 1962. Free monosaccharides in soil organic matter. Nature 194: 896–897.

Park, D. 1956. Effect of substrate on a microbial antagonism, with reference to soil conditions. Trans. Brit. Mycol. Soc. 39: 239–259.

Stevenson, I. L. 1956. Antibiotic activity of actinomycetes in soils as demonstrated by direct observation techniques. J. Gen. Microbiol. 15: 372–380.

Stover, R. H. 1958. Influence of soil fungitoxins on behavior of Fusarium oxysporum f. cubense in soil extracts and diffusates. Can. J. Botany. 36: 439–453.

Tribe, H. T. 1960. Decomposition of buried cellulose film, with special reference to the ecology of certain soil fungi. In The ecology of soil fungi, pp. 246–256. Liverpool University Press.

Wager, H. G. 1954. Analyst 79: 34–38.

SYMPOSIUM VI

EFFECT OF CHEMICAL AND BIOLOGICAL CONTROL MEASURES ON SOIL MICRO-ORGANISMS

Chairman: H. KATZNELSON

H. L. JENSEN

The Influence of Herbicidic Chemicals on Soil Metabolism and on the Zymogenic Soil Microflora

C. A. I. GORING

Control of Plant Pathogenic Micro-organisms in Soil

R. H. STOVER

The Use of Organic Amendments and Green Manures in the Control of Soil-Borne Phytopathogens

KENNETH F. BAKER

Control of Phytopathogenic Micro-organisms in Soil by Management Practices

N. A. KRASSILNIKOV

The Role of Micro-organisms in Plant Life

CHAIRMAN'S REMARKS

H. KATZNELSON

Microbiology Research Institute
Canada Department of Agriculture
Ottawa, Canada

THE SUBJECTS to be discussed in this symposium bring together areas of work which have become particularly important and have aroused a great deal of interest and concern during recent years. Moreover, they deal with aspects of agricultural microbiology—plant pathology, pesticide residues and biological control—which will receive relatively little attention at this Congress despite its emphasis on topics of agricultural interest.

The increasing use of a wide variety of potent pesticidal and herbicidal chemicals (millions of pounds on millions of acres of soil) has aroused serious concern not only because of their potential hazard to man and animal but also because of their possible harmful effects on soil microorganisms and on fundamental soil processes from organic matter decomposition to nitrogen fixation. In consequence it is necessary to know how readily these substances are broken down in the soil and by what organisms. The nature of the breakdown products is also important since some of these may be even more toxic than the original substances used.

In regard to the control of soil-borne plant pathogenic organisms such as fungi and nematodes there are a number of approaches. Perhaps the most common is the use of chemicals, with their attendant problems as mentioned. Another important method, shown to be very effective in the control of wheat rust, is breeding resistant varieties of plants. Since this aspect of control is not essentially microbiological in nature, it was not included in the symposium. A third means of combating microbial pests—biological control—has not perhaps received the attention it warrants. However, in the light of residue and related hazards involved in the use of agricultural chemicals, I expect that this method will become increasingly important.

Biological control is concerned primarily with the creation of a microbiological environment which is inimical to the soil-borne pathogen. This may be achieved in several ways. The microbial population of the soil can be modified by physical methods such as flooding and steaming. The addition of organic matter such as green manures or other plant and animal residues can cause a marked shift in the microbiological equilibrium of the soil to the detriment of the parasite. The use of specific microbial antagonists particularly as seed inoculants represents still another approach to the problem, and one which appears to have met with some success in the U.S.S.R. The mechanism of biological control, be it the production of antibiotics in soil, competition for nutrients or overgrowth of the pathogen by actively multiplying organisms in response to a given treatment, is another area of work requiring detailed investigation and one which soil microbiologists should relish.

I have tried to point out briefly the scope and significance of the subjects to be discussed and I shall now turn to the symposium speakers for their more detailed contributions.

THE INFLUENCE OF HERBICIDIC CHEMICALS ON SOIL METABOLISM AND THE ZYMOGENIC SOIL MICROFLORA

H. L. JENSEN

Government Laboratory for Soil and Crop Research
Lyngby, Denmark

It is probably not unscientific to suggest that somewhere or other some organism may exist which can, under suitable conditions, oxidize any substance which is theoretically capable of being oxidized. E. F. GALE (1951)

THE USE OF CHEMICALS for eradication of noxious weeds is far from new but has not until the last fifteen years aroused widespread interest among soil biologists. The change is largely due to the discovery in the late 1940's of a class of selective herbicides with exceptional potentialities: the "hormone herbicides" typified by 2,4-dichlorophenoxyacetic acid (2,4-D). Many new synthetic products have since been added and several others of old standing have held their ground, so that today close to a hundred substances, mostly organic, are in use as herbicides (Crafts, 1961). During the same short span of our "age of synthesis" a wide range of other chemicals have come into use as fungicides and insecticides for crop protection. Synthetic detergents, waste products of the chemical industries, etc., make a further addition and thus an increasing amount of "nature-foreign" and partly very poisonous substances find their way into the two major sites of biological dissimilation: the soil and natural waters. Herbicides and other pesticides added to the soil may be partly inactivated by adsorption to the soil colloids, but this is a process that cannot go on indefinitely. Others may be removed by leaching, but this only means transfer to some other locality. Short of chemical instability their ultimate destruction and removal from the biological cycle can only be mediated through the microbial world with its almost infinitely varied adaptability and powers of dissimilation. On the way to their final disappearance the substances may affect microbiological soil conditions in several ways, for instance, (a) by inhibiting desirable processes, (b) by causing partial sterilization, a beneficial effect if its victims include plant-pathogenic fungi or animal parasites, (c) by acting as metabolic stimulants, or (d), most important of all, by becoming food material for the soil microbes and giving rise to a detoxicating zymogenic microflora.

In this paper I shall limit myself to the herbicides and among these to a few examples chosen for diversity of biological properties rather than quantitative or economic importance. The literature is already very voluminous and has been well reviewed in four recent articles by Audus (1960), Fletcher (1960), Gustafson (1960) and Bollen (1961). The appended list of references includes mainly recent publications not covered by these reviews.

EFFECT AND FATE OF SOME HERBICIDES IN SOIL

The "Hormone Herbicides"

Most interest has naturally centred around two world-important compounds: 2,4-dichlorophenoxyacetic acid (2,4-D) and 2-methyl-4-chlorophenoxyacetic acid (MCPA). The general consensus of opinion seems to be that they are far less toxic to micro-organisms as a whole than to higher plants and that normal field doses have little effect upon the soil microflora (Fletcher, 1960). Research on their biological detoxication was initiated long ago by Audus (1960) whose studies revealed a sequence of events that is generally characteristic of "exotic" substances introduced into the soil: a slight initial reduction of biological activity may arise from adsorption of the substance to the soil colloids; next follows a lag or latency period, more or less protracted according to the nature and concentration of the substance; this lasts until an active zymogenic flora has arisen and then a rapid decomposition of the added substance ensues. Repeated application now results in immediate decomposition. Micro-organisms able to decompose the added substance *in vitro* may be isolated from the enriched soil and their activity "*in terra*" under varying external conditions may be verified by adding an inoculum of their cells together with the compound in question to a non-enriched soil: if active under the conditions at hand, the inoculum will abolish the otherwise normal lag period.

The active soil microflora that arises in response to 2,4-D and related compounds consists typically of non-spore-forming and mostly gram-negative bacteria (cf. Audus, 1960): *Flavobacterium, Achromobacter, Arthrobacter* (?) and *Mycoplana* (?), but no actinomycetes or fungi as far as we know.

The mechanism of hormone decomposition is clearly mediated by inducible enzymes, but otherwise the intricate pathways of dissimilation are outside this present topic. Yet it is worth noticing that intermediate products sometimes seem to arise that are either stimulatory or even more toxic to test plants than the original herbicide (Audus & Symonds, 1955).

Bell (1960), Alexander and Aleem (1961) and Burger *et al.* (1962) have recently discussed the significance of molecular structure for liability to biological decomposition. A most striking feature is the number and particularly the position of halogen substituents which are conducive to decomposability in the para-position but have the opposite effect in the meta-position. Another factor is the length of the aliphatic side chain in α-substituted compounds; thus a *Flavobacterium* studied by Burger *et al.* would attack 4-(2,4-dichlorophenoxy)-butyric acid and several analogues but not 2,4-D.

Nitro-Substituted Phenols

The herbicides of this group, 4,6-dinitroortho-cresol (DNOC) and 4,6-dinitrobutylphenol (DNBP) have attracted much less notice than the hormones, although DNOC has a longer past as a selective herbicide and both possess important physiological properties. They are, *inter alia*, considerably more toxic to microbial life than the hormones; indeed the inhibitory effect of nitrophenols on assimilatory processes through uncoupling of oxidative phosphorylation is too well known to need comment. Further they sometimes show rather enigmatic stimulatory effects on plant growth (cf. Bruinsma, 1960) and finally our knowledge of their microbiological transformation (like that of organic nitro-compounds in general) is recent and still very incomplete.

It is known that both substances slowly lose their phytotoxic effect in soil. From DNOC-treated soil we (Gundersen & Jensen, 1956) isolated a variety of *Arthrobacter simplex* that utilized DNOC and several related substances with release of the excess nitrogen as nitrite. Only compounds with a nitrogroup in para-position to hydroxyl were attacked, and this with two exceptions: 3,5-dinitrosalicylic acid and, more surprisingly, DNBP (a case of the length of the side chain controlling decomposability?). In fact we have not yet in spite of many attempts succeeded in finding aerobic organisms that will utilize DNBP. The only case on record seems to be a brief preliminary communication by Dourus and Reid (1956). We did, however, find growing cultures of *Clostridium butyricum* to reduce this and several other aromatic nitro-compounds to still unidentified colourless substances, probably amines. Such processes have been observed before, for example, in bacteria that reduce 2,4-dinitrophenol (Radler, 1955; Lehmberg, 1956), and liver xanthine-oxidase is stated to reduce several nitro-organic compounds, especially the para-substituted ones, to the corresponding amines with reduced diphosphopyridine-nucleotide as electron donor (Kielly, 1956).

The butyric acid bacteria doubtless exist at times as vegetative cells in the soil and may contribute to the slow disappearance of added DNBP—which indeed would presuppose a supply of organic matter other than the herbicide itself. This transformation, however, is essentially different from the oxidative breakdown, inasmuch as the DNBP-molecule only serves as electron acceptor without any evidence that it otherwise enters the metabolism of the bacteria.

The toxicity of nitrophenols is known to be markedly pH-dependent, the undissociated molecules being more active than the anions. Gundersen and I found, in agreement with this, that our *A. simplex* only attacked the weak acid DNOC (pK 4.4) at pH 7.3 to 8.3, but the strong picric acid (pK 0.8)

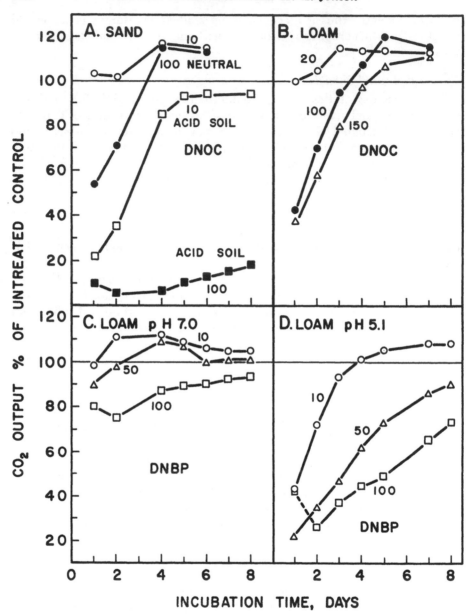

FIG. 1. Influence of herbicides on carbon dioxide production from 0.5 per cent lucerne meal in soils. *A* and *B*—dinitro-ortho-cresol: *A* in sand soil (pH 4.8–5.0) and limed to pH 6.5–7.0; *B* in loam soil, pH 7.0–7.3; *C* and *D*—dinitrobutylphenol: *C* in loam soil of pH 7.0; *D* in loam pH 5.1. Figures represent concentration of herbicide in ppm.

was attacked over practically the whole pH-latitude (approx. 5.5 to 8.5) where growth took place at all. Corresponding effects were seen in some experiments at Lyngby (hitherto unpublished), where we measured the output of carbon dioxide from soil incubated with basal addition of 0.5 per cent lucerne meal and the two herbicides in concentrations from 1 to 150 ppm, the smallest being comparable to normal field application.

Fig. 1 shows some of the results found with DNOC in a sandy field, at its original pH about 5 and also limed to pH about 6.6. CO_2 production is at first strongly inhibited by 10 ppm, but after 5 days it reaches the level of DNOC-free control soil; smaller doses from 1.0 to 5.0 ppm had a similar smaller effect. The heavy dose of 100 ppm depresses the process to a very low level with extremely slow recovery. The state of affairs at near-neutral reaction is totally different: 10 ppm causes no inhibition but a definite early stimulation, and 100 ppm also results in stimulation after a strong but transient depression. Another experiment in a neutral loam soil gave similar results; even the enormous dose of 150 ppm causes inhibition for 4 to 5 days only, and the subsequent stimulation is still in evidence. DNBP showed essentially the same effects in loam soil of pH 5.1 and 7.0 (Fig. 1).

The stronger inhibition at low pH is most probably an effect of the dissociation of the herbicide molecules. DNOC with pK 4.4 would be almost completely ionized in neutral soil, while nearly 20 per cent would remain undissociated at pH 5.0. The pK of DNBP does not seem to be known but is probably not very different.

The mechanism that causes stimulation is more obscure but might well be a combination of "partial sterilization" and increased dissimilation. It is easily imagined that the herbicides would immediately depress the metabolism of the more sensitive members of the soil microflora, and that the proportion would increase with increasing concentration of both nitro-compound and hydrogen ions. The field is then left to the more resistant fraction of the microflora whose respiration is intensified owing to suppressed assimilation of the metabolized organic carbon. It is too early to say if such an acceleration of the soil metabolism is a contributing factor in the stimulated plant growth that sometimes follows DNOC-treatment.

Chlorinated Aliphatic Acids

A few simple compounds of this class have found some use in recent years, viz., 2,2-dichloropropionate (Dalapon), trichloroacetate (TCA) and the less important monochloroacetate (MCA), all mostly as sodium salts. Field doses seem to have no striking influence on soil metabolic processes except perhaps some inhibition of nitrification (Fletcher, 1960), but all three compounds may induce higher bacterial numbers including zymogenic organisms with ability to use them as food substances. Several such organisms have been described by Magee and Colmer (1959), Hirsch and Alexander (1961) and Jensen (1959; see also Audus (1960)). At Lyngby we found the fungus *Trichoderma viride* very active in the decomposition of MCA in acid soil, but the two more important herbicides seem to fall prey to bacteria only, viz., *Pseudomonas, Alcaligenes, Agrobacterium* (?), *Arthrobacter* (?) and *Nocardia*. The length of the latency period before active breakdown increased according to the sequence: MCA < Dalapon < TCA.

We also found Dalapon and TCA to remain practically stable for four months in soil of pH 4.5, TCA also at pH 5.4, which further suggests immunity to attack by fungi.

Allyl Alcohol and Sulphamic Acid

These two minor herbicides may be cited as typifying simple substances of extremely divergent biological availability. Very little has until recently been known about biological transformation of allyl alcohol. Experiments at Lyngby (Jensen, 1961) showed that its phytotoxic effect in soil could disappear so rapidly (within two to eight days) that inoculation with active bacteria sometimes failed to accelerate the detoxication. The zymogenic flora was restricted to a very few types: *Nocardia corallina*, *Trichoderma viride* and particularly *Pseudomonas fluorescens* which under favourable conditions could multiply within a couple of days to such an extent as to comprise 80–90 per cent of all the colonies that developed on selective agar medium. *Trichoderma viride* showed a correspondingly profuse vegetative growth in acid soil (pH 5.7).

Sulphamic acid forms a striking contrast to allyl alcohol as being rather immune to biological attack. A preliminary statement by Bollen (1961) seems to be the only reference to its transformation in soil. It is described as neither nitrifiable nor particularly inhibitory to nitrification (Quastel & Scholefield, 1951) nor reducible by *Vibrio desulphuricans* (Postgate, 1953). Our experiments confirmed this and also failed to give evidence that its nitrogen was available to the soil flora in glucose or straw decomposition. Likewise many pure cultures of bacteria, actinomycetes and fungi failed to utilize sulphamate nitrogen, with two exceptions. A randomly isolated *Flavobacterium* sp. used it as a mediocre nitrogen source about equal to nitrate, and a very recently found variety of *Pullularia pullulans* (?) produced a slow but eventually vigorous growth on glucose-sulphamate agar.

GENERAL IMPRESSIONS

These few random examples cover only a very small section of a vast field, yet they show how varied is the behaviour of herbicidic substances in the soil. There are highly efficient compounds fairly susceptible to dissimilation and otherwise with little effect on the soil microflora, like the hormone herbicides. There are the nitrophenols which are used in similar small concentrations but can exert strong effects on soil metabolism, both stimulation and inhibition. There are simple compounds, of which some are only slightly toxic to the microflora and decomposed with moderate ease (the halogenated aliphatic acids), while another is metabolized with extreme ease (allyl alcohol) and yet another is remarkably inaccessible (sulphamic acid). In addition we may quote simazin (Guillemat *et al.*, 1960) as a substance of complicated structure, great but not absolute biological resistance and little or no harmful effect on the soil microflora.

We are still a long way from being able to predict liability to biological dissimilation from molecular structure, although a few guiding principles have emerged, such as the importance of para- and meta-substitution and the length of the side-chain in aromatic compounds. Similarly in the halogen-aliphatic acids double or triple substitution at a carbon atom seems to make for increased resistance, perhaps because such compounds rarely occur as natural metabolites (cf. Petty, 1961).

The numbers of soil inhabitants able to adapt themselves to some "unnatural" nutrient or other may be very limited, and adaptation may take place only after long intervals of time, as evidenced by the often very protracted latency period that precedes the active breakdown of pesticides and similar substances. Even then the biological elimination may proceed at a very slow rate, although, as Audus (1960) puts it, there are probably few organic compounds altogether immune to ultimate bacterial attack. We may agree with Gale (1951) in his opinion quoted at the heading of this article and we may also extend "oxidation" to other types of decomposition but should not forget the proviso "under suitable conditions"—which stresses the immense importance of environmental factors.

REFERENCES

Alexander, M., and M. I. H. Aleem. 1961. Effect of chemical structure on microbial decomposition of aromatic herbicides. Agric. and Food Chem. 9: 44–47.

Audus, L. J. 1960. Microbial breakdown of herbicides. *In* Herbicides and the soil, ed. E. K. Woodford and G. R. Sagar, pp. 1–17. Blackwell Scientific Publications, Oxford.

Audus, L. J., and K. V. Symonds. 1955. Further studies on the breakdown of 2:4-dichlorophenoxyacetic acid by a soil bacterium. Ann. Appl. Biol. 42: 174–182.

Bell, G. R. 1960. Studies on a soil Achromobacter which degrades 2,4-dichlorophenoxyacetic acid. Can. J. Microbiol. 6: 325–337.

Bollen, W. B. 1961. Interaction between pesticides and soil microorganisms. Ann. Rev. Microbiol. 15: 69–92.

Bruinsma, J. 1960. The action of 4,6-dinitro-o-cresol (DNOC) in soil. Plant and Soil 12: 249–258.

Burger, K., J. C. McRae, and M. Alexander. 1962. Decomposition of phenoxyalkyl carboxylic acids. Soil Sci. Soc. Am. Proc. 26: 243–247.

Crafts, A. S. 1961. The chemistry and mode of action of herbicides. Interscience Publishers, New York and London.

Douros, J. D., and J. J. Reid. 1956. Decomposition of certain herbicides by soil microflora. Bacteriol. Proc. 1956: 23–24.

Fletcher, W. W. 1960. The effect of herbicides on the soil micro-organisms. *In* Herbicides and the soil, ed. E. K. Woodford and G. R. Sagar, pp. 20–62. Blackwell Scientific Publications, Oxford.

Gale, E. F. 1951. The chemical activities of bacteria. University Tutorial Press, London.

Guillemat, J., M. Charpentier, P. Tardieux, and J. Pochon. 1960. Interactions entre une chloro-amino-triazine herbicide et la microflore fongique et bactérienne du sol. Ann. Epiphytes 11: 261–290.

Gundersen, K., and H. L. Jensen. 1956. A soil bacterium decomposing organic nitro-compounds. Acta Agr. Scand. 6: 100–114.

Gustafson, M. 1961. Bekämpningsmedelrester i gröda och jord (Residues of pesticides in plants and soil). J. Royal Swedish Acad. Agr. For. Suppl. No. 4.

Hirsch, P., and M. Alexander. 1961. Microbial decomposition of halogenated propionic and acetic acids. Can. J. Microbiol. 6: 241–249.

Jensen, H. L. 1959. Biological decomposition of herbicides in the soil (I). (Danish with English summary.) Tidsskr. Planteavl 63: 470–499.

Jensen, H. L. 1961. Biological decomposition of herbicides in the soil (II). (Danish with English summary.) Tidsskr. Planteavl 65: 185–198.

Kielly, R. 1956. Discussion of paper by A. Nason. *In* A symposium on inorganic nitrogen metabolism, ed. W. D. McElroy and B. Glass, pp. 205–207. Johns Hopkins University Press, Baltimore.

Lehmberg, C. 1956. Untersuchungen über die Wirkung von Ascorbinsäure, Stoffwechselgiften und anderen Faktoren auf den Stoffwechsel von *Clostridium butyricum* Prazm. Arch. Mikrobiol. 24: 323–346.

Magee, L. A., and A. R. Colmer. 1959. Decomposition of 2,2-dichloropropionic acid by soil bacteria. Can. J. Microbiol. 5: 255–260.

Petty, M. R. 1961. An introduction to the origin and biochemistry of microbial halometabolites. Bact. Rev. 25: 111–130.

Postgate, J. R. 1953. The reduction of sulphur compounds by *Desulphovibrio desulphuricans*. J. Gen. Microbiol. 5: 725–738.

Quastel, J. H., and P. G. Scholefield. 1951. Biochemistry of nitrification in soil. Bact. Rev. 15: 1–53.

Radler, F. 1955. Untersuchungen über den Verlauf von Stoffwechselerscheinungen bei *Azotobacter chroococcum* Beij. Arch. Microbiol. 22: 335–367.

CHEMICAL CONTROL OF PLANT PATHOGENIC MICRO-ORGANISMS IN SOIL

C. A. I. GORING

The Dow Chemical Company
Agricultural Chemical Research
Seal Beach, California, U.S.A.

THE HISTORY OF MANKIND teaches us that discovery of disease is soon followed by a search for means of control. The biologist frequently looks for chemicals that can serve this purpose. His assault on plant pathogenic micro-organisms in soil, which has been going on for over two hundred years, has been no exception.

Highly effective disease control agents for application to soil have, however, been developed only within the last fifty years. The progress that has been made can be largely attributed to the growth of organic chemistry which is providing the enormous variety of compounds that are being tested.

The biologist is traditionally concerned not only with the discovery of toxic chemicals, but also with the practical means of contacting and controlling the disease organisms. Many different kinds of compounds are being used (17, 23, 24, 27, 32, 33, 40). Some are very volatile, others are essentially non-volatile. Some are quite soluble in water, others are not. Developing suitable methods of application for each new pesticide has been a very important and continuing task.

The purpose of this presentation is to (*a*) review briefly the history of the current pesticidal arsenal and the important disease problems that are being controlled; (*b*) mention the methods of pesticide application; and (*c*) anticipate future trends.

The chemicals at present being employed can be conveniently, if somewhat arbitrarily, divided into three categories (*a*) the soil disinfectants, (*b*) the nematocides and (*c*) the fungicides.

Soil Disinfectants

Disinfection of soil with chemicals is an old practice (2, 16, 18, 28, 29). The chemicals at present being used include methyl bromide, chloropicrin, sodium methyldithiocarbamate, carbon disulphide, formaldehyde, allyl alcohol, 3,5-dimethyltetrahydro-1,3,5,2H-thiadiazine-2-thione, methyl isothiocyanate and propargyl bromide. Only the first three materials are currently of major importance.

The oldest soil disinfectant of significance is carbon disulphide. In the latter part of the nineteenth century, it was used extensively for control of Phylloxera on grapes in France until the introduction of resistant root-stocks. Over the years it has enjoyed limited use as a soil insecticide and to some extent as a control measure for perennial weeds. It is not a very active nematocide or fungicide but nevertheless has been shown to be effective against *Armillaria* root-rot of citrus and peaches. The control of *Armillaria* was not due to the toxicity of the chemical to the organism, but was the result of antibiotic action by *Trichoderma viride* growing vigorously in the fumigated soil. Because of its low toxicity to most organisms, carbon disulphide never achieved popularity as a fumigant for greenhouse soils.

Chloropicrin was developed during the First World War. Shortly thereafter, many investigators established its high toxicity to many kinds of organisms. It was first used extensively in pineapple soils in Hawaii because it was found to be effective in controlling the disease complex and restoring yields of pineapples. It has since been replaced by better and less expensive fumigants. Currently, it is being applied as a preplant fumigant for various plant beds, floral crops, and especially for control of *Verticillium* on strawberries.

Methyl bromide was employed as a space fumigant in vaults and greenhouses prior to its use as a soil fumigant. In the 1940's, its value as a general eradicant when applied to soil under a plastic cover became generally known and accepted. It is at present being used extensively for this purpose on tobacco, vegetables, forest tree and other plant beds, strawberries, old and new turf areas and planting sites for trees and shrubs.

Sodium methyldithiocarbamate and 3,5-dimethyltetrahydro-1,3,5,2H-thiodiazine-2-thione were being generally tested as early as 1955 and were both shown to be highly effective general biocides. Sodium methyldithiocarbamate is a water-soluble salt which is ordinarily formulated and sold as a liquid concentrate. 3,5-Dimethyltetrahydro-1,3,5,2H-thiadiazine-2-thione is a relatively insoluble solid and is formulated as a water-dispersable material. Both chemicals break down in soil to give various gases including methyl isothiocyanate, a highly toxic fumigant.

Sodium methyldithiocarbamate was intensively tested in two ways: (*a*) when injected into the soil and (*b*) when diluted with water and drenched onto the soil. More reliable results were generally obtained by using the latter method. 3,5-Dimethyltetrahydro-1,3,5,2H-thiadiazine-2-thione is dusted or drenched onto the surface of the soil and then raked in thoroughly. Neither chemical performs as consistently as does methyl bromide. Both chemicals are recommended as disinfectants for ornamental and nursery stock, vegetable plant beds, turf renovation and planting sites for trees and shrubs, but sodium methyldithiocarbamate appears to be the more extensively used.

Formaldehyde has been employed as a seed, soil and space disinfectant for many years. It was first recommended as a dust for control of smut of cereals and then later as a soil drench. Like carbon disulphide, and because of its low activity, it was never used extensively for any purpose in soil.

Allyl alcohol is a somewhat more popular soil disinfectant than formaldehyde. Water solutions of the material are being utilized as drenches for controlling weed seedlings and damping-off in tobacco seed beds. It is often fortified with ethylene dibromide or 1,3-dichloropropene to ensure good nematode control. Actually, allyl alcohol is a good fungicide and nematocide but is ordinarily dissolved and applied in minimal amounts of water and therefore gives pest control only in the surface layers of soil.

Few new soil disinfectants are on the horizon. The appearance of methyl isothiocyanate can be regarded as a development that was inevitable in view of the mode of action of sodium methyldithiocarbamate and 3,5-dimethyltetrahydro-1,3,5,2H-thiadiazine-2-thione. Currently, it is still more or less an experimental chemical. Propargyl bromide is at present being marketed as an ingredient of a fumigant mixture which also contains chloropicrin and methyl bromide. It appears to be the most generally toxic soil fumigant.

Nematocides

The discovery of the nematocidal properties of dichloropropane-dichloropropene mixtures in the early 1940's ushered in a new era in soil fumigation and stimulated a considerable amount of research on nematode control (1, 6, 13, 36, 37). The main active component of the mixture, 1,3-dichloropropene, is highly toxic to plant parasitic nematodes and relatively non-toxic to other organisms. The discovery and development of ethylene dibromide as a nematocide followed shortly thereafter. It is even more toxic to nematodes than 1,3-dichloropropene, but is less toxic to fungi and weed seeds.

The outstanding feature of these two fumigants is that, because of their relatively low volatility and high toxicity to nematodes, they can be applied economically without the use of a plastic cover. They are at present employed as preplant fumigants for the control of most of the important plant parasitic nematodes on a wide variety of crops. Ethylene dibromide is somewhat more specific than 1,3-dichloropropene and is, for example, essentially ineffective on cyst-forming nematodes.

The most recent nematocide of major importance is 1,2-dibromo-3-chloropropane. It was developed in the late 1950's and is not only the most active nematocidal fumigant at present known but is also the first to be used with general success on growing crops. This has been a particularly important development with respect to fruit and vine crops such as citrus, pineapples, bananas and grapes.

The three fumigant chemicals previously described are certainly the nematocides of major importance. However, the development of 0-2,4-dichlorophenyl 0,0-diethyl phosphorothioate in 1955 represented an interesting departure from the soil fumigant type of chemical. It had already been shown that organic phosphorus insecticides such as demeton and parathion were somewhat nematocidal and thus the arrival of 0-2,4-dichlorophenyl 0,0-diethyl phosphorothiate was not entirely unexpected. It was, of course, necessary to mix it with or drench it onto the soil because of its lack of volatility. However, it could be applied around living plants and thus it has found a small niche for itself as a postplant nematocide for certain ornamentals and turf.

As one might suspect, the trail does not end here. In recent years other active organic phosphorus compounds have been sampled and are being developed, for example 0,0-diethyl 0,2-pyrazinyl phosphorothioate. This chemical appears to be much more active than 0-2,4-dichlorophenyl 0,0-diethyl phosphorothioate and has been used successfully in row treatments on certain crops at dosages lower than those used for soil fumigants. It seems likely that in the future new nematocides of this type possessing even greater potency will be developed.

Fungicides

The treatment of seeds with fungicidal chemicals in order to protect them from the ravages of seed- and soil-borne pathogenic micro-organisms while they are germinating is an old practice dating back several hundred years (11, 19, 20, 21, 38). Copper sulphate was the first inorganic chemical that showed real promise for control of cereal smuts. It was followed a hundred years later by formaldehyde, the first organic chemical to be used. Even today copper carbonate is still employed on a limited scale although the industry is now completely dominated by the newer organic materials.

The organic mercurials are the most widely used seed protectants in the current versatile arsenal that also includes tetramethylthiuramdisulphide; N-trichloromethyl mercapto-4-cyclohexene-1,2-dicarboximide; 2,3,5,6-tetrachloro-1,4-benzoquinone; 2,3-dichloro-1,4-naphthoquinone; hexachlorobenzene and pentachloronitrobenzene.

The mercurials are used primarily on wheat, oats, barley, rye, flax, sorghums, rice and cotton. Hexachlorobenzene is used on wheat, and pentachloronitrobenzene on wheat and cotton. The remaining materials are used principally on vegetables and corn.

The principal organisms controlled are the smut fungi on the cereal crops, *Pythium* on corn, *Rhizoctonia* on cotton and *Pythium, Fusarium,* and *Rhizoctonia* on vegetables.

The development of fungicides for soil treatment (16, 18) does not seem to have fared nearly as well as the development of fungicides for seed treatment. All of the chemicals used for seed treatment and some used primarily as foliage fungicides, zinc ethylenebisdithiocarbamate and zinc, iron and manganese salts of dimethyldithiocarbamate, have been extensively tested as soil fungicides with very limited success. Practically speaking, most of the fungicides have been used in soil principally as drenches on turf, seedling flats, and soil for ornamentals.

A chemical that seems to have carved a special niche for itself in soil treatment is pentachloronitrobenzene. Its activity as a fungicide has been known for a long time, but its commercial development has been quite recent. It is highly insoluble in water, essentially non-volatile and stable for long periods in soil. It is quite specific, controlling only certain genera, notably *Sclerotinia, Sclerotium, Rhizoctonia, Streptomyces*, and *Plasmodiophora*. Generally, it is recommended that the material be mechanically mixed with the soil prior to or at the time of planting. However, for control of post-emergence damping-off of cotton, which is its most important use, the material, formulated in combination with N-trichloromethyl mercapto-4-cyclohexene-1,2-dicarboximide as a dust, is mixed with the seed in the hopper box just prior to planting.

METHODS OF APPLICATION

The zone of soil through which plant pathogenic micro-organisms are controlled depends not only on the availability of highly active chemicals but also on the properties of these chemicals and the methods by which they are applied.

Volatile, relatively water-insoluble chemicals such as carbon disulphide, methyl bromide, chloropicrin, 1,3-dichloropropene, ethylene dibromide and 1,2-dibromo-3-chloropropane are usually allowed to disperse themselves through soil. Some of the first applications of carbon disulphide involved injection into holes 20 inches apart or spraying in the furrow while plowing. Hand injection or application has largely given way to application by tractor equipment using pressure or gravity flow delivery from the bottom of a plow or suitably spaced shanks.

The less volatile fumigants such as chloropicrin, 1,3-dichloropropene, 1,2-dibromo-3-chloropropane and ethylene dibromide are usually applied without a soil cover. However, the value of sealing the soil after injection is well recognized and so for some uses (pineapples in Hawaii) partial sealing with tar paper and more recently polyethylene is of considerable value and an established practice.

For a more volatile fumigant such as methyl bromide, a soil cover is mandatory. The chemical was at first introduced into soil by allowing it to vaporize under a raised polyethylene film. Finally a machine was developed that would simultaneously inject the fumigant into the soil and lay a polyethylene film over the soil surface. By eliminating the air space between the ground and the polyethylene film the pesticidal efficiency of the fumigant was approximately doubled.

Using the chemical with maximum efficiency is a most important goal in soil fumigation. Over the years there has been a continuing effort to develop an understanding of all of the factors influencing the efficiency of fumigants. A substantial amount of information has been accumulated, reviewed (1, 5,

6, 13, 16, 27, 28, 29, 36, 37) and welded together into a reasonably comprehensive discussion of the principles of soil fumigation (13).

Suitably formulated fumigants may also be applied to soil in water as may other non-fumigant chemicals. Injected fumigants can give pest control to depths as great as 6–10 feet and are usually expected to give control to a depth of at least 1½–2 feet. Chemicals applied in water seldom penetrate the soil to a depth of more than 3–4 inches per inch of water applied and frequently are sorbed in the surface layers of soil.

Currently, a number of chemicals are being applied to soil in water. 1,2-Dibromo-3-chloropropane is applied postplant to crops such as cotton, citrus and grapes for nematode control. Sodium methyldithiocarbamate and allyl alcohol are being used as soil disinfectants. All three of these chemicals are not highly sorbed by soil and in addition are sufficiently volatile to diffuse through the soil to varying degrees on their own account. The depth to which they give pest control will depend on the dosage and the amount of water in which they are applied but it could be as much as 4–6 inches for every inch of water.

The seed protectant and foliage fungicides that are being applied to soil in water are either so insoluble or so strongly sorbed that their use as drenches invariably involves control of disease organisms in the soil surface. In order to control micro-organisms to various depths beneath the surface, intimate mixing of chemicals of this type with the soil would be required. Even 3,5-dimethyltetrahydro-1,3,5,2H-thiadiazine-2-thione, which decomposes in soil to give a pesticidal fumigant, is sufficiently insoluble and non-volatile that raking it into the soil is recommended to ensure proper treatment.

Intimate mixing of chemicals with soil in the field is a difficult problem mechanically and not a very suitable method for treating much of the soil volume in which plant roots may be expected to grow. When chemicals are mixed into the soil it is usually in the plant row and to a depth of no more than 6 inches. Pentachloronitrobenzene is sometimes applied in this manner.

A simpler method of application is the spraying or dusting of the chemical in the furrow at the time of planting, thus treating an even smaller portion of the soil zone in which the plant will grow. Pentachloronitrobenzene, mixtures of this material with N-trichloromethyl mercapto-4-cyclohexene-1,2-dicarboximide, and zinc ethylenebisdithiocarbamate have been used in this manner to control post-emergence damping-off of cotton. However, even this mode of application has proven to be a burden for the busy cotton farmer at planting time and so mixing the chemical and the seed together in the hopper box, although less effective, now appears to be a more popular practice than spraying or mixing the chemical in the furrow.

The oldest and simplest method of application is the coating of seed with fungicides. This procedure more or less disinfects the seed and at the same time ensures that while it is germinating there is a thin protective barrier between it and the soil. Dust formulations were the first to be used, but later the industry switched to slurry formulations that were somewhat less noxious to handle. At the present time, several of the mercurial formulations are clear, water-dilutable liquids which are applied by machines approaching the ultimate in safety and efficiency.

FUTURE TRENDS

There appears to be general optimism among phytopathologists regarding the probability of discovering much more effective chemicals for control of plant pathogens in soil than those at present used (9, 18, 25, 37). Certainly past success provides a firm basis for such optimism. Nevertheless, the future is not without its problems. It has been forcefully pointed out (39) that the development of an agriculture biocide now costs over $1,000,000 and certainly this figure will go much higher. An investment such as this will ordinarily be made only for a problem of commensurate size. It seems likely that to an increasing extent new chemicals will be developed principally for control of the disease problems of greatest economic importance, and that control of less important disease problems concurrently achieved with these same chemicals could well be fortuitous.

Chemicals of increasing specificity can certainly be anticipated, not just because in many instances this may be a desirable biological characteristic but also because specificity is frequently associated with an unusually high degree of activity against the organism in question. Nevertheless, specificity has its pitfalls. p-Dimethylamino benzenediazosodium sulphonate is specific and highly effective mainly against *Pythium*. It remains to be seen whether control of *Pythium* constitutes a worthwhile target for this seed and soil fungicide. Pentachloronitrobenzene does not control *Pythium* and *Fusarium*. Thus, although *Rhizoctonia* is the primary disease organism attacking cotton seedlings, pentachloronitrobenzene is applied in admixture with N-trichloromethyl mercapto-4-cyclohexene-1,2-dicarboximide which does control *Pythium* and *Fusarium*. Successful specific chemicals will of necessity have to be specific for major targets. Even so they will be used in conjunction with other chemicals where the problem is not a single organism but a complex of many organisms.

It is probable that new seed protectants will loom on the horizon from time to time, but unless they exhibit unique activity (for example, systemic control of early post-emergence diseases) they will not easily replace the present excellent pre-emergence protectants.

Greater progress should be made in discovering more active chemicals suitable for Band application to soil at the time of planting to give early partial control of nematodes, seedling rots caused by *Pythium* and *Rhizoctonia*, basal stem rots caused by *Pythium*, *Phytophthora*, *Fusarium*, *Sclerotinia*, *Helminthosporium*, and *Sclerotium*, and shallow root rots caused by *Aphanomyces*.

However, certain formidable problems constitute a barrier to further progress in controlling the root pathogens such as *Meloidogyne, Pratylenchus, Tylenchulus, Heterodera* and other plant parasitic nematodes as well as *Fusarium, Verticillium, Armillaria, Phytophthora, Phymatotrichum* and other pathogenic fungi that attack plants mainly at soil depths below 3 inches and also throughout the growing season. Treating a few inches of soil to protect the young roots often is inadequate. Usually the organism must be eliminated from a major portion of the soil profile if the root system of the plant is to thrive.

Fumigants appear to be the most practical way to do this job although chemicals that will penetrate the soil when drenched onto it in water may be excellent alternatives. Pre- or postplant application may be feasible. The alternative is a preplant mix with the soil of a highly sorbed or water-insoluble chemical. Mechanically, this is a very difficult type of application.

Significantly, a random selection of organic chemicals will consist of many more of the latter than of the former types, although at this point in history quite the opposite is true as far as commercially useful chemicals for the control of root pathogens are concerned. Unfortunately, it is unlikely that discovery of new valuable fumigants will continue indefinitely. We will surely exhaust the feasible structures in this field first. The search for chemicals that can be applied in water may hold more promise.

To many phytopathologists control of plant disease by chemotherapy is the ultimate goal towards which they are striving and so it is not surprising that a considerable amount of attention has been devoted to this subject (3, 4, 7, 8, 9, 10, 12, 14, 15, 22, 26, 30, 31, 34, 35, 41). Basically there are three ways in which chemotherapeutants might work: (*a*) direct action against the pathogen; (*b*) inactivation of vivotoxins; (*c*) by increasing the resistance of the plant to disease. The latter mechanism of action seems to hold the most promise for a spectacular breakthrough because of the extraordinary sensitivity of various plants to growth regulators, and the subtle biochemical differences that distinguish disease-resistant from susceptible varieties of plants. Applications to soil or foliage are envisaged as feasible means of introducing the chemical into the plant. To date, practical success in this field has been very limited.

If the outlook for new chemicals seems promising, the future for many of the chemicals now in use is even more promising. As farming becomes more intensive with accompanying increases in yields and crop values per acre, the disease problems originating in the soil will assume increasing importance. Treatment of soil for disease control will become a standard agricultural practice on many additional acres. Diseases which are not being controlled now will ultimately fall before the chemical onslaught. The food requirements of mankind are increasing at a staggering pace. It is unlikely that soil diseases will be permitted to stand in the way of fulfilling these requirements.

REFERENCES

1. Allen, M. W. 1960. Nematocides. *In* Plant pathology, vol. 2, The pathogen, ed. J. G. Horsfall and A. E. Dimond, pp. 603–638. Academic Press, Inc., New York and London.
2. Bollen, W. B. 1961. Interaction between pesticides and soil microorganisms. Ann. Rev. Microbiol. *15*: 69–92.
3. Brian, P. W. 1952. Antibiotics as systemic fungicides and bactericides. Ann. Appl. Biol. *39*: 434–438.
4. Brian, P. W. 1957. Effects of antibiotics on plants. Ann. Rev. Plant. Physiol. *8*: 413–426.
5. Burchfield, H. P. 1960. Performance of fungicides on plants and in soil—physical, chemical and biological considerations. *In* Plant pathology, vol. 3, The diseased population, ed. J. G. Horsfall and A. E. Dimond, pp. 447–520. Academic Press, Inc., New York and London.
6. Christie, J. R. 1959. Plant nematodes, their bionomics and control. H. and W. B. Drew Co., Jacksonville, Florida.
7. Crowdy, S. H. 1952. The chemotherapy of plant disease. Empire J. Exptl. Agr. *20*: 187–194.
8. Dickson, J. G. 1959. Chemical control of cereal rusts. Botan. Rev. *25*: 486–513.
9. Dimond, A. E. 1959. Plant chemotherapy. *In* Plant pathology, problems and progress, 1908–1958, ed. C. S. Holton, *et al.*, pp. 221–228. University of Wisconsin Press, Madison.
10. Dimond, A. E., and J. G. Horsfall. 1959. Plant chemotherapy. Ann. Rev. Plant. Physiol. *10*: 257–276.
11. Fischer, G. W., and C. S. Holton. 1957. Biology and control of the smut fungi. Ronald Press Co., New York.
12. Ford, J. H., W. Klomparens and C. L. Hamner. 1958. Cycloheximide (acti-dione) and its agricultural uses. Plant Disease Reptr. *42*: 680–695.
13. Goring, C. A. I. 1962. Theory and principles of soil fumigation. *In* Advances in pest control research, ed. R. L. Metcalf, vol. 5: 47–84. Interscience Publishers, Inc., New York. In press.
14. Horsfall, J. G., and A. E. Dimond. 1951. Plant chemotherapy. Ann. Rev. Microbiol. *5*: 209–222.
15. Howard, F. L., and J. G. Horsfall. 1959. Therapy. *In* Plant pathology, vol. 1, The diseased plant, ed. J. G. Horsfall and A. E. Dimond, pp. 563–604. Academic Press, Inc., New York and London.
16. Kendrick, J. B., Jr., and G. A. Zentmyer. 1957. Recent advances in control of soil fungi. *In* Advances in pest control research, ed. R. L. Metcalf, *1*: 219–275. Interscience Publishers, Inc., New York.
17. van der Kerk, G. J. M. 1959. Chemical structure and fungicidal activity of dithiocarbamic acid derivatives. *In* Plant pathology, problems and progress, 1908–1958, ed. C. S. Holton, *et al.*, pp. 280–290. University of Wisconsin Press, Madison.
18. Kreutzer, W. A. 1960. Soil treatment. *In* Plant pathology, vol. 3, The diseased population, ed. J. G. Horsfall and A. E. Dimond, pp. 431–476. Academic Press, Inc., New York and London.
19. Leukel, R. W. 1936. The present status of seed treatment with special reference to cereals. Botan. Rev. *2*: 498–527.
20. Leukel, R. W. 1948. Recent developments in seed treatment. Botan. Rev. *14*: 235–269.
21. Leukel, R. W. 1953. Treating seeds to prevent diseases. *In* Plant diseases, U.S. Dept. Agr. Yearbook, pp. 134–145.

22. Livingston, J. E., and M. T. Hilborn. 1959. The control of plant diseases by chemotherapy. Econ. Botany *13*: 3–29.
23. Ludwig, R. A., and G. D. Thorn. 1960. Chemistry and mode of action of dithiocarbamate fungicides. *In* Advances in pest control research, ed. R. L. Metcalf, *3*: 219–252. Interscience Publishers, Inc., New York.
24. McCallan, S. E. A., and L. P. Miller. 1958. Innate toxicity of fungicides. *In* Advances in pest control research, ed. R. L. Metcalf, *2*: 108–134. Interscience Publishers, Inc., New York.
25. McNew, G. L. 1959. Landmarks during a century of progress in use of chemicals to control plant diseases. *In* Plant pathology, problems and progress, 1908–1958, ed. C. S. Holton *et al.*, pp. 42–54. University of Wisconsin Press, Madison.
26. Mitchell, J. W., B. C. Smale and R. L. Metcalf. 1960. Absorption and translocation of regulators and compounds used to control plant diseases and insects. *In* Advances in pest control research, ed. R. L. Metcalf, *3*: 359–436. Interscience Publishers, Inc., New York.
27. Moje, W. 1960. The chemistry and nematocidal activity of organic halides. *In* Advances in pest control research, ed. R. L. Metcalf, *3*: 181–217. Interscience Publishers, Inc., New York.
28. Newhall, A. G. 1946. Volatile soil fumigants for plant disease control. Soil Sci. *61*: 67–82.
29. Newhall, A. G. 1955. Disinfestation of soil by heat, flooding and fumigation. Botan. Rev. *21*: 189–250.
30. Pramer, D. 1959. The status of antibiotics in plant disease control. Advances in Appl. Microbiol. *1*: 75–85.
31. Pramer, D. 1959. Discussion of chapter xxi. *In* Plant pathology, problems and progress, 1908–1958, ed. C. S. Holton *et al.*, pp. 229–230. University of Wisconsin Press, Madison.
32. Rich, S. 1960. Fungicidal chemistry. *In* Plant pathology, vol. 2, The pathogen, ed. J. A. Horsfall and A. E. Dimond, pp. 553–602. Academic Press, Inc., New York and London.
33. Sisler, H. D., and C. E. Cox. 1960. Physiology of fungitoxicity. *In* Plant pathology, vol. 2, The pathogen, ed. J. G. Horsfall and A. E. Dimond, pp. 507–552. Academic Press, Inc., New York and London.
34. Stoddard, E. M., and A. E. Dimond. 1949. The chemotherapy of plant diseases. Botan. Rev. *15*: 345–376.
35. Tanner, F. W., Jr., and S. C. Beesch. 1958. Antibiotics and plant diseases. Advances in Enzymol. *20*: 383–406.
36. Taylor, A. L. 1951. Chemical treatment of the soil for nematode control. *In* Advances in agronomy, ed. A. G. Norman, *3*: 243–264. Academic Press, Inc., New York.
37. Taylor, A. L. 1959. Progress in chemical control of nematodes. *In* Plant pathology, problems and progress, 1908–1958, ed. C. S. Holton *et al.*, pp. 427–434. University of Wisconsin Press, Madison.
38. Walker, J. C. 1950. Plant pathology, 1st ed. McGraw-Hill Book Co., Inc., New York.
39. Wellman, R. H. 1959. Commercial development of fungicides. *In* Plant pathology, problems and progress, 1908–1958, ed. C. S. Holton *et al.*, pp. 239–245. University of Wisconsin Press, Madison.
40. Woodcock, D. 1959. The relation of chemical structure to fungicidal activity. *In* Plant pathology, problems and progress, 1908–1958, ed. C. S. Holton *et al.*, pp. 267–279. University of Wisconsin Press, Madison.
41. Zaumeyer, W. J. 1958. Antibiotics in the control of plant diseases. Ann. Rev. Microbiol. *12*: 415–440.

THE USE OF ORGANIC AMENDMENTS AND GREEN MANURES IN THE CONTROL OF SOIL-BORNE PHYTOPATHOGENS

R. H. STOVER

Plant Pathology Department
Vining C. Dunlap Laboratories
Tela Railroad Co., La Lima, Honduras

SINCE THE FIRST REPORTS of suppression of potato scab by antagonistic micro-organisms, there has developed a large literature under the title of "biological control" on the deleterious action of decomposing organic matter on soil-borne pathogens. This subject has been reviewed by Garrett (1939) and Clark (1942) with special reference to take-all disease of wheat and *Phymatotrichum* root-rot of cotton. More recent and extensive reviews are those of Sanford (1946, 1959), Wood and Tveit (1955), Brian (1957, 1960), and Kendrick and Zentmyer (1957). In addition to the above diseases, the following have been suppressed by organic amendments: *Rhizoctonia* on potatoes (reviewed by Sanford, 1946, 1959), lettuce (Wood, 1951), and beans (Davey & Papavizas, 1959, 1960); strawberry root-rot (Hildebrand & West; West & Hildebrand, 1941); *Helminthosporium* and *Fusarium culmorum* root-rots of cereals (Tyner, 1940; Chinn *et al.*, 1953, 1961); *Fusarium* on cotton (Pinckard & Leonard, 1944), beans (Snyder

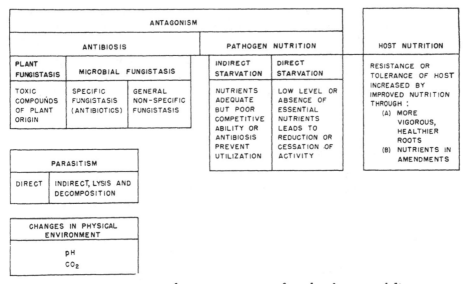

FIG. 1. How organic amendments may suppress fungal pathogens and disease.

et al., 1959; Mitchell & Alexander, 1961), and bananas (Sequeira, 1962; Stover, 1962); *Verticillium* on tomatoes (Wilhelm, 1951); *Phytophthora* on avocado (Zentmyer, 1953); *Aphanomyces* on peas (Davey & Papavizas, 1961).

With the exception of extensive field studies with potato scab, cotton root-rot, and cotton and banana wilts, most observations were made in the laboratory and greenhouse often using amendments in quantities and physical states seldom found under field conditions. Nevertheless, many organic amendments consisting of crop remains or manures do suppress pathogens under field conditions even though practical control of disease in the absence of rotations of several or more years is uncommon.

Undoubtedly amendments in the form of roots and refuse of non-host crops contribute to the frequently successful biological control of fungal pathogens by rotations. Thus, studies of the short-term action of organic amendments, frequently under highly artificial conditions, also contribute to an understanding of disease control by rotations.

MECHANISMS OF CONTROL OF SOIL-BORNE FUNGAL PATHOGENS BY ORGANIC AMENDMENTS

In Fig. 1, I have outlined under three topics—antibiosis, pathogen nutrition, and host nutrition—how organic amendments may suppress pathogen and disease development. Antibiosis was aptly defined by Sanford (1959) as "The complete or partial suppression of the growth or pathogenicity of a pathogen by direct parasitism, by lysis, or by toxic metabolites of associated organisms, or by fungitoxins in the soil." It is one aspect of the general phenomenon of antagonism among soil fungi as discussed by Park (1960). The other major facet of antagonism is microbial influence on pathogen nutrition. In addition to antagonistic factors, host nutrition and root vigor, as influenced by organic amendments, can play a role in suppression of disease.

Antibiosis

Antibiosis resulting from toxic metabolites of microbial origin may be divided into two types: a non-specific widespread soil fungistasis (Dobbs & Hinson, 1953) and a specific fungistasis associated with chemically defined metabolites called antibiotics. Antibiotics are produced in soil in decomposing plant residues, and in situations where manipulation of the soil environment leads to the predominance of a single antibiotic-producing species such as *Trichoderma* (Wright, 1952, 1956; Stevenson, 1956; Brian, 1957). In general, however, attempts to establish specific antibiotic producers on organic amendments in natural soils have been unsuccessful. Nonetheless, with increasingly sensitive bioassay and chromatographic techniques of identification, Wright's demonstration that high concentrations of an antibiotic can be produced in and around particles of organic matter in natural soils will likely be extended to a variety of micro-organisms and soil microhabitats. Also, more information on the chemical and physiological basis of the widespread non-specific soil fungistasis will undoubtedly help to elucidate the role of specific antibiotics in antagonism. Until more information is available, however, the role of chemically defined antibiotics in soil-borne disease control with organic amendments still remains obscure.

The widespread soil fungistasis is associated with the activity of the soil flora (Dobbs *et al.*, 1960; Lingappa & Lockwood, 1961). What role the soil flora associated with decaying organic amendments may have in intensifying or reducing soil fungistasis is unknown. The problem remains of determining whether stimulation of pathogen growth by amendments is due primarily to added nutrients or to a suppression of fungistasis. If, as postulated by Park and Barton (1960), fungistasis is akin to staling in pure cultures, then increased microbial activity should result in increased fungistasis. Lingappa and Lockwood (1961) attributed stimulation of microbial activity in the vicinity of fungal structures as contributing to general soil fungistasis. They presented evidence, based on an assay procedure using water agar, that a reserve of fungitoxins was not maintained in soils; fungistasis was dependent on stimulation of microbial growth on the assay substrate and diffusion of the fungistatic metabolites through layers of agar or synthetic films. The possibility of the inactivation or adsorption by water agar of certain fungitoxins demonstrated by others to be present in the soil solution was not considered.

Since fungistasis is associated with microbial activity, it is likely that some types of amendments could increase fungistasis more than others and thus account for differing pathogen response. However, with the high levels of available nutrients in some amendments, fungistasis may no longer be adequate or develop rapidly enough to prevent a germination level of assimilation. Germination could then occur while microbial activity was still in the relatively low–fungitoxin or low–antibiotic lag phase. In addition Park (1960) has suggested that "the amendment provides a fresh physical substratum in which there is no accumulated level of antibiotic substances."

Antibiosis may also involve fungistatic organic compounds of plant origin released into the soil by leaching and decay (Winter, 1955).

Antibiosis may result from pathogen sensitivity to increased carbon dioxide levels (Garrett, 1939; Blair, 1943) or changes in the pH especially in microhabitats associated with amendments. It is unlikely that these factors would be critical in the dormant stage. During germination and active growth, however, retardation might be sufficient to allow competitors to dominate.

Direct parasitism as typified by *Trichoderma* and other fungi attacking and colonizing *Rhizoctonia* (Boosalis, 1956) is of less significance in comparison with the general and widespread lysis of soil fungi by bacteria and actinomycetes (King *et al.*, 1934; Chudiakov, 1935; Park, 1956; Carter and Lockwood, 1957). Although hyphae are much more susceptible to lysis than dormant spores, even the latter can be destroyed (Subramanian, 1946; Park, 1956). There is considerable evidence that lysis is increased by decomposing organic amendments. Direct observations (Mitchell *et al.*, 1941; Subramanian, 1946; Chinn *et al.*, 1953; Park, 1956) and the recent work on the role of sucrose and sugarcane (Sequeira, 1962) and chitin (Mitchell and Alexander, 1961) in suppressing fusarial wilts indicate that disease suppression is associated with pathogen destruction by bacteria- and actinomycete-induced lysis. Large structures such as sclerotia and rhizomorphs are also decomposed (King *et al.*, 1934; Mitchell *et al.*, 1941).

Pathogen Nutrition

Organic amendments frequently provide sufficient nutrients to stimulate germination of resting structures (Mitchell *et al.*, 1941; Chinn *et al.*, 1953). Germ tubes and hyphae are more sensitive to antibiosis than spores or sclerotia. Indeed, antibiosis may even be intensified by stimulation of microbial activity on and around the hyphae (Novogrudsky, 1948). The development of resting spores or infection processes may cease after germination because of their inability to compete successfully for nutrients or, more likely, susceptibility to increasing toxic metabolites and lysis associated with the flora of decomposing amendments. Inability to compete because of an inherently slow rate of assimilation or because of reduced efficiency in assimilation as a result of fungitoxins is an indirect form of starvation.

Although there are likely sufficient nutrients in the soil solution to maintain resting structures (Park, 1960), deficiencies could easily develop when dormancy is broken. Resting structures are often imbedded in debris or root and stem fragments in various stages of decay. It is conceivable that the flora associated with these decaying substrates could deplete nitrogen or some other essential compound *in the vicinity of the germinating spore* to such an extent that the pathogen is critically weakened by starvation. The amount and type of nitrogen sometimes determine whether pathogens are stimulated or suppressed by amendments (Wilhelm, 1951; Garrett, 1956, p. 158; Snyder *et al.*, 1959; Papavizas & Davey, 1961). However, the role of competition *per se* for nitrogen and other nutrients, and of fungitoxins or antibiotics in pathogen behavior cannot easily be separated. Nutrient levels may be critical, mainly in the sense that they determine whether reproduction and/or pathogenesis will proceed in the presence of fluctuating levels of fungitoxins. Brown's (1922) tenet that inhibitory substances have their greatest effect when the energy of growth is small and increasing nutrients may enable an organism to overcome fungistasis is basic to an understanding of antibiosis phenomena associated with organic amendments. Even after a growth-inhibiting level of fungistasis is overcome by added nutrients, the pathogen must quickly conclude reproduction, colonization or infection before the level again becomes inhibiting.

Competition for nutrients where fungistasis is not the controlling factor cannot always be invalidated as a cause of antibiosis as suggested by Park (1960). The development of a vigorous thallus requires an optimum nutrient level and if certain nutrients or growth factors become limiting, a slow-growing, weak thallus will result. Certainly a weak thallus is more prone to destruction or failure in pathogenesis than its robust, well-fed counterpart.

Host Nutrition

The addition of organic amendments, especially stable manures, can reduce disease by improving the health and vigor of the host. Thus, Stumbo *et al.* (1942) and Clark (1942) stressed the influence of nitrogen present in manure on the host rather than on the pathogen. Improved host nutrition increased resistance or tolerance to *Ophiobolus graminis*. Similarly, Pinckard and Leonard (1944) attributed the tolerance of heavily manured cotton to fusarial wilt infection to improved host nutrition. Even a partial reduction in pathogenic activity that may not be reflected in above-ground symptoms could increase root vigor resulting in increased metabolic activity and resistance to infection.

Organic amendments may also be detrimental to host nutrition and vigor by injuring the root system (Cochrane, 1949), thereby reducing resistance to pathogen attacks.

WHY ORGANIC AMENDMENTS USUALLY FAIL TO PROVIDE DISEASE CONTROL

Failure of organic amendments to provide disease control can be attributed to the following: (i) lack of contact betwen pathogen and amendment due to uneven distribution; (ii) the short duration of peak biological activity in decomposing organic matter; (iii) protection of the pathogen within host tissue and debris; (iv) variation in soils; (v) increase of disease by some amendments.

Perhaps the greatest problem in attempting to control disease by soil amendments is the difficulty of achieving adequate contact between the pathogen and the amendment. Even assuming pathogen distribution in the top 12 inches of the soil profile (it is frequently much deeper), the tremendous soil mass involved creates formidable problems. Hulbert and Menzel (1953) showed that two operations with a rotary tiller were necessary to mix the soil uniformly to a 6-inch depth. Plowing left most of the tracer material used in the lower part of the tilled section. Even with uniform mixing, a large volume of soil and debris particles would not be in close contact with amendment particles.

When organic amendments are mixed with soil, peak microbial activity is reached and declines within one or two months. Repeated sowings of susceptible crops in amended soil have shown that any benefit to the first crop is much reduced or non-existent with subsequent crops. Thus, intensified antagonism is associated with the peak period of biological decomposition. Escape from and tolerance of this relatively short period of intense antagonism is too general to yield adequate or prolonged disease control.

Many soil-borne pathogens are harbored within pieces of root, stems, and organic debris. Presumably survivors within this material have reached a *modus vivendi* with their neighbors which provides some protection and buffering from a surrounding antagonistic flora. Thus, many pathogens escape the action of temporarily intensified antagonism.

Individual crops are frequently grown over a range of soil conditions differing physically, chemically, and biologically. Thus, as amply demonstrated with potato scab, control measures effective in one soil type or location are ineffective in another owing to one or more limiting soil factors that preclude the development of a sufficiently antagonistic flora.

Although most organic amendments suppress or have no effect on pathogen activity, there are examples of pathogen stimulation, sometimes attributed to the addition of readily utilizable nitrogen present in green plant residues (Boyle, 1956; Davey & Papavizas, 1959; Snyder *et al.*, 1959).

ELUCIDATING THE ACTION OF ORGANIC AMENDMENTS IN DISEASE CONTOL

Evidence to date indicates that the major factors involved in pathogen suppression by organic amendments are: (i) germination is stimulated but the pathogen starves through inherent or fungistasis-induced inability to compete for or rapidly assimilate ephemeral nutrients; (ii) microbial lysis and decomposition is increased, sometimes as a result of germination of resting structures; (iii) amendment decay results in an increase in general fungistasis and antibiotics. All of these factors are interrelated and dependent on nutritional stimulation of microbial activity. Plant residues provide such stimulation. A better understanding of what takes place after incorporation of amendments requires a co-ordinated approach by soil microbiologists, plant pathologists, and biochemists. More intensive rather than extensive observations are needed. Multiple techniques of *direct observations* of organic debris and soil microhabitats (Stevenson, 1956; Chesters, 1960; Tribe, 1960) should be accompanied by increasingly sensitive bioassays and chromatographic analyses. Direct observation should also be supplemented with floral studies of various successions in organic amendments. The "antibiotic-index" (McGahen, 1951) of the changing flora should be related to pathogen behavior rather than disease incidence. All aspects of pathogen response to a changing microhabit need study, especially the relative prevalence of dormant and active stages, not just the amount of population or disease decline. Combined microbiological-biochemical studies would help to define mechanisms of lysis (auto- or heterolysis) and the role of exoenzymes, antibiotics and other products of microbial growth. If investigations of broad floral changes and disease incidence involving a multiplicity of amendments or cropping practices in a variety of soils were channeled into an intensive microbiological-biochemical study of one or two contrasting amendments in natural soil under defined conditions, much greater progress would be made in understanding why pathogens are or are not controlled by organic amendments.

REFERENCES

Barton, R. 1960. Antagonism amongst some sugar fungi. *In* The ecology of soil fungi, pp. 160–167. Liverpool Univ. Press.

Blair, I. D. 1943. Behaviour of the fungus *Rhizoctonia solani* Kühn in the soil. Ann. Appl. Biol. *30*: 118–127.

Boyle, Lytton. 1956. The role of saprophytic media in the development of southern blight and root rot on peanuts. Phytopath. Abst. *46*: 7.

Boosalis, M. 1956. Effect of soil temperature and green-manure amendment of unsterilized soil on parasitism of *Rhizoctonia solani* by *Penicillium vermiculatum* and *Trichoderma* sp. Phytopathology *46*: 473–478.

Brian, P. W. 1957. The ecological significance of antibiotic production. Microbial Ecology Symposium, Soc. Gen. Microbiol., pp. 168–188. Cambridge Univ. Press.

Brian, P. W. 1960. Antagonistic and competitive mechanisms limiting survival and activity of fungi in soil. *In* The ecology of soil fungi, pp. 115–127. Liverpool Univ. Press.

Brown, W. 1922. On the germination and growth of fungi at various temperatures and in various concentrations of oxygen and carbon dioxide. Ann. Bot. N.S. *36*: 257–283.

Carter, H. P., and J. L. Lockwood. 1957. Lysis of fungi by soil micro-organisms and fungicides including antibiotics. Phytopathology *47*: 154–158.

Chesters, C. G. C. 1960. Certain problems associated with the decomposition of soil organic matter by fungi. *In* The ecology of soil fungi, pp. 223–228. Liverpool Univ. Press.

Chinn, S. H. F., R. J. Ledingham, B. J. Sallans and P. M. Simmonds. 1953. A mechanism for the control of common rootrot of wheat. Phytopathology *43*: 701.

Chinn, S. H. F., and R. J. Ledingham. 1961. Mechanisms contributing to the eradication of spores of *Helminthosporium sativum* from amended soil. Can. J. Bot. *39*: 739–748.

Chudiakov, J. P. 1935. The lytic action of soil bacteria on parasitic fungi. Microbiologia *4*: 193–204.

Clark, F. E. 1942. Experiments toward the control of the take-all disease of wheat and the *Phymatotrichum* root rot of cotton. U.S. Dept. Agr. Tech. Bull. 835.

Cochrane, V. W. 1949. Crop residues as causative agents of root rots of vegetables. Conn. Agr. Exp. Sta. Bull. 526.

Davey, C. B., and G. C. Papavizas. 1959. Effect of organic soil amendments on the *Rhizoctonia* disease of snap beans. Agron. J. *51*: 493–496.

Davey, C. B., and G. C. Papavizas. 1960. Effect of dry mature plant materials and nitrogen on *Rhizoctonia solani* in soil. Phytopathology *50*: 522–525.

Davey, C. B., and G. C. Papavizas. 1961. Aphanomyces root rot of peas as affected by organic and mineral soil amendments. Phytopathology *51*: 131.

Dobbs, C. G., and L. H. Hinson. 1953. A widespread fungistasis in soils. Nature *172*: 197–199.

Dobbs, C. G., W. H. Hinson and Joan Bywater. 1960. Inhibition of fungal growth in soils. *In* The ecology of soil fungi, pp. 130–147. Liverpool Univ. Press.

Garrett, S. D. 1939. Soil-borne fungi and the control of root disease. Imp. Bur. Soil Sci. Tech. Comm. 38.

Garrett, S. D. 1956. Biology of root-infecting fungi. Cambridge Univ. Press.

Hildebrand, A. A., and P. M. West. 1941. Strawberry root rot in relation to microbiological changes induced in root rot soil by the incorporation of certain cover crops. Can. J. Res. C19: 183–198.

Hulbert, W. C., and R. G. Menzel. 1953. Soil mixing characteristics of tillage implements. Agr. Engin. 34: 702–708.

Kendrick, J. B., Jr., and G. A. Zentmyer. 1957. Recent advances in control of soil fungi. *In* Advances in pest control research, ed. R. L. Metcalf, 1:219–275. Interscience Pub. Inc., New York.

King, C. J., C. Hope, and E. O. Eaton. 1934. Some microbiological activities affected in manurial control of cotton root rot. J. Agr. Res. 49: 1093–1107.

Lingappa, B. T., and J. L. Lockwood. 1961. The nature of the widespread soil fungistasis. J. Gen. Microbiol. 26: 473–485.

McGahen, J. W. 1951. Soil amendments in relation to the actinomycete population and the antibiotic index of sugar-cane soil. Phytopath. Abst. 41: 25.

Mitchell, R. B., D. R. Hooton and F. E. Clark. 1941. Soil bacteriological studies on the control of the *Phymatotrichum* root rot of cotton. J. Agr. Res. 63: 535–547.

Mitchell, R., and M. Alexander. 1961. The mycolytic phenomenon and biological control of *Fusarium* in soil. Nature 190:110.

Mitchell, R., and M. Alexander. 1961. Chitin and the biological control of *Fusarium* diseases. Plant Disease Reptr. 45: 487–490.

Novogrudsky, D. M. 1948. The colonization of soil bacteria on fungal hyphae. Mikrobiologia 17: 28–35.

Papavizas, G. C., and C. B. Davey. 1960. *Rhizoctonia* disease of bean as affected by decomposing green plant materials and associated microfloras. Phytopathology 50: 516–522.

Papavizas, G. C., and C. B. Davey. 1961. Saprophytic behaviour of *Rhizoctonia* in soil. Phytopathology 51: 693–699.

Park, D. 1956. Effect of substrate on a microbial antagonism, with special reference to soil conditions. Trans. Brit. Myc. Soc. 39: 239–259.

Park, D. 1960. Antagonism—the background to soil fungi. *In* The ecology of soil fungi, pp. 148–159. Liverpool Univ. Press.

Pinckard, J. A., and O. A. Leonard. 1944. Influence of certain soil amendments on the yield of cotton affected by the Fusarium-Heterodera complex. Agron. J. 36: 829–843.

Sanford, G. B. 1946. Soil-borne diseases in relation to the microflora associated with various crops and soil amendments. Soil Sci. 61: 9–21.

Sanford, G. B. 1959. Root-disease fungi as affected by other soil organisms. *In* Plant Pathology, Problems and Progress, 1908–1958, ed. C. S. Holton *et al.*, pp. 367–376. University of Wisconsin Press.

Sequeira, Luis. 1962. Influence of organic amendments on survival of *Fusarium oxysporum* f. *cubense* in the soil. Phytopathology 52: 976–982.

Snyder, W. C., M. W. Schroth and T. Christou. 1959. Effect of plant residues on root rot of bean. Phytopathology 49: 755–756.

Stevenson, I. L. 1956. Antibiotic activity of actinomycetes in soil as demonstrated by direct observation techniques. J. Gen. Microbiol. 15: 372–380.

Stover, R. H. 1962. Fusarial wilt (Panama disease) of bananas and other Musa species. Phytopathological Paper No. 4. Commonwealth Mycological Institute, Kew.

Stumbo, C. R., P. L. Gainey and F. E. Clark. 1942. Microbiological and nutritional factors in the take-all disease of wheat. J. Agr. Res. 64: 653–665.

Subramanian, C. V. 1946. Some factors affecting growth and survival of *Fusarium vasinfectum* Atk., the cotton wilt pathogen, in the soil with special reference to microbiological antagonism. J. Indian Bot. Soc. *25*: 89–101.

Tribe, H. T. 1960. Decomposition of buried cellulose film, with special reference to the ecology of certain soil fungi. *In* The ecology of soil fungi, pp. 246–256. Liverpool Univ. Press.

Tyner, L. E. 1940. The effect of crop debris on the pathogenicity of cereal root-rotting fungi. Can. J. Res. C*18*: 289–306.

West, P. M., and A. A. Hildebrand. 1941. The microbiological balance of strawberry root rot soil as related to the rhizosphere and decomposition effects of certain cover crops. Can. J. Res. C*19*: 199–210.

Wilhelm, S. 1951. Effect of various soil amendments on the inoculum potential of the *Verticillium* wilt fungus. Phytopathology *41*: 684–690.

Winter, G. 1955. Untersuchungen über Vorkommen und Bedeutung von antimikrobiellen und antiphytotischen Substanzen. Z. Planzenern., Düng., Bodenkunde *69*: 224–233.

Wood, R. K. S. 1951. The control of diseases of lettuce by the use of antagonistic organisms. II. The control of *Rhizoctonia solani* Kühn. Ann. Appl. Biol. *38*: 217–230.

Wood, R. K. S., and M. Tveit. 1955. Control of plant diseases by use of antagonistic organisms. Botan. Rev. *21*: 441–492.

Wright, J. M. 1952. Production of gliotoxin in unsterilized soil. Nature *170*: 673.

Wright, J. M. 1956. The production of antibiotics in soil. III. Production of gliotoxin in wheatstraw buried in soil. IV. Production of antibiotics in coats of seeds sown in soil. Ann. Appl. Biol. *44*: 461–466, 561–566.

Zentmyer, G. A. 1953. Diseases of the avocado. U.S. Dept. Agr. Yearbook: 875–881.

CONTROL OF PHYTOPATHOGENIC MICRO-ORGANISMS IN SOIL BY MANAGEMENT PRACTICES

KENNETH F. BAKER

Department of Plant Pathology
University of California
Berkeley, California, U.S.A.

IN THE EARLY DEVELOPMENT of agriculture, control of plant disease depended largely on empirical management practices, owing to lack of information and funds. Because of the drawbacks inherent in such unsophisticated controls (Stevens, 1960), the emphasis shifted to chemicals and disease resistance as soon as knowledge and economics permitted, and interest in management practices accordingly declined (Stevens, 1940). The success of these measures has led subtly to the unwarranted assumption by many plant pathologists that disease control by altered cultural practices has been outgrown or is unimportant. The fact that there is usually nothing to sell in management practices, whereas massive promotional organizations are behind chemicals, has intensified this prevalent idea. Furthermore, it is difficult for extension workers to promote the control of a disease by management practices because this usually requires intimate knowledge of the life history of the pathogen and its predisposing environmental conditions. As a result, control by altered culture is utilized more in forest pathology (because often little else can be done, for physical and economic reasons), cereal pathology (because the low economic return restricts other methods), and pathology of ornamentals (because the environment can be controlled, and returns justify the expense), than in the pathology of fruits or vegetables.

This modern lack of appreciation of management practices ignores several phytopathological axioms:

(*a*) The probability of dependable control of a plant disease is progressively enhanced by application of several varied procedures; only rarely is a single technique continuously satisfactory. In terms of the old adage, don't put all your eggs in one basket. Van der Plank (1960) has provided a mathematical basis for this fact with respect to the accumulative effect of several control procedures. The supplemental controls are usually management practices.

(*b*) A plant disease always involves a variable host and its unpredictable environment, usually also an adaptable parasite, and sometimes a mobile insect. Control methods are known which operate through each of these factors, and should be concurrently used when applicable. The resistance of the host may be increased. Once the critical factors of the environment are known, they may be increased or decreased by management practice. Chemicals may be used to destroy or inhibit the parasite or control the vector.

(c) The environment of the plant includes many physical and biological factors, each of the critical ones supplying one or more possibilities for disease control by management practices. Potential control procedures by altered culture are thus both numerous and varied.

(d) The host and the soil are, in the last analysis, the sources of inoculum of plant pathogens, and the soil is the ultimate reservoir of them (Baker, 1962). Control procedures should include measures aimed at these primary sources of inoculum.

(e) The elimination of a pathogen from a given site or location is frequently better and less costly than constantly combating it (Baker, 1957). This axiom has been effectively applied by many nurseries and is the basis for production of pathogen-free propagules.

SOIL MICRO-ORGANISMS

Although the soil population consists of many species of micro-organisms, only relatively few may be actively growing at any given period. Most of the time they are dormant, then they pass quite rapidly through a growth phase, formation of resting structures, and back into dormancy. Whether the growth phase occurs at any given time is determined by (a) the genetic potentiality and level of vigor of the micro-organism, (b) the available organic and inorganic substrates, (c) the physical environment, particularly soil moisture, temperature, carbon dioxide and oxygen level, and pH, and (d) the associated micro-organisms which may compete for substrate, produce antibiotics, or be parasitic. Three of these four factors may be strikingly affected by cultural practices.

Most of the management practices for control of root disease are aimed at the period of active growth of the pathogen. For example, controlling the amount and time of irrigation, use of mixed plantings as opposed to monoculture, roguing of diseased plants, trenching around infested spots, growing crops on raised beds, altering pH of soil, using proper methods of applying nitrogen fertilizer, use of trap crops, alteration of time or place of planting, poisoning of stumps, and production of plants with strong root systems, are effective in the period of germination of resting bodies and subsequent growth of the fungus. On the other hand, modified forest cutting practices and elimination of surface debris are aimed more at the period of cessation of growth and slow or rapid formation of resistant structures. Crop rotation, flood fallowing, and deep plowing are aimed at the dormant micro-organism.

Have we overlooked weak spots in the life cycle of root pathogens during the time of declining vigor and dormancy? During the period of decreasing growth and development of resting bodies there is a sharp decline in the number of viable units of a pathogen. The cessation of growth from exhaustion of nutrients or intervention of unfavorable environment is accompanied by rapid decline of antibiotic production and corresponding rapid destruction of mycelia and conidia of fungi, for example. Resting structures are produced, and the number of these promptly begins to decline from microbial attack (Burges, 1958). Application of materials (e.g., nitrogen and readily decomposable organic matter) to stimulate antagonistic microorganism activity should be at the time growth of the pathogen ceases, or just before the host is replanted and dormancy again broken. These would often be the periods of greatest vulnerability and lowest population, respectively, of the pathogen. It is usually just before planting that chemical treatments are applied to soil, and this may well contribute to their successful use. In the period just after harvest, when resting bodies are being formed, usually nothing is done to decrease inoculum.

Probably the eventual answer to the control of root diseases will be found in mild treatment of the soil, greater emphasis on management practices which minimize development of any pathogen that escapes and which favor saprogens, and planting with pathogen-free propagules which are as resistant as practicable. Some management practices have been reviewed by Burges (1958), Newhall (1955), and Stevens (1960).

EFFECT OF MANAGEMENT PRACTICES

Management practices for control of root diseases are frequently tried without careful analysis of what the fundamental objective of the practice may be. Crop rotation, one of the commonest and oldest cultural controls, seems often to be based on the reasoning that, since the parasite attacks the host, in the absence of the host it will die out and the crop may then be replanted. This oversimplification ignores the fact, for example, that the pathogen may live, without producing symptoms, in the roots of other crops or weeds (*Verticillium alboatrum* on nightshade in strawberry fields—Wilhelm, 1961) or in the rhizosphere of unrelated plants (*Pseudomonas tabaci* of tobacco—Valleau *et al.*, 1943), or that the resting structures may be extremely resistant in some conditions (*Verticillium alboatrum* in California), or that the beneficial effect may be from trapping action of the alternate crop (*Crotalaria spectabilis* in peach orchards—Mcbeth & Taylor, 1944). These and other variables have contributed to the frequently inconclusive results from crop rotation. When properly applied, rotation forces the parasite to compete with the saprophytic flora or to remain in a state of dormancy, and in either case its population declines. If means could be found to cause resting bodies to break dormancy during the rotation, would its effectiveness be greatly increased? The chemical stimulus to hatching of

Heterodera rostochiensis cysts (Franklin, 1951) suggests that it may have a wider application.

The use of trap crops was for many years based on the idea that a highly susceptible host should be planted, to be removed and destroyed once the nematodes had entered it. Since this entailed the danger that delay or poor timing would permit an actual increase of inoculum, the method never caught on. Barrons (1939) discovered that nematodes penetrated resistant about as well as they did susceptible roots but failed to complete their cycle in the uncongenial host. Mcbeth and Taylor (1944) demonstrated that *Crotalaria spectabilis* greatly reduced the population of root knot nematode and even decreased host injury when interplanted in peach orchards. Although efforts in this direction ceased when low-cost nematocides were developed, the method may yet prove useful in special cases.

Rigolen is an old practice of Dutch bulb growers which involves inverting, by hand spading, the top 30–36 inches of soil immediately after digging the bulbs and applying manure. This is done every third year, or oftener if soil-borne disease has been found (Drayton, 1929). It is not known whether control results simply by moving the inoculum below the root zone, from increased moisture from the relatively high water table, from altered gas exchange, or from antagonistic micro-organisms. The same basic method, mechanized by large plows, has recently been utilized for control of mint Verticillium in Indiana (Green, 1958).

AERATED STEAM

There has been increasing and wider use of chemical soil treatment for control of root pathogens during the last thirty years. The first materials to be generally used (e.g., chloropicrin and methyl bromide) were wide-spectrum lethal fumigants which destroyed most of the soil micro-organisms. It was soon apparent that the enhanced development of any reintroduced pathogen (recontamination) was the central problem in the use of such treatments. Emphasis is shifting from the development and use of treatments which destroy most of the micro-organisms to those which kill or inhibit pathogens, with minimal effect on saprogenous micro-organisms (Baker, 1961, 1962). We have, then, come nearly full circle in our thinking, and the gap is slowly closing between the use of chemicals and management practices. The definition of management as the "judicious use of means to accomplish an end; guidance by careful or delicate treatment" accurately presents this new approach.

Heat treatment of soil is undergoing similar moderation. Although it was realized that soil treatment with steam at 212 F for 30 minutes was unnecessarily drastic, the only way to obtain a lower temperature was by heating continuously moving soil, a costly and restrictive method. With the development and use of aerated steam treatment (Baker, 1957; Baker &

Olsen, 1960; Baker, 1962), it became possible to treat soil at any desired temperature. The 212 F temperature of the water vapor (steam) is lowered by dilution with air which has been moisture-saturated from evaporation of water drops carried in the steam. The space between molecules of B.t.u.-carrying water vapor is increased, and the condensation point lowered accordingly. Therefore, the soil is heated to the temperature determined by the ratio, air : steam, of the mixture, and does not increase with time. Aerated steam moves through soil in the same manner and velocity as regular steam and with equal or better thermal efficiency. Exposure to 140 F for 30 minutes now seems approximately right, as the following effects indicate: (*a*) Plant pathogenic fungi, nematodes, bacteria, and most viruses are destroyed. (*b*) Saprogenic micro-organisms sustain minimal reduction. Many of the residual ones are antagonistic to pathogens, and tend to reduce the activity of parasites accidentally reintroduced. The dormancy of ascospores of some saprophytic fungi is broken by treatment at 140 F, and the number of these antagonistic fungi in the soil is thus increased. (*c*) The phytotoxicity of some soils following steaming at 212 F seems to be prevented by treatment at 140 F. This toxicity can be avoided in container culture by choice of inert growing media, but for field use the treatment must not produce toxins. This obstacle to field steaming is thus removed. (*d*) The cost of treatment is greatly reduced, since the temperature is increased only about half as much. A second obstacle to field steaming is thus removed.

Obviously, the margin of safety for effective treatment is reduced from that at 212 F, and final recommendation of temperature must await further study. However, at least six commercial nurseries in Australia have been using aerated steam at 140–150 F in vaults and pipe-grid boxes for nearly a year, with excellent results. Recontamination, toxicity, and cost have been reduced. Aerated steam has been applied to field soil in California with a moving steam blade, but tests to determine the practical effects have yet to be made.

The studies thus far indicate that the aerated steam technique may answer the drawbacks that have largely restricted 212 F steam to use in containers.

PATHOGEN-FREE PROPAGULES

Seeds, bulbs, transplants, and other propagules are one of the most common media for infesting soil with root pathogens. The more nearly sterile the soil, the greater is the injury from the contaminant pathogens on the propagule. Ferguson (1958) showed that inoculum of *Fusarium oxysporum* f. *gladioli* added to pathogen-free gladiolus corms was much more effective in augmenting disease following planting than greater amounts added to either steamed or raw soil. Furthermore, planting infected corms in treated soil gave greater disease than planting in raw soil.

Methods for obtaining and maintaining pathogen-free propagules are beyond the scope of this paper, and have been reviewed elsewhere (Baker & Committee, 1956; Baker, 1957). The important point here is that the use of pathogen-free stock is highly significant in the control of root disease. The planting of pathogen-free propagules in clean soil, and the application of management practices (e.g., sanitation) to keep them in that state, will ensure freedom from root diseases (Baker, 1957). The addition of even a modest level of host resistance will strengthen the protection. Even if one of the practices is not perfectly executed (e.g., a few propagules carry the pathogen, or a few bits of inoculum in the soil escaped destruction), the other restrictive measures will minimize the losses. This is the value of applying multiple control measures.

EPILOGUE

The proper utilization of management practices in control of root disease has been handicapped by a tendency to test each of them as a complete control in itself, rather than as supplemental to other procedures. The accumulative effect of several modest procedures might well be as great as, and probably much more stable than, a single, wide-spectrum, lethal soil fungicide. There is excessive preoccupation today with single-shot control procedures, and many excellent supplemental practices are probably discarded because they failed in solo tests. After all, the individual voices in a chorus need not have solo quality or volume to produce an excellent concert. If a fraction of the expense and effort now devoted to developing effective fungicidal controls for root diseases under any environmental condition was spent on studies of combinations of fugicidal treatment of soil with management practices, and perhaps a modest level of resistance, greater progress would be made.

Most management practices are the reverse image of the effect of some environmental factor on the incidence of root disease. Thus, water-mold root rots, favored by very wet soils, may be decreased in severity by reduced irrigation, use of raised beds, or improved drainage. Increased emphasis on the biology and ecology of the parasitic and saprophytic micro-organisms involved in a root disease might indicate new means of control by altered culture. If these were tested in conjunction with other procedures, better and more reliable control might be attained. Furthermore, this analytical approach might be more fun than fungicide testing!

REFERENCES

Baker, K. F., and Committee. 1956. Development and production of pathogen-free propagative material of ornamental plants. Plant Dis. Rep. Suppl. 238: 57–95.

Baker, K. F. (editor). 1957. The U.C. system for producing healthy container-grown plants. Calif. Agr. Exp. Sta. Manual 23: 1–332.

Baker, K. F., and C. M. Olsen. 1960. Aerated steam for soil treatment (Abstract). Phytopathology 50: 82.

Baker, K. F.   1961.   Control of root-rot diseases. Proc. IX Internat'l Bot. Congress *1*: 486–490.

Baker, K. F.   1962.   Principles of heat treatment of soil and planting material. J. Austral. Inst. Agr. Sci. *28*: 118–126.

Barrons, K. C.   1939.   Studies on the nature of root knot resistance. J. Agr. Res. *58*: 263–272.

Burges, A.   1958.   Micro-organisms in the soil. Hutchinson and Co., London. 188 pp.

Drayton, F. L.   1929.   Bulb growing in Holland and its relation to disease control. Sci. Agr. *9*: 494–509.

Ferguson, J.   1958.   Reducing plant disease with fungicidal soil treatment, pathogen-free stock, and controlled microbial colonization. Thesis, Univ. of Calif., Berkeley. (Also in Phytopathology *45*: 693.)

Franklin, M. T.   1951.   The cyst-forming species of Heterodera. Commonwealth Agr. Bur., Farnham Royal. 147 pp.

Green, R. J.   1958.   "Deep plowing" for controlling Verticillium wilt of mint in muck soils. Phytopathology *48*. 575–577.

Mcbeth, C. W., and A. L. Taylor.   1944.   Immune and resistant cover crops valuable in root-knot-infested peach orchards. Proc. Am. Soc. Hort. Sci. *45*: 158–166.

Newhall, A. G.   1955.   Disinfestation of soil by heat, flooding and fumigation. Botan. Rev. *21*: 189–250.

Stevens, N. E.   1940.   Recent trends in plant disease control. Trans. Illinois State Acad. Sci. *33*: 66–67.

Stevens, R. B.   1960.   Cultural practices in disease control. *In* Plant pathology, ed. J. A. Horsfall and A. E. Dimond, 3: 357–429. Academic Press, Inc., New York and London.

Valleau, W. D., E. M. Johnson, and S. Diachun.   1943.   Angular leafspot and wildfire of tobacco. Kentucky Agr. Exp. Sta. Bull. *454*: 1–60.

van der Plank, J. E.   1960.   Analysis of epidemics. *In* Plant pathology, ed. J. A. Horsfall and A. E. Dimond, 3: 229–289. Academic Press, Inc., New York and London.

Wilhelm, S.   1961.   Diseases of strawberry. Calif. Agr. Exp. Sta. Circ. *494*: 1–26.

THE ROLE OF MICRO-ORGANISMS
IN PLANT LIFE

N. A. KRASSILNIKOV

Institute of Microbiology, Academy of Sciences
Moscow, U.S.S.R.

OUR KNOWLEDGE of the part which microbes play in plant life has made tremendous progress during the past two decades. This is especially true in regard to the relationship of soil micro-organisms and higher plants. The results obtained so far warrant the conclusion that the microbes of the soil are a fundamental factor in the development of plants, and must not be ignored by the practical plant-grower or soil specialist.

Of the manifold effects that micro-organisms have on plants, two seem most important: (1) the role of micro-organisms in plant nutrition; (2) the influence of microbes and their metabolites on the growth and development as well as on the quality of the yield of plants.

Micro-organisms are known not only to supply plants with mineral elements, which involves decomposition of organic matter, but also to feed them directly with metabolites. They synthesize compounds that are by all standards essential for the normal growth and development of plants and there is every reason to believe that without microbes plants could not develop normally and give adequate yields.

The few biologically active microbe-generated compounds already known include vitamins, auxins, gibberellins, studied relatively in detail; growth-promoting factors, such as Z-, X-, and P-factors, spermin and spermidin, studied in less detail, and antibiotics, amino acids, hormones, and some other metabolites studied least. The effects of these substances on plants have also been investigated. Numerous data are available on the beneficial effects of auxins (heteroauxins) in practical plant- and fruit-growing and amenity-planting and on their intracellular action (Bentley, 1960; Hepden and Hawker, 1961; Linser-Kiermayer, 1957; Bachrach & Cohen, 1961). Many effects of gibberellins on plant growth have been studied. They were shown to elongate cells, especially in the stalks of plants (peas, etc.), activate enzyme systems, induce flowering and fruit ripening (Conference on gibberellin research results, 1961, Moscow; Abstract of the fourth meeting of Japan Gibberellin Research Association, 1961, Tokyo), and stimulate the synthesis of various substances. In addition, many micro-organisms of the soil form substances quite different from gibberellins but also able to affect plants. Some of these metabolites increase the growth and yield of plants

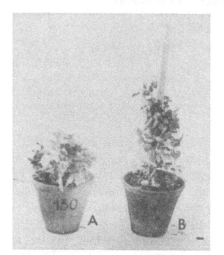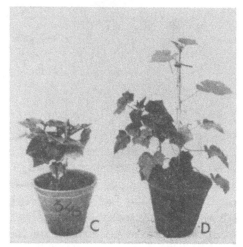

FIG. 1. Growth stimulation in plants by microbial metabolites. (A and B) Effect of preparation "D," obtained from yeasts, on the growth of dwarf peas: (A) control; (B) experimental. (C and D) Effect of preparation "P," obtained from organisms of the genus Pseudomonas, on the growth of cucumbers: (C) control; (D) experimental.

by 50–100 per cent or more (Fig. 1) but the nature of their effects is different from those of gibberellins.

Antibiotics. Some microbial metabolites exert tremendous influence on plants without providing nutrients, as in the case of antibiotics. The effects of these substances as medicines are generally known. They are also used in the field for plant disease control, in fruit and vegetable growing, amenity-planting, etc. (Klinkowski, 1954; Krassilnikov, 1958; Rubin & Ladygina, 1961; Symposium on the application of antibiotics in plant-growing (summaries of papers), 1958, Erevan).

Toxins. According to many researchers, soils harbour numerous bacteria, actinomyces, and fungi which form phytotoxins that inhibit the growth and development of plants as well as other micro-organisms which may themselves be antagonists and antibiotic producers. The phytotoxins differ in degree of activity. Some sharply inhibit plant growth, seeds soaked in them either do not germinate at all (Fig. 2) or very slightly, in small numbers, and mostly die out soon afterwards. Other toxins are not so active and only arrest seed germination and seedling growth. The degree of inhibition also depends on the concentration of the toxin. Some phytotoxins cause very weak, almost unnoticeable, inhibitions of plant growth yet they affect the biochemical processes in the tissues of the plants. Nitrogen metabolism and amino acid relationships in the plants undergo considerable changes. In the presence of toxins the content of lysine, threonine, alanine, valine and methionine, phenylalanine, etc. decreases in the plant tissues (Mirchink & Aseeva, 1959).

There are toxins that inhibit chlorophyll synthesis. The plants may either have acute chlorosis or chlorophyll synthesis may be completely inhibited.

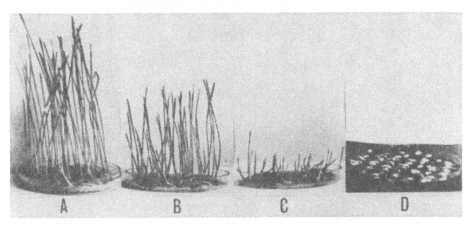

FIG. 2. Effect of toxic substances on the growth of wheat: (A) control, seeds treated with water; (B) weak toxin, formed by *Bacterium* sp.; (C) moderate toxin, obtained from *Act. griseus*; (D) strong toxin from *Penicillium cyclopium*.

Such toxins were obtained from fungi of the genus *Fusarium* (Krassilnikov & Kublitskaya, 1956; Kublitskaya, 1955) and from actinomyces (Krassilnikov, 1958; Ladygina, 1960; Rubin & Ladygina, 1961).

A decreased vitamin content is observed in plants in the presence of toxins. With toxins of *Penicillium cyclopium*, the tissues of wheat contained 1.7 mg thiamine, 12.5 mg pantothenic acid, and 0.09 mg biotin per gram dry weight as against the control 3.6 mg, 34.7 mg, and 0.7 mg, respectively (Table 1).

TABLE 1

EFFECTS OF PHYTOTOXINS ON VITAMIN CONTENT OF THE TISSUES
OF WHEAT
(mg per g of dry mass)

	Vitamins		
Toxins	Thiamin	Pantothenic acid	Biotin
Control	3.6	34.7	0.7
Penicillium cyclopium	1.7	12.5	0.09
B. subtilis	2.1	8.7	0.4
Act. griseus	3.4	11.4	0.09

The data concerning negative and positive effects of these substances on plants were obtained experimentally with isolated and purified preparations, often under strictly artificial conditions. It may therefore be relevant to ask: What is the biological function, under natural conditions, of the organisms that produce physiologically active substances in the laboratory? Some authors (Waksman, 1959–61) deny the biological significance of the microbe-generated active metabolites, alleging that these substances are not synthesized in the soil.

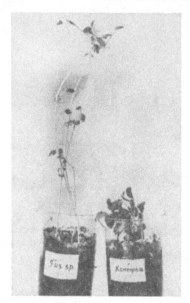 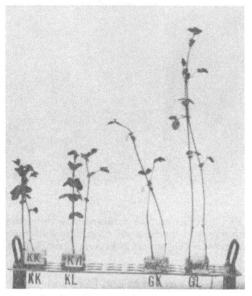

FIG. 3. Effect of gibberellin, formed by fungus in soil. Peas were grown in soil in which *Fusarium* sp., a gibberellin producer, had developed. Control on right.

FIG. 4. Effect of gibberellin absorbed from the soil by peas. KK, extract from the *roots*, and KL, extract from the *leaves*, of normal peas added to soil. GK, extract from the *roots*, and GL, extract from the *leaves*, of peas grown in soil containing gibberellin.

Our viewpoint is different. The observations and tests we have made for years show that all micro-organisms that produce metabolites in the laboratory do likewise in natural substrates. This is borne out by experiments with antibiotics, gibberellins, toxins, and other compounds produced by soil micro-organisms (Krassilnikov, 1958; Khristeva, 1961; Wright, 1952; Brian, 1957; Stevenson, 1956; Gottlieb, 1952; Khudyakova & Zueva, 1959; etc.). Antibiotics may remain in soils for a long time, ranging from several hours to several weeks or even months. Similar data were obtained in experiments with gibberellins. It was synthesized in soil by fungi—*Fusarium fujikuroi*—if conditions were favourable. From the soil the metabolite is taken up through the roots. The peas sown on soil inoculated with the fungus were manifestly tall, their stalks expanded and thin, leaves elongated and pale green (Fig. 3); in short, all the plants appeared as though they had been treated with pure gibberellin. It was also shown that the tissues of plants grown in soil rich in gibberellin-producing fungi contained gibberellin in large amounts. If extracts are made from these plants and added into the substratum in which pea seeds germinate the peas grow as tall as in the presence of gibberellin (Fig. 4). Consequently, gibberellin is produced in the soil and taken up through the root system of the plant in which it may accumulate in various tissues and in various quantities.

TABLE 2

EFFECTS OF JUICE FROM PEAS GROWN IN TOXIN-CONTAINING SOIL FOR 4 TO 7 WEEKS
ON THE GROWTH OF WHEAT SEEDLINGS
(Lengths in cm.)

Test soils	Juice from above-ground parts				Juice from pea roots			
	4 weeks		7 weeks		4 weeks		7 weeks	
	Leaves	Roots	Leaves	Roots	Leaves	Roots	Leaves	Roots
Control no toxin	2.8	1.0	3.2	0.5	6.6	5.2	6.9	6.5
Soil + toxin "cyc"	2.4	0.5	2.0	0.0	4.1	0.0	7.0	6.5
Soil + toxin "pur"	2.5	0.1	2.1	0.0	4.1	0.4	5.0	3.9

What is true of antibiotics and gibberellins is equally true of toxin formation in natural soil substrates. Fungi, actinomyces, and bacteria produce phytotoxins not only in artificial media but also in the soil. It was shown experimentally that toxin formation and toxication of a soil vary according to the type of soil, seasonal changes, and variety of micro-organisms. By using sensitive test-microbes (*Azotobacter*) we were able to isolate soil toxins in quantities from 1–2 to 300 and more units per gram. Soil toxins are taken up into plants through the roots. If the concentration of soil toxin is high the plants either develop slowly or die. They are concentrated chiefly in the roots. As with pure toxins from fungus cultures, these soil toxins affect biochemical processes such as nitrogen metabolism (see above) (Krassilnikov, 1958, 1962). Absorbed toxins may be extracted from plant tissues and their quantity precisely determined either by microbial assay or by plant height (Table 2). According to these data, having concentrated in the roots the toxin proceeds into the above-ground part where it accumulates more than in the roots.

Toxins produced in the soil by microbes were analysed chemically, chromatographically (Fig. 5), and biologically. Soil extracts and lysimetric water were chemically purified, fractionated by paper chromatography, and then compared with one another. It was shown that the toxins taken up into plants coincided with individual toxins in the soil, in which the corresponding microbe-inhibitors had developed, as well as with the toxins produced by the same microbes in pure culture in artificial media. By the above methods for identifying and differentiating toxins we were able to compare toxins of different soils (Fig. 6). We made a study of Pamir soils (primitive, Alpine) chernozems, chestnuts, and turf podzols. The toxins of the soils were found to differ in composition and biological spectrum. Toxins may also differ according to the vegetative cover as shown in Table 3.

ADSORPTION OF METABOLITES BY SOIL

The substances produced by microbes are not wholly absorbed by plants but are partly, perhaps mostly, inactivated, destroyed, or transformed. To some extent they are adsorbed by soil. We made a special study of the

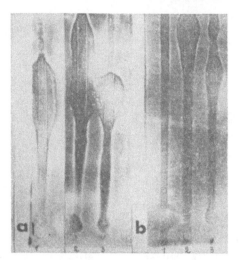

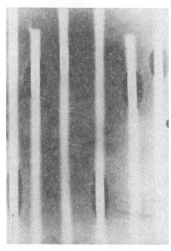

FIG. 5. Chromatogram of the toxins of different forest soils: (*a*) under a pine grove, (*b*) under a spruce grove. 1, acetone; 2, water; 3, methanol.

FIG. 6. Chromatograms of the toxin produced by *Penicillium cyclopium* on Czapek's agar (*left*) and in soil (*right*). Solvents, left to right, are benzene, butanol, and butanol–acetic acid. Test organism, *Azotobacter.*

TABLE 3

ANTIMICROBIC SPECTRUM OF TOXINS IN SOILS UNDER VARIOUS VEGETATION COVER.
TURF-PODZOL SOIL
(Chashnikov Experiment Station near Moscow)

Test microbes	Extracts from soils			Lysimetric water		
	Birches	Firs	Pines	Birches	Firs	Pines
Staph. aureus	+	+	++	+++	+++	+++
Bact. prodigiosum	+++	+++	+++	+++	−	−
Mycob. violaceum	−	+	+	−	+++	+
B. subtilis	+++	+++	+++	−	+	+
Act. globisporus	++	−	−	−	+++	++
Act. violaceus	−	++	+++	++	+++	+++

+ small zone of inhibition (0.5–1 mm).   +++ large zone (5–8 mm).
++ moderate zone (2–4 mm).   − no inhibition, normal growth.

adsorption of microbial metabolites. Antibiotics, gibberellins, toxins, and amino acids were adsorbed by soils in various quantities depending on the nature of the substance, the soil, and the season. We studied the adsorption by soils of streptomycin, aureomycin, terramycin, subtilin, penicillin, etc. Some of these are adsorbed in large amounts, some in small; some soils adsorb strongly, some weakly (Krassilnikov, 1958; Khudyakova & Zueva, 1959). The adsorbed metabolites may be demonstrated by biological methods and by means of fluorescence microscopy directly in soil, a method which we have recently developed (Krassilnikov & Zvyagintsev, 1958;

[Zvyagintsev, 1959–61;] Khudyakova & Zvyagintsev, 1961). Adsorbed gibberellin is readily identified with the help of pea seedlings, which react to gibberellin even in minute dosage (the vestiges left on soil particles after washing)—elongation of internodes and etiolation of leaves (Fig. 3) (Khudyakova & Zueva, 1959). Adsorbed toxins and antibiotics are identifiable either by test-microbes or by sensitive plants. It was shown that soils adsorbed and held fast many, if not all, microbial metabolites such as amino acids, vitamins, enzymes, various hormones, etc. The degree of fixation of these substances differs according to their chemical affinity and the soil properties. The same gibberellin is washed out of a humus-enriched chernozem less readily than out of turf podzol.

One may say in conclusion that the data cited cover only individual aspects of microbial effects on plants. In fact, the microbial factor plays a far more diverse and complex part in the life of higher plants. Microbes causing positive and negative effects are in complex interrelations, which may be either antagonistic or metabiotic in nature. As a consequence of this struggle definite microbial cenoses come into being. Within the cenoses microbial varieties undergo changes according to the changing soil conditions, cultivation, fertilization, vegetation cover, etc. The soil population must be a very important factor in soil fertility. The study of the interrelation between plants and soil micro-organisms, especially as far as the rhizosphere is concerned, is a very important problem.

CONCLUSIONS

Individual aspects are elucidated of the effects of soil micro-organisms on plants. Two problems have come under scrutiny: (a) the role of micro-organisms in the additional nutrition of plants, and (b) the immediate effects of their metabolites on the growth and development of plants.

1. It was shown that the microbes directly feed the plants with their metabolites, of which biologically active substances, such as vitamins, amino acids, gibberellins, and other growth-promoting factors are especially significant. These substances impart to the plants peculiar properties, not only improving their growth but also the quality of their yields.

2. The micro-organisms synthesize biologically active metabolites, antibiotics, gibberellins and gibberellin-like substances, toxins, etc. not only in artificial media but also in soil.

3. The microbial metabolites are absorbed by soil particles and accumulate in the soil in various quantities depending on the composition and type of soil.

4. From the soil, microbial metabolites penetrate through the roots into plants and accumulate in different tissues.

5. The plant may assimilate the microbial metabolites, which are adsorbed by soil particles.

REFERENCES

Bachrach, U. and J. Cohen. 1961. Spermidine in the bacterial cell. J. Gen. Microbiol. *26*: 1–9.

Bentley, J. 1960. J. Mar. Biol. Assoc. UK *39*(3).

Brian, P. 1957. Ann. Rev. Plant Physiol. 8: 413.

Hepden, P. M. and L. E. Hawker, 1961. A volatile substance controlling early stages of zygospore formation in *Rhizopus sexualis*. J. Gen. Microbiol. *24*: 155–164.

Gottlieb, D. 1952. Phytopathology *42*: 493.

Khristeva, L. 1961. Trudy Inst. Mikrobiol. Moscow *11*: 34.

Khudyakova, U. and J. Zueva. 1959. Proc. Symposium. Itogi i zadachi izucheniya roli mikroorganizmov (Results and problems in the study of the role of micro-organisms). Leningrad.

Khudyakova, U. and D. Zvyagintsev. 1961. Proc. Symposium. Timiryazev. Selskokhoz. Akad. (Timiryazev Academy of Agriculture), Moscow 3: 51.

Klinkowski, M. 1954. Die Antibiotica und ihre Bedeutung in der Phytopathologie. Leipzig.

Krassilnikov, N. 1958. Soil micro-organisms and higher plants. Moscow.

Krassilnikov, N. 1962. Vestnik Moscow State University No. 3.

Krassilnikov, N. and M. Kublitskaya. 1956. Doklady Akad. Nauk USSR *110*(4).

Krassilnikov, N. and D. Zvyagintsev. 1958. Doklady Akad. Nauk USSR *123*(2).

Kublitskaya, M. 1955. Paraziticheskii khloroz vinogradnikov v Tsentralnoi Azii (The parasitic chlorosis of vines in Central Asia) Dissertation, Tashkent.

Ladygina, M. 1960. O prirode deistviya streptomitsina (On the nature of the action of streptomycin). Dissertation, Moscow.

Linser-Kiermayer, M. 1957. Methoden zur Bestimmung planzlicher Wuchstoffe. Wien.

Mirchink, T. and I. Aseeva. 1959. Nauchnye Doklady Vyshchei Shkoly. Biological Series 2.

Rubin, B. and M. Ladygina. 1961. Uspekhi Sovremennoi Biologii 4.

Stevenson, I. 1956. Antibiotic activity of actinomycetes in soil as demonstrated by direct observation techniques. J. Gen. Microbiol. *15*: 372–380.

Waksman, S. 1959–61. The Actinomycetes, I, II, III.

Wright, I. 1952. Nature, *170*: 672.

Zvyagintsev, D. 1952. Nauchnye Doklady Vyshchei Shkoly. Biological Series 2: 212.

PANEL DISCUSSION 1

GENETICS APPLIED TO INDUSTRIAL MICROBIOLOGY

Chairman: G. PONTECORVO

S. G. BRADLEY

Genetics of Actinomycetes: Mechanisms and Significance

FRANCIS J. RYAN

Bacterial Variation

J. A. ROPER

Mechanisms of Recombination in Certain Filamentous Fungi

HERSCHEL ROMAN

Sources of Variability in Vegetative Yeast Cultures

CHAIRMAN'S REMARKS

G. PONTECORVO

Genetics Department
The University, Glasgow, Scotland

THE ADVANCES of the last fifteen years in the genetics of micro-organisms, and the success in applying genetics to breeding more productive crop plants, contrast strangely with the apathy in applying genetics to strain improvement of industrial micro-organisms.

The main reason is that while the farmer would not dream of becoming his own plant breeder—an activity concentrated in a few specialized centres, mainly government-run—each industrial fermentation firm thinks that it can carry out with success its own programme of strain improvement. This fragmentation of effort, and its concomitant exclusiveness, narrow the scope of genetic research in industrial fermentation laboratories to the point that specialists of the right calibre are not attracted by them. The result is that strain improvement is still based almost exclusively on induced mutations and selection, and the potentialities of the far more powerful tool of recombination are ignored.

Yet an obvious feature that distinguishes the genetics of micro-organisms from that of higher plants is precisely the versatility of the mechanisms of recombination. In this Symposium we shall have a review of the genetics of the bacteria, of the actinomycetes, and of the fungi. We shall see the variety of ways by which micro-organisms recombine their genetic material. Strain improvement is essentially the art of making use of recombination in the synthesis of desirable combinations of genes. It requires a background of genetics no less than the background of chemistry required for the successful synthesis of new valuable compounds.

GENETICS OF ACTINOMYCETES:
MECHANISMS AND SIGNIFICANCE

S. G. BRADLEY

Department of Microbiology
University of Minnesota, Minneapolis, U.S.A.

THE PROCESSES which bring diverse genetic material together thereby permitting gene recombination to occur in microbes may be divided into three categories: gametic-gametangial conjugation, somatic conjugation and transduction. Gametic-gametangial conjugation, in which differentiated sexual elements fuse, is found in many fungi, algae and protozoa but is generally considered to be absent in the bacteria and actinomycetes. Somatic conjugation, which involves fusion of undifferentiated vegetative elements, is one stage of the parasexual process and of bacterial "sexuality," and occurs throughout the microbial world. Transduction, defined broadly, refers to the transfer of a limited amount of genetic information from a disrupted cell to an intact cell; deoxyribonucleic acid–mediated transformation and phage-mediated transduction have been demonstrated for many bacteria.

Genetic evidence for somatic conjugation has been reported for many actinomycetes, including *Streptomyces violaceoruber* or *S. coelicolor* as it was formerly designated (Sermonti & Spada-Sermonti, 1956; Bradley, 1957; Braendle & Szybalski, 1957; Hopwood, 1959), *S. griseus* (Bradley & Lederberg, 1956), *S. vinaceus* (Bradley & Anderson, 1960), *S. fradiae* (Braendle & Szybalski, 1957), *S. rimosus* (Alikhanian *et al.*, 1959), *S. griseoflavus* (Saito, 1958), *S. aureofaciens* (Alikhanian & Borisova, 1961; Anderson, personal communication) and *Nocardia erythropolis* (Adams, personal communication). After hyphae of two complementary auxotrophic (growth-factor dependent) strains join, a prototrophic (growth-factor independent), heterogenomic mycelium may be established; however, hyphal anastomosis as determined cytologically does not lead invariably to an interaction between the genomes of the fusing strains. A recombinant mycelium can be maintained indefinitely by subculture of long hyphal strands although selective conditions may be needed to prevent dissociation.

Spores borne by heterogenomic mycelia of *S. griseus* rarely perpetuated the recombinant, prototrophic character; a chain of spores usually contained conidia of each auxotrophic, parental type. *S. violaceoruber* spores from prototrophic colonies which arose by joining of hyphae of complementary auxotrophs, were primarily prototrophic even when the selective medium was supplemented with one of the growth factors needed by each parent. Initially the recombinants usually displayed the dominant characteristics:

drug sensitivity over resistance; prototrophy over auxotrophy; phage sensitivity over resistance; sporulation over asporogeny; and blue pigmentation over pink. From the primary recombinants both parental types could be recovered as clones derived by serially subculturing spores from single colonies. Non-parental types also were found during testing of spores from purified, prototrophic recombinants. Some of these were stable with respect to one characteristic but remained heterogeneous with respect to other characteristics. Another non-parental class, which was rarely encountered, was stable for all expressions studied. Additionally, a few recombinants displayed nutritional requirements not recognized in either parental strain. Recovery of non-parental types has been achieved, after allowing for phenomic lag, by selecting for one or more recessive expressions, for example, phage immunity and resistance to streptomycin. Many of these recombinants were stable, non-parental types. With the streptomycetes no recombinants were found until the parental strains had been grown together for three days, but *N. erythropolis* may be crossed on minimal medium (Bradley, 1962).

Hopwood, using richly supplemented minimal medium (50μg growth factor/ml in contrast to 10 μg/ml), has reported isolation of all possible combinations of auxotrophic markers on appropriately fortified medium. The complementary types were found in nearly equal numbers. Accordingly, Hopwood has assigned many genes controlling drug susceptibility and nutritional requirements to one of two linkage groups.

S. violaceoruber 199 produces an antibiotic pigment which is similar to but not identical with actinorhodin. This antibiotic inhibits growth of gram-positive bacteria but not gram-negative bacteria, yeasts or molds. Mutants having more or less antibacterial activity than the wild type strain have been isolated. Recombinants formed by the interaction of a strain that made antibiotic and one that did not were able to synthesize antibiotic. Antibiotic yields by recombinants resulting from a cross between a low producing mutant and a high producing mutant were usually intermediate between those of the parents; however, clones with decreased and increased productivity were encountered. Infrequently, recombinants from a cross between two non-producing mutants gave antibiotics yields comparable to the wild type. Alikhanian *et al.* (1959, 1961) have obtained similar results with chlorotetracycline production by *S. aureofaciens* recombinants and with oxytetracycline production by *S. rimosus* recombinants. In addition, these workers have shown that qualities such as foaming are subject to genetic control (Mindlin *et al.*, 1961).

Although most genetic studies with streptomycetes have been carried out with descendants of a single clone, intraspecific recombination between strains having different origins has been successful. Moreover, recombinants between mutants of two distinctly different species have been found. The base composition of the deoxyribonucleic acid of the streptomycetes, nocardia and micromonospora are all approximately the same (72–74 per cent guanine + cytosine); therefore, sufficient genetic homology may exist within the group to permit extensive interspecific hybridization. Recovery of recombinants, however, is limited by genetic and environmental considerations. No recombinants have been found among mutants of S. *violaceoruber* grown on peptone-yeast-extract medium although they occur abundantly when this medium is supplemented with glucose. Genetic interaction is also restricted by a compatibility system, which, unlike the F-factor of *Escherichia coli*, is not transmissible on contact. The combinations A + A, A + B, B + B, B + C, C + C are compatible but A + C is not compatible.

Alikhanian *et al.* (1960) have reported that genetic information can be transferred by actinophages of *Streptomyces olivaceus*. Auxotrophic mutants were transformed to prototrophy by actinophage grown on the prototrophic wild type strain but not by actinophages grown on the homologous auxotroph.

The streptomycetes have proven to be quite amenable to genetic manipulation. Within the near future, recombination should take its place along with mutation and selection as a powerful tool for strain improvement.

REFERENCES

Alikhanian, S. I., S. Z. Mindlin, S. U. Goldat and A. V. Vladimizov. 1959. Genetics of organisms producing tetracyclines. Ann. N.Y. Acad. Sci. *81*: 914–949.

Alikhanian, S. I., T. S. Iljina and N. D. Lomovskaya. 1960. Transduction in actinomycetes. Nature *188*: 245–246.

Alikhanian, S. I., and L. N. Borisova. 1961. Recombination in *Actinomyces aureofaciens*. Microbiologiya *30*: 214–220 (Russian).

Bradley, S. G. 1957. Heterokaryosis in *Streptomyces coelicolor*. J. Bacteriol. *73*: 581–582.

Bradley, S. G. 1962. Parasexual phenomena in micro-organisms. Ann. Rev. Microbiol. *16*: 35–52.

Bradley, S. G., and D. L. Anderson. 1960. Preferential compatibility in *Streptomyces violaceoruber*. J. Gen. Microbiol. *23*: 231–241.

Bradley, S. G., and J. Lederberg. 1956. Heterokaryosis in streptomyces. J. Bacteriol. *72*: 219–225.

Braendle, D. H., and W. Szybalski. 1957. Genetic interactions among streptomycetes: Heterokaryosis and synkaryosis. Proc. Nat. Acad. Sci. (U.S.) *43*: 947–955.

Hopwood, D. A. 1959. Linkage and the mechanism of recombination in *Streptomyces coelicolor*. Ann. N.Y. Acad. Sci. *81*: 887–898.

Mindlin, S. Z., S. I. Alikhanian, A. V. Vladimirov and G. R. Mikhailova. 1961. A new hybrid strain of an oxytetracycline-producing organism, *Streptomyces rimosus*. Appl. Microbiol. *9*: 349–353.

Saito, H. 1958. Heterokaryosis and genetic recombination in *Streptomyces griseoflavus*. Can. J. Microbiol. *4*: 571–580.

Sermonti, G., and I. Spada-Sermonti. 1956. Gene recombination in *Streptomyces coelicolor*. J. Gen. Microbiol. *15*: 609–616.

BACTERIAL VARIATION

FRANCIS J. RYAN

Department of Zoology
Columbia University, New York, U.S.A.

AMONG HIGHER ORGANISMS the immediate cause of observed variation is a re-assemblage of genes, through sexual reproduction and its attendant cytological processes. Such heterogeneity is restricted by the amount of genetic variation, cryptic and overt, in the reproducing population and this, in turn, is dependent eventually upon the processes of mutation. In bacteria no one really knows the extent to which sexual conjugation and the infectious transmission of genes takes place; the role played by the exchange of genes cannot be assessed quantitatively. It is clear, however, that large populations of bacteria frequently exist, especially in laboratories, and that the component members of these populations are usually haploid. The result is that rare mutants are easily found so that, even though the rates are low, the role played by mutation can be assessed.

Bacterial mutants are readily secured since, by virtue of rapid growth, selective forces can sometimes be imposed which result in explosive changes in the composition of the population that contains them. Witness the selection for streptomycin-resistant mutants on streptomycin-containing medium, for prototrophs on medium devoid of the relevant growth factor; or conversely, for streptomycin non-requiring mutants on medium without streptomycin, or for auxotrophs on medium without the growth factor but with penicillin which kills the growing prototrophs. Many other examples could be cited but, so far as I know, they have been of most interest to the academic investigator. Industry has been largely concerned with mutants which accumulate some desired product, and no doubt many interesting methods are locked in company files.

A variety of mutagenic agents have been employed—heat, radiation, and chemicals. It is true that various genes respond differently to different agents but, with the exception of certain non-chromosomal factors, none have responded in any organism so uniquely as to provide an instance, even quantitatively, of elective mutation. Specific, directed mutation must have been the aim of students of mutation from the first. With the advent of a better knowledge of structure of the gene the hope of attainment of specific mutation seemed to fade away. The functional gene is considered at present to be a long tract of some thousand nucleotide pairs in DNA, their sequence conferring specificity on the unit. Since each nucleotide pair—A:T, T:A, G:C, and C:G—must be represented many times in all genes, the hope does not exist that a mutagen specific for one of them would mutate only one gene. No one has, in this default, come forward with an idea as to how to use the chemical reactivity of the whole gene sequence to induce mutation electively.

But the same course of events which led to this discouragement now promises a way out. Although it was not appreciated at the time, the path opened up when it was shown that certain chemicals could induce point mutations. Mundry and Gierer (1958) showed that nitrous acid, which oxidatively deaminates adenine, guanine, and cytosine, induced mutations in the RNA of tobacco mosaic virus with a kinetics that indicated one chemical event to be sufficient. Later, comparisons of the kinetics of deamination and mutation induction by Vielmetter and Schuster (1960) and by Ephrussi-Taylor and Litman (see Litman, 1961) showed that the transformation of a particular adenine into hypoxanthine was sufficient to cause the mutation observed. The event, in DNA, was imagined to proceed as follows:

$$
\begin{array}{l}
\text{A:T} \\
\quad\downarrow\!\!-\!\!-\text{HNO}_2 \\
\text{H:T} \\
\quad\downarrow \\
\text{H:C} \\
\quad\downarrow \\
\text{G:C}
\end{array}
$$

This change of the DNA *in vitro* was paralleled by changes *in vivo* after the incorporation of certain base analogues. Freese and Benzer (see Freese, 1961) employed such analogues as 5-bromouracil (BU) and 2-amino-purine (AP) with the rII mutants of phage T4 and developed a theory of mutagenesis based upon incorporation followed by erroneous pairing. For example:

$$
\begin{array}{ll}
\text{A:T} \leftrightharpoons \text{BU} \qquad & \text{AP} \leftrightharpoons \text{A:T} \\
\quad\downarrow & \qquad\qquad\downarrow \\
\text{A:BU} & \text{AP:T} \\
\quad\downarrow & \qquad\downarrow \\
\text{G:BU} & \text{AP:C} \\
\quad\downarrow & \qquad\downarrow \\
\text{G:C} & \text{G:C}
\end{array}
$$

These basic suppositions were amply confirmed by Rudner (1961) and Strelzoff (1962) who worked with synchronized populations of *Salmonella typhimurium* and *Escherichia coli*. They also showed, as Freese and Benzer had further postulated, that mutations occurred not only according to the patterns described above, with a constant chance per replication, but also by erroneous incorporations in other mutants where the needed transitions were from G:C to A:T. For example:

$$
\begin{array}{ll}
\text{G:C} \leftrightharpoons \text{BU} \qquad & \text{AP} \leftrightharpoons \text{G:C} \\
\quad\downarrow & \qquad\qquad\downarrow \\
\text{G:BU} & \text{AP:C} \\
\quad\downarrow & \qquad\downarrow \\
\text{A:BU} & \text{AP:T} \\
\quad\downarrow & \qquad\downarrow \\
\text{A:T} & \text{A:T}
\end{array}
$$

The mutations required the replication of DNA for the incorporation of the analogue, and subsequent DNA replications for the transition to be completed. All the results were consistent with the notion that simple transitions of base pairs were required for the mutations, in one or the other direction according to the particular mutant under investigation.

Meanwhile a completely independent line of investigation, undertaken by Nagata (1962, 1963), showed that some of the parameters of DNA replication, generally believed to be true, did, in fact, operate. He synchronized the division of populations of *E. coli* and measured the time-course of increase in the prophage λ which they contained. In two different *Hfr* strains of *E. coli*, where the prophage was located in quite different positions, the number of the prophages per cell increased abruptly at a time during DNA replication which was in accordance with that location. In an *F⁻* strain, where the chromosome is thought to be continuous, the prophage, like the mutations studied by Strelzoff (1962), increased continuously in proportion to the increase in DNA. All experiments were consistent with the notion that the chromosomes (molecules of DNA) of *E. coli* were synchronously replicating, but that only in *Hfr* strains, where the chromosome is linear, did the molecule begin to replicate at the end where the *F* factor is located; this replication proceeds to the other end in unison, doubling the prophage while passing its locus. Thus DNA seems to replicate with a polarity and all molecules in a population can be made to do this in synchrony.

A logical consequence of these findings is that a base analogue might be pulsed into a synchronously replicating population of bacteria at various times. If the DNA is replicating in synchrony and with a polarity, there will be one specific time when the analogue can be incorporated in and mutagenic for a given locus. In proportion to the smallness of the interval during which the analogue is available to the cell, relative to the length of the DNA replicative cycle, induced mutation can be made specific. This is the only known approach to elective mutation.

The use to which elective mutation is put will depend upon those who are interested in humanity, dollars, or service on behalf of the national product—to wit, the medical, agricultural, and industrial biologists.

REFERENCES

Freese, E. 1961. The molecular mechanisms of mutation, Symp. V Inter. Congress Biochem. Moscow.

Litman, R. M. 1961. Genetic and chemical alterations in the transforming DNA of Pneumococcus caused by ultraviolet light and by nitrous acid. J. Chimie phys. 58: 997–1004.

Mundry, K. W., und A. Gierer. 1958. Die Erzengung von Mutationen des Tobakmosaik-virus durch chemische Behandlung seiner Nucleinsaure *in vitro*. Z. Vererbungslehre 89: 614–630.

Nagata, T. 1962. Polarity and synchrony in the replication of DNA molecules of bacteria. Biochem. Biophys. Res. Com. 8: 348–351.

Nagata, T. 1963. The molecular synchrony and sequential replication of DNA in *Escherichia coli*. Proc. Nat. Acad. Sci. U.S. 49: 551–559.

Rudner, R.   1961.   Mutation as an error in base pairing. Z. Vererbungslehre 92: 336–379.

Strelzoff, E.   1962.   DNA synthesis and induced mutations in the presence of 5-bromouracil. Z. Vererbungslehre *93*: 287–318.

Vielmetter, W., and H. Schuster.   1960.   The base specificity of mutation induced by nitrous acid in phage T2. Biochem. Biophys. Res. Com. 2: 324–328.

MECHANISMS OF RECOMBINATION IN CERTAIN FILAMENTOUS FUNGI

J. A. ROPER

Department of Genetics
The University, Sheffield, England

SEGREGATION AND RECOMBINATION are the foundation stones on which genetics and experimental breeding are built. Mutation provides the units of hereditary variation but, by itself, mutation is an extremely inefficient way of deriving combinations of these units. Only when mutation and recombination are combined is there hope of exploiting the full scope of available hereditary variation. Without segregation and recombination, rigorous genetic analysis and planned breeding are impossible. It is in this context that we must consider any advances which permit recombination in organisms, or under conditions where it previously appeared impossible.

Less than twenty years ago the sexual cycle was the only known means for achieving gene recombination. In certain microbial species, recombination, and mechanisms by which it might occur, were unknown. Since that time a variety of processes have been discovered in viruses, bacteria and fungi which lead to recombination, but which differ from the sexual cycle in one or more respects.

The present account deals with some mechanisms of recombination in certain Ascomycetes and allied imperfect fungi. Mechanisms of recombination via heterokaryosis, via the sexual cycle and, in particular, via the parasexual cycle are surveyed.

RECOMBINATION VIA HETEROKARYOSIS

This can be considered by reference to some clear-cut examples in the homothallic ascomycete *Aspergillus nidulans*. Heterokaryons are formed by anastomoses between hyphae carrying nuclei of different genotypes. The nuclear types are segregated out when the heterokaryon produces its uninucleate vegetative spores (conidia). The almost universal experience is that each conidium is of one or other parental genotype and phenotype. However, there are exceptions, apparently rare, to this situation (Roper, 1958). For example, from a heterokaryon between a strain of genotype A and abnormal morphology and a strain of genotype B, normal morphology, the conidia yield the parental types and, sometimes, one or more classes with genotype B and abnormal morphology. There has been no nuclear fusion and no exchange of known genic markers; by sharing a common cytoplasm the two types have interacted so as to yield recombinants.

The mechanism responsible for this cytoplasmic transmission of heredi-tary information is not yet known. Whatever the mechanism, it leads to a type of recombination. Present experience suggests a limited application of this approach. However, we shall be better able to assess its potentialities and limitations when the mechanism is elucidated fully.

THE SEXUAL CYCLE

The cardinal features of the sexual cycle, nuclear fusion and meiosis, appear to be identical in fungi and in higher organisms. Fungal species with a perfect stage are open to classical genetic analysis and planned breeding. Certain groups may, of course, require special approaches such as those devised by Pontecorvo (1949) for homothallic species.

THE PARASEXUAL CYCLE

The parasexual cycle was first demonstrated in *Aspergillus nidulans*, some ten years ago. The cycle offers an alternative to the sexual cycle for segregation and recombination. Both cycles lead to essentially the same end results, but by different routes. *A. nidulans* has been thoroughly studied by conventional genetical analysis (Pontecorvo, Roper, Hemmons, Mac-donald & Bufton, 1953). Linkage maps have been constructed and some centromere positions determined. This has made it possible to elucidate the major features of the parasexual cycle in this species. We now know that the parasexual cycle, or something very like it, occurs in a variety of imperfect species (for review see Roper, 1962); it seems reasonable to sup-pose that the processes occurring in the imperfect species closely parallel those found for *A. nidulans*.

Occurrence of the standard sexual cycle is readily detected by the presence of distinctive structures. The processes of the parasexual cycle occur at low frequency and special techniques are required to facilitate their detection and use.

Formation of "Zygotes"

A heterokaryon is prepared between two strains which differ from wild type, and from each other, in a number of mutant alleles. In *A. nidulans*, for example, one strain might have yellow conidia (wild type are green) and growth requirements for p-amino benzoic acid and biotin while the other strain might have white conidia and requirement for adenine. Since the mutant alleles determining conidial colour are autonomous, the hetero-karyon carries a mixture of white and yellow conidia of parental types. However, as a rare, but regular, event pairs of nuclei fuse in the vegetative cells (Roper, 1952). When two unlike nuclei fuse the result is a heterozygote and, since most mutant alleles are recessive, the heterozygous diploid is generally phenotypically wild type. Such diploid nuclei are fairly stable at mitosis and their mitotic descendents may form conidia. These conidia may be detected, in a case such as this, as a rare green sector in the yellow/white mosaic of the heterokaryon. If the heterozygotes are not seen, they can be selected by plating conidia on a minimal medium deficient in the growth requirement of the haploid parents.

In this way it is a simple matter to synthesize a heterozygote of any required genotype. Thus, through a rare karyogamy, occurring in the mycelium, a persistent "zygote," relatively stable at mitosis, is obtained.

Recombination in Diploids

The genotype of the diploid in the above example is as follows:

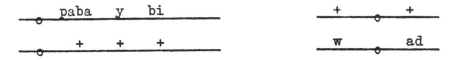

Diploid colonies of this genotype carry mainly green conidia. However, there are occasional colonies, sectors or patches carrying white or yellow conidia. Isolates from such patches are tested for ploidy (by conidial size) and for nutritional requirements.

These yellow and white recombinant classes arise by three types of rather rare mitotic "accidents" whose details are now well understood.

1. *Mitotic non-disjunction.* This results in diploid nuclei homozygous for one pair of homologous chromosomes but still heterozygous for the other chromosome pairs (Pontecorvo & Käfer, 1958).

2. *Mitotic crossing-over.* This occurs at the 4-strand stage and is exactly reciprocal (Roper & Pritchard, 1955). At any one event, crossing-over is almost invariably confined to one chromosome arm (Pontecorvo & Käfer, 1958). The subsequent segregation of strands is mitotic in form. Appropriate segregation leads to homozygosis for all alleles linked in coupling and distal to the cross-over. Markers proximal to the cross-over, and markers on other chromosome arms, remain heterozygous. In the present example all the yellow diploids which arose by this process would require biotin and a proportion would also require p-amino benzoic acid.

3. *Haploidization.* Haploids arise by infrequent breakdown of the diploid nuclei. There is rarely, if ever, coincident crossing-over (Pontecorvo, Tarr Gloor & Forbes, 1954). The haploids arise mainly through aneuploidy by successive loss of chromosomes (Käfer, 1957, 1960, 1961). For example, from the above diploid, haploidization would produce, among others, haploids of genotypes *paba y bi*; *w ad* and +++; ++.

Of the three processes, (2) and (3) are, for most purposes, the important ones. Individually, they bring about restricted recombination limited in (2) to all or part of a chromosome arm and in (3) to recombination of whole chromosomes. These limitations may, in some genetically complex systems, prove advantageous.

The steps of the parasexual cycle, and a comparison with those of the standard sexual cycle, are summarized below:

SEXUAL CYCLE	PARASEXUAL CYCLE
1. Nuclear fusion in specialized structures.	1. Rare nuclear fusion in vegetative cells.
2. Zygote usually persists one nuclear generation only.	2. "Zygote" persists through many mitoses.
3. Recombination by meiosis.	3. Recombination by rare "accidents" at mitosis.
4. Meiotic products readily recognized and isolated.	4. Recombinants occur among vegetative cells. Recognized by use of suitable genetic markers.

It should be added that laboratory use of the parasexual cycle is less laborious than has been implied above. Techniques are now available which facilitate recognition and isolation of recombinants (Roper & Käfer, 1957; Pontecorvo, 1958; Morpurgo, 1961).

DISCUSSION

Recombination *via* heterokaryosis is difficult, at present, to assess. It may have strictly limited application. The parasexual cycle of fungi is now well elucidated. It is known to occur in at least two species which have a perfect stage, *A. nidulans* and *A. rugulosus*. In these it provides valuable additional approaches in genetic analysis. The parasexual cycle has now been discovered in a number of imperfect species (for review see Roper, 1962). Its discovery in such species raises important evolutionary considerations (Pontecorvo, 1954; Roper, 1962). In addition, the parasexual cycle offers the only available approach to the genetic analysis of imperfect species. Not only that, the way is now open for a study of the genetic control of industrially important biosyntheses in some asexual species, and the planned breeding of improved strains has already started.

REFERENCES

Käfer, E. 1957. Genetics of *Aspergillus*. Carnegie Inst. Wash. Ybk. *56*: 376–378.

Käfer, E. 1960. High frequency of spontaneous and induced somatic segregation in *Aspergilus nidulans*. Nature *186*: 619–620.

Käfer, E. 1961. The processes of spontaneous recombination in vegetative nuclei of *Aspergillus nidulans*. Genetics *46*: 1581–1609.

Morpurgo, G. 1961. Somatic segregation induced by p-flouro-phenylalanine. *Aspergillus* News Letter 2: 10.

Pontecorvo, G. 1949. Genetical techniques for self-fertile (homothallic) species. Proc. 8th Int. Congr. Genet.: 642–643.

Pontecorvo, G. 1954. Mitotic recombination in the genetic systems of filamentous fungi. Caryologia *6* (suppl.): 192–200.

Pontecorvo, G.   1958.   Trends in genetic analysis. Columbia University Press, New York.

Pontecorvo, G., and E. Käfer.   1958.   Genetic analysis based on mitotic recombination. Advances in Genet. 9: 71–104.

Pontecorvo, G., J. A. Roper, L. M. Hemmons, K. D. Macdonald and A. W. J. Bufton.   1953.   The genetics of *Aspergillus nidulans*. Advances in Genet. 5: 141–238.

Pontecorvo, G., E. Tarr Gloor and E. Forbes.   1954.   Analysis of mitotic recombination in *Aspergillus nidulans*. J. Genet. 25: 226–237.

Roper, J. A.   1952.   Production of heterozygous diploids in filamentous fungi. Experientia 8: 14–15.

Roper, J. A.   1958.   Nucleo-cytoplasmic interactions in *Aspergillus nidulans*. Cold Spring Harbor Symp. Quant. Biol. 23: 141–154.

Roper, J. A.   1962.   Genetics and microbial classification. *In* Microbial classification, XIIth Symp. Soc. Gen. Microbiol., ed. G. C. Ainsworth and P. H. A. Sneath, pp. 270–288. University Press, Cambridge.

Roper, J. A., and E. Käfer.   1957.   Acriflavine resistant mutants of *Aspergillus nidulans*. J. Gen. Microbiol. 16: 660–667.

Roper, J. A., and R. H. Pritchard.   1955.   The recovery of the complementary products of mitotic crossing over. Nature 175: 639.

SOURCES OF VARIABILITY IN VEGETATIVE YEAST CULTURES

HERSCHEL ROMAN

Department of Genetics, University of Washington
Seattle, U.S.A.

FOR WHATEVER REASON the industrial microbiologist wishes to use yeast, whether for its enzyme content, for its contribution to taste, or for its nutritional qualities, he first selects the strain most suited to his purpose and then hopes that the strain will be stable and maintain the characteristics for which it was selected. He is aided in choosing the strain by the genetic variability which is an intrinsic feature of all living organisms, yeast included, and he is hindered in maintaining the strain by this same variability. It is with reference to certain aspects of the problem of the maintenance of constancy that the following remarks are addressed.

We shall take as an example a heterothallic yeast which is used extensively in our laboratory and elsewhere for experimental purposes and which is akin to *Saccharomyces cerevisiae* in its morphology and life cycle. It may seem unfair to compare this yeast with industrial yeasts since our yeast has been subjected to rather special treatment in the laboratory and has been selected for properties particularly useful in genetic research. The comparison nevertheless is justified inasmuch as the mechanisms which will be discussed are found in a wide variety of organisms and should certainly apply to other yeasts. At the least, a study of the behavior of laboratory yeast should tell us what we might expect to find in industrial yeast of similar type.

We shall start with the haplophase, with a culture of cells derived from a single ascospore. Each cell has the minimal number of chromosomes essential to viability. It has not been possible to determine this number by direct cytological examination but it is now known, as a result of linkage studies, that there are at least 12 chromosomes in the haploid set (Hawthorne and Mortimer, 1960; Hawthorne, personal communication). A spore culture of this type is of one or another of two mating types, *a* and *α* (Lindegren & Lindegren, 1943). Mating occurs and the diplophase is restored when cells of opposite mating type are brought together.

A number of events may occur in a haplophase culture which will markedly alter its cellular composition. In a culture of cells of mating-type *a*, for example, mutation may occur at the mating-type locus to produce haploid cells of mating-type *α* (Ahmad, 1952). Such mutated cells will now mate with the neighboring *a* cells and a diploid cell of mating type composition aa will result. The diploid cell frequently multiplies at a more rapid rate than its haploid neighbors and after several cell generations the culture which was originally haploid has become largely diploid. Diploidization may also take place as the result of endomitotic doubling, that is, the doubling in chromosome number without a corresponding doubling in cell number. The result here also is a diploid cell but in this case the cell contains two a genes. The haploid culture with which we started can be envisaged, after a certain time in continuous culture, as being a composite (Fig. 1) of haploid a cells, diploid aa cells, and diploid $a\alpha$ cells (Roman & Sands, 1953).

The two diploid types are distinguishable in the following ways: (1) The $a\alpha$ cell, like its haploid progenitor, will mate with a cell of mating type α, whereas the aa cell is incapable of mating, or mates only very rarely, when confronted with cells of either mating type a or α; (2) the $a\alpha$ cell is capable of sporulation whereas the aa cell is not; (3) the pattern of budding is different in the two types (Townsend & Lindegren, 1954).

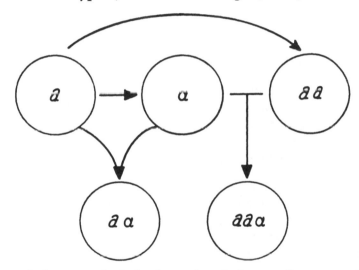

Fig. 1. Diploidization in haploid culture of mating-type a, due to mutation at the mating-type locus and to endomitotic doubling. The triploid $aa\alpha$ is also expected, as a secondary result.

The same events occur in haplophase culture of mating-type α. Mutation at the mating-type locus to a and subsequent fusion of a and α cells produce the $a\alpha$ diploid. There is no reason to doubt that endomitotic doubling occurs here also but the $\alpha\alpha$ cells found in these cultures can arise by a second means, not found in a cultures in our experience (D. C. Hawthorne, personal communication), namely the fusion of two α cells. The fusion of α cells occurs quite rarely, about twice as often as mutation at the mating-type locus or perhaps of the order of one in 10^7 cells. The diploid $\alpha\alpha$ will mate with a or aa cells and, like its aa counterpart, is incapable of sporulation. Its budding pattern is like that of aa cells.

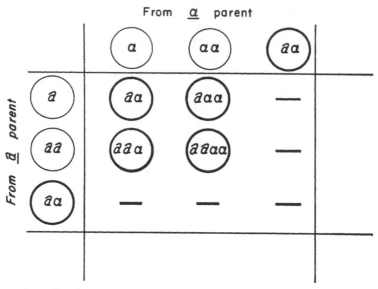

FIG. 2. The cell types expected from a cross of two strains which have undergone diploidization. The heavy circles designate cells capable of sporulation.

An interesting consequence of the instability of haplophase cultures as described above, and one which the yeast geneticist must take into account, is the wide variety of cell types (Fig. 2) which would result from a mixture of the two cell populations just described, when two supposedly haploid cultures of opposite mating types are mixed to make a cross between the two strains. In addition to the two types of *aa* cells already present, each of which would reflect the properties of the strain in which it arose, a third *aa* type would result from the mating of *a* and *α* haploid cells in the parental strains and this would combine the properties of the two strains. Triploid cells would also be formed, either *aaα* or *aαα*, owing to the mating of *aa* cells with *α* cells and of *αα* cells with *a* cells, respectively. We would also obtain tetraploid cells, *aaαα*, from the mating between *aa* and *αα* cells (Roman, Phillips, & Sands, 1955). If this mixture is now induced to sporulate, the six cell types which possess at least one *a* gene and one *α* gene will each produce spores.

The asci which are thus obtained are generally four-spored. The *aa* diploids and the *aaαα* tetraploid produce chiefly haploid and diploid spores, respectively, and are highly fertile, that is, the four spores in the asci from these are likely to be viable. This is not true of the triploids, the asci of which only infrequently have four viable spores. The sterility of the triploids is the consequence of chromosomal segregation during meiosis and the resulting distribution of unbalanced chromosomal sets to the spores. Thus, a spore is viable if it has a haploid or a diploid set of chromosomes but it may be less viable or even inviable if its chromosome number is somewhere between the haploid and diploid number. The diploids, triploids, and tetraploids can be distinguished one from the other also by the characteristic segregations for mating type among the spores. Further, the three types of diploids are separable by genetic analysis if the two strains involved in the cross were different in their genetic properties.

We shall turn now to what can happen in a diploid culture maintained under vegetative conditions of growth. The diploid is *aa* with reference to the mating type alleles and is heterozygous as well for other genes affecting the various properties of the yeast in question. It has been demonstrated in yeast (James & Lee-Whiting, 1955), and in organisms as diverse as *Aspergillus* and *Drosophila*, that genetic recombination can take place in diploid cells without the intervention of meiosis. The consequences of mitotic recombination, as this is called, are shown in Fig. 3. An exchange occurring

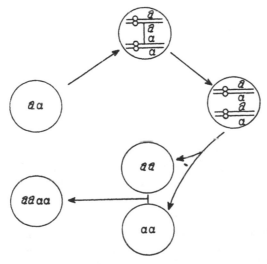

Fig. 3. Evolution of tetraploid cells from diploid cells by mitotic recombination.

between the centromere of the chromosome and the locus of the gene in heterozygous condition will result in two dyads each heterozygous for the gene in question. The appropriate separation of the chromatids in each dyad during mitosis can result in daughter cells which are now homozygous for one or the other of the two allelic forms of the gene. Since the two homozygotes may each be different in property from the heterozygote and from each other, the culture is now heterogeneous with reference to cell types. The degree of heterogeneity will depend on the number of genes in heterozygous condition and this in turn depends on the original composition of the culture and the occurrence of mutation during the growth of the culture. The frequency of recombination between centromere and gene depends on the distance of the gene from the centromere. We have found frequencies of the order of one such event per chromosome per 10,000 cells undergoing division, a rate which is sufficient to alter rapidly the genetic make-up of a culture.

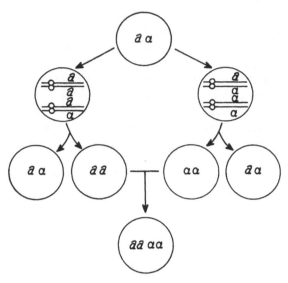

FIG. 4. Evolution of tetraploid cells from diploid cells by gene conversion.

We encounter in yeast a second type of mitotic recombination, called gene conversion (Lindegren, 1949), or allelic recombination (Roman & Jacob, 1958), which also results in the production of homozygous cells from heterozygous cells. In this type of recombination, illustrated in Fig. 4, one of the dyads remains homozygous and the other becomes heterozygous for reasons which are not yet well understood. The result of such an event is the production of a daughter cell in which one or the other of the genes in heterozygous condition becomes homozygous. The frequency with which allelic recombination occurs is a characteristic of the allelic pair in question and may be as high as one in 10^4 or 10^5 cells undergoing division.

In addition to variation in genotype as a result of gene mutation and mitotic recombination, variation in chromosome number, in the form of tetraploidy, has been observed in diploid cultures. Tetraploids are in fact expected, from endomitosis and from mitotic recombination. Cells homozygous at the mating-type locus, *aa* and *αα*, are obtained from the latter and tetraploids are the result of the subsequent mating of such cells.

The foregoing discussion has dealt with variation in heterothallic yeast. Homothallic yeast, such as *Saccharomyces chevalieri*, differs from heterothallic yeast in the following way. In heterothallic yeast mating within a haploid spore culture occurs very rarely, as a result of infrequent mating-type mutation, or, in the case of *a* cultures, fusion of cells of like mating type. In homothallic yeast, cell matings occur frequently and within a few divisions after spore germination. Winge and Roberts have shown (1949), by crossing *Saccharomyces cerevisiae* and *Saccharomyces chevalieri*, that the difference between heterothallism and homothallism in these yeasts is attributable to a "diploidization" gene present in *S. chevalieri*. This gene segregates independently of the *a* and *α* genes. Hawthorne has more recently found (personal communication) that the effect of the diploidization gene is to increase enormously the mutation rate of *a* to *α* and *α* to *a* and that the matings observed in homothallic cultures are actually matings between *a* and *α* cells. For example, a spore of mating-type *a* germinates to produce cells of mating-type *a* and these in turn produce, with a very high frequency, cells of mating-type *α*. The diploidization gene ceases to be operative in *aα* diploids and the diploid is therefore stable, subject to the kinds of variation which we have already discussed. We can therefore regard homothallism as a special case of heterothallism and can be confident that the types of genetic behavior described above are applicable to both.

Thus, because of mutation, either genic or cytoplasmic (see Ephrussi, 1953), the recombination of mutations, and variation in chromosome number, any sizable population of yeast cells growing vegetatively is certain to be genetically heterogeneous. The frequency with which such events occur is high enough to be worrisome for the purpose of long-term culture yet low enough to be manageable for the maintenance of a reasonable constancy. Quality control requires the periodic purification of the strain by re-isolation, preferably from single cells, of subcultures which possess the characteristics for which the strain was originally selected.

ACKNOWLEDGMENTS

Some of the investigations reported in this paper were supported by Grant No. E-328 of the National Institutes of Health, U.S. Public Health Service. The permission of Dr. D. C. Hawthorne to quote from his unpublished work is gratefully acknowledged.

REFERENCES

Ahmad, M. 1952. Single-spore cultures of heterothallic *Saccharomyces cerevisiae* which mate with both the tester strains. Nature *170*: 546–547.

Ephrussi, B. 1953. Nucleo-cytoplasmic relations in micro-organisms. Clarendon Press, Oxford.

Hawthorne, D. C., and R. K. Mortimer. 1960. Chromosome mapping in Saccharomyces: Centromere-linked genes. Genetics *45*: 1085–1110.

James, A. P., and B. Lee-Whiting. 1955. Radiation-induced genetic segregations in vegetative cells of diploid yeast. Genetics *40*: 826–831.

Lindegren, C. C. 1949. The yeast cell, its genetics and cytology. Educational Publishers, Saint Louis.

Lindegren, C. C., and G. Lindegren. 1943. Segregation, mutation, and copulation in *Saccharomyces cerevisiae*. Ann. Missouri Bot. Garden *30*: 453–468.

Roman, H., and F. Jacob. 1958. A comparison of spontaneous and ultraviolet-induced allelic recombination with reference to the recombination of outside markers. Cold Spring Harbor Symp. Quant. Biol., *23*: 155–160.

Roman, H., M. M. Phillips, and S. M. Sands. 1955. Studies of polyploid Saccharomyces. I. Tetraploid segregation. Genetics *40*: 546–561.

Roman, H., and S. M. Sands. 1953. Heterogeneity of clones of Saccharomyces derived from haploid ascospores. Proc. Natl. Acad. Sci. (U.S.) *39*: 171–179.

Townsend, G. F., and C. C. Lindegren. 1954. Characteristic growth patterns of the different members of a polyploid series of Saccharomyces. J. Bacteriol. 67: 480–483.

Winge, O., and C. Roberts. 1949. A gene for diploidization in yeasts. Compt. R. Lab. Carlsberg, Ser. Physiol. 24: 341–346.

PANEL DISCUSSION 2

MICROBIAL PRODUCTION
OF AMINO ACIDS

Chairmen
T. ASAI
M. J. THIRUMALACHAR

EUGENE L. DULANEY

Industrial Implications of Microbial Production of Amino Acids

T. ASAI

General Aspects of Amino Acid Fermentation in Japan

S. KINOSHITA

Production of Amino Acids with Special Consideration of the
Function of Biotin

H. S. MOYED

The Regulation of Biosynthetic Reactions

R. A. LATIMER

Comparison of Analytical Methods for the Determination of
Amino Acids

CHAIRMAN'S REMARKS

T. ASAI

Tokyo, Japan

METABOLISM of amino acids has been a subject of intensive study during the last few decades and a considerable amount of information and knowledge concerning this subject has accumulated in the fields of biochemistry and physiology as well as microbiology. Although the extracellular accumulation of small amounts of certain amino acids by micro-organisms had been known for many years, no one would have imagined ten years ago the realization of the successful microbial production of some amino acids in large quantities similar to alcohol or organic acid fermentations. The direct fermentative production of glutamic acid, that is, the extracellular accumulation of large quantities of glutamic acid, was achieved in 1956 by Japanese workers at Kyôwa Fermentation Co. Ltd. and at the University of Tokyo, and attracted the attention of microbiologists all over the world.

The so-called "amino acid fermentation" implies the accumulation of certain amino acids extracellularly in large quantities and may be understood as a result of unbalanced amino acid metabolism of micro-organisms. The abnormal accumulation of amino acids probably results from some complicated interrelationships among various activities of microbial cells and amino acids, such as biosynthesis, degradation, incorporation, mobilization and excretion.

Initial studies on amino acid fermentation were directed towards the selection of microbial strains which accumulated amino acids in abnormally large quantities when grown in the presence of excess inorganic nitrogen, mainly ammonium salts, as a result of an imbalance between carbohydrate metabolism and nitrogen assimilation. The utilization of mutants requiring amino acids and feed-back control mechanisms has been introduced recently in this field and has contributed to the successful production of other amino acids than glutamic acid.

The VIIIth International Congress of Microbiology, to my great pleasure, has taken up this newly developed field of "Microbial Production of Amino Acids" as a topic for panel discussion and, to my great honour and gratitude, has asked me and Dr. Thirumalachar to be moderators of the discussion. Five lectures to be given in this morning's session will cover both the scientifically and the industrially important aspects. I should like to ask all of you to participate in an earnest discussion and in frank and active expressions of opinions.

Finally, I should like to use this opportunity to mention the Association of Amino Acid Fermentation formed three years ago in Japan. This Association holds two symposia a year on various problems of amino acid fermentation and publishes an official journal, *Amino Acids*.

INDUSTRIAL IMPLICATIONS OF MICROBIAL PRODUCTION OF AMINO ACIDS

EUGENE L. DULANEY

Merck, Sharp & Dohme Research Laboratories
Rahway, U.S.A.

THE RECENT INDUSTRIAL INTEREST in microbial production of amino acids, except for glutamic acid, arose primarily from the need for some of these compounds as dietary supplements. Amino acid supplementation of diets must be preceded by a demonstration of such a need. Once such a need is established and the required amino acid balance is known, the goals can be met efficiently by addition of pure amino acids. This general problem is outside the scope of this discussion but the case for supplementation of pure amino acids has been presented in part by Howe (1961). My discussion will be directed to microbial processes for amino acids.

The microbial processes, however, must compete with synthetic processes. White (1961) has recently discussed synthesis and costs of essential amino acids. His long-range estimates of selling prices of individual amino acids at an arbitrary level of 5,000,000 pounds per year are tabulated below. Included also are some current costs taken or calculated from prices listed in *Chemical and Engineering News* for May 7, 1962.

Howe (1961) is somewhat more optimistic than White. He estimates that given a sufficiently large market any of the L-amino acids eventually might

TABLE 1
FUTURE ESTIMATES AND CURRENT COSTS OF AMINO ACIDS

Amino acid	Dollars per pound	
	Estimates from White	Current costs from Chem. Eng. News
L-lysine HCl	2.06–3.50	4.50
DL-threonine (75% assay)	1.75–3.10	
DL-threonine		50.0
DL-tryptophan	4.70–8.00	
L-tryptophan		140.60
DL-leucine	0.90–1.60	
L-leucine		19.00
DL-phenylalanine	1.05–1.80	29.50
DL-valine	0.85–1.45	
L-isoleucine/D-alloisoleucine	1.05–1.80	
DL-isoleucine		29.26
DL-methionine		1.43
Glutamic acid		1.65–1.80
Monosodium glutamate		0.79–0.86

be made to sell for $1.00 to $4.00 per pound. Thus it is quite clear that, in order to compete, microbial processes must convert a lot of cheap carbon to amino acids with a high efficiency. That this can be done is shown by the present microbial production of glutamic acid and lysine.

In the following discussion of individual amino acids, glutamic acid, isoleucine, valine and ornithine are omitted as these will be treated by Dr. Asai. The four amino acids most commonly deficient in dietary proteins, i.e., methionine, threonine, tryptophan and lysine, are treated plus some amino acids of lesser immediate interest.

Methionine

Several million pounds of DL-methionine are used each year as a feed supplement, primarily for chickens which are also capable of using the D-isomer (Gordon & Sizer, 1955). This demand is met by synthetic DL-methionine selling at approximately $1.40 per pound. Thus any proposed microbial methionine process has strong competition. There apparently, however, have been no developments towards a microbial process. Reports of methionine accumulation in extracellular metabolism solutions are rare. Failure of methionine to accumulate may be due to its synthesis being controlled by negative feedback (Cohn, Cohn, & Monod, 1953). However, one of our leucine-requiring auxotrophs of *Ustilago maydis* was found to accumulate approximately 6 mg/ml methionine in a synthetic medium (Dulaney, Jones, & Dulaney).

Threonine

Microbial processes for this essential amino acid have been directed to the use of auxotrophs for threonine accumulation and to the conversion of homoserine to threonine.

Of the *Escherichia coli* auxotrophs screened, Huang (1960a, 1960b, 1961b) found only the diaminopimelic acid–requiring strain D of Work (Meadow, Hoare, & Work, 1957) to accumulate threonine. This culture accumulated 100–300 μg/ml. Ultraviolet light treatment of strain D yielded No. 1307 which yielded No. 13070 by subsequent ultraviolet light treatment. These two strains accumulated approximately 2 mg/ml threonine but differed in optimum requirements for maximum accumulation. The addition of sucrose or beet molasses singly or sucrose plus cornsteep liquor to medium resulted in increased threonine accumulation. Strain No. 13070 accumulated 3.7 mg/ml threonine with optimum concentrations of supplements.

Shimura *et al.* (1959) studied cell suspensions of a number of organisms for ability to convert homoserine to threonine and found a variant of *Bacillus subtilus* to be superior. From 12 mg/ml DL-homoserine, 3.7 mg/ml L-threonine was obtained for a conversion efficiency of 60 per cent of the L-homoserine.

Fermentation variables of this process have been studied in detail by

Hayashiba *et al.* (1959). The best threonine accumulation was between two and three mg/ml.

Tryptophan

Studies on this amino acid have been concerned with conversion of precursors.

Aida *et al.* have studied transamination (1958) and reductive amination (1959) of 3-indolepyruvic acid. Dried cells of a number of bacteria were capable of transaminating this precursor in 0.1M phosphate buffer at pH 7.6 plus appropriate amino donors. A strain of *B. megaterium* yielded 67.5 per cent conversion, *E. coli*, 67.1 per cent, and *Aerobacter aerogenes* 52.6 per cent from a substrate charge of 17.5 mg. Aspartic and glutamic acids were superior amino donors.

Most cultures tested could reductively aminate 3-indolepyruvic acid, species of *Serratia* and *Micrococcus* being superior. *M. lysodeikticus* yields a 55 per cent conversion with NH_4Cl as the nitrogen source, while *M. luteus* cells gave a 61.8 per cent conversion with urea as the nitrogen source.

Tryptophan has also been produced by condensation of indole and serine. Malin and Westhead (1959) studied this coupling in detail using *Claviceps purpurea*. A yield of 1.5 mg/ml tryptophan was obtained from 550 µg/ml indole charged. Added serine caused no significant increase in tryptophan production. This process has been patented (Malin, 1961).

In another process, anthranilic acid or indole requiring auxotrophs of *E. coli* are used to couple indole and serine (Indian Patent Specification No. 61235). This patent reports that 10.4 g of L-tryptophan are obtained from two liters of whole broth charged with 6 g of indole and 12 g of DL-serine.

The conversion of anthranilic acid to tryptophan has been studied by Terui and Enatsu (1960) using an isolant of *Candida*.

Lysine

The screening studies of Richards and Haskins (1957) revealed that *Ustilago maydis* was capable of accumulating several hundred µg/ml of lysine. In later studies, Haskins and Spencer (1959) obtained 1.9 mg/ml lysine, plus 1.9 mg/ml glutamic acid and 3 mg/ml arginine from *U. maydis* culture broths.

Niosaka and Shimura (1959) found that yeast cells accumulated lysine when grown with a-aminoadipic acid. Conversion of precursors such as 5-formyl-2-oxovaleric acid (Broquist & Brockman, 1960), a-ketoadipic acid and a-aminoadipic acid (Broquist & Stiffey, 1959; Broquist, Stiffey & Albrecht, 1961) have also been investigated. *Saccharomyces cerevisiae* gave molar conversion of 50 per cent of 10 mg/ml a-aminoadipic acid added to a complex cornsteep liquor medium. Conversions of 50–70 per cent were obtained with 1–5 mg/ml a-ketoadipic acid. *Torulopsis utilis* affected conversion of 63.2 and 71.2 per cent from 1 and 5 mg/ml a-aminoadipic acid respectively, and of 83.5 and 56.8 per cent from 1 and 5 mg/ml a-ketoadipic acid.

Lysine-requiring auxotrophs of *E. coli* that accumulate diaminopimelic acid have been used in a lysine process (Davis, 1952; Casida, 1956; Kita & Huang, 1958; Huang, Griffin & Fried, 1960; Nubel, 1961). Diaminopimelic acid is decarboxylated by another culture or by release of an intracellular decarboxylase from the producing culture. Refinements of this process resulted in 23.65 mg/ml diaminopimelic acid from a medium with 80 mg/ml crude beet molasses and 7 per cent glycerol by volume as the carbon sources.

Kinoshita *et al.* (1958a) and Nakayama *et al.* (1961a; 1961b) found that several types of auxotrophs of *Micrococcus glutamicus* accumulate lysine. An auxotroph responding to homoserine or threonine plus methionine was superior and was used to develop the process. In a medium with 50 mg/ml glucose and 10 mg/ml NH₄Cl, 28 mg/ml lysine HCl was accumulated after 72 hours incubation (Kinoshita *et al.*, 1958).

Alanine

This amino acid occurs commonly in broths of various types of micro-organisms, but bacteria have been used mainly in process studies.

New species of *Brevibacterium, B. pentoso-aminoacidicum* and *B. pentoso-alanicum* were found by Yamada and Hirose (1960a) to be superior alanine accumulators with pentoses or glucose as the carbon source. The former culture gave a 40 per cent yield of alanine from glucose, and 25 per cent alanine plus 15 per cent glutamic acid from xylose (Yamada & Hirose, 1960b; Hirose & Yamada, 1960c).

Samejima *et al.* (1960e; 1960f) studied an unidentified bacillus that accumulated 17–18 mg/ml alanine from 100 mg/ml glucose. The probable route to alanine was via reductive amination of pyruvic acid. Okumura *et al.* (1960) screened bacteria from cheese, soil and sewage and found a number of isolants to yield 40–55 per cent alanine from glucose. Superior isolants belonged to *Brevibacterium* and *Corynebacterium*.

We have found a nicotinic acid–requiring mutant of *U. maydis* to accumulate 20 mg/ml alanine in a synthetic medium with 100 mg/ml glucose (Dulaney, Jones & Dulaney).

Homoserine

Homoserine accumulation has been studied by Kinoshita and collaborators (Samejima *et al.*, 1960a, 1960b, 1960c, 1960d; Kinoshita *et al.*, 1960a, 1960b) using an auxotroph of *M. glutamicus* that requires biotin and threonine. The mutant accumulated 13–15 mg/ml homoserine and 9 mg/ml lysine in a synthetic medium with glucose at 100 mg/ml and (NH₄)₂SO₄ at 20 mg/ml. Production of homoserine was less in the above medium plus peptone or N-Z-amine owing probably to the methionine present in the complex materials. DL-methionine at 200 μg/ml and greater decreases homoserine and increases lysine accumulation though the total amount of the two compounds was usually fairly constant (Samejima *et al.*, 1960c, 1960d).

Phenylalanine and Tyrosine

Shibuya *et al.* (1960) reported soil isolants capable of accumulating 500–900 µg/ml phenylalanine. Tyrosineless auxotrophs of *E. coli* (Huang, 1961b) and M. *glutamicus* (Nakayama *et al.*, 1961a) also accumulate phenylalanine. The *E. coli* mutant produced 2 mg/ml phenylalanine with sorbitol or glycerol as the carbon source (Huang, 1961a).

Phenylalanine and tyrosine have also been produced by amination of phenylpyruvic acid and p-hydroxyphenylpyruvic acid respectively (Asai *et al.*, 1959). Dried cells of a number of bacteria could convert phenylpyruvic acid to phenylalanine in buffered reaction mixtures with glutamic and aspartic acid as amino donors. *Alcaligenes faecalis* yielded 63.5 per cent phenylalanine from 14.3 mg substrate whereas *Pseudomonas cruciviae, P. aeruginosa, A. aerogenes* and *E. coli* showed 53 per cent conversion or better. Quantitative results on p-hydroxyphenylpyruvic acid conversion to tyrosine were not given. Different cultures, however, were best at affecting the two conversions.

Aspartic Acid

Aspartic acid can be made from fumaric acid. In *Chemical and Engineering News* for July 16, 1962, the price of fumaric acid is given as 20.5¢ lb in carload drums.

Kinoshita *et al.* (1958b) found growing cultures of a number of micro-organisms could accumulate 1 to 5 mg/ml of aspartic acid from 10 mg/ml fumaric acid. The best culture, *B. megaterium*, on further study was able to yield 80 per cent aspartic acid from 3 per cent fumaric acid.

Kisumi *et al.* (1959; 1960) also found *Bacillus* species *E. coli* and *P. fluorescens* to be superior convertors of fumaric to aspartic acid. Both *P. fluorescens* and *E. coli* carried out the reaction with efficiencies in excess of 95 per cent.

S. marcescens, E. coli and *Bacterium succinicum* were superior in this transformation for Kitahara *et al.* (1959a; 1959b). In a 100 ml reaction mixture containing 1 per cent dried *E. coli* cells and 50 per cent fumaric acid (as ammonium fumerate) buffered to pH 7.2–7.4, the conversion to aspartic acid was 99.4 per cent after 24 hours incubation at 37 C with slow agitation.

SUMMARY

The extracellular metabolism solutions of micro-organisms frequently contain free amino acids but the accumulation of one or more amino acid in large amount is unusual. By the use of mutation, or natural selection, auxotrophs with changed reaction rates and shifts in metabolic pathways have been obtained which accumulate quantities of one or more amino acids. Glutamic acid is produced microbially on a large scale in Japan and this country. Of the four amino acids, i.e., lysine, methionine, threonine and tryptophan, commonly found deficient in part in common dietary proteins, only lysine is produced microbially. Synthetic DL-methionine is so inexpensive that microbial processes would have difficulty in competing. Processes for threonine and tryptophan need development, however. Yields of a number of other amino acids, i.e., alanine, homoserine, ornithine and valine, are such that possibilities for microbial process development are good should they be needed. Still other amino acids, such as arginine, glycine, proline, histidine, leucine and serine have not been reported to occur in extracellular metabolism solution in promising amounts, except possibly arginine at 3 mg/ml (Haskins & Spencer, 1959).

Auxotroph study may yield accumulators of some of these amino acids but negative feedback must be overcome in some instances. Indeed, a procedure to screen mutants for loss of negative feedback would be of great help.

REFERENCES

Aida, K., T. Asai, T. Kajiwara, and K. Iizuka. 1958. On the preparation of L-tryptophan by bacterial transaminase. J. Gen. Appl. Microbiol. *4*: 200–202.

Aida, K., T. Asai, K. Iizuka, and T. Kajiwara. 1959. Studies on amino acid fermentation. VI. Preparation of L-tryptophan by microbial reductive amination. Amino Acids *1*, paper No. 13.

Asai, T., K. Aida, and K. Oishi. 1959. On the enzymatic preparation of L-phenylalanine. J. Gen. Appl. Microbiol. *5*: 150–152.

Broquist, H. P., and A. V. Stiffey. 1959. Biosynthesis of lysine from adipic acid precursors by yeast. Fed. Proc. *18*: 198.

Broquist, H. P., and J. A. Brockman. 1960. Production of lysine. U.S. Patent No. 2,965,545. Dec. 20.

Broquist, H. P., A. V. Stiffey, and A. M. Albrecht. 1961. Biosynthesis of lysine from α-ketoadipic acid and α-aminodipic acid. Appl. Microbiol. 9: 1–5.

Casida, L. E. 1956. Preparation of diaminopimelic acid and lysine. U.S. Patent No. 2,771,396. Nov. 20.

Cohn, M., G. M. Cohn, and J. Monod. 1953. Specific inhibitory effect of methionine in the formation of methionine synthetase with *Escherichia coli*. Compt. Rend. *236*: 746–748.

Dulaney, E. L., C. A. Jones, and D. D. Dulaney. Amino acid accumulation, principally alanine, by auxotrophs of *Ustilago maydis*. Unpublished research.

Davis, B. D. 1952. Biosynthetic interrelations of lysine, diaminopimelic acid, and threonine in mutants of *Escherichia coli*. Nature *169*: 534–536.

Gordon, R. S., and I. W. Sizer. 1955. The biological equivalence of methione hydroxy analogue. Poultry Sci. *34*: 1198.

Haskins, R. H., and J. F. T. Spencer. 1959. Production of lysine, arginine, and glutamic acids. U.S. Patent No. 2,902,409. Sept. 1.

Hayashibe, M., T. Sugihashi, Y. Saeki, A. Ichiba, Y. Fujii, K. Shimura, and T. Uyemura. 1959. Preparation of L-threonine by fermentation. Amino Acids *1*, paper No. 10.

Hirose, Y., and K. Yamada. 1961. Studies on the fermentation of amino acids from pentose. II. Fermentation and accumulation of amino acids by *Brevibacterium pentoso-aminoacidicum*. Amino Acids 3, paper No. 2.

Howe, E. E. 1961. Summary of progress on the use of purified amino acids in foods. *In* Progress in meeting protein needs of infants and preschool children. Publication 843, National Academy of Sciences, National Research Council, Washington, D.C.

Huang, H. T. 1960a. Production of L-threonine. U.S. Patent No. 2,937,121. May 17.

Huang, H. T. 1960b. Production of L-threonine. U.S. Patent No. 2,937,122. May 17.

Huang, H. T. 1961a. Fermentation process. U.S. Patent No. 2,973,304. Feb. 28.

Huang, H. T. 1961b. Production of L-threonine by auxotrophic mutants of *Escherichia coli*. Appl. Microbiol. 9: 419–424.

Huang, H. T., J. M. Griffin, and J. H. Fried. 1960. Improved fermentation process for the production of diaminopimelic acid. U.S. Patent No. 2,955,986. Oct. 11.

Indian Patent Specification No. 61235. Process for preparing tryptophan. July 25, 1957. Charles Pfizer & Co.

Kinoshita, S., K. Nakayama, and S. Kitada. 1958a. L-lysine production using microbial auxotroph. J. Gen. Appl. Microbiol. 4: 128–129.

Kinoshita, S., K. Nakayama, and S. Kitada. 1958b. Production of aspartic acid from fumaric acid by microorganisms. Hakkô Kyôbaishi 16: 517–520. Chem. Abstr. 53: 11514.

Kinoshita, S., H. Samejima, C. Fujita, and T. Nara. 1960a. L-homoserine fermentation. Amino Acids 2, paper No. 6.

Kinoshita, S., H. Samejima, K. Nakayama, T. Nara, and C. Fujita. 1960b. L-homoserine fermentation. J. Gen. Appl. Microbiol. 6: 193–195.

Kisumi, M., Y. Ashikaga, and I. Chibata. 1959. Studies on the fermentative preparation of L-aspartic acid from fumerate. Amino Acids 1, paper No. 15.

Kisumi, M., Y. Ashikaga, and I. Chibata. 1960. Studies on the fermentative preparation of L-aspartic acid from fumaric acid. Bull. Agr. Chem. Soc. Japan 24: 296–305.

Kita, D. A., and H. T. Huang. 1958. Fermentation process for the preparation of L-lysine. U.S. Patent No. 2,841,532. July 1.

Kitahara, K., S. Fukui, and M. Misawa. 1959a. Preparation of L-aspartic acid by bacterial aspartase. J. Gen. Appl. Microbiol. 5: 74–77.

Kitahara, K., S. Fukui, and M. Misawa. 1959b. Enzymatic preparation of L-aspartic acid from fumerate. Amino Acids 1, paper No. 14.

Malin, B. 1961. Method of producing L-tryptophan. U.S. Patent No. 2,999,051. Sept. 5.

Malin, B. and J. Westhead. 1959. Production of L-tryptophan in submerged culture. J. Biochem. Microbiol. Technol. Eng. 1: 49–57.

Meadow, P., D. S. Hoare, and E. Work. 1957. Interrelationships between lysine and a,ϵ-diaminopimelic acid and their derivatives and analogues in mutants of *Escherichia coli*. Biochem. J. 66: 270–282.

Nakayama, K., S. Kitada, Z. Sato, and S. Kinoshita. 1961a. Induction of nutritional mutants of glutamic acid bacteria and their amino acid accumulation. J. Gen. Appl. Microbiol. 7: 41–51.

Nakayama, K., S. Kitada, and S. Kinoshita. 1961b. Studies on lysine fermentation. I. The control mechanism on lysine accumulation by homoserine and threonine. J. Gen. Appl. Microbiol. 7: 145–154.

Niosaka, K. and K. Shimura. 1959. Studies on lysine synthesis. Amino Acids 1, paper No. 11.

Nubel, R. C. 1961. Amino acid and process. U.S. Patent No. 2,968,594. Jan. 17.

Okumura, S., H. Okada, A. Ozaki, K. Kono, and K. Sakaguchi. 1960. Studies on alanine fermentation, III. Amino Acids 2, paper No. 4.

Richards, M., and R. H. Haskins. 1957. Extracellular lysine production by various fungi. Canad. J. Microbiol. 3: 543–546.

Samejima, H., T. Nara, C. Fujita, and S. Kinoshita. 1960a, b, c, d. L-homoserine fermentation. I. Quantitative determination of L-homoserine and accumulation of L-homoserine by microorganisms. II. L-homoserine production in a natural medium. III. L-homoserine production in chemically defined media. IV. Effect of DL-methionine and L-threonine on homoserine accumulation. Nippon Nôgeikagaku Kaisi *34*: 750–754, 750–754, 824–828, 828–832. Abstracted Bull. Agr. Chem. Soc. Japan *24*: A67, A68, A74.

Samejima, H., T. Nara, C. Fujita, and S. Kinoshita. 1960e, f. L-alanine fermentation. I. L-alanine fermentation by No. 483 strain. II. Enzymatic aspects of L-alanine fermentation by No. 483 strain. Nippon Nôgeikagaku Kaishi *34*: 832–838, 838–844. Abstracted Bull. Agr. Chem. Soc. Japan *24*: A75.

Shibuya, J., S. Suzuki, Y. Fujii, and S. Namura. 1960. L-phenylalanine production by bacteria. Amino Acids *2*, paper No. 5.

Shimura, K., Y. Watanabe, Y. Fujii, and S. Konishi. 1959. Synthesis of L-threonine from homoserine. Amino Acids *1*, paper No. 8.

Terui, G., and T. Enatsu. 1960. Metabolism of anthranilic acid and production of tryptophan. Amino Acids *3*, paper No. 8.

White, H. C. 1961. Practical synthetic routes to the essential amino acids. *In* Progress in meeting protein needs of infants and preschool children. Publication 843, National Academy of Sciences, National Research Council, Washington, D.C.

Yamada, K., and Y. Hirose. 1960a. Studies on the amino acids fermentation of pentose materials. I. Isolation of strains capable of producing amino acids from pentose and their taxonomical studies. Bull. Agr. Chem. Soc. Japan. *24*: 621–627.

Yamada, K. and Y. Hirose. 1960b. Amino acid fermentation using pentose as the carbohydrate source. Amino Acids *2*, paper No. 2.

GENERAL ASPECTS OF AMINO ACID FERMENTATION IN JAPAN

TOSHINOBU ASAI

Suita Laboratory
The Brewing Science Research Institute
Asahi Breweries, Tokyo, Japan

I. HISTORICAL DEVELOPMENT OF THE STUDIES ON AMINO ACID FERMENTATION

It has been known for many years that micro-organisms accumulate free amino acids extracellularly, and this phenomenon has been studied by a number of workers. But the fact that they accumulate some "specific" amino acids in large quantities in media under certain conditions was not known until recently. When this last phenomenon is used for the production of amino acids, specific amino acids can be manufactured in the L-forms and in large quantities. This method of production combines the oxidation of sugars with the assimilation of nitrogen through micro-organisms, resulting in the production of amino acids. Although amino acid production from biosynthetic precursors through one or several enzymatic steps using microbial cells cannot be called fermentation in its strict sense, the expression "amino acid fermentation" is used here to represent all methods of amino acid production using micro-organisms.

In 1956 the production of glutamic acid by fermentation was invented by the Kyôwa Fermentation Co. and attracted attention all over the world. Since then the progress has been remarkable and many papers and patents concerning glutamic acid as well as other amino acids have been published in Japan and in other countries.

II. PROBLEMS IN THE GLUTAMIC ACID FERMENTATION

1. *Micro-organisms.* The Kyôwa Fermentation Co. succeeded in producing glutamic acid on an industrial scale for the first time using *Micrococcus glutamicus* (Kinoshita *et al.*, 1957 b, c). Glutamic acid–producing strains isolated by Asai's group in an early stage of study also belonged to the genus *Micrococcus* (Asai *et al.*, 1957). The genus *Brevibacterium* then came into the limelight as a strong glutamic acid producer (Yamada & Su, 1959; Ogawa *et al.*, 1959; Okumura *et al.*, 1959; Ota & Tanaka, 1959; Kobayashi *et al.*, 1959; Yoshino *et al.*, 1960; Yamada & Hirose, 1960). This genus was newly adopted in the 7th edition of Bergey's *Manual of Determinative Bacteriology*, and many of the active glutamic acid–producing strains reported so far belong to this genus. Some active strains of *Microbacterium* have also been reported (Doi & Kaneko, 1960).

Interestingly enough, although the majority of strains reported as active glutamic acid producers belong to *Micrococcus* or *Brevibacterium*, all efforts to find an active strain among the organisms previously assigned to these two genera have failed (Iizuka & Komagata, 1959).

2. *Media and cultural conditions*. Glucose (or acid hydrolysate of starch) is the most common carbon source in industrial production. Molasses may also be used. Pentoses (Hirose & Yamada, 1961), α-ketoglutarate (Otsuka *et al.*, 1957), acetate (Tsunoda *et al.*, 1961) and γ-aminobutyrate (Tsunoda *et al.*, 1959) have been used successfully as carbon sources in laboratory scale production of glutamic acid. Urea and ammonia are considered the best nitrogen sources and are commonly used. The pH is maintained between 6.0 and 8.5 and these nitrogen sources act as buffers and prevent the lowering of pH as a result of acid production. Successive additions of the nitrogen source form a currently adopted method for efficient production of glutamate. Growth-promoting substances, such as cornsteep liquor, bran extract, casein hydrolysate, polypeptone, yeast extract and NZ-amine, are added to media. The biotin content in the culture medium is important. Tanaka *et al.* (1960) reported that the glutamic acid accumulation was most marked when biotin was present in a concentration suboptimal for growth.

Okumura *et al.* (1962 a, b, c) reported that biotin could be replaced by biotin analogues; DL-desthiobiotin, biotin sulfoxide, biocytin and 7, 8-diaminopelargonic acid were almost as effective as biotin. 7,8-diketopelargonic acid could also replace biotin, though it was not as effective as others.

Recently Miyai *et al.* (1962 a) reported the stimulative effect of cystine on glutamic acid accumulation using *Microbacterium ammoniaphilum*. According to them (1962b) sorbitanmonooleate and trioleate were also effective for the accumulation. Some plant hormones, such as indole-3-acetic acid and 2,4-dichlorophenoxy acetic acid, may also substitute for biotin in glutamic acid fermentation although not as effectively as biotin (Kinoshita *et al.*, 1962).

Aeration and agitation are other important problems. The Kd optimal for high glutamic acid production was reported to lie around 4.5 to 5.0 × 10⁻⁶ by many workers.

Details of the production of L-glutamic acid by *Brevibacterium divaricatum* on a pilot plant scale have been reported by Su and Yamada (1960).

3. *Mechanism of glutamic acid fermentation*. A considerable amount of work has been done on the pathways by which glutamic acid is formed and accumulated (Tanaka *et al.*, 1959; Shiio *et al.*, 1959, 1960 a, b, 1961 a, b; Aida *et al.*, 1960 a, b; Yata *et al.*, 1961; Su *et al.*, 1961 a, b). This has been summarized in Fig. 1 and also in the figure of Dr. Kinoshita's paper (Fig. 2).

4. *Interconversion of glutamic acid fermentation and succinic acid fermentation*. Okada *et al.* (1961) found with *Brevibacterium flavum* that when the aeration rate was reduced or when the concentration of cornsteep

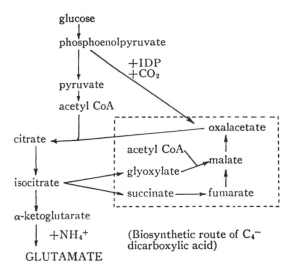

glucose
↓
phosphoenolpyruvate

+IDP
+CO₂

pyruvate
↓
acetyl CoA

citrate ← oxalacetate

acetyl CoA
↓ malate
glyoxylate

isocitrate ← succinate → fumarate

α-ketoglutarate

↓ +NH₄⁺   (Biosynthetic route of C₄⁻
            dicarboxylic acid)
GLUTAMATE

FIG. 1. Main pathway of glucose metabolism and glutamate biosynthesis in *Brev. flavum.*

liquor (CSL) in the medium was increased a considerable amount of succinic acid was accumulated instead of glutamic acid. The conditions optimal
for succinic acid formation were Kd at 0.4 to 0.7 $\times$ 10⁻⁶ and a concentration
of 1.0 to 2.0 per cent CSL. The yield of succinic acid was 30 per cent of
the sugar consumed. Oishi *et al.* (1961) observed a similar phenomenon
with *B. divaricatum.* The role of CSL was shown to be due to the biotin
present. According to experiments with radioactive isotopes, succinic acid
is formed reductively from fumaric acid not only under poor aeration but
also at a high concentration of biotin. Both the total DPN content (both
oxidized and reduced) and the DPNH/DPN ratio were found to be much
higher in "biotin-rich" cells than in "biotin-deficient" cells and they concluded that these differences were responsible for the accumulation of
succinic acid under biotin-rich conditions (Oishi *et al.*, 1962).

III. STUDIES ON THE MICROBIAL PRODUCTION OF OTHER AMINO ACIDS

1. *Ornithine.* Kinoshita *et al.* (1957a) reported a successful ornithine
fermentation: arginine- or citrulline-requiring mutants of *Micrococcus
glutamicus* accumulated 26 mg ornithine per ml. In the presence of a large
amount of arginine in the medium the same organism accumulated glutamate
instead of ornithine (Udaka & Kinoshita, 1958a).

Ornithine fermentation has set an important milestone by introducing
into amino acid fermentation the utilization of nutritional mutants and
feedback control mechanisms.

2. *Valine.* This amino acid has often been detected along with glutamic
acid, alanine, leucine and isoleucine in amino acid–producing media since
the early phase of amino acid fermentation studies. Udaka and Kinoshita

TABLE 1
MICROBIAL PRODUCTION OF OTHER AMINO ACIDS

Amino acids	Micro-organisms	Substrates (concent.)	Yields[a]	References[b]
Alanine	*Streptomyces coelicolor*	Glucose 2%	6 (DL)	Yazaki (1958)
	Brevibacterium alanicum	Glucose 5%	12	Ogawa (1959)
	Brevibacterium monoflagellum	Glucose 10%	50 (DL)	Ozaki (1960)
	Corynebacterium gelatinosum, strain 483	Glucose 10%	17.5 (L)	Samejima (1960)
Threonine	*B. subtilis*	Glucose 5% Homoserine added	2.9	Hayashibe (1959a)
Homoserine	*M. glutamicus* mutant (requiring threonine)	Glucose 10%	13–14[c]	Kinoshita (1960)
Aspartic acid	*B. megaterium* *E. coli* *S. marcescens* *Bact. succinicum* *B. megaterium*	NH_4-fumarate 3% Fumaric acid 50% (NH_4 Salt) (by dried cells)	24 560 *ca* 90% yield	Kinoshita (1958a) Kitahara (1959)
	Ps. fluorescens	NH_4-fumarate 6.5%	50	Kisumi (1959)
Lysine	*M. glutamicus* mutant (requiring homoserine or methionine and threonine)	Glucose 5%	15	Kinoshita (1958b)
	B. subtilis	Starch and fish soluble	2.5	Aida (1958b)
Tyrosine	*M. glutamicus* mutant (requiring phenylalanine)	Glucose 2%	0.6	Nakayama (1961b)
Phenyl-alanine	*Alc. faecalis*	Phenylpyruvic acid and amino acid mixt. (asp. glut. acid and leucine)	78% (by dried cells)	Asai (1959)
	M. glutamicus mutant (requiring tyrosine)	Cerelose 7.5%	1.3	Nakayama (1961a)
Tryptophan	*B. megaterium*	3-Indolpyruvic acid and glutamic acid or aspartic acid	70% (by dried cells)	Aida (1958a)
	M. lutens *M. lysodeikticus*	3-Indolpyruvic acid and inorganic NH_4 salts	55–62% (by dried cells)	Aida (1959)
	Candida sp.	Glucose 6% and anthranilic acid 0.05%	0.3	Terui (1961)

[a]Grams per litre unless otherwise stated.
[b]First author only given.
[c]Lysine amounting to 9–10 g/l was also produced.

(1958b) reported the accumulation of valine up to 15 mg/ml by a strain of *Paracolobactrum coliforme*. According to them one of the mechanisms for the accumulation of valine was ascribed to the action of an active acetolactate-forming enzyme which is not suppressed by valine itself.

Sugisaki (1959) isolated *Aerobacter* strains which accumulated valine up to 13 per cent of sugar added in a medium containing 10 per cent glucose. Nakayama *et al.* (1960) found, among the isoleucine- or leucine-requiring mutants of *M. glutamicus*, several strains which accumulated up to 8 g of valine per litre and reported that by changing the concentrations of required amino acids and biotin these strains accumulated either valine, glutamic acid or lactic acid.

3. *Isoleucine*. Since the isolation of isoleucine from protein hydrolysate is made difficult by the presence of concomitant leucine, a good fermentation method for the production was desired. Hayashi *et al.* (1959b), working with a strain of *Bacillus subtilis*, obtained an accumulation of up to 7 g isoleucine per litre, and Chibata *et al.* (1960) isolated a strain of *Pseudomonas aeruginosa* which accumulated 14 g isoleucine per litre in the presence of α-aminobutyric acid. Later, the same authors (1962) reported

TABLE 2

AMINO ACID PRODUCTION IN JAPAN

Amino acids	Production, tons/year		Processes of manufacture	Uses
	1961	1962 (expected)		
DL-Alanine	10	10	S (F)	sp
L-Alanine		0.5	H (F)	r
L-Arginine-HCl (L-Arginine)	8	20	H	p
L-Aspartic acid	0.6	6	H F	ps
L-Cystine	0.1	0.2	H	p
Glycine	20	25	S	sp
L-Glutamine	0.3	1.2	S	p
L-Glutamic acid (Monosodium glutamate)	29,000	35,000	H F (S)	sp
L-Histidine-HCl	3	8	H	ps
L-Hydroxyproline	0.1	0.3	H	r
*L-Isoleucine	0.1	0.2	H F	r
*L-Leucine	1	3	H	p
L-Leucine and L-Isoleucine (2:1 mixture)	8	14	H	p
*L-Lysine-HCl	50	90	H F S	fp
DL-Methionine	100	100	S	pf
*L-Methionine	5	7	S	p
*L-Phenylalanine	4	8	H (S F)	p
L-Proline	0.4	0.7	H	r
L-Serine	0.2	0.4	H	r
D,L-Threonine	3	4	S	p
*L-Threonine	3	6	S H	p
*L-Tryptophan	1	3	S	p
L-Tyrosine	0.5	0.8	H	r
*L-Valine	3	6	S H F	p

*Essential amino acids.

Abbreviations: S, chemical synthesis; H, hydrolysis of proteinous materials; F, fermentation; s, seasoning; p, pharmaceutical; f, food fortifier and feed; r, reagent; ( ), indicates possible method.

a fairly good yield of isoleucine (8 mg/ml) in a D-threonine–containing glucose medium using a strain of *Serratia marcescens*. Recent works on the microbial production of other amino acids have been listed in Table 1.

IV. INDUSTRIAL PRODUCTION OF AMINO ACIDS IN JAPAN, AND THE STATUS OF THE MICROBIOLOGICAL METHODS THEREIN

In the early history of amino acid fermentation amino acids such as glutamic acid, alanine and valine were easily produced in large quantities in growth media after simple isolation of organisms from natural environment and improvement of cultural conditions. In the microbiological production of ornithine, lysine, threonine and isoleucine, however, new techniques have been introduced, such as the addition of specific metabolic precursors or the use of various nutritional mutants. The present status of amino acid production in Japan is summarized in Table 2. It might be mentioned that of world production in 1960 of 42,300 tons of mono-sodium glutamate, Japan produced 22,300 tons, the United States 9,000, Western Europe 8,000 and other countries 3,000 tons.

A combination of negative feedback control mechanism and of mutants with defective amino acid synthesizing systems will probably lead to the development of new amino acid fermentations. Another important future problem in industrial production of amino acids is mechanization and the introduction of continuous fermentation processes. It is also necessary to explore new markets for amino acids; study of the production of synthetic fibers through polymerization of amino acids is an example of effort in this direction. Chemical synthesis is already catching up with fermentation with the production of glutamic acid from acrylnitrile. If the fermentation industry is to keep ahead of petro-chemical industrial developments a better understanding of the characteristics of microbiological reactions and their application to practical aspects of fermentation is essential.

REFERENCES

Aida, K., T. Asai, T. Kajiwara, and K. Iizuka. 1958a. On the preparation of L-tryptophan by bacterial transaminase. J. Gen. Appl. Microbiol. 4: 200–202.

Aida, T., and T. Uemura. 1958b. Studies on L-lysine fermentation. I. Presented at the Annual Meeting of Agr. Chem. Soc. Japan, May.

Aida, K., T. Asai, K. Iizuka and T. Kajiwara. 1959. On the preparation of L-tryptophan by bacterial reductive amination (in Japanese). Amino Acids 1: 94–98.

Aida, K., K. Oishi and T. Asai. 1960a. Studies on amino acid fermentation. II. On the mechanism of L-glutamic acid fermentation (in Japanese). Nippon Nôgeikagaku Kaishi 34: 70–77.

Aida, K., K. Oishi, K. Shimizu, and T. Asai. 1960b. Studies on amino acid fermentation. V. On the mechanism of L-glutamic acid fermentation (2) (in Japanese). Nippon Nôgeikagaku Kaishi 34: 77–83.

Asai, T., K. Aida and K. Oishi. 1957. On L-glutamic acid fermentation. Bull. Agr. Chem. Soc. Japan 21: 134–135.

Asai, T., K. Aida and K. Oishi. 1959. On the enzymatic preparation of L-phenylalanine. J. Gen. Appl. Microbiol. 5: 150–152.

Chibata, I., M. Kisumi and Y. Ashikaga. 1960. Studies on the fermentative production of L-isoleucine, I (in Japanese with English summary). Amino Acids 2: 90–96.

Chibata, I., M. Kisumi, Y. Ashikaga and J. Kato. 1962. Studies on the fermentative production of L-isoleucine, II (in Japanese with English summary). Amino Acids 5: 76–91.

Doi, S., and Y. Kaneko. 1960. A glutamic acid–producing bacterium (in Japanese). Amino Acids 2: 25–30.

Hayashibe, M., T. Sugihashi, N. Saeki, A. Ichiba, Y. Fujii, K. Shimura and T. Uemura. 1959a. Fermentative production of L-threonine (in Japanese). Amino Acids 1: 80–84.

Hayashi K., Y. Watanabe, Y. Fujii and K. Shimura. 1959b. Studies on the isoleucine fermentation, I (in Japanese). Amino Acids 1: 89–98.

Hirose, Y., and K. Yamada. 1961. Studies on the amino acids fermentation of pentose materials. II. Amino acids formation by Brevibacterium pentosoaminoacidicum nov. sp. (in Japanese). Amino Acids 3: 21–25.

Iizuka, H., and K. Komagata. 1959. Amino acid accumulation and bacteria (in Japanese). Amino Acids 1: 111–115.

Kinoshita, S., K. Nakayama and S. Udaka. 1957a. The fermentative production of L-ornithine. J. Gen. Appl. Microbiol. 3: 276–277.

Kinoshita, S., K. Tanaka, S. Udaka and S. Akita. 1957b. Glutamic acid fermentation. Proc. Intern. Symposium Enzyme Chem. (Tokyo and Kyoto): 464–468.

Kinoshita, S., S. Udaka and M. Shimono. 1957c. Production of L-glutamic acid by various microorganisms. Presented at the Annual Meeting of Agr. Chem. Soc. Japan, April.

Kinoshita, S., K. Nakayama and S. Kitada. 1958a. Production of aspartic acid from fumaric acid by microorganisms (in Japanese). Hakkô Kyôkai Shi 16: 38–41.

Kinoshita, S., K. Nakayama and S. Kitada. 1958b. L-lysine production using microbial auxotroph. J. Gen. Appl. Microbiol. 4: 128–129.

Kinoshita, S., H. Samejima, T. Nara and C. Fujita. 1960. L-homoserine fermentation (in Japanese). Amino Acids 2: 125–132.

Kinoshita, K., T. Shiio, K. Narui, T. Tsuchiya and T. Tsunoda. 1962. Effect of plant hormone for glutamic acid fermentation (in Japanese with English summary). Amino Acids 5: 48–52.

Kisumi, M., Y. Ashikaga and I. Chibata. 1959. Studies on the fermentative preparation of L-aspartic acid from fumaric acid (in Japanese). Amino Acids 1: 102–110.

Kitahara, K., S. Fukui and M. Misawa. 1959. Preparation of L-aspartic acid by bacterial aspartase. J. Gen. Appl. Microbiol. 5: 74–77.

Kobayashi, K., N. Nunoko, K. Sato and N. Ogawa. 1959. Studies on the L-glutamic acid fermentation of beet molasses, I (in Japanese). Hakkô Kôgaku Zasshi 37: 440–449.

Miyai, K., I. Tsuruo, R. Kodaira, S. Hayakawa, Y. Akimoto and K. Gotô. 1962a. The stimulative effect of cystine on the glutamic acid fermentation. Presented at 6th Symposium on Amino Acid Fermentation (Sendai), April.

Miyai, K., K. Gotô, I. Tsuruo, R. Kodaira and Y. Akimoto. 1962b. The stimulative effect of some surface active agents on the glutamic acid fermentation. Presented at 6th Symposium on Amino Acid Fermentation (Sendai), April.

Nakayama, K., S. Kitada and S. Kinoshita. 1960. L-valine production using microbial auxotroph (in Japanese). Amino Acids 2: 77–85.

Nakayama, K., Z. Sato and S. Kinoshita. 1961a. L-phenylalanine accumulation by tyrosine-less mutant of glutamic acid–producing bacteria (in Japanese). Nippon Nôgeikagaku Kaishi 35: 142–145.

Nakayama, K., Z. Sato and S. Kinoshita. 1961b. L-tyrosine accumulation by phenylalanine-less mutant of glutamic acid–producing bacteria (in Japanese). Nippon Nôgeikagaku Kaishi 35: 146–150.

Ogawa, C., T. Oide and Y. Midorikawa. 1959. Studies on alanine and glutamic acid production by *Brevibacterium alanicum* nov. sp. (in Japanese). Amino Acids 1: 45–49.

Oishi, K., K. Aida and T. Asai. 1961. Studies on amino acid fermentation. VIII. On the mechanism of conversion of L-glutamic acid fermentation to succinic acid fermentation (I). J. Gen. Appl. Microbiol. 7: 213–226.

Oishi, K., K. Aida and T. Asai. 1962. Studies on amino acid fermentation. IX. On the mechanism of conversion of L-glutamic acid fermentation to succinic acid fermentation, II (in Japanese). Nippon Nôgeikagaku Kaishi 36: 172–176.

Okada, H., I. Kameyama, S. Okumura and T. Tsunoda. 1961. L-glutamic acid and succinic acid fermentation by *Brevibacterium flavum* No. 1996. J. Gen. Appl. Microbiol. 7: 177–191.

Okumura, S., T. Togawa, T. Tsunoda, T. Matsui and K. Kono. 1959. On glutamic acid–producing bacteria. II. On *Micrococcus, Brevibacterium* and *Corynebacterium*. Presented at 192th Monthly Meeting of Agr. Chem. Soc. Japan, May.

Okumura, S., R. Tsugawa, T. Tsunoda and A. Kitai. 1962a. Studies on the L-glutamic acid fermentation. II. Activity of d-biotin and the biotin group compounds as a growth factor (in Japanese). Nippon Nôgeikagaku Kaishi 36: 197–203.

Okumura, S., R. Tsugawa, T. Tsunoda and S. Motozaki. 1962b. Studies on the L-glutamic acid fermentation. III. Activities of the various pelargonic acid compounds to promote the fermentation (in Japanese). Nippon Nôgeikagaku Kaishi 36: 204–211.

Okumura, S., K. Kinoshita, R. Tsugawa, H. Okada and T. Tsunoda. 1962c. Studies on the L-glutamic acid fermentation. IV. The biotin activity of 7,8-diaminopelargonic acid (in Japanese with English summary). Amino Acids 5: 33–40.

Ota, S., and M. Tanaka. 1959. Taxonomic studies on *Brevibacterium aminogenes* nov. sp. (Studies on glutamic acid fermentation, I; in Japanese). Amino Acids 1: 50–52.

Otsuka, S., H. Yazaki, H. Nagase and K. Sakaguchi. 1957. Fermentative production of L-glutamic acid from a-ketoglutaric acid and ammonium salt. J. Gen. Appl. Microbiol. 3: 35–53.

Ozaki, A., K. Kôno, S. Okumura, H. Okada and K. Sakaguchi. 1960. Studies on alanine fermentation, III. Presented at the 2nd Symposium on Amino Acid Fermentation, April.

Samejima, H., T. Nara, C. Fujita and S. Kinoshita. 1960. L-alanine fermentation by No. 483 strain (in Japanese). Nippon Nôgeikagaku Kaishi 34: 832–838.

Shiio, I., S. Otsuka and T. Tsunoda. 1959, 1960a, 1960b. Glutamic acid formation from glucose by bacteria. I. Enzymes of the Embden-Meyerhof-Parnas pathway, the Krebs cycle, and the glyoxylate bypass in cell extracts of *Brevibacterium flavum* No. 2247. III. On the pathway of pyruvate formation in *Brevibacterium flavum* No. 2247. IV. Carbon dioxide fixation and glutamate formation in *Brevibacterium flavum* No. 2247. J. Biochem. 46: 1303–1311; 47: 414–421; 48: 110–120.

Shiio, I., S. Otsuka and M. Takahashi. 1961a. Significance of α-ketoglutaric dehydrogenase on the glutamic acid formation in *Brevibacterium flavum*. J. Biochem. *50*: 164–165.

Shiio, I., S. Otsuka and M. Takahashi. 1961b. Effect of growth substrates on levels of glyoxylate by-pass enzymes in a glutamate forming bacterium, *Bacterium flavum* No. 2247. J. Biochem. *49*: 262–263.

Su, Y. C., and K. Yamada. 1960. Studies on L-glutamic acid fermentation. Pilot plant scale test of the fermentative production of L-glutamic acid by *Brevibacterium divaricatum* nov. sp. Bull. Agr. Chem. Soc. Japan *24*: 525–529.

Su, Y. C., N. Tanaka and K. Yamada. 1961a, b. Studies on L-glutamic acid fermentation. IV. Metabolism of L-glutamic acid and glycolytic enzymes of the E.M.P. pathway in cell-free extracts of *Brevibacterium divaricatum* nov. sp. V. The enzymes of the tricarboxylic acid cycle and glyoxylate bypass in cell-free extracts of *Brevibacterium divaricatum*. Agr. Biol. Chem. *25*: 553–558; *25*: 685–692.

Sugisaki, Z. 1959. Studies on L-valine fermentation. I. Production of L-valine by *Aerobacter* bacteria. J. Gen. Appl. Microbiol. *5*: 138–149.

Tanaka, K., S. Akita, K. Kimura and S. Kinoshita. 1959. Studies on glutamic acid fermentation. IV. Mechanism of glucose metabolism in *Micrococcus glutamicus* (in Japanese). Amino Acids *1*: 62–70.

Tanaka, K., T. Iwasaki and S. Kinoshita. 1960. Studies on L-glutamic acid fermentation. V. Biotin and L-glutamic acid accumulation (in Japanese). Nippon Nôgeikagaku Kaishi *34*: 593–600.

Terui, G., and T. Enatsu. 1961. On the metabolism of anthranilic acid and the production of tryptophan by microorganisms (in Japanese with English summary). Amino Acids *3*: 71–79.

Tsunoda, T., R. Aoki, K. Kinoshita and Y. Kondo. 1959. Formation of L-glutamic acid from γ-aminobutyric acid by bacteria (in Japanese). Nippon Nôgeikagaku Kaishi *33*: 221–224.

Tsunoda, T., I. Shiio and K. Mitsugi. 1961. Bacterial formation of L-glutamic acid from acetic acid in the growing culture medium, I, II. J. Gen. Appl. Microbiol. *7*: 18–29, 30–40.

Udaka, S., and S. Kinoshita. 1958a. Studies on L-ornithine fermentation. II. The change of fermentation product by a feedback type mechanism. J. Gen. Appl. Microbiol. *4*: 283–287.

Udaka, S., and S. Kinoshita. 1958b. The fermentative production of L-valine by bacteria. J. Gen. Appl. Microbiol. *5*: 157–174.

Yamada, K., and Y. Su. 1959. Studies on L-glutamic acid production by *Brevibacterium divericatum* nov. sp. (in Japanese). Amino Acids *1*: 38–44.

Yamada, K., and Y. Hirose. 1960. Taxonomical studies on *Brevibacterium pentoso-aminoacidicum* nov. sp. and *Brevibacterium pentoso-alanicum* nov. sp. which are capable of producing amino acids from pentose (in Japanese). Amino Acids *2*: 36–41.

Yata, F., Y. Kaneko and S. Doi. 1961. Studies on the glutamic acid fermentation. II. On the mechanism of L-glutamic acid fermentation (in Japanese with English summary). Amino Acids *3*: 14–20.

Yazaki, H., S. Otsuka and M. Takahashi. 1958. On alanine formation by *Streptomyces*. Presented at the Annual Meeting of the Agr. Chem. Soc. Japan, April.

Yoshino, D., W. Hashida, S. Kida, Y. Nakagiri, H. Jose and S. Teramoto. 1960. The effects of agitation and aeration on glutamic acid production (in Japanese). (Studies on the fermentative production of glutamic acid and its application, I). Hakkô Kôgaku Zasshi *38*: 116–123.

PRODUCTION OF AMINO ACIDS WITH SPECIAL CONSIDERATION OF THE FUNCTION OF BIOTIN

SHUKUO KINOSHITA

Tokyo Research Laboratory
Kyowa Hakko Kogyo Co., Ltd.
Tokyo, Japan

SINCE THE DISCOVERY of high glutamate-producing micro-organisms (Kinoshita *et al.*, 1957a), the commercial production of glutamate by the fermentation method has received considerable attention.

As a result of the intense research activities that have been focused on this field, quite an amount of knowledge has been accumulated. In this regard, the role of biotin in glutamate fermentation is of great interest because of its effect both on formation of glutamate and on growth of the organism. Attention must also be paid to the fact that all strains of high glutamate-producing capacity, so far reported, require biotin at least as a growth factor (Kinoshita, 1959a). Although the opposite is not always true, biotin does play an important role in glutamate accumulation. Its dual function in growth promotion and metabolic control indicates that the physiological activities of the micro-organism are linked closely with the process of cell multiplication.

EFFECTS OF BIOTIN ON GLUTAMIC ACID FERMENTATION

The various effects of biotin on glutamic acid fermentation will be reviewed briefly. *Micrococcus glutamicus No. 541** was used as the test organism. This strain requires about $10 \sim 25$ μg biotin/l in a synthetic medium to give maximum growth and the growth response is proportional to the biotin content of the medium.

When the actual fermentation is carried out, in bottle fermentors, the biotin content of the medium affects the amount of glutamate produced to a considerable extent (Fig. 1).

The most favourable biotin level for glutamate production lies in the range of $1 \sim 5.0$ μg/l which is suboptimal or deficient for growth. At the higher level of biotin, cell multiplication proceeds vigorously but glutamate yield is very poor. On the contrary, at a too low level, poor growth gives a poor yield. At the high level of biotin, glucose is consumed very rapidly and an appreciable amount of lactate is accumulated in the broth, together

*This organism may be better called *Corynebacterium Glutamicum*.

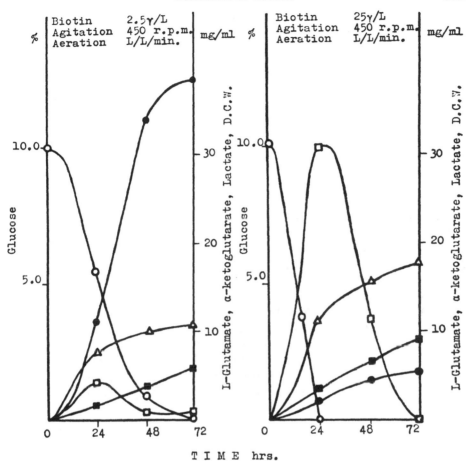

T I M E hrs.

FIG. 1. Chemical changes during glutamic acid fermentations. The basal medium consisted of 10 per cent glucose, 0.05 per cent KH_2PO_4, 0.05 per cent K_2HPO_4, 0.025 per cent $MgSO_4.7H_2O$, 0.001 per cent $FeSO_4.7H_2O$, 0.001 per cent $MnSO_4.4H_2O$, 0.5 per cent urea: △—△ D.C.W., ○—○ Glucose, □—□ Lactate, ●—● L-Glutamate, ■—■ α-ketoglutarate.

with other organic acids, such as acetic and succinic. These acids are normally consumed after the glucose disappears. The metabolic activities of cells from media of high and suboptimal biotin levels were also compared. Cells from biotin-rich media oxidized substrates such as glucose, acetate, pyruvate, succinate, fumarate and malate very actively; the oxygen consumption of biotin-rich cells using glucose as a substrate was 70 per cent of the theoretical amount. Cells from biotin-deficient media, however, were relatively inactive.

In contrast with the above fact, the oxygen absorption of the cells was almost negligible when the tricarboxylic acids, citric and isocitric, were used as substrates. Nevertheless these acids can be converted efficiently to the glutamate in the presence of ammonium ions by homogenized cells from either biotin levels. These results indicate that the effect of biotin on the

TABLE 1

COMPARISON OF OXIDIZING ABILITY FOR VARIOUS SUBSTRATES OF CELLS OF *M. glutamicus*
GROWN IN BIOTIN-RICH AND -DEFICIENT MEDIA

	QO_2 by biotin-deficient cells		QO_2 by biotin-rich cells	
	Intact cells	Homogenized cells	Intact cells	Homogenized cells
Glucose	58	43	65	58
Pyruvate	14	9	23	15
Lactate	35	22	44	45
Acetate	11	9	41	39
Oxalacetate	19	13	25	18
Citrate	negligible	negligible	negligible	negligible
Cis-aconitate	,,	,,	,,	,,
α-ketoglutarate	,,	,,	1.0	0.7
Succinate	1	3	29	15
Fumarate	9	8	20	10
Malate	11	9	18	11

Reaction mixture: Substrate 25 μmole, phosphate 150 μmole, intact cells or homogenized cells 20 mg, final volume 2.0 ml, pH 7.8, 30 C.

metabolic activity of cells lies mainly in their ability to oxidize various substrates, with the exception of the tricarboxylates (Table 1). This organism also oxidizes α-ketoglutarate to a very limited extent although the amount oxidized increases with an increase in biotin level. However this low activity towards α-ketoglutarate should favour the formation of glutamate during glucose metabolism. The activity of isocitritase, which is known as the key enzyme in the glyoxylate bypath, was next examined (Table 2). Activity of isocitritase was demonstrable only when acetic acid was provided as the sole carbon source. This conforms with other investigators' results that the enzyme is adaptive for acetic acid (Kornberg

TABLE 2

PRODUCTS OF CITRATE METABOLISM BY CELLS OF *M. glutamicus*
GROWN ON DIFFERENT LEVELS OF BIOTIN (A) IN THE PRESENCE
AND (B) IN THE ABSENCE OF SEMICARBAZIDE
(Expressed as μmoles)

	Biotin conc. in medium	Glycollate	Glyoxylate	α-Ketoglutarate
A	20 μg/L	0.00	2.42	0.55
	10	0.00	2.21	0.65
	5	0.00	0.27	0.83
	2.5	0.00	0.00	0.77
	0.5	0.00	0.00	0.15
B	20 μg/L	0.60	0.00	2.74
	10	0.58	0.43	1.94
	5	0.07	0.12	1.06
	2.5	0.00	0.00	0.92
	0.5	0.00	0.00	0.11

Reaction mixture: Na₃ citrate 50 μmole, TPN 1 μmole, phosphate 100 μmole, Fe^{++} 0.2 μmole, Mn^{++} 0.2 μmole, Mg^{++} 4 μmole, dialysed cell-free extract 5 mg as protein, with or without semicarbazide HCl neutralized 250 μmole, final volume 2.5 ml, pH 7.0. Stationary, 30 C, 3 hr.

& Elsden, 1961). In glucose medium, when biotin was present in high level, isocitritase activity was demonstrable in the cells, but the activity decreased with a decrease of biotin level. It is interesting to note that at the biotin level optimal for glutamate fermentation, no isocitritase activity could be shown. The results indicate that the glyoxylate bypath will operate only in biotin-rich cells, while in normal cells the metabolic stream will proceed quantitatively to glutamate formation. The appearance of isocitritase activity in biotin-rich cells is probably due to its formation adaptively as a result of the accumulation of acetate during the rapid oxidation of glucose by such cells.

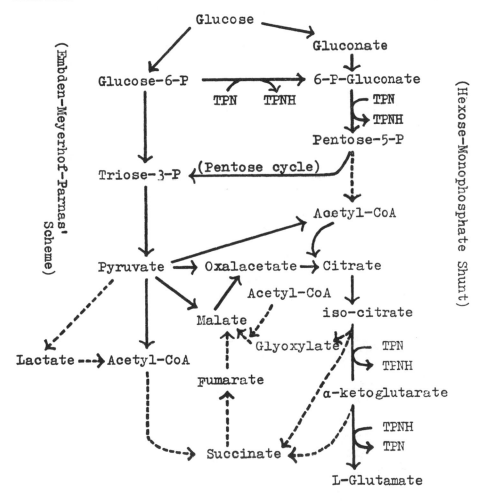

Glutamate

Biosynthesis by Micrococcus glutamicus.

Fig. 2. Pathway of glucose metabolism and glutamate biosynthesis by *Micrococcus glutamicus*.

In the synthesis of glutamate (Fig. 2), the mechanism of ammonium ion uptake is of interest. In a previous report it was pointed out that glutamic dehydrogenase was concerned in glutamate formation. Other papers support this view (Aida *et al.*, 1960; Yada *et al.*, 1961).

This problem was also studied to clarify whether other nitrogen uptake mechanisms may occur at different biotin levels. Enzymes, such as aspartase, L-alanine dehydrogenase and L-leucine dehydrogenase, which are considered responsible for nitrogen uptake were present in small amount or were absent in all tests. However, glutamic dehydrogenase activity was strong at all biotin levels. Transaminase activities were also compared at different biotin levels although these enzymes will contribute to the synthesis of various amino acids from glutamate rather than to the synthesis of glutamate itself. The activity of the transaminases present in any amount (aspartase, alanine, valine and leucine) was only slightly improved by high levels of biotin.

Another interesting difference between high (25 μg/l) or suboptimal (2.5 μg/l) biotin levels is the amount of amino acids inside or outside of the cells. The amount of glutamate excreted into the medium was much higher when biotin was low, whereas the over-all amount of amino compounds synthesized at each biotin level was almost comparable. From these results it can be assumed that in biotin-deficient cells glutamate can rapidly flow out of the cell, but in biotin-rich cells glutamate once syn-

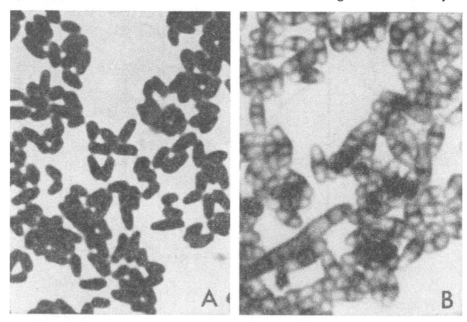

FIG. 3. Cell forms of *M. glutamicus*. (A) Grown in a glucose bouillon-medium, 9 hr. culture, stained with methylene blue. (B) Septated form grown in a biotin-deficient medium for glutamate production, cell wall strain.

thesized is used for the synthesis of other amino acids or cell proteins. There is also a marked difference in the free amino acid pool in the cells. In biotin-deficient cells the amino acid pool was very low, especially in glutamate, as compared with biotin-rich cells. The methionine, lysine, proline and histidine content of biotin-deficient cells was also low. This may indicate that the cell permeability is changed according to biotin content.

These various physiological effects are very interesting when considered along with the fact that the morphology varies with the biotin content of the medium (Kinoshita & Itagaki, 1959b). Cells grown in suboptimal levels of biotin tend to be elongated, septated and swollen in contrast to the ellipsoidal or short rod shape in biotin-rich media (Fig. 3). It might be mentioned that biotin is absorbed very rapidly by the cell; it soon disappears even from a biotin-rich medium and may be found inside the cells.

From all these experiments it may be concluded that biotin has a role not only in connection with the synthetic pathway of glutamate but also with protein synthesis in the cells. By these complicated processes biotin seems to regulate the versatile metabolic reactions and possibly cell permeability.

EFFECTS OF BIOTIN ON OTHER AMINO ACID FERMENTATIONS

It was found that a homoserine-requiring mutant of M. glutamicus can accumulate an appreciable amount of L-lysine in the medium (Kinoshita et al., 1958). Since this mutant requires biotin, as does its parent culture, it was of interest to see whether biotin had any effect on lysine fermentation.

Experiments showed that at concentrations of biotin below a certain level glutamic acid was produced but very little lysine. The best yield of lysine was obtained when high levels of biotin were used in conjunction with limited amounts of homoserine. The inhibition by high amounts of homoserine can be explained by a feedback control mechanism.

A similar phenomenon was also observed with the ornithine fermentation (Kinoshita et al., 1957b). The organism requires biotin and arginine. When sufficient arginine is provided, but biotin is limited, glutamate is produced. However, when arginine is limited but adequate biotin is provided, ornithine is produced. A similar tendency has been noted with the homoserine fermentation (Kinoshita et al., 1960).

SUMMARY

A series of amino acid fermentations using M. glutamicus and its mutants has revealed the remarkable properties of biotin. The vitamin is not only a simple growth factor but also affects the activities of various enzymes and the composition of the cell. It seems that cell multiplication and physiology are closely linked and biotin functions as a controlling agent.

REFERENCES

Aida, K., K. Oishi and T. Asai. 1960. Studies on amino acid fermentation. II. On the mechanism of L-glutamic acid fermentation (1). J. Agr. Chem. Soc. Japan, *34*: 70–77.

Kinoshita, S., K. Tanaka, S. Udaka and S. Akita. 1957a. Glutamic acid fermentation. Proc. Intern. Symposium Enzyme Chem. (Tokyo): 464–468.

Kinoshita, S., K. Nakayama and S. Udaka. 1957b. The fermentative production of L-ornithine. J. Gen. Appl. Microbiol., *3*: 276–277.

Kinoshita, S., K. Nakayama and S. Kitada. 1958. L-lysine production using microbial auxotroph. J. Gen. Appl. Microbiol. *4*: 128–129.

Kinoshita, S. 1959a. The production of amino acids by fermentation processes. *In* Advances in applied microbiology *1*: 201–214. Academic Press, New York.

Kinoshita, S., and S. Itagaki. 1959b. Studies on cell elongation phenomena of glutamic acid producing organisms; Symposia on cell multiplication. Institute Appl. Microbiol. (Tokyo) *1*: 146–172.

Kinoshita, S., H. Samejima, K. Nakayama, T. Nara and C. Fujita. 1960. L-homoserine fermentation. J. Gen. Appl. Microbiol. *6*: 193–195.

Kornberg, H. L., and S. R. Elsden. 1961. The metabolism of 2-carbon compounds by microorganisms. Advances in Enzymol. *23*: 401–470.

Yada, F., Y. Kaneko and S. Doi. 1961. Studies on the glutamic acid fermentation. II. The mechanism of glutamic acid fermentation. Amino Acids *3*: 26–30.

THE REGULATION OF BIOSYNTHETIC REACTIONS

H. S. MOYED

Department of Bacteriology and Immunology
Harvard Medical School, Boston, U.S.A.

BACTERIAL BIOSYNTHESIS is characterized by great economy and precision. *Escherichia coli*, the favorite representative of the bacteria, synthesizes several grams of cells per liter of a medium containing glucose and ammonium sulphate as the carbon and nitrogen sources. Half of this cell substance is protein. A quarter of it is nucleic acid. The organism must therefore synthesize considerable amounts of amino acids, purines, and pyrimidines. Nevertheless, only traces of these metabolites are overproduced and excreted into the medium. Even the intracellular pools of the amino acids and bases are small in comparison to the amount of material that flows through them.

This tight coupling of the synthesis and utilization of low molecular weight metabolites is, of course, economical for the bacterium. For the fermentation industry it is a barrier that must be overcome in order to achieve microbial synthesis of valuable metabolites in excess of the microorganism's own needs. For bacterial physiology the problem has been to learn how this coupling or balanced metabolism is maintained.

The solution to this problem started with the discoveries that bacteria utilize an exogenous source of low molecular weight metabolites in preference to synthesizing their own supply (Cowie, Burton, & Sands, 1951). Such observations led to the idea that a metabolite might be able to shut off its own synthesis through feedback mechanisms as its internal level becomes excessive. Experimental evidence followed shortly thereafter for two such feedback loops either of which might be responsible for metabolic regulation.

The first of these phenomena is now known as repression. The end-product of a biosynthetic pathway is able to repress or prevent the formation of each enzyme of the sequence. Fig. 1 is an abbreviated description of some of the current proposals concerning a mechanism of repression in a typical pathway (Jacob & Monod, 1961). The end-product itself is thought not to be the active form of the repressor, but rather is imagined to be activated by combining with an aporepressor, the product of a regulatory gene. The regulatory gene and its product are highly specific, affecting only a single pathway. The inhibition of the enzyme-forming mechanism by the repressor is readily reversible. Thus when the end-product concentration drops, and

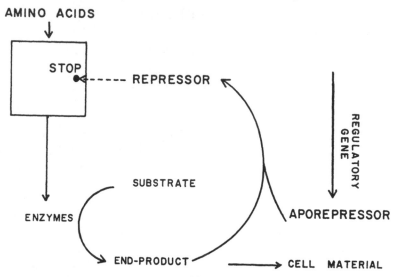

FIG. 1. Repression of biosynthetic enzymes.

thereby reduces the concentration of repressor, the enzyme-forming mechanism can resume operation. The formation of the active repressor can be prevented by several strategems. In that case there is unrestrained synthesis of these enzymes and their levels increase by as much as a thousand fold over normal. This is the so-called derepressed state.

The typical end-product not only represses enzyme formation, but also inhibits enzyme action. The earliest examples of such inhibition were found in isoleucine biosynthesis (Umbarger, 1956) and in pyrimidine biosynthesis (Yates & Pardee, 1956). This phenomenon is diagrammed in Fig. 2. The upper-case letters represent the intermediates of a pathway, and the lower-case letters indicate the enzymes responsible for the stepwise conversion of the intermediates to the end-product. In contract to repression, which affects the *formation* of all the enzymes in a pathway, end-product inhibition of *activity* involves only the first enzyme. This location for end-product inhibition would prevent excessive production of not only the end-product

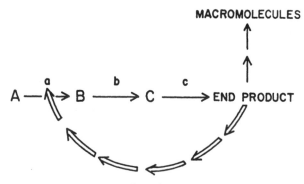

FIG. 2. End-product inhibition.

itself but the intermediates as well. End-product inhibition should permit the internal pool of the end-product to remain small but constant even though the demands on it for macromolecule synthesis may fluctuate.

The discoveries of end-product inhibition and repression invited a number of questions. First of all it was necessary to know whether these mechanisms were in fact as well as in theory responsible for the control of biosynthesis. It seemed that this question might be readily answered if the following assumptions proved to be correct: an enzyme that is inhibited by its eventual end-product might also be a target for inhibition by a structural analogue of the end-product. If the analogue, having shut off synthesis of the end-product, cannot be used in place of the end-product for the production of active macromolecules it would be bacteriostatic. Mutants selected for resistance to an analogue of this kind might produce an enzyme with altered sensitivity not only to the analogue but hopefully also to the end-product itself. With such a mutant in hand it should be possible to make a comparative study of the consequences associated with an altered regulatory system.

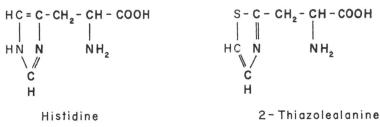

Histidine   2 - Thiazolealanine

Fig. 3. An end-product inhibitor and its structural analogue.

2-Thiazolealanine, an analogue of histidine, was ideally suited for this approach. These compounds have a considerable area of structural similarity (Fig. 3), which permits thiazolealanine to mimic histidine as an inhibitor of the first step in histidine synthesis. However, the analogue cannot be used in place of histidine for the synthesis of proteins and is therefore bacteriostatic. In a mutant of *E. coli* selected for resistance to bacteriostasis by the analogue the first enzyme of histidine synthesis was found to be insensitive to inhibition not only by the analogue but also by the end-product itself, histidine. However, sensitivity to the repressive effect of histidine was retained, but in the face of the loss of end-product inhibition repression by itself could not prevent the mutant from excreting histidine during growth. This illustrates the point that the regulatory mechanisms are barriers to excessive synthesis of metabolites. A more important indication of disrupted regulation was the mutant's inability to utilize an exogenous supply of histidine in preference to making its own. If repression as well had been lost the resulting high enzyme levels acting without the restraint of end-product inhibition would have converted approximately half the carbon source to histidine (Moyed, 1961).

The other questions one might ask about end-product inhibition and repression have to do with the underlying mechanisms. The former process presents mainly a problem of enzyme chemistry. The end-product-inhibited reaction might be as many as eight or nine steps removed from the end-product. Thus, the end-product and the substrate of the first enzyme often have totally dissimilar structures yet they are generally competitive. It was difficult to understand how a protein could recognize a compound structurally unrelated to that recognized by the enzymatic site. It is now apparent that there are separate substrate and inhibitor binding sites (Gerhart & Pardee, 1962; Changeux, 1961. It remains to find out how the two sites interact.

By contrast the problem of understanding the mechanism of repression seems far more difficult. It is probably inseparable from the problems posed by protein synthesis and the transcription phase of gene action. In considering again the currently accepted model for repression we see that the repressor itself is still conceptual, its chemical nature still a subject for speculation. Only the end-product or co-repressor is known.

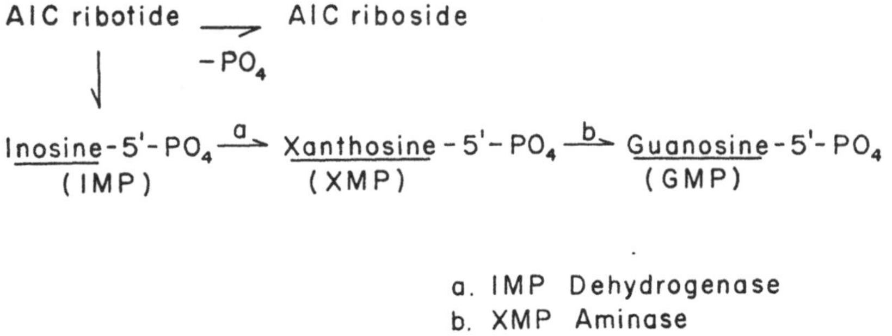

AIC ribotide $\longrightarrow$ AIC riboside

$$\downarrow \quad -PO_4$$

Inosine-5'-PO_4 $\xrightarrow{a}$ Xanthosine-5'-PO_4 $\xrightarrow{b}$ Guanosine-5'-PO_4
(IMP)   (XMP)   (GMP)

a. IMP Dehydrogenase
b. XMP Aminase

FIG. 4. Terminal steps of guanine synthesis.

An obvious approach to the problem is to study the chemical events that take place when repression is antagonized under conditions in which the chemical nature of both the aporepressor and the antagonist is known. Several unexpected observations made during an attempt to increase the yield of an enzyme furnished Dr. Shigezo Udaka (Udaka & Moyed, 1962) with a specific tool for this approach to the problem. He found that aminoimidazolecarboxamide riboside (AIC riboside) antagonizes repression of the terminal part of the guanine pathway. The relationship of the riboside to this pathway is shown in Fig. 4. AIC riboside is a dephosphorylation product of AIC ribotide. The reverse reaction, or phosphorylation, does not occur in *E. coli*. Therefore, AIC riboside is a by-product rather than an intermediate in the synthesis of guanosine-5-PO_4. The riboside causes growing cells to produce five-fold elevated levels of both IMP dehydrogenase and *XMP* aminase. Operationally it is therefore an inducer of these enzymes. The effect might be considered an example of *positive feedback*, but it is somewhat marred by the fact that the riboside is not an intermediate. A similar phenomenon occurs in the arginine pathway, but there, too, its physiological role is questionable as only a small part of the pathway is affected (Gorini, 1960).

The mechanism of the induction is our immediate concern. The aminase and the dehydrogenase are coordinately repressed by a derivative of GMP. Measurements made with AIC riboside and external sources of guanine show that the riboside induces by counteracting this repressive effect. Two possible explanations for the antagonism were eliminated: the riboside does not act (1) by inhibiting the synthesis of the co-repressor, guanosine-5′-P, or (2) by preventing the entry of its precursors such as guanine or guanosine. A remaining possibility is that AIC riboside interferes at some step in the formation of the active repressor from the co-repressor. If this working hypothesis is correct, a demonstrable effect on the metabolism of guanine derivatives might be expected to accompany induction by AIC riboside. To test this hypothesis a strain of *E. coli* that can synthesize neither AIC riboside nor guanosine-5′-PO$_4$ was exposed to radioactive guanine both with and without the addition of the riboside (Table 1). The riboside

TABLE 1

The Effect of AIC Riboside on the Utilization of Guanine-8-C^{14}

			Radioactivity of cell fractions	
Guanine-8-C^{14} µg/ml×15′	AIC riboside µg/ml	IMP deH'ase Specific activity	Nucleic acids counts per min.	Intracellular pool counts per min.
0.1	None	1.0	67,000	5,650
0.1	10	4.9	72,500	3,120

caused a five-fold induction of IMP dehydrogenase. There was no effect on the incorporation of guanine-8-C^{14} into the nucleic acid fraction. However, AIC riboside decreased incorporation into the intracellular pool fraction by about 30 per cent. Further examination of the pool by paper chromatography revealed that the decrease is selective. Guanine is incorporated into three separable components of the pool. AIC riboside reduced the incorporation into two of the components by about 60 per cent but did not affect the third. The compounds with reduced incorporation may be intermediates or by-products of the synthesis of an active repressor; thus, their identification might offer leads to this pristine area of regulatory metabolism.

The conclusion of this paper was originally intended to be a consideration of how current theory might be applied to by-passing the regulatory processes as these are obviously barriers to the extensive synthesis of amino acids and other metabolites. In retrospect, however, this particular juxtaposition of theory and application seems presumptuous. The fermentation industry has been successful in overcoming such barriers for thousands of years without detailed knowledge of biological regulation. To cite a recent example of the art consider the various amino acid fermentations by *Micrococcus glutamicus*. This organism was isolated without the application of theories of regulation; on the other hand inquiry into the reasons for its extensive excretion of ornithine has contributed to our understanding of regulatory mechanisms (Udaka & Kinoshita, 1958).

ACKNOWLEDGEMENTS

This work was supported by Grant No. RG 6059 from the United States Public Health Service and by a United States Public Health Service Career Development Award.

REFERENCES

Changeux, J. 1961. The feedback control mechanism of biosynthetic L-thrionine deaminase by L-isoleucine. Cold Spring Harbor Symp. Quant. Biol. *26*: 313–318.

Cowie, D. B., E. T. Bolton and M. K. Sands. 1951. Sulfur metabolism in *Escherichia coli*. II. Competitive utilization of labeled and nonlabeled sulfur compounds. J. Bacteriol. *62*: 63–74.

Gerhart, J. C., and A. B. Pardee. 1962. The enzymology of control by feedback inhibition. J. Biol. Chem. *237*: 891–896.

Gorini, L. 1960. Antagonism between substrate and repressor in controlling the formation of a biosynthetic enzyme. Proc. Natl. Acad. Sci. U.S. *46*: 682–690.

Jacob, F., and J. Monod. 1961. Genetic regulatory mechanisms in the synthesis of proteins. J. Mol. Biol. *3*: 318–356.

Moyed, H. S. 1961. Interference with feedback control of enzyme activity. Cold Spring Harbor Symp. Quant. Biol. *26*: 323–329.

Udaka, S., and S. Kinoshita. 1958. Studies on L-ornithine fermentation. II. The change of fermentation product by a feedback type mechanism. J. Gen. Appl. Microbiol. *4*: 283–287.

Udaka, S., and H. S. Moyed. 1962. Antagonism of repression in the guanine parthway. Unpublished observations.

Umbarger, H. E. 1956. Evidence for a negative-feedback mechanism in the biosynthesis of isoleucine. Science *123*: 343.

Yates, R. A., and A. B. Pardee. 1956. Control of pyrimidine biosynthesis in *Escherichia coli* by a feedback mechanism. J. Biol. Chem. *221*: 757–770.

COMPARISON OF ANALYTICAL METHODS
FOR THE DETERMINATION OF
AMINO ACIDS

R. A. LATIMER

John Labatt Ltd.
London, Canada

THE NEED FOR THE DEVELOPMENT of methods of analysis for the determination of amino acids dates back perhaps to the last decade in the nineteenth century when Rubner recognized the fact that proteins of different origin were not of equivalent value in nutrition. Later investigations into the feeding of protein hydrolysates led to the now accepted idea that protein nutrition is essentially amino acid nutrition.

Of the known amino acids, twenty-four are generally thought to be protein constituents. Some of the amino acids are synthesized by the animal body while others must be in an available form and supplied in the diet. Rose (1938) classified amino acids as dispensable or indispensable on this basis and defined an indispensable amino acid as one which could not be synthesized from materials ordinarily available at a rate commensurate with the demands of normal growth. The term "indispensable," however, when referred to an amino acid has a significance only when qualified as to nutritional state.

Herein lie some of the main reasons for the importance of determining amino acid concentrations in a variety of biological systems. Analytical methods are required which are accurate, reproducible and sensitive enough to detect amino acids down to concentrations of 10^{-9} moles or better. Over the last sixty or so years sample preparation techniques and analytical methods have shown a diversity and ingenuity which are tributes to the so-called "wet" chemists and more lately to the instrumental analysts.

The choice of a method of analysis for any particular amino acid or group of amino acids depends mainly on the purpose of the analysis, the degree of accuracy required and the equipment available. Time taken to obtain the result is also important, especially in process control. In many cases the sample size available will determine the method used.

The analyst is concerned with accuracy, sensitivity of the method and the amount of time he has to spend on a given number of samples. He is concerned also with sample preparation or the clean-up procedures required before the actual determination. In many cases the clean-up may be more exacting than the actual determination itself, as is often the case with instrumental analysis.

On the other hand, the research worker is normally concerned only with the results of a particular analysis and not necessarily with the detailed procedure of obtaining these results. He may be interested in the statistical significance of a difference in results after manipulation of some variable but he is not generally interested in, say, the concentration of ninhydrin used as the final developing agent.

Collaboration with the research analyst has long since been accepted practice and in the realm of amino acid analysis this has produced remarkable results. While it is very commendable that the biochemist, who is vitally concerned with elucidating, say, the amino acid sequence of proteins and protein fragments, frequently spends a considerable portion of his research time exploring the vagaries of some new analytical technique designed to improve quantitation, this represents a dilution of effort and perhaps not always the most rewarding answer.

As a summation of this line of reasoning and without discussing the problem at greater length, it may be said that for continued advances in analytical chemistry, of which amino acid analysis is necessarily a part, industry, government and educational institutions must accept the responsibility of providing the facilities for producing research analysts who are equipped to solve the analytical problems which are being presented by the increasing tempo of researches into the life sciences.

AMINO ACID ANALYSES

Purely chemical procedures for the determination of amino acids were used almost entirely for the first forty years of the present century. The amino acid was either isolated and weighed or reacted specifically with a compound to form a coloured product. The intensity of the coloured product was estimated by comparative colorimetry. These and other laborious methods alone provided the information during this period on the amino acid composition of proteins.

The mass spectrograph has been used to measure the proportion of radioactive nitrogen to normal nitrogen after isotopic dilution of a pure sample of amino acid which has been isolated from a protein hydrolysate. This method, while purported to be a most accurate method, is limited by the availability of equipment and the technical ability required. Recently published work by Biemann and co-workers who have used mass spectrometry to measure amino acids after conversion to their ethyl esters indicates progress in this area (Biemann, Seibl & Gapp, 1959; Biemann & Vetter, 1960).

Biological methods for amino-acid analysis have been in use since 1914, and since 1943 these methods using micro-organisms and specific enzyme systems have been developed for the routine estimation of all known amino acids. Determinations of lysine, methionine and threonine have been made recently by microbiological assay on 0.2 ml of rat plasma (McLaughlan *et al.*, 1961).

Microbiological assays are tedious and time-consuming and the results often are not commensurate with the amount of work involved. The bulk of this type of assay is being used for the determination of vitamins and other growth factors and not for amino acids.

Since about 1950 the procedures mentioned above have been largely replaced by chromatographic methods and some startling advances have appeared. The purpose of this presentation is primarily to discuss two chromatographic procedures: gas liquid partition chromatography (G.L.P.C.) and automated column-chromatography.

Paper chromatography has found wide use and hundreds of articles are to be found in the literature dealing with the many applications of this technique. While it is not intended to discuss here the paper chromatographic determination of amino acids, these procedures probably include a great proportion of the routine and comparative determinations being carried out at the present time. The introduction in 1941 of paper chromatography by Martin and Synge for the determination of amino acids completely revolutionized the approach to the biochemical field. Many modifications (Consden et al., 1948) have been made since that time to the techniques of paper chromatography for amino acid analysis including even assays carried out entirely under the microscope (Lakshminarayanan, 1954).

The exciting advances have grown through the use of column chromatography and subsequent automation. G.L.P.C. analysis of amino acids, which I shall discuss first, also offers interesting possibilities.

The G.L.P.C. system of analysis of an amino acid mixture can be outlined as follows: Sample Preparations*—Injection—Column—Detector—Readout. "Sample Preparation" can be expanded to include: Protein*—Hydrolysate—Reaction*—Derivative. The critical points are asterisked, the most critical point being the sample preparation. If the problems associated with preparation of protein hydrolysates are omitted as being common to all analyses of this type, and the elimination of proteins and carbohydrates is assumed, then we are left with the basic problem of the preparation and purification of the volatile amino acid derivatives.

For quantitative results the detector output (A) as shown by the readout system for the separated derivative must be proportional to the original amino acid concentration (c). Therefore $A = Kc$ where K is a constant made up of the product of the instrument factor K' and the reaction factor K''. We may assume that the instrument factors have been made constant by the manufacturers and the analyst and we are left with the reaction factors. After choice of a suitable volatile derivative and a knowledge of the side reactions involved, the most important consideration remaining becomes "constancy of yield" of the amino acid derivative. If the yield of product varies from one determination to another then our K is not constant and the detector output does not reflect the true concentration of the amino acid in the original sample. If the yield is consistently low, sensitivity is lost. Apart from the usual variables which beset an organic reaction—temperature, concentration of reagents (other than amino acids in this case), pH, etc.—the formation of derivatives from an amino acid mixture for G.L.P.C. analysis presents at least three other variables which can influence constancy and percentage yield.

The first of these variables represents the effect that the concentration of one (or more) amino acid will have on the derivative formation of the other amino acids present. This difficulty appears to exist for the most accurate work only and probably depends upon the particular derivative used.

The second but perhaps the most annoying variable is introduced by the use of impure reagents. The chemical manufacturers are assisting greatly by further purifying "Reagent Grade" chemicals for G.L.P.C. work, but the analyst usually learns by bitter experience to check all reagents and purify them, if necessary, before use so that minute amounts of contaminants may be removed.

The third variable which effects the constancy of yield in derivative formation is the operator who may be unskilled in the manipulative techniques of synthetic organic chemistry. Here we have another problem which is amenable to solution.

It has been reported in the literature that a number of different amino acid derivatives have been analysed successfully by G.L.P.C. but the methods are not in wide use as yet (Youngs, 1959; Zlatkis *et al.*, 1960; Bayer *et al.*, 1957; Weygand & Geiger, 1956). Much work remains to be done in simplifying the schemes for derivative preparation and in the selection of derivatives which lead to quantitative results. The recent work of Johnson, Scott and Meister (1961) who used N-acetyl amino acid n-amyl esters shows considerable promise. The problems do not appear insurmountable and G.L.P.C. analysis of amino acids has advantages over some of the other methods. Some of these advantages are: relatively low instrumentation cost; flexibility; sensitivity; the short time required for complete analysis; and the possibility of process control applications.

I feel certain that amino acid analysis by G.L.P.C. will be in a much stronger position in the near future. Research analysts who are first good instrumentationalists with a solid grounding in the chemical disciplines must find time to develop this important analytical problem.

The determination of amino acids by column chromatography on ion exchange resins, as published by Moore and Stein in 1951, paved the way for the advent of automated column-chromatography. Spackman, Stein and Moore (1956) presented a simplified chromatographic separation of amino acids together with an automatic recording apparatus for measuring ninhydrin colour density. Many improvements have appeared since and a significant contribution to the precise determination of amino acids in protein hydrolysates and other biological systems has been made. Complete automatic amino acid analysers are manufactured by several companies and their wide distribution testifies to the general acceptance of this type of instrumental analysis. Although the instruments may appear complex, examination of the flow diagrams reveals the logic and the ingenuity of the various systems available. The instruments may be obtained as completely enclosed units or in modular form. In all cases the protein hydrolysate or amino acid mixture is applied to the column and after separation and reaction the results are presented by suitable readout.

The advantages and disadvantages of the automatic analysers over other methods of amino acid determinations may be summarized as follows:

Reproducibility: The instruments have inherent accuracy by virtue of the remarkably stable pumps and flow systems. Operator variable also is reduced to a minimum.

Sensitivity: It is claimed that by recent improvements 10^{-8} moles of amino acid may be determined with an accuracy of about 1 per cent. Detection to 10^{-9} moles is possible.

Resolution: About fifty amino acids have been resolved using a single column and pH-gradient elution.

A disadvantage could be the relatively high initial cost—$9,000–$15,000 in Canada—but the precision obtained can in most cases justify this expenditure.

The time taken to complete a single analysis by this system at present could be considered a drawback also; however, it has been intimated that in the very near future analysis of a number of samples in the same time through the use of multiple columns will be possible. By combining multiple columns and storage coils the output may be increased considerably.

Improvements in the gradient elution cell, the particle size distribution and type of ion exchange resin, and the use of improved colorimeters promise increases in resolution and sensitivity for amino acid determinations.

It was reported recently (Schilling et al., 1961) that ninhydrin can react with keto acids to give coloured products which appear as peaks on automatically produced chromatograms. The difficulties raised by these extra peaks are at present under study and probably will be resolved by the automatic production of other amino acid derivatives at some point in the reaction chain.

In the brewing industry we are interested in the relationships between the nitrogen spectrum and flavour factors in the finished product. Routine methods which are rapid and accurate are required for amino acid determinations at various points during the production process. In flavour work we are interested not only in the concentrations of particular amino acids, but the relative concentrations of certain groups of amino acids.

Methods of analysis by G.L.P.C. are being investigated, but to date have not been applied on a routine-quantitative basis.

In a sample of beer, produced by the continuous fermentation process and analysed by automatic amino acid analysis, forty amino acids were detected, twenty-seven of which have been identified tentatively. It is evident then that a whole research programme is necessary to unravel this information so that process variables may be studied. It is felt that at the present time such investigation could not be carried out without the aid of this type of equipment.

In conclusion it may be said that the automatic analyser system represents the brightest star in the analytical sphere today. Significant advances in instrumentation, precision and facility have been obtained and exciting developments are promised for the very near future.

G.L.P.C. analysis is making headway but a great deal more work by competent analysts is required before general acceptance can be expected.

ACKNOWLEDGMENT

I wish to acknowledge the technical assistance of Technicon Controls, Inc. in obtaining the automatic amino acid analyses.

REFERENCES

Bayer, E., K. H. Reuther, and F. Born. 1957. Analysis of amino acid mixtures by vapour-phase chromatography. Angew. Chem. *69*: 640–642.

Biemann, K., J. Seibl, and F. Gapp. 1959. Mass spectrophotometric identification of amino acids. Biochem. Biophys. Res. Commun. *1*: 307–311.

Biemann, K., and W. Vetter. 1960. Quantitative amino acid analysis by mass spectrometry. Biochem. Biophys. Res. Commun. *2*: 93–96.

Consden, R., A. H. Gordon, and A. J. P. Martin. 1948. Separation of acidic amino acids by means of a synthetic anion exchange resin. Biochem. J. (London) *42*: 443–447.

Johnson, D. E., S. J. Scott, and A. Meister. 1961. Gas-liquid chromatography of amino acid derivatives. Anal. Chem. *33*: 669–673.

Lakshminarayanan, K. 1954. Microchromatography. I. A technique for separation and identification of traces of amino acids, sugars, etc. Arch. Biochem. Biophys. *51*: 367–370.

McLaughlan, J. M., F. Noel, A. B. Morrison, and J. A. Campbell. 1961. Blood amino acid studies. I. Micro method for the estimation of free lysine methionine and threonine. Canad. J. Biochem. Physiol. *39*: 1669–1674.

Martin, A. J. P., and R. L. M. Synge. 1941. A new form of chromatogram employing two liquid phases. I. A theory of chromatography. II. Application to the microdetermination of the higher monoamino-acids in proteins. Biochem. J. (London) *35*: 1358–1368.

Moore, S., and W. H. Stein. 1951. Chromatography of amino acids on sulfonated polystyrene resins. J. Biol. Chem. *192*: 663–681.

Rose, W. C. 1938. The nutritive significance of the amino acids. Physiol. Rev. *18*: 109–136.

Rubner, M. Quoted from Black, R. J., and K. W. Weiss. 1956. Amino acid handbook, p. 3. Charles C. Thomas, Springfield, Ill.

Schilling, E. D., P. T. Burchill, J. R. Coffman, and R. A. Clayton. 1961. Keto acids confuse amino acid picture. Chem. Eng. News *26*: 36–38.

Spackman, D. H., W. H. Stein, and S. Moore. 1956. Automatic recording apparatus for use in chromatography of amino acids. Fed. Proc. *15*: 358.

Weygand, F., and R. Geiger. 1956. N-trifluorazetyl Aminosaeuren. IV. Mitteil. N-trifluorazetylierung von Aminosaeuren in wasserfreier Trifluoressigsaeure. Chem. Ber. *89*: 647–652.

Youngs, C. G. 1959. Analysis of mixtures of amino acids by gas phase chromatography. Anal. Chem. *31*: 1019–1021.

Zlatkis, A., J. F. Oro, and A. P. Kimball. 1960. Direct amino acid analysis by gas chromatography. Anal. Chem. *32*: 162–164.

PANEL DISCUSSION 3

EVOLUTIONARY OPERATION AND HORIZONS IN INDUSTRIAL MICROBIOLOGY

Chairman: J. C. SYLVESTER

EDWIN F. WHITING

Evolutionary Operation in Industrial Microbiology

RICHARD W. JACKSON

Horizons in Fermentation as Viewed by the Development Engineer

T. O. WIKEN

Horizons in Industrial Microbiology as Viewed by the Microbiologist

CHAIRMAN'S REMARKS

J. C. SYLVESTER

Abbott Laboratories
North Chicago, U.S.A.

THE FIRST USE by man of a controlled microbial process to produce something that improved his standard of living is lost in the pages of history. Undoubtedly this first use resulted in an end-product that was either a food or a beverage. Many thousands of years passed, after that first directed fermentation, before the genius of Pasteur elucidated the fundamental nature of fermentation processes and opened the door for man to begin utilizing the abilities of micro-organisms for his direct benefit. Almost a hundred more years passed by before the fermentation industry was really launched in the 1920's with the production of such fermentation products as ethanol, acetone, n-butanol, citric acid and enzymes on a large scale. In the 1930's additional materials such as organic acids, vitamins, sorbose and more enzymes became significant fermentation products. Since then, tremendous progress in the utilization of micro-organisms has been made and a wide variety of valuable microbial products added to the list. Today micro-organisms provide us with life-saving antibiotics, steroids, amino acids, industrial chemicals, plant growth factors, poultry pigmentors, to mention just a few of the developments of the last twenty years.

Despite the great strides we have made thus far in using the living microbial cell for man's benefit, we have, I firmly believe, only scratched the surface of the tremendous potential of fermentation processes. I am sure that we shall witness in the years ahead an accelerating use of cell systems and that fifty years from now the list of microbial products of great value to man will be many times longer than it is today. Recent discoveries in microbial genetics portend the "creation" of organisms for special purposes. Advances in the cultivation of plant and animal cells indicate that these will be added to the yeast, mold, bacterial and algal cell systems now being utilized. The potential of the "little bags of enzymes" to synthesize chemicals seems almost infinite, and man's use of them will only be limited by his degree of success in understanding them. I have no fear that our success will not be great, and expect that compounds yet undreamed of will continually be added to the list of microbial products in the years ahead.

In the discussion in this panel we hope not only to summarize the fermentation processes of today, but to explore the potential of this exciting field and to attempt to forecast some of the developments of the future. We have a panel of distinguished scientists, each of whom will discuss the field of fermentations from a different viewpoint.

Dr. E. F. Whiting will discuss evolutionary operations in industrial microbiology and will bring out, I am sure, a philosophy of utilizing production operations to generate valuable technical information to increase efficency and productivity. Dr. Whiting is associated with the Upjohn Company of Kalamazoo, Michigan, and has applied the concept of evolutionary operations proposed by Dr. George E. P. Box in 1955 to their fermentation processes. He has had considerable experience in this field and has presented a number of discussions on the subject.

Dr. R. W. Jackson, Chief, Fermentation Laboratory, Northern Utilization Research and Development Division, Peoria, Illinois, will consider industrial microbiology from the standpoint of the chemical engineer. He will cover the subject of substrate materials and the use of enzymes for synthesis. The use of new types of substrates, i.e., petroleum products, is of great interest today and undoubtedly will be an area of significant developments.

Dr. T. O. Wiken, head of the famous laboratory for microbiology of the Technische Hogeschool, Delft, Holland, will discuss industrial microbiology from the standpoint of the microbiologist. Dr. Wiken will present some aspects of the trend of the future, and the developments in industrial microbiology in the years ahead.

EVOLUTIONARY OPERATION IN INDUSTRIAL MICROBIOLOGY

EDWIN F. WHITING

The Upjohn Company, Kalamazoo, Michigan, U.S.A.

TRADITIONALLY, the course of research changes markedly as a process (of any type) proceeds from conception to completion. The basic scientific method continues throughout, but with considerable alteration in emphasis.

The "basic researcher" studies broad aspects such as: What raw materials shall be tried? Which samples will provide activity against certain organisms? What chemical structures are involved? In considering these questions, the scientist is looking for new products and processes, and much effort in industry is directed toward this end.

The scientific worker in the development area then is responsible for turning the laboratory process into a practical, operable, controllable, plant operation which will yield the desired product in sufficient quantity, suitable purity, and with maximum profit to the company. The "developer" is concerned with the problems of scale-up, and he becomes more cost conscious and dependent on the assistance of an engineering function to overcome the difficulties involved in scaling his process to plant size.

Once the process has reached the plant and is on stream, the prime objective is to turn out the desired product of acceptable quality and in sufficient quantity to satisfy the requirements. Experimentation, in the traditional sense, is frowned upon since subquality material is costly to rework and inventories could be affected. Although there may be exceptions, most plant managers will resist any efforts to tamper with their processes unless sufficient data have been generated by research and development people to warrant such a move.

PLANT IMPROVEMENTS

But further effort is usually necessary on the plant process, for it is a rare process indeed that operates at its optimum early in its history.

Frequently, new ideas are generated in the research and pilot plant areas either from the efforts of their staff or from suggestions of production people, and, after suitable testing in smaller equipment, plant trials are called for. If the plant data are favorable, the change to new operating conditions is made and possibly the process benefits.

Another way to experiment in the plant is through the plant foreman himself via small changes in the plant procedure which, he hopes, will improve the situation. If the change is beneficial it is usually incorporated into the S.O.P. (Standard Operating Procedure), while any negative results (no change or an adverse effect) merely become part of the "natural process variation."

Both techniques for process improvement are severely handicapped by the large variation commonly associated with microbiological reactions. As often as improvements are made there must be many more times when at least one of the following occurs: (1) A beneficial effect is masked by the error variation and discarded. (2) A beneficial effect appears to injure the process and is discarded with warnings not to try again. (3) A harmful effect actually appears to be an improvement over the existing S.O.P.; in this case, the true situation is usually noted after a time, and the process is restored to its original form. Any combination of these factors gives rise to the vast accumulation of folklore and "old wives' tales" that surround every plant process and serve mostly to confuse further optimization.

A third method for obtaining valuable information about a process involves the analysis of plant records. Whether by the "eyeball" technique of production and development personnel or the sophisticated approach of the statistician, the idea is to go back into the past history of the plant and try to find some assignable causes for the various shifts in process operation. Quite often this PARC analysis (*p*ractical *a*ccumulated *r*ecords and *c*alculations), as the statisticians call this approach (Hunter, 1960), is fruitful and the leads uncovered are exploited on the large scale.

EVOLUTIONARY OPERATION

What we would really like to have is a method for forcing the production process to provide information about how to improve itself while the product stream continues. This method should be simple to apply, readily interpreted and administered by production personnel, sparing of technical manpower and time, and above all should not interfere with the normal flow of product output and quality. Other important features of this method should be that it is operated on a regular basis and that the information obtained is immediately applicable in the plant.

The evolutionary operation concept satisfies all these requirements by making small changes in the plant process, establishing a new set of operating conditions, and repeatedly alternating these changes with the old S.O.P. in cyclic fashion. Although the immediate effect of the change is usually obscured by process variability, the "better" of the two possibilities is simple to detect after continued repetition, and the choice can be strengthened by the use of simple statistical tools. The improved conditions are then established in the plant, and a new cycle of small, repeated changes is instituted as before.

In his original paper in 1957, G. E. P. Box describes his EVOP as a "more powerful and concentrated form of the naturally occurring evolutionary process which goes on in all manufacture." Since we must proceed under a strict DO NOT TAMPER WITH THE PROCESS (Whitwell, 1959) atmosphere, which dictates only small changes in conditions, the power of EVOP stems from its ability to detect effects which would otherwise *not* be obvious because of the large process variation. Actually, EVOP should become a normal production method wherein, ideally, every step of every process in the plant is being investigated constantly.

To make this concept work in practice, the entire responsibility should rest within the production area. The plant supervisor should have the prime power to administer EVOP, and plant personnel should make the necessary calculations to maintain the programs. To the latter end, Box (1957) and Box and Hunter (1959) have simplified the calculations and constructed work forms and tables which can be handled, easily, by the average plant operator after only a short indoctrination.

To illustrate how EVOP works, consider an example. Suppose the plant foreman is concerned with an antibiotic production process whose fermentation he wishes to study. Prior research and his own data indicate that two variables, the air rate and the temperature, are likely to be important. In addition, past experience has shown that small changes around the S.O.P. levels of these variables (say ± 15 per cent for air and ± 2 F for temperature) are not only tolerable but normal for the usual plant operation. Two responses are important: (1) the yield, as represented by the harvest biological assay, and (2) the quality, as determined by a papergram assay.

A convenient representation for the program started in the plant is given in Fig. 1a with the five sets of operating conditions making up a cycle of the EVOP program. One complete fermentation is run at each of the five points and all the runs are completed within a cycle before the next cycle begins. The points are numbered for computation purposes as well as for

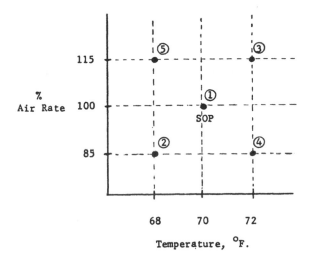

FIG. 1a

reference, and do not necessarily indicate the order in which the trials are made. When the cycle is completed, the proper calculations are made on the worksheets, and the completed data are entered on an information board. The information board is an essential feature of EVOP, since it displays, in simple fashion, the up-to-date picture of the program for all to follow. If another cycle is run, calculations are again performed and the information board is revised to reflect the new data. Since the plant foreman is constantly observing the board, he is in a position to make one or more of many possible decisions: he can run another cycle; if he feels that one of the points represents an improvement he can terminate this phase of the program, move his process to the more favorable location, and set up another cycle of changes around the new point; conversely, if unfavorable conditions exist he can move away from them; if he has run many cycles and no particular advantage can be seen, he might terminate this phase and either broaden the experimental range or select some new variables for study.

If we let Fig. 1b represent one portion of the information board for our

INFORMATION BOARD

	YIELD (Bio-assay - mcg./g.)			QUALITY (% X)	
⑤ 1044		③ 1054	⑤ 80.8		③ 85.6
	① 1042 SOP			① 85.7 SOP	
② 1045		④ 1059	② 89.2		④ 93.3

Temp.	+12	± 34.4	+4.4	± 5.3	
Air	- 3	± 34.4	-8.1	± 5.3	
Int'n. (Air x temp.)	- 2	± 34.4	+0.4	± 5.3	
Change-in-mean	+ 7	± 30.6	+1.2	± 4.7	

FIG. 1b

example, after six cycles, the plant foreman might view the data in the following fashion:

1. The upper part shows the running averages for each response at each point. No particular yield differences from the S.O.P. are apparent, but it does look as if superior quality has resulted from operating at the lower level of air rate. Furthermore, the combination of higher air–lower temperature (upper left) seems to produce poorer quality material than does the S.O.P.

2. The lower part of the board is concerned with the average effects of changing the variables, plus an expression of the reliability of these effects. In the case at hand, these data seem to support the general conclusions drawn from observing the averages themselves.

What should the plant foreman do after assessing the situation? There is no clear-cut answer to this question. He should consider his prior knowledge of the process; the opinions of any colleagues with whom he may choose to consult; plant restrictions on how much he can change his variables; and other pressing production problems he may face. Whatever his decision is, though, he will have a simple method of measuring its worth. If it was a good move his process will improve. If he was in error, his next cycles will reveal this and enable him to reverse himself and choose a new course. This flexible feature of EVOP is particularly appealing to most production people.

Two references cited herein (Box & Hunter, 1959; Barnett, 1960) provide examples of the calculation worksheets, and they contain comprehensive discussions of calculation techniques for 2- and 3-variable programs.

OPERATION OF EVOP

The emphasis so far has been on the role of plant personnel in managing EVOP. To reap the greatest benefits, however, all pertinent information about a process should be available to the plant manager, and the information generated by the plant should be readily accessible to other interested parties. An EVOP committee (Box, 1957), either formal or informal, is an excellent mechanism to achieve these goals. With the production man at the head, this committee could include: key production people involved; research and development men with knowledge of the process; someone from quality control who is interested in product purity; and a sympathetic statistician to help with the indoctrination and advise on suitable experimental designs and the interpretation of data.

The EVOP committee also fulfils an important "feedback" function. The more people who view the plant data, the greater the probability that new ideas will be generated, either for plant studies or for further work in research and development.

Experience has shown, also, that EVOP is most effective when the experimental designs are simple and the number of controlled variables being studied is limited, say, to two or three. Programs that are too complicated lead to confusion and are almost certain to terminate EVOP for good.

The real key to the success of EVOP, however, lies in the genuine enthusiasm for, and the belief in, EVOP of the production personnel responsible for the programs. Where these qualities do not exist, EVOP will fail. This brings up the important problem of developing a proper climate for EVOP, since there are many people who will not be impressed merely with the type of exposition given in the previous sections. A proper discussion of this subject is beyond the scope of this paper, but "climate" is detailed in two excellent articles by L. F. VanEck (1958, 1962), which are recommended reading for anyone interested in starting EVOP.

EVOP IN OPERATION

There is really no limit to the type of variables that can be investigated via EVOP techniques. They can be continuous (time, temperature, pH, amount of nutrient, etc.) as well as discontinuous (different raw materials, an ingredient is either present or absent, etc.) in nature, and are subject to two main limitations: there should be some degree of control over the levels of the variables; and some meaningful response should be available to evaluate the changes made. In addition, the continuity and quality of product, the safety of personnel and equipment, and the physical limitations of the plant are all fundamental restrictions that are part of the basic philosophy of EVOP.

In our plant, we have not limited our studies to fermentation alone. Variables associated with beer filtration, extraction and crystallization lend themselves very well to the EVOP concept.

EVOP BENEFITS

The most powerful argument for the adoption of any new idea comes from the money it might save the company that uses it. Especially in recent times, when cost reduction in our plants has become more and more essential, a technique with the appeal and potential of Evolutionary Operation should be of great value financially. This has proven to be the case in the past for many chemical plants (including our own), and we can report "significant" dollar savings from the use of EVOP in our fermentation plant, also.

There are also several indirect benefits from EVOP: improved performance and decreased variability quite often result when the plant process is constantly under surveillance instead of being looked at only when in trouble; processes that are out of control lend themselves well to a trouble-shooting role for EVOP; the approach to a new process might change in a plant where EVOP has been adopted—instead of trying to pinpoint the exact optimum conditions in the pilot plant and then transferring to production, which could be very time-consuming, the development effort could rather be aimed at determining a general operating range for the key variables, and at this point, the process could be put into the plant immediately with a considerable saving in time.

Finally, one of the major contributions of EVOP, in my opinion, has been to provide a means of extracting meaningful information from processes which have always been labelled as "too variable to work with." We are constantly being told that the fermentation plant is no place to get reliable data. If this be so, what is actually implied is: there are variables operating that we know nothing about; or, there are variables operating that we are aware of but cannot control. Now, those who are really concerned with improving their plants will be quick to recognize the value of Evolutionary Operation in their fight against these formidable problems.

REFERENCES

Barnett, E. H. 1960. Introduction to evolutionary operation. Ind. Eng. Chem. 52(6): 500–503.

Box, G. E. P. 1957. Evolutionary operation: A method for increasing industrial productivity. Applied Statistics 6(2): 3–23. (This is the finest exposition of EVOP. It is written in simple language and should be required reading for those interested in the subject.)

Box, G. E. P. and J. S. Hunter. 1959. Condensed calculations for evolutionary operation programs. Technometrics 1(1): 77–95.

Hunter, J. S. 1960. Optimize your chemical process with evolutionary operations. Chem. Eng. 67(19): 193–202.

VanEck, L. F. 1958. Management's role in an evolutionary operations program. Proceedings of the Second Stevens Symposium on Statistical Methods. Chemical Industry 57 (January 25)

VanEck, L. F. 1962. Evolutionary operations: A path to more effective use of process data. Ind. Qual. Control 19(2): 8–10.

Whitwell, J. C. 1959. Practical applications of evolutionary operation. Transactions, 13th Annual Convention, Amer. Soc. Qual. Control: 603–616.

HORIZONS IN FERMENTATION AS VIEWED BY THE DEVELOPMENT ENGINEER

RICHARD W. JACKSON

Northern Regional Research Laboratory
U.S. Department of Agriculture
Peoria, Illinois, U.S.A.

THE DEVELOPMENT of fermentations for use on a large scale involves three principal elements: the substrate, the technique of conversion by enzymes or enzyme systems, and the product. In discussing horizons, I shall restrict my remarks to potential raw materials and to less traditional means for their economic conversion.

Inasmuch as carbohydrate is a principal item in many fermentations, the cost of carbohydrate itself may be decisive. My colleague, Mr. V. E. Sohns of our engineering staff, has projected, as shown in Table 1, the approximate costs of starting materials and other charges per unit of product for a number of fermentations. As expected, the cost of carbohydrate as percentage of total "cost to make" is much larger in those fermentations that are used to prepare chemicals in bulk, namely, solvents, acids and polymers.

TABLE 1
RELATIONSHIP OF COST OF CARBOHYDRATE AND OTHER ITEMS TO TOTAL "COST TO MAKE" FOR A VARIETY OF FERMENTATION PROCESSES

	"Cost to Make" of Product							
	Grain alcohol		Sodium gluconate		Microbial polymer B-1459		Vitamin B$_{12}$	
Item	¢/gal.	% of cost	¢/lb.	% of cost	¢/lb.	% of cost	$/gram	% of cost
Raw material								
Carbohydrate	26.5[a]	56.4	6.84	58.1	7.0	20.4	1.67	6.2
Other raw materials	2.9[b]	6.2	0.84	7.1	5.0	14.4	4.63	17.2
Utilities	5.2	11.1	0.96	8.1	11.0	32.1	6.40	23.8
Labor and supervision	5.6	11.9	0.98	8.3	4.1	11.9	5.30	19.7
Maintenance	1.8	3.8	0.59	5.0	2.0	5.8	2.39	8.9
Fixed charges	5.0	10.6	1.58	13.4	5.3	15.4	6.51	24.2
TOTAL	47.0	100.0	11.8	100.0	34.4	100.0	26.90	100.0
Plant capacity	54,000 gal./day[c]		3×10^6 lbs./yr.		5×10^6 lbs./yr.[d]		28.5 grams/day[e]	

[a]Corn, at $1.20 per bu. less credit of 48.6¢ per bu. for byproduct feed.
[b]Converting agent, fungal amylase and malt.
[c]Yield of alcohol 2.7 gal. 95 per cent alcohol per bu. (20,000 bu.).
[d]Industrial grade product.
[e]Grams of contained B$_{12}$ in dried fermentation solids.

Despite the inroads of the petrochemical industry, lactic acid is still manufactured by fermentation.* Gluconic acid can be made by chemical reactions but is actually obtained through fermentation. A great deal of molasses has been imported in recent years into the United States for production of industrial alcohol. Although this molasses was obtained at a special price for this particular use we have proof here that, if the cost of the carbohydrate substrate is low enough, fermentation alcohol can be made and sold on the market.

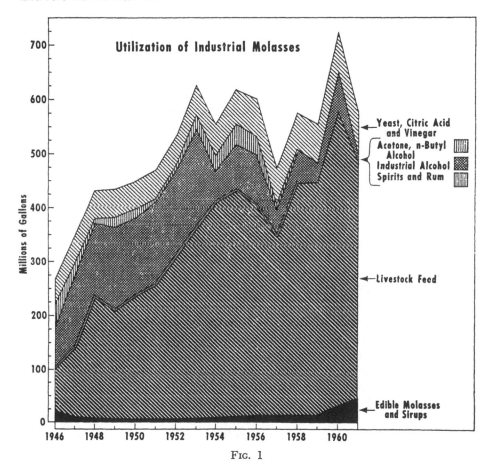

FIG. 1

CARBOHYDRATE SUBSTRATES

Molasses, long the cheapest source of crude sugar in concentrated form, costs more now, owing to competition for it by the feed industry. Figures are not available to show the end uses for the world supply of molasses but those (8) for the United States may be used to indicate the trends (see Fig. 1). Between 1946 and 1961, annual consumption of molasses doubled,

*An announcement has since been made in financial columns of plans to erect a chemical plant for the production of lactic acid.

reaching a peak of 700 million gallons in 1960, of which more than 500 million went into feeds. Over the same period, the amount of molasses used each year for making yeast, citric acid and vinegar increased somewhat and has since held steady at 70 million gallons, but the volume of molasses for industrial alcohol, butanol and acetone has dwindled very drastically from a former annual range of 100 to 200 million gallons. It is apparent that molasses as a source of fermentative sugar is subject to great shifts in competing uses, availability, price and even quality as the sugar producer squeezes more and more sugar out of his residual materials.

Because the utilization of grains is a principal goal of our Laboratory at Peoria, some of us are especially interested in the utilization of grains by fermentation. Distillers' solubles and cornsteep liquor are important in many fermentations, but starch, comprising two-thirds of the grain, is our main consideration. In some processes, for example those for making butanol and citric acid, it is possible to employ an organism that does its own saccharification of the starch. Otherwise it is necessary to supply sugar in some state of purity. Our engineers have estimated that glucose for use in fermentation processes can be obtained through enzymatic hydrolysis in 10 per cent solution at a cost of 3.7¢ per pound. The calculation is based on corn at 2¢ per pound and credit is taken for feed recovered. The sugar solution also contains valuable nutrients. It appears possible in these times for crude sugar from grain to compete with molasses at its current price plus cost of purification by ion-exchange or other procedure.

Cellulose is the most abundant available organic substrate, and a vast amount of research on cellulose-degrading organisms has revealed perhaps a dozen different end-products including cellobiose, glucose, methane, organic acids and alcohol. Yet, today, apparently there are no commercial plants for the primary production of any of these chemicals from cellulose by fermentation. The great difficulties experienced in plants designed to hydrolyze cellulose by chemical means emphasize the desirability of getting at cellulose by the enzyme route, that is, by fermentation. The known processes are too slow, and the products are too diverse and dilute for efficient recovery. It has been noted (4) that the amount of cellulose that can be fermented in a period of a few days is usually less than 2 grams per litre. Perhaps a novel method for the physical manipulation of the cellulose, a superior combination of cultures or a new powerful enzyme preparation will provide the means for efficient fermentative use of cellulose.

PETROLEUM PRODUCTS AS POSSIBLE SUBSTRATE

Hydrocarbon, rich in energy and carbon, is the means by which the chemical industry was able to undercut the fermentative production of industrial solvents. We are now learning that it is possible for microorganisms to convert hydrocarbon into attractive oxygenated products. For example, Raymond and Davis (5) showed that a *Nocardia* species consumed

52 of 80 grams of octadecane added in a 2-litre fermentation over 112 hours and produced 50 grams of dried cells of which lipid accounted for 60 per cent. Interestingly, an appreciable fraction of the lipid consisted of waxes, such as octadecyl palmitate or octadecyl stearate. I think this experiment is quite remarkable.

Certainly substrates that are insoluble in water medium present an extra fermentation problem. This has been solved for the conversion of 1 or 2 per cent concentrations of steroids in the production of high-priced drug products. One can use dispersing solvents and detergents, as well as a high rate of agitation, to increase contact between the substrate and the organism with its enzyme systems. Perhaps more can be done with emulsions. At all events, we may conclude that the possibility of commercial use of hydrocarbon as fermentation substrate is on the horizon. Also we should take note that such material as alcohol, glycerol and acetic acid derived from petroleum *via* the petrochemical industry can serve as fermentation substrates.

SPECIAL SUBSTRATES

I wish now to leave the area of general substrate materials such as starch and sugar, and cellulose, and dwell a little on special substrate chemicals that have been found to undergo simpler types of chemical reaction, for instance, the reduction of a ketone to an alcohol. A survey of the literature made a few years ago (10) revealed a total of more than 700 different reactions and more than 700 different products from more than 400 different substrates. If we eliminate glucose and the rather specialized steroids as starting materials, we still have about 350 different substrates yielding more than 500 different products by various reactions, ranging from oxidation and reduction to dismutation and polymerization.

One is struck by this great variety of known fermentative "type" reactions —but almost as much by the relatively few commercial applications. The production of sorbose from sorbitol, the decarboxylation of diaminopimelic acid in the synthesis of lysine and hydroxylation of steroids loom large among the applications, but the list is not a long one. Greater flexibility is needed in fermentative conversion. Some has been attained in recent years by means of mutants possessing abnormal patterns of metabolism; but it appears that the maximum flexibility will be established only when the enzyme mechanism, or one of the possible enzyme mechanisms, is well known and its elements can be derived economically from micro-organisms.

USE OF ENZYMES FOR SYNTHESIS: DEXTRAN AN EXAMPLE

I shall therefore next project some ideas relative to the probable future use of enzymes, especially microbial enzymes, for the synthesis of organic compounds. I shall consider the synthesis of polysaccharide by a cell-free system and select for the moment the synthesis of dextran as a prototype.

$$x \text{ Sucrose} \longrightarrow \text{Glucose}_x + x \text{ Fructose}$$

This relatively simple transfer type of reaction is catalyzed by the enzyme, dextransucrase (3).

The enzyme production of dextran entails several advantages. In the first place, we found, by study of nutritional and environmental factors, that the organism *Leuconostoc mesenteroides* could be made to increase its production of dextransucrase (7). In fact, the resulting enzyme was sufficiently potent that it could be diluted for use. It was also possible to remove the cells before there was enough dextran polymer present to make the solution viscous and difficult to handle. The process was later operated on a commercial scale. Industry has long used hydrolytic enzymes, but here we have a process in which an enzyme was employed to synthesize a product—in any amount desired. It was further found that the molecular weight of the dextran product was dependent on the concentration of substrate, concentration of enzyme, temperature and the primer substance used (6). By proper regulation of these factors, we were able to produce a large proportion of the product in the desired range of 75,000 (for blood plasma replacement) rather than of the several million obtained ordinarily. Thus, in the illustration, an enzyme preparation was more effective than the whole culture as measured by quantity and quality of product.

PROJECTION OF MORE COMPLEX ENZYME PROCESSES

The enzyme system just described admittedly has relatively simple characteristics. First, the enzyme may be obtained in high concentration in the cell-free fermentation liquor. Further, the synthesis is uncomplicated with regard to energy, which is sufficient in the glucose-fructose bond of the sucrose substrate to drive the reaction. The situation is in contrast, for example, to the phosphorylation of glucose as a starting point in many biochemical reactions of this substrate. Finally, no expensive coenzyme is required at dollars per gram.

Realizing that it would be very easy to over-speculate about the potential commercial use of microbial enzymes for the synthesis of organic compounds, I shall nevertheless venture a little and discuss a synthetic system which my colleague, Dr. M. E. Slodki, and I have projected from the literature (*inter alia* 2, 9). It is more complex than the dextran-producing system and, as far as we know, has not been operated on a similarly large scale. It involves a series of coupled enzyme reactions whereby we would be able to start with two cheap substrate materials, starch and inorganic phosphate, to employ enzymes that are obtainable from yeast or in one instance from potato, to limit the expensive coenzyme to an initial catalytic amount, and thus to synthesize two products, 6-phosphogluconic acid and L-glutamic acid (Fig. 2).

The points of equilibrium of the four basic reactions are all favorable, and the over-all process certainly appears technically feasible. We might need

Cell-Free Coupled Production of
L-Glutamic Acid and 6-Phosphogluconic Acid

(1) Starch + P_i $\xrightarrow{\text{Phosphorylase (potato or yeast)}}$ Glucose-1-P

(2) Glucose-1-P $\xrightarrow{\text{Mutase (yeast)}}$ Glucose-6-P

(3) Glucose-6-P + TPN^+ + H_2O $\xrightarrow{\text{Dehydrogenase(yeast) "Zwischenferment"}}$ 6-PGA + TPNH + H^+

(4) α-KG + NH_3 + TPNH + H^+ $\xrightarrow{\text{Glutamic Dehydrogenase(yeast)}}$ L-Glutamic + TPN^+ + H_2O

---

(5) Starch + P_i + α-KG + NH_3 $\xrightarrow{\hspace{3cm}}$ 6-PGA + L-Glutamic

FIG. 2

to use enzyme to linearize the amylopectin of the starch, and we doubtless would find it necessary to remove or sequester phosphate from Reaction 1 that would be inimical to Reaction 2. But such problems and their solution are not unusual in the development of new processes and products. It appears that such a process could be operated on a large scale. We might anticipate the neat situation of making two useful chemicals simultaneously.

These illustrations show how the use of enzymes would contribute to flexibility of process and economy in cost. Enzymes could be obtained from different sources—as a rule from micro-organisms—and recombined as needed in the particular system.

What are some of the obvious difficulties that will be encountered in making greater use of enzymes for synthetic work?

It will be necessary to prepare many enzymes from cells, since the agents are not released into the fermentation liquor, and large quantities of cells will have to be ruptured by either physical or chemical means or both. For this we have an increasing variety of tools. For instance, there are pressure cells and adjustable colloid mills, which can be modified for semi-continuous flow, to effect mechanical breakup. There is also ultrasonic disruption, which can be applied on a continuous basis. Finally, we have lyozyme available to degrade cell walls.

Another problem will be the amount of enzyme available in the cell for liberation or extraction. The concentration may well be less than that necessary for a going process. Here again we have considerable basis for thinking that in many cases, if not in all, the yield of enzyme obtainable *from within* the cell can be increased. I refer, of course, to the discoveries that have been made with regard to the "inducer" or "repressor" actions of substrate material or of metabolic product and to the operation of the feedback mechanism as it controls the production of enzyme (1). Increases of fifteen- to a thousandfold have been obtained by this technique.

It is supposed that in many instances crude preparations of enzymes will be used and that side reactions brought on by the presence of unwanted enzymes may require some degree of enzyme fractionation, or perhaps differential destruction of the offender. Complicated and extremely expensive procedures will hardly qualify for large-scale work.

Finally, we have the frequent requirement for rare and expensive coenzymes such as ATP and TPN. One answer to that problem, as shown in the example, would be the use of coupled reactions. Otherwise, separate steps or reactions would have to be incorporated to regenerate the costly item by oxidation or photosynthesis.

One could speculate further about the possibility of obtaining the proper RNA template and synthetic system to make the desired enzyme for large-scale use, but I refrain from more than mention of that possibility. These are some thoughts that come to me as I think about the horizons of the fermentation industry. Such developments in the use of microbial enzymes may come gradually, but we surely should expect them.

REFERENCES

1. Cold Spring Harbor, New York, The Biological Laboratory. 1961. Cellular regulatory mechanisms, 408 pp. *In* Cold Spring Harbor symposia on quantitative biology, vol. 26. Long Island Biological Association.
2. Colowick, S. P., and E. W. Sutherland. 1942. Polysaccharide synthesis from glucose by means of purified enzymes. J. Biol. Chem. *144*: 423–437.
3. Hehre, E. J. 1951. Enzymic synthesis of polysaccharides: A biological type of polymerization. *In* Advances in enzymology, ed. F. F. Nord, *11*: 297–337. Interscience Publishers, New York.
4. McBee, R. H. 1950. The anaerobic thermophilic cellulolytic bacteria. J. Bacteriol. *14*: 51–63.
5. Raymond, R. L., [and J. B. Davis]. 1961. Microbial oxidation of n-paraffinic hydrocarbons. *In* Developments in industrial microbiology 2: 23–32. Proc. 17th Gen. Meeting Soc. Ind. Microbiol., 1960. Plenum Press, New York.
6. Tsuchiya, H. M., N. N. Hellman, H. J. Koepsell, J. Corman, C. S. Stringer, S. P. Rogovin, M. O. Bogard, G. Bryant, V. H. Feger, C. A. Hoffman, F. R. Senti, and R. W. Jackson. 1955. Factors affecting molecular weight of enzymatically synthesized dextran. J. Am. Chem. Soc. 77: 2412–2419.
7. Tsuchiya, H. M., H. J. Koepsell, J. Corman, G. Bryant, M. O. Bogard, V. H. Feger, and R. W. Jackson. 1952. The effect of certain cultural factors on production of dextransucrase by *Leuconostoc mesenteroides*. J. Bacteriol. *64*: 521–526.
8. U.S. Department of Agriculture, Agricultural Marketing Service. 1956–62. Molasses (annual market news summary). AMS-79.
9. Wachsman, J. T. 1956. The rôle of α-ketoglutarate and mesaconate in glutamate fermentation by *Clostridium tetanomorphum*. J. Biol. Chem. *223*: 19–27.
10. Wallen, L. L., F. H. Stodola, and R. W. Jackson. 1959. Type reactions in fermentation chemistry. U.S. Dept. Agr. Bull. ARS-71-13, 496 pp. Northern Regional Research Laboratory, Peoria, Illinois.

HORIZONS IN INDUSTRIAL MICROBIOLOGY AS VIEWED BY THE MICROBIOLOGIST

T. O. WIKÉN

Laboratory of Microbiology
Technological University
Delft, The Netherlands

. . . since Pasteur's startling discoveries of the important role played by microbes in human affairs, microbiology as a science has always suffered from its eminent practical implications. By far the majority of the microbiological studies were undertaken to answer questions either directly or indirectly connected with the well-being of mankind. A. J. KLUYVER, April, 1954

THE WORLD POPULATION undergoes a rapid expansion. At present it amounts to about 3 milliard (3×10^9) mouths and will at the end of this century very probably reach a figure of 6 milliard. The rate of population growth is particularly high in the Far East and in Latin America, while in Europe it seems to have been calmed down by the blessings of industrialization. Some optimists hold the view that the increase of the earth's human population will take place according to the well-known S-formed curve representing the microbial multiplication in a batch culture and other growth processes in more or less closed systems of constant space and limited supply of nutrients. Mankind is supposed to enter the phase of exponential growth just now and to reach the maximum stationary phase around the year 2200 at a world population figure of about 11 milliard. However that may be, experts are aware that some two-thirds of the present population are under-fed, and they realize that, in view of the average annual increase of about 35 million human beings, undoubtedly greater food supplies, particularly in the form of proteins and fats, will be needed in the future, the next fifty years being considered an especially critical period for several reasons (1, 2).

From time immemorial man has settled by lakes and rivers, and during all the ages large municipalities have been concerned with their water supplies. Water is used for drinking; for bathing and washing; for sprinkling of gardens, lawns and streets; for recreational purposes in swimming pools, fountains and cascades; for the protection of life and property against fire; for moving turbines; for transferring heat and generating steam power; and for numerous other industrial processes. In this connection it should be pointed out that the food industries require unpolluted water suitable for human consumption. Residential and industrial communities use tremendous quantities of water, and, notwithstanding the efforts of sanitary engineering to solve the interdependent problems of water supply and disposal of sewage and wastes, the increasing industrialization, illustrated particularly well in Western Europe, has resulted in a shortage of both drinking water and water for industrial purposes.

Processes, brought about by enzymes, have been used by man through the ages to leaven bread and to prepare cheese, wine, beer and vinegar. Nowadays, sixty-five years after the epoch-making discovery by Buchner that alcoholic fermentation does not require the presence of intact yeast cells but may be performed by yeast juice, not only enzymes associated with living cells but also cell-free preparations of these catalysts find so many diverse applications in various industries that I do not hesitate to state that every modern household in the world uses an ever increasing number of products in the manufacture of which one or more enzymes were utilized (3, 4, 5).

The general social advance is accompanied by an increasing demand for attractively-flavoured soft drinks and for the stimulating beverages which in all tongues are known by names suggesting spirits and vitality and are used for enhancing sociability and the pleasure of life. Flavour and taste chemicals which render the commonplace staple dishes as well as the courses of the banquet appealing to the palate of man are today being produced commercially on a scale which means an important contribution to the economy of the countries concerned.

Since the discovery of the antibacterial action of penicillin, which undoubtedly is one of the most exciting events in the history of science, the production of antibiotics, started during the Second World War, has grown to a vast industry. Penicillin was followed by streptomycin, aureomycin, chloromycetin, terramycin, bacitracin, tyrothricin, neomycin, achromycin, griseofulvin, blasticidin, and numerous other miracle drugs with bacteriostatic or fungistatic, bactericidal or fungicidal action against a more or less wide range of the respective microbes. Today, thirty-three years after the first observations made by Fleming on the inhibiting action of a mold colony and the culture filtrate of this mold on gram-positive bacteria, the antibiotics manufactured annually in the United States for human and veterinary uses, and for animal feed supplementation, food preservation and crop protection are valued at 350 to 400 million dollars, which is said to correspond to more than 60 per cent of all medicinal chemicals produced yearly in that country (6).

After the finding by Kendall, Hench and co-workers in 1949 that cortisone has a dramatically beneficial effect in the treatment of chronic rheumatoid arthritis and acute rheumatic fever, this and other adrenocortical steroids or derivatives thereof are produced commercially. Although some early exaggerated hopes of the clinical value of cortisone were ill founded, this hormone and its analogues are of the greatest importance in therapeutics, and during the last ten to fifteen years steroid chemistry has been dominated by the search for biological methods of converting the currently marketed hormones into new and better analogues (7–10).

In 1926 the effectiveness of liver preparations in the dietary treatment of pernicious anaemia, which until then was incurable and fatal, was described. The active agent was called the "liver factor" or the "antipernicious anaemia principle." Two years later the administration of gastric juice from a normal human stomach along with meat was found to avert the symptoms of the same disease. The success of this treatment was supposed to be due to the combined action of two agents: the "intrinsic factor" in the gastric juice and the "extrinsic factor" in the meat. In attempts made during the Second World War to raise poultry on purely vegetable protein rations the birds failed to grow at a normal rate. On feeding animal or fish wastes as supplements to the vegetable diets an appreciable increase in growth was obtained. The essential substance missing from the vegetable feeds was named the "animal protein factor." In 1947 and 1948 an examination of the growth factor requirements of *Lactobacillus lactis* Dorner in synthetic media revealed that a substance present in tomato juice and in liver extract was essential for development of the organism. This substance was termed the "Lactobacillus lactis Dorner factor." Finally, in 1948, the four lines of investigation mentioned on human, animal and microbial nutrition converged and led to the discovery of vitamin B_{12}, a member of a biologically extremely important family of complex co-ordination compounds with a central cobalt atom. In 1959 and 1960 the annual production in the United States of all grades of this vitamin amounted to about 1000 pounds, representing a value of 20 to 60 million dollars depending on the market price (6, 11, 12).

During the last few years mankind has entered an era of extraterrestrial exploration which may culminate in placing a man on the moon. In view of the great achievements already performed in developing space craft it seems likely that in the not too distant future there will be manned space flights having a duration of months or years, and perhaps even long-term extraterrestrial habitation by man on orbiting stations and on fixed stations on the moon or on planets like Mars and Venus. In the course of long-term operations by means of space vehicles as well as during missions of relatively extended duration on extraterrestrial stations man will face the problems of everyday existence on a magnified scale. On earth he has at least for the present comparatively little difficulty in obtaining an adequate supply of food appealing to his palate or of gaseous oxygen essential for respiration, and in disposing of the wastes. Under the special conditions of space travel and extraterrestrial habitation, however, attempts to transport and store a year's supply of food for a crewman or two will meet with great difficulties because the mass as well as the volume of a manned or unmanned space cabin should of necessity be kept at a minimum. Now a system simultaneously providing food and free oxygen and disposing of wastes may be constructed on the basis of our knowledge of the metabolism of the various terrestrial and marine ecosystems making up the biosphere on earth. Such a regenerative biological life-support system for use in extraterrestrial operations implies, in addition to man representing the consumers, creatures of

three types: producers like the green plants, and decomposing and transforming organisms like the bacteria and fungi. In this biological microcosm,
which as a matter of fact represents an artificial symbiosis between a fixed
number of organisms with well-known physiological activities, the cycles of
carbon, nitrogen, oxygen, hydrogen, sulphur and other essential elements
should function in principle as in the biosphere on earth and at rates balanced
to maintain man's ability to exist and to perform his duties for extended
periods of time under the particular conditions of space flights and extraterrestrial habitation (13, 14).

So far we have briefly discussed a few industrial products helping to
satisfy man's material needs, including those for health and pleasure. Some
of these products are of such commercial importance that their manufacture
influences the economy of the countries concerned. We shall next turn our
attention to the forms of life known as microbes and, in just a few words,
touch upon those of their biochemical and physiological properties which
may be of interest to industry.

Since the animalcules were discovered 288 years ago the microbiologists
have made us acquainted with an immense number of different types of
organisms capable of utilizing the most diverse chemical compounds as
substrates for the assimilatory and dissimilatory processes involved in their
growth and multiplication and resulting in the formation of an enormous
variety of extracellular metabolic products in addition to the numerous
compounds constituting the cell material. This diversity of substrates used
and of metabolic products formed in building up and maintaining the living
substance of microbial cells covers a spectrum of biochemical and physiological properties far surpassing that normally considered by the biologists
dealing with larger plants and animals (15). These microbes were isolated
from a great many natural sources such as air, water, mud, soil and sewage
sludge; grains and malt sprouts; grapes and fruits; spoiled must, wine and
beer; fermenting cucumber and olive brines; samples of fresh and spoiled
food materials like milk and fermented milk preparations; butter and cheese;
meat, fish and vegetables; or various parts of the intestinal tract of insects,
birds, ruminants and other animals, etc. etc. In the attempts to isolate
specific micro-organisms from such sources the ecological approach, introduced by Winogradsky and developed further by Beijerinck, has been
applied with amazing success. It is well known among microbiologists as the
principle of elective or enrichment cultures and sometimes designated as the
principle of selective or differential media. The microbial strains thus isolated and subsequently maintained in our pure culture collections as stock
cultures on various substrates may undergo spontaneous mutation. In consequence, a single-cell culture after several transfers in the course of months
or years may be found to contain one or more new types of organisms in
addition to the original isolate, and it even happened that after some months
of subculturing this isolate, owing to the process of selection following

spontaneous mutation, was completely replaced by one or more mutants (15). In such cases the phenomenon of mutation mostly had unpleasant consequences as the new microbial strains had lost the capacity of the original isolates to form one or more commercially valuable products in high yields. On the other hand, the method of deliberately inducing mutation by the aid of irradiation or mutagenic chemicals has nowadays become the routine means of obtaining strains producing antibiotics and other complex organic substances in enormously increased yields as compared to the parent strains, or showing nutritional deficiencies and therefore being of great value as test organisms in the elucidation of biosynthetic pathways and in the assays of amino acids, vitamins, etc. As a matter of fact, analytical microbiology is a branch of science with ever increasing importance in research in general and applied biology, chemistry and biochemistry as well as in routine testing and screening in industry (16).

In view of the facts just outlined it is no wonder that the number of industries based on the metabolic activities of microbes is expanding year by year as new processes are developed and new microbial strains are tamed for the service of mankind. As is well known, microbes nowadays are or may be utilized for production of simple or relatively simple organic compounds: the hydrocarbon methane; alcohols such as ethanol, isopropanol and n-butanol, 2,3-butanediol, glycerol and mannitol; organic acids like acetic, propionic and n-butyric acids, lactic acid, fumaric and citric acids, gluconic, itaconic and kojic acids, a-ketoglutaric, 2-ketogluconic and 5-ketogluconic acids, gallic acid; ketones like acetone and dihydroxyacetone; amino acids such as L-glutamic acid, L-lysine, L-ornithine and L-valine. Furthermore, micro-organisms are or may be used on an industrial scale for production of relatively or highly complex organic compounds: ustilagic acid; substances with stimulating effects in higher plants like gibberellic acid; vitamins such as riboflavin and cyanocobalamin; provitamins like ergosterol and β-carotene; compounds used in vitamin synthesis, such as sorbose; antibiotics such as penicillin, streptomycin, chlortetracycline, oxytetracycline and tetracycline; steroid hormone analogues; enzymes like amylases, cellulase, pectinase, lactase and invertase, proteases, penicillinase, glucose oxidase and numerous specially prepared and highly specific enzyme reagents which are used to an increasing extent in qualitative and quantitative analyses as well as for therapeutic and diagnostic purposes; polysaccharides like dextrans and levans; and alkaloids such as ergotamine, ergosine, ergocristine, ergocornine, ergocryptine and ergobasine, agroclavine, elymoclavine, secaclavine, penniclavine, triseclavine and lysergic acid amide. Several microbes particularly rich in protein or fat were cultivated on a technical scale and used as food for man or as fodder for animals (17, 18, 19). In addition, micro-organisms are utilized extensively in the anaerobic and aerobic treatment of sewage and industrial wastes, including the reduction of the biological oxygen demand of effluents (20, 21). On the other hand, industries nowadays must be well informed about the microbes which are detrimental in manufacturing processes or destructive to raw materials and end-products, and they must be well versed in the methods applied in combating such microbes. Indeed, the branch of microbiology studying the deterioration of various materials—for example the breakdown of cellulose and lignin in wood, the proteins of skin, and the polymers, plasticizers and other ingredients of plastics; the degradation of cotton and natural rubber; the decay of fruits and vegetables, etc.—is assuming an important position in industrial research owing to its economic implications (22–27).

After this brief survey of some chemical compounds useful to man, and of the capacities of microbes to produce these compounds on a technical scale, I should like to call your attention to some particular questions which might be of importance for the developments that, in view of the extremely rapid advances made in industrial microbiology during the last few years, undoubtedly may be expected in this branch of science in the near future. These questions are the following.

As previously mentioned, the great value of microbes to industry is closely connected with the vast diversity of chemical conversions which may be brought about by these organisms, and, furthermore, with the existence of several microbes in whose metabolism a certain conversion occupies a predominant position which in turn results in the formation and accumulation of a particular end-product. In view of this it may be said without overstatement that the most valuable working capital of a microbiological institution is its collection of stock cultures of microbial strains constant in their ability to produce useful compounds in high yields. Consequently, the hunt for new microbial strains with the property of synthesizing new substances of so far unknown chemical structure, or already known substances which are difficult to prepare by chemical means, will even in the future remain the clue to rapid progress in industrial microbiology. As a matter of fact, I consider improvements of the conventional laboratory screening techniques as one of the most urgent tasks of modern microbiology. Once you have succeeded in isolating a microbe capable of forming a certain compound in fairly great amounts, it is usually a relatively easy affair to increase the yield to an economically satisfactory level by producing mutants of the strain concerned and by varying the composition of the medium or other conditions of growth and production, such as temperature, aeration and agitation.

In connection with the statements just made I should like to stress that the microbiologists responsible for planning the large screening projects carried out all over the world for various purposes should not restrict the studies to the classical objects of industrial microbiology, viz. the bacteria, actinomycetes, yeasts and molds, but should for several reasons extend their efforts to the algae and higher fungi, and even to protozoa and other microscopic invertebrate animals. Because of their ability to convert carbon dioxide into organic matter by means of light energy, the algae, like other plants containing chlorophyll, occupy a key position in the carbon cycle in nature. The total amount of carbon dioxide assimilated per year by the marine plankton algae has by various authors been estimated at 330 milliard tons, corresponding to 90 milliard tons of carbon or 225 milliard tons of glucose, while the total quantity of carbon dioxide consumed annually in the photosynthesis of the terrestrial plants amounts to only about 60 milliard tons, equivalent to approximately 16 milliard tons of carbon or 40 milliard tons of glucose. According to these estimations the microscopic algae of the oceans would contribute more than four-fifths of the total amount of carbon dioxide fixed yearly on earth in organic compounds through the process of photosynthesis (28–30).

The dry substance of the cells of microscopic green algae such as members of the genus *Chlorella*, grown in presence of an adequate source of nitrogen, has been found to contain 45 to 50 per cent or more of protein. On cultivation under conditions of nitrogen starvation cells of the same algae with a lipid content as high as 80 to 85 per cent have been obtained, while cells harvested from cultures raised on substrates of normal composition do not contain more than 20 to 25 per cent of such material. Furthermore, nearly all important vitamins are known to be present in the algal cell substance at reasonably high levels. Moreover, it has been stated that suspensions of microscopic green algae under the proper environmental conditions utilize the light-energy much more efficiently than most field cultures of higher plants. In addition, the introduction of algal cultures would imply a possibility of rational utilization of land which owing to unfavourable climate and soil conditions, etc., is not suited for classical agriculture. In view of these and other advantages of microscopic algae over higher plants and with regard to the need of the world for additional sources of human food, animal feed and industrial raw materials rich in protein, lipid and vitamins, it is not surprising that the possibility of growing *Chlorella pyrenoidosa*, *Scenedesmus obliquus* and other microscopic algae on a large scale has been considered seriously, particularly in countries with overpopulated areas. Experiments performed about ten years ago on the growth of unicellular and simple coenobic green algae in pilot plants with natural illumination have shown conclusively that mass cultivation of these organisms is technically feasible and that average yields of 20 g of algal dry substance per square metre per day could be realized under favourable climatic conditions. This corresponds to approximately 45 tons of dry cell substance per hectare per year, which, in view of the high protein content of the algal cells and the crying need for more protein in the world, undoubtedly justifies further investigation of the problems involved irrespective of the conventional economic considerations. In this connection it may be worth while to recall the fact that algae are rich in chlorophyll used as a deodorant and a colouring matter, xanthophyll used as a poultry feed supplement, and many other pigments, and therefore constitute a promising source of such substances. Further, it is encouraging to note that an institution in Japan, established with governmental funds for research on algae, is said to be self-supporting from the sale of a dried product and an extract of *Chlorella* cells, the latter being used in the commercial preparation of yogurt as an agent stimulating the development of the lactic acid bacteria and thus reducing fermentation time and production costs (31–38).

As is well known, the formation of organic substance through photosynthesis in aerobic organisms is associated with uptake of carbon dioxide and liberation of gaseous oxygen. These characteristics of the carbon dioxide assimilation in green plants point towards the application of microscopic green algae to maintain adequate living conditions for man during long-term space flights and extraterrestrial habitation. An essential part of the recycling or regenerating biological self-support systems considered to serve such purposes is an algal culture unit for production of food or food supplements rich in protein and vitamins, for removal of certain waste components including carbon dioxide formed in man's respiration, and for supply of free oxygen utilized in that process. The balance between man's requirement of food and oxygen and the recycling of these requisites of life in the algal gas exchanger, which in addition prevents the accumulation of carbon dioxide in toxic concentrations, has already been the subject of much subtle speculation and experimental work; and such delicate problems as that of the nutritive value of fecal amino acids and fecal pyrolysis gases for algae have been studied by several workers. In summary, it does not matter whether we would like to leave earth for the moon or prefer to stay on earth, in any case the algae are most certainly of increasing importance as objects of research in general and applied microbiology (13, 14, 39–44).

Edible mushrooms or fleshy fungi were highly appreciated as delicacies by epicures among the old Greeks and Romans, and these fungi represent undoubtedly one of man's earliest foods. The mass cultivation of mushrooms, belonging to the genus *Agaricus*, on beds of horse manure in the open started in Europe, probably in France, in the seventeenth century and spread to other European countries and to the United States. Although mushrooms generally are considered a luxury food, their cultivation has developed to a large industry, the production in the United States alone amounting to between 75 and 100 million pounds annually. The classical techniques of growing mushrooms on a large scale, using beds of horse manure or mixtures of this rare material with straw, corn fodder, brewer's grains, etc., is time-consuming and expensive. As a large proportion of the mushrooms are pulped and used in the manufacture of soups, gravies and flavourings, the idea arose of applying the method of submerged cultures in order to produce mycelium rather than sporophores. Such mycelium might also serve as inoculum or spawn for seeding manure beds intended for growing the latter bodies. In the experiments performed rapid growth and high yields of mushroom mycelium were obtained in aerated liquid media prepared with a wide range of nitrogen, carbon and energy sources, and the protein, vitamin and mineral contents of this mycelium compared favourably with those of the tissue of commercially produced sporophores. Unfortunately the mycelium of *Agaricus* strains did not possess the typical flavour of fresh mushrooms. However, the mycelia of *Morchella* strains grown in such cultures quite readily developed distinct flavours suggestive of those characteristic of the respective fruiting bodies. The research on the growth of higher basidiomycetes and ascomycetes in submerged cultures and on the chemical nature of the mycelium and the extracellular compounds formed seems to be accelerated and rightfully so (45–47).

A situation similar to that just described also holds for the commercial production of ergot alkaloids synthesized by strains of various species of ascomycetes classified in the genus *Claviceps*. Up till now these alkaloids have been extracted from sclerotia of *Claviceps purpurea* grown in parasitic field cultures on rye. During recent years successful investigations have been performed on the growth of pure *Claviceps* strains and on the formation and accumulation of various ergot alkaloids by such strains on laboratory scale in stationary cultures with surface mycelium and in shaken cultures with submerged mycelium as well as on a semitechnical scale in fermentors with aeration. The results obtained show conclusively that strains of various *Claviceps* species under the proper nutritional conditions are capable of synthesizing and accumulating considerable amounts of ergot alkaloids, both in the mycelium and in the liquid medium, in cultures of the types mentioned. In view of these findings it seems quite likely that the classical agricultural method will be replaced in the future by modern fermentation techniques using saprophytic cultures. An increase in the demand for the alkaloids or their derivatives would most certainly accelerate such a development (19, 48–50).

We know that enzymes have several unique advantages over conventional chemical reagents including most catalysts originating from other sources than cells of organisms visible or invisible to the naked eye. By way of example the enzymes are highly specific in their action, and this usually takes place at a maximum rate under moderate conditions of temperature, pressure and pH. In addition, the enzymes are active even at very low concentrations, and they may, as soon as the desired reaction is completed, be inactivated by applying relatively mild conditions. Moreover, they are non-toxic, a property of particular significance in the food industry. No wonder that the commercial preparation of enzymes for various purposes is steadily increasing. It may be that the large-scale production of these organic catalysts from macroscopic plants and animals still exceeds that from microscopic organisms. However, I do not hesitate to state that in the future enzymes of microbial origin will be of increasing importance as compared with those from the former sources. This prophecy seems justified for several reasons, a few of which may be briefly considered here. In the first place, the number of enzymes obtainable in bulk from the bodies of larger plants and animals is comparatively small, whereas the microbial cells because of their unparalleled flexibility may form an enormous variety of these biocatalysts, on the one hand against a constant genetic background, on the other in response to changes in the genotype of the cell. Secondly, if enzymes are to be prepared from larger plants and animals in an economically feasible way, they will mostly have the status of industrial by-products, which might result in a supply inadequate to meet a sudden or steady increase in the demand for these catalysts. The manufacture of enzymes based on microbial activity has the great advantage of being highly flexible as regards productive capacity and, therefore, seems to be more suited to meet such fluctuations in the market requirements. Finally, the great potentiality of microbes to produce induced enzymes, including the adaptive ones, implies almost unlimited possibilities of providing for the most specialized and subtle needs of industry, diagnostics and therapeutics for biocatalysts of high substrate specificity (3–5, 51).

As pointed out by several authors, some traditional fermentations yielding simple or comparatively simple organic molecules such as ethanol, isopropanol, n-butanol, glycerol, acetone, acetic acid, n-butyric acid and racemic lactic acid, have been or are being replaced by pure chemical processes in which products of the petro-chemicals industry and other sources serve as raw materials. On the other hand, a great many new microbial processes have been introduced for the manufacture of compounds with a relatively or highly complex chemical structure such as antibiotics, provitamins, vitamins, polysaccharides and enzymes. This revolutionary change in the pattern of the industry is mainly the result of economic competition. Many fermentations are based on the use of corn, potatoes, grain, molasses and other carbohydrate sources as raw materials, and these are, at least in the countries of the Western world, at present too expensive to serve economically as substrates for commercial production of the simple molecules mentioned. In addition, the market prices of some simple fermentation products may become too high owing to the heavy cost of recovering and purifying these products from the fermented culture media. However, citric and gluconic acids, as well as the optically active forms of lactic acid, will most certainly for years ahead be manufactured by fermentation; and the microbial production of the L-isomers of certain amino acids such as glutamic acid, lysine, ornithine, tryptophan and valine, which has been realized on the basis of pioneer work by Japanese scientists, is a rapidly expanding branch of industry (6, 31, 36, 52–55).

The phenomenon of reciprocal or bilateral growth stimulation between microbes has been known for a long time. It has been shown that this in many cases involves a mutual exchange of vitamins, amino acids and other growth factors, one organism being heterotrophic with regard to a factor synthesized by the other, and vice versa. Such interrelationships undoubtedly play a significant role in microbial associations occurring in nature and utilized in industry, and an intensified study of the artificial symbiosis between micro-organisms with known growth factor requirements in mixed cultures and in systems of dialysis cells might be of importance for the elucidation of the mechanism of the stepwise breakdown of complex organic substances like carbohydrates, proteins and fats in sewage sludge digestion. Such a study would also yield results that could be applied in the utilization of agricultural and industrial wastes poor in vitamins and other growth factors (56–58).

During the last ten years several workers have studied the action of lysozyme and other enzymes and the effect of metabolic disturbance on a number of bacteria, yeasts and molds, with special regard to changes produced in the shape of the cells concerned. It was found that in an osmotically balanced medium the entire cell wall, or the part of this responsible for the rigidity, may be removed with formation of globular bodies, the so-called protoplasts and spheroplasts, respectively. In addition, it was demonstrated that these forms, which still possess the cytoplasmic membrane, are capable of various activities characteristic of life: respiration in the sense of an uptake of gaseous oxygen; fermentation; incorporation of nutrients such as glucose, acetic acid, amino acids and nucleic acid components; synthesis of constitutive and induced enzymes; fixation of gaseous nitrogen; and growth as manifested by increase in dry weight and volume. It is true that the spherical forms so far prepared, particularly the protoplasts, are extremely sensitive to osmotic shock, but nevertheless the question quite naturally arises whether intact microbial cells could be replaced by protoplasts or spheroplasts as biochemical agents in industrial production of compounds incapable of penetrating the cell wall or capable of passing through this barrier only at a low rate (59, 60).

In trying to forecast the next trends of development in industrial microbiology one is confronted inevitably with the problem of microbial nitrogen fixation which is of the greatest importance not only to agriculture but also to industry. In the last two years encouraging results have been obtained in preparing active cell-free extracts containing the nitrogen-fixing enzyme systems of several bacteria and blue-green algae. In view of this remarkable progress it seems worth while to ponder the question whether the enzymatic fixation of atmospheric elementary nitrogen in absence of cells might be developed to an industrial process and, furthermore, whether such a method actually would have some advantages over a method based on the use of intact whole cells (61).

In summary, our allies among the animalcules have contributed substantially to the progress of industry in times past, and we may safely state that they will continue doing so for all time to come, on earth and even on the moon, Mars and Venus.

REFERENCES

1. Virtanen, A. I. 1961. Ernährungsmöglichkeiten der Menschheit und die Chemie. Naturwiss. Rundschau *14*: 371–379.
2. Woodbine, M. 1959. Microbial fat: Micro-organisms as potential fat producers. *In* Progress in industrial microbiology, *1*: 179–245, ed. D. J. D. Hockenhull. Heywood & Company Ltd., London.

3. Beckhorn, E. J. 1960. Production of industrial enzymes. Wallerstein Lab. Comm. *23*: 201–212.
4. Hoogerheide, J. C. 1954. Microbial enzymes other than fungal amylases. *In* Industrial fermentations, *2*: 122–154, ed. L. A. Underkofler and R. J. Hickey. Chemical Publishing Co., Inc., New York.
5. Underkofler, L. A. 1954. Fungal amylolytic enzymes. *Ibid.*, *2*: 97–121.
6. Perlman, D. and Ch. Kroll. 1962. Fermentation, CW Report. Chemical Week *90*: 97–104.
7. Klyne, W. 1960. The chemistry of the steroids. *In* Methuen's Monographs on Biochemical Subjects, ed. R. Peters and F. G. Young. Methuen & Co., Ltd., London.
8. Shoppee, Ch. W. 1958. Chemistry of the steroids. *In* Organic Chemistry Monographs, ed. J. W. Cook and M. Stacey. Butterworths Scientific Publications, London.
9. Stanley, A. R., and R. J. Hickey. 1954. Miscellaneous fermentations. *In* Industrial fermentations, *2*: 387–416, ed. L. A. Underkofler and R. J. Hickey. Chemical Publishing Co., Inc., New York.
10. Whitmarsh, J. M. 1958. Transformation of steroids. *In* British fermentation industries, pp. 112–128. Sir Isaac Pitman & Sons, Ltd., London.
11. Smith, E. L. 1960. Vitamin B_{12}. *In* Methuen's Monographs on Biochemical Subjects, ed. R. Peters and F. G. Young. Methuen & Co., Ltd., London.
12. Whitmarsh, J. M. 1958. Vitamin B_{12} (Cyanocobalamin). *In* British Fermentation Industries, pp. 76–83. Sir Isaac Pitman & Sons, Ltd., London.
13. Krall, A. R., and Kok, B. 1960. Studies on algal gas exchangers with reference to space flight. *In* Developments in industrial microbiology, *1*: 33–44, ed. B. M. Miller. Plenum Press, New York.
14. Phillips, J. N. 1962. Closed ecological systems for space travel and extraterrestrial habitation. *In* Developments in industrial microbiology, *3*: 5–13, ed. Ch. F. Koda. Plenum Press, New York.
15. Kluyver, A. J. and C. B. van Niel. 1956. The microbe's contribution to biology. Harvard University Press, Cambridge, Mass.
16. Sokolski, W. T. and O. S. Carpenter. 1959. Microbiological assay. *In* Progress in industrial microbiology, *1*: 93–135, ed. D. J. D. Hockenhull. Heywood & Company Ltd., London.
17. Duddington, C. L. 1961. Micro-organisms as allies. Faber and Faber, London.
18. Prescott, S. C. and C. G. Dunn. 1959. Industrial microbiology, 3rd ed. McGraw-Hill Book Company, Inc., New York.
19. Rose, A. H. 1961. Industrial microbiology. Butterworths Scientific Publications, London.
20. Buswell, A. M. 1954. Fermentations in waste treatments. *In* Industrial fermentations, *2*: 518–555, ed. L. A. Underkofler and R. J. Hickey. Chemical Publishing Co., Inc., New York
21. Porges, N. 1960. Newer aspects of waste treatment. *In* Advances in applied microbiology, *2*: 1–30, ed. W. W. Umbreit, Academic Press Inc., New York.
22. Beraha, L., M. A. Smith and W. R. Wright. 1961. Control of decay of fruits and vegetables during marketing. *In* Developments in industrial microbiology, *2*: 73–77, ed. S. Rich. Plenum Press, New York.
23. Berard, W. N., Ethel K. Leonard, and W. A. Reeves. 1961. Cotton made resistant to microbiological deterioration using formic acid colloid of methylolmelamine. *Ibid.*, *2*: 79–91.
24. Cordon, Th. C. 1960. Some aspects of protein degradation in leather processing. *In* Developments in industrial microbiology, *1*: 137–145, ed. B. M. Miller. Plenum Press, New York.

25. Duncan, Catherine G. 1960. Deterioration of wood by terrestrial ascomycetes and fungi imperfecti. *Ibid.*, *1*: 148–156.

26. Klausmeier, R. E. and W. A. Jones. 1961. Microbial degradation of plasticizers. *In* Developments in industrial microbiology, 2: 47–53, ed. S. Rich. Plenum Press, New York.

27. Roddy, W. T. 1960. Microbial deterioration of skin proteins. In Developments in industrial microbiology, *1*: 133–136, ed. B. M. Miller. Plenum Press, New York.

28. Loomis, W. L. 1949. Photosynthesis: An introduction. *In* Photosynthesis in plants, ed. J. Franck and W. E. Loomis, pp. 1–17. Iowa State College Press, Ames, Iowa.

29. Rabinowitch, E. I. 1945. Photosynthesis and related processes, *1*: 5–11. Interscience Publishers, Inc., New York.

30. Stocker, O. 1952. Grundriss der Botanik. Springer-Verlag, Heidelberg.

31. Anderson, R. 1962. Fermentation, CW Report. Chemical Week *90*: 105–112.

32. Anonymous. 1953. Pilot-plant studies in the production of Chlorella. *In* Algal culture; From laboratory to pilot plant, ed. J. S. Burlew, pp. 235–272. Carnegie Institution of Washington Publication 600, Washington, D. C.

33. Burlew, J. S. 1953. Current status of the large-scale culture of algae. *Ibid.*, pp. 3–23.

34. Fisher, A. W. 1953. Microscopic algae as industrial raw materials. *Ibid.*, pp. 311–315.

35. Fisher, A. W., and J. S. Burley. 1953. Nutritional value of microscopic algae. *Ibid.*, pp. 303–310.

36. Foster, J. W. 1961. Microbiological process discussion: A view of microbiological science in Japan. Appl. Microbiol. 9: 434–451.

37. Milner, H. W. 1953. The chemical composition of algae. *In* Algal culture; From laboratory to pilot plant, ed. J. S. Burlew, pp. 285–302. Carnegie Institution of Washington Publication 600, Washington, D. C.

38. Mituya, A., T. Nyunoya, and H. Tomiya. 1953. Pre-pilot-plant experiments on algal mass culture. *Ibid.*, pp. 273–281.

39. Dyer, D. L., and R. D. Gafford. 1962. The use of *Synechococcus lividus* in photosynthetic gas exchangers. *In* Developments in industrial microbiology, 3: 87–97, ed. Ch. F. Koda. Plenum Press, New York.

40. Gafford, R. D., and D. E. Richardson. 1960. Mass algal culture in space operations. J. Biochem. Microbiol. Techn. Eng. 2: 299–311.

41. Gray, W. D. 1962. Microbial protein for the space age. *In* Developments in industrial microbiology, 3: 63–71, ed. Ch. F. Koda. Plenum Press, New York.

42. Lancaster, J. H., R. G. Tischer, and Rebecca J. Long. 1962. Human feces as a nitrogen source for some green algae. *Ibid.*, 3: 25–34.

43. Tischer, R. G., B. P. Tischer, and D. Cook. 1962. Human feces as a nutrient for algae in closed space ecologies. *Ibid.*, 3: 72–86.

44. Winders, W. H., and R. G. Tischer. 1962. The nutritive value for algae of fecal pyrolysis gases. *Ibid.*, 3: 14–24.

45. Humfeld, H. 1948. The production of mushroom mycelium (*Agaricus campestris*) in submerged culture. Science *107*: 373.

46. Wikén, T., H. G. Keller, C. L. Schelling, and A. Stöckli. 1951. Ueber die Verwendung von Myzelsuspensionen als Impfmaterial in Wachstumsversuchen mit Pilzen. Experientia 7: 237–239.

47. Robinson, R. F., and R. S. Davidson. 1959. The large-scale growth of higher fungi. *In* Advances in applied microbiology, *1*: 261–278, ed. W. W. Umbreit. Academic Press Inc., New York.

48. Abe, M. 1960. A consideration concerning the biosynthesis of the ergot alkaloids. Osaka.
49. Arcamone, F., C. Bonino, E. B. Chain, A. Ferretti, P. Pennella, A. Tonolo, and Lidia Vero. 1960. Production of lysergic acid derivatives by a strain of *Claviceps paspali* Stevens and Hall in submerged culture. Nature *187*: 238–239.
50. Kobel, H., R. Brunner, and A. Brack. 1962. Vergleich der Alkaloidbildung von *Claviceps purpurea* in parasitischer und saprophytischer Kultur. Experientia *18*: 140–141.
51. Underkofler, L. A., R. R. Barton, and S. S. Rennert. 1958. Production of microbial enzymes and their applications. Appl. Microbiol. *6*: 212–221.
52. Butlin, K. 1962. Prospects in industrial microbiology. New Scientist, No. 281, pp. 804–806.
53. Humphrey, A. E. and F. H. Deindoerfer. 1961. Fermentation; An I/EC unit processes review. Ind. Eng. Chem. *53*: 934–946.
54. Kinoshita, S. 1959. The production of amino acids by fermentation processes. *In* Advances in applied microbiology, *1*: 201–214, ed. W. W. Umbreit. Academic Press Inc., New York.
55. Kinoshita, S., K. Tanaka, S. Udaka, and S. Akita. 1958. Glutamic acid fermentation. *In* Proceedings of the International Symposium on Enzyme Chemistry, Tokyo and Kyoto, 1957. I. U. B. Symposium Series, *2*: 464–468. Pergamon Press, London.
56. Kögl, F., and N. Fries. 1937. Ueber den Einfluss von Biotin, Aneurin und Meso-Inosit auf das Wachstum verschiedener Pilzarten. Hoppe-Seyler's Ztschr. physiol. Chemie *249*: 93–110.
57. Nurmikko, V. 1957. Microbiological determination of vitamins and amino acids produced by microorganisms, using the dialysis cell. Appl. Microbiol. *5*: 160–165.
58. Schopfer, W. H. 1949. Plants and vitamins. Chronica Botanica Company, Waltham, Mass.
59. Islam, M. F., and J. O. Lampen. 1962. Invertase secretion and sucrose fermentation by *Saccharomyces cerevisiae* protoplasts. Biochim. Biophys. Acta *58*: 294–302.
60. McQuillen, K. 1960. Bacterial protoplasts. *In* The Bacteria, *1*: 249–359, ed. I. C. Gunsalus and R. Y. Stanier. Academic Press Inc., New York.
61. Mortenson, L. E., H. F. Mower, and J. E. Carnahan. 1962. Nitrogen fixation by enzyme preparations. Bact. Rev. *26*: 42–50.

SYMPOSIUM VII

MECHANISMS OF IMMUNITY
IN INFECTIOUS DISEASE

Chairman: MORRIS POLLARD

JONAS SALK

Mechanisms of Immunity in Virus Infections

A. A. MILES

Mechanisms of Immunity in Bacterial Infections

NIELS K. JERNE

Mechanisms of Immunity in Infections Associated with Exotoxins

CHAIRMAN'S REMARKS

MORRIS POLLARD

Lobund Laboratory
University of Notre Dame
Notre Dame, U.S.A.

EPIDEMIOLOGISTS have recorded a dramatic decline in morbidity during the past one hundred years. The decline in incidence of communicable diseases has been attributed to many specific facets of biological phenomena. Such factors as housing, nutrition, vector control, and social improvements have had prominent roles in the improvement of man's status with regard to communicable diseases. Of more direct influence have been developments in immunization and the use of antibiotic drugs, both prophylactical and therapeutical.

When I studied at the university, I had the impression that immunology was of fading importance in biology; and that it consisted of serological procedures for diagnosis of disease, and the use of several bacterial and few viral immunizing preparations. Immunology has manifested a renaissance in which (1) increasing numbers of viral diseases are controlled by immunization, (2) diseases once identified as organic are now immunologic dyscrasias, and (3) the immunogenic process is being analysed from a physiological and biochemical viewpoint. Immunology, once relegated by students to extinction, has had a resurgence of interest, and through such methodologies as immunochemistry and molecular biology its role as a biological phenomenon is growing significantly. This is evident to scientists who recruit additions to staff positions. Immunologists are scarce.

The three participants in this symposium represent viewpoints in virology, in bacteriology, and in the latter with special regard to toxins. We hope that they will orientate us to the trends along which immunologists are moving.

MECHANISMS OF IMMUNITY IN VIRUS INFECTIONS*

JONAS SALK†

School of Medicine
University of Pittsburgh
Pittsburgh, U.S.A.

THE USEFULNESS of the phenomenon of immunity has greatly increased as we better understand how it works and not merely that something happens under certain circumstances. Each new observation adds depth to the clarifying patterns; each helps define what we do not yet know, and what we still need to know.

It may be stated, in general, that immunity to infection or disease is the consequence of multiple molecular interactions and that each immunologic effect is determined by specific quantitative reactions. For example, the amount of antibody induced in an animal is related not only to the number of molecules of antigen involved but to the number of molecules capable of being induced at each stage in the antibody formation sequence.

In the process of infection, interaction between antibody and virus can occur at any point where the two specific reactants meet; the outcome, for the individual or for the community, depends upon the specificity and the quantity of antibody present, or upon the time of its appearance in relation to the sequence of transmission from cell to cell, or from host to host.

Much of our understanding of immunity mechanisms has come about in the course of attempting to simulate the natural immunizing process. The particular immunologic factors that are operative in a particular disease often have not become clearly defined until such deliberate attempts have been made. I should like to present certain relevant observations, made in the course of such studies, which have led to an appreciation of the importance of quantitative considerations for understanding the nature of the immunity mechanism in certain virus diseases.

RELATIONSHIP BETWEEN ANTIBODY AND IMMUNITY

Not all antibodies induced by a virus are related functionally to the process of immunity to infection. The problem is further complicated by the existence of minor as well as major differences in antigenic constitution among certain infectious agents that produce indistinguishable clinical syndromes, and significant differences exist among antigens in their capacity to induce antibody formation.

*Aided by a grant from The National Foundation.
†Present address: The Salk Institute for Biological Studies, San Diego, California.

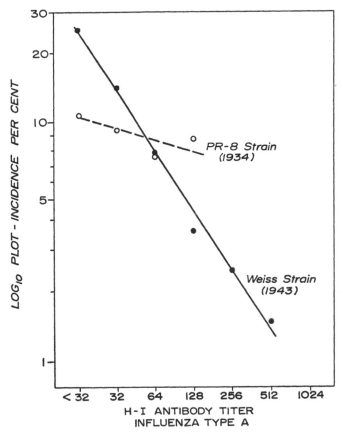

FIG. 1. Relationship between antibody level and illness rate (influenza A, 1943).

An example of the quantitative relationship between antibody level and immunity to disease is shown in Fig. 1, where, in an epidemic of influenza, illness rate was clearly influenced by serum antibody level. However, a striking difference was observed in slope of the correlation line when two different strains of influenza virus type A were used as indicators for antibody in the serum. As is evident a high degree of correlation was observed when measurements were made with a then recently isolated strain (Weiss, 1943) whereas with a strain isolated about a decade earlier (PR8, 1934) it appeared that there was little, if any, correlation between antibody level and resistance.

It is clear from the data that influenza virus infection may develop even in the presence in the serum of what appears to be highly specific antibody. This is true because the influenza virus attaches to and multiplies in the superficial cells of the respiratory tract unless prevented by readily available antibody in superficial secretions. Francis has shown that the amount of antibody available superficially is dependent, in part, on the level of antibody in the serum.

The relationship of antibody to the prevention of a paralyzing poliovirus infection should be expected to be, and is different from that of influenza. The reason for this difference is that for the central nervous system infection the poliovirus is transported via the blood stream to the deeper target area. For this reason, virus is intimately exposed to antibody and therefore relatively low serum antibody levels are effective for interception of virus. However, as in influenza, higher levels of serum antibody are required for prevention of the more superficial intestinal infection and here there appears to be a similar kind of correlation between antibody level and resistance to intestinal infection with poliovirus as for the superficial infection with influenza virus.

MECHANISM OF IMMUNITY INDUCED BY NON-INFECTIOUS ANTIGENS

Studies of immunization against influenza and poliomyelitis have provided an opportunity to clarify the nature of the mechanisms of immunity to these diseases and to deepen our understanding of the role of humoral factors in immunity. As has already been explained, the data in Fig. 1 have revealed the relationship between antibody level and clinically recognizable influenza, illustrating the degree of correlation between antibody and immunity when infection is superficial and the agent does not traverse the bloodstream en route to the target area. Fig. 2 illustrates in a somewhat indirect way certain relationships for an infectious agent that passes through the bloodstream en route to the deeper site of infection.

Fig. 2 shows the relationship of paralytic rate to number of doses of vaccine as was observed in the 0–4 year old segment of the population in the United States in the years 1959 and 1961. These data suggest that the frequency of paralysis in vaccinated groups is inversely related to the number of doses of vaccine administered. This linear relationship suggests that a critical antibody level is attained in some after the first dose and in additional individuals after subsequent doses, and that following each dose the proportion of susceptibles converted to the immune state was the same. Linear relationships such as this are seen in biological and physical inactivation processes of an irreversible nature such as in destruction of activity of a virus or an enzyme, or in radioactive decay. Does this mean that immunization against paralysis induced by means of a non-infectious polio vaccine involves a critical event? Does this also mean that the immunizing effect as measured against the paralytic disease is irreversible?

If the answer is in the affirmative, the data in Fig. 2 suggest that a single dose of vaccine would have sufficed and that multiple doses would have been needless if the antigen content of vaccine in general use was sufficient to convert a large enough proportion to the immune state upon the first injection. This is different from the problem posed by influenza where more than one dose is required to effect the high levels of antibody indicated in Fig. 1; such high levels can be induced only by the booster phenomenon.

Although it appears that the booster phenomenon is not required for effective immunity to polio, the phenomenon has been studied with this virus and it has been shown that the antibody level attained after a

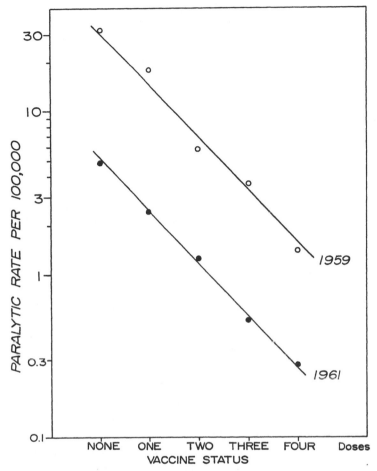

FIG. 2. Paralytic rate in 0–4 age group.

secondary, or booster, dose is strongly influenced by the concentration of antigen used for the primary dose; the larger the primary dose the greater will be the response to a given booster dose.

A further effect attributable to the mass of antigen employed for the first dose is in the degree and the level of persistence of measurable antibody. From studies on persistence of antibody in human subjects who have been observed for more than eight years, the indications are that highly durable effects can be induced; and from field experiences with individuals who have no demonstrable antibody by the usual laboratory methods, it appears that the phenomenon of immunologic conditioning may play an important role in the persistence of immunity to paralysis.

Attention was drawn to the possibly important role of immunologic conditioning in the mechanism of immunity in poliomyelitis when it appeared that a prior natural infection with type II poliovirus afforded relative immunity to type I paralysis, whereas a prior natural type III infection seemed to have no such effect.

An independent observation that suggested the significance of the foregoing was the finding of greater type I antibody responsiveness following
vaccination in those who had a prior type II natural infection, as compared
with those who had had a prior type III natural infection or those with no
prior experience with any of the polioviruses. This suggests that a prior,
naturally acquired, type II infection induces cross-immunity to type I
paralysis, even though the degree of cross-immunity that exists is not
directly apparent serologically, but is revealed by the immunologic response
to vaccination. Although immunity to type I paralysis in persons who have
had prior type II infection may be due to the presence of a less than
demonstrable level of antibody, it is also possible that a sufficiently
heightened conditioning of the immunologic mechanism, for a sufficiently
rapid response after infection, is the mechanism whereby the CNS is
protected in such individuals. For the present considerations, the point of
interest is the possibility of the existence of immunity to paralysis although
antibody is not demonstrable, and that the immune effect is mediated by
the prior immunologic conditioning induced by whatever degree of immunologic crossing exists between types I and II polioviruses.

If one could imagine that two sets of opposing forces are at play, those
of pathogenesis and of immunogenesis, then the effect of immunologic
conditioning can be imagined to be mediated through an acceleration of
antibody responsiveness sufficient to create a balance in favor of the host.
The outcome for the host would then depend upon the rate of immunologic
reactivity, in relation to the rate of aggression of the pathogen. This suggests that, in polio at least, a prior immunologic experience, sufficient to
accelerate the specific antibody responding mechanism, may be all that
is required for persistence of the protective effect against paralysis. This
implies that immunity to paralysis may persist even in the absence of a
demonstrable level of antibody. It further suggests that escape from paralysis under natural circumstances, and without prior vaccination, may be due,
in some instances, to a naturally speedy immunologic responsiveness to
infection as compared to the rate of aggression of the pathogen. It would
follow from this that the minimal requirement for protection of the individual is the initial conditioning of enough antibody forming cells to
accelerate sufficiently the rate of immunogenesis over pathogenesis. It would
also follow that this could be accomplished by a single dose sufficiently
potent to affect essentially all who are so treated.

IMMUNIZATION AND THE VIRUS RESERVOIR

The ideal to be attained through the use of vaccine is not merely protection of the vaccinated individual but the prevention of exposure to virus
that would result from the elimination of the agent itself. By what mechanism can this be brought about and what are the minimal requirements for
such an effect? What has been the experience thus far?

In the six-year period, 1949–1954, preceding the introduction of vaccination in the United States, an average of approximately 25,000 cases of paralytic polio occurred annually. After 1955, and by 1960, slightly more than 50 per cent of the population under age 60 had received three or more doses of vaccine. Considering the age distribution of those who had received vaccine, vaccination could have been expected to have brought about a reduction of about 65 per cent in the average incidence from the pre-vaccine period, i.e., a decline from 25,000 to about 9,800. However, in 1960 and 1961, respectively, 2,551 and 918 cases occurred, a difference suggesting a decline of 90 per cent and 97 per cent, respectively, from the incidence of the pre-vaccine period. This suggests that vaccination had a greater effect than was expected if the assumption is made that vaccine is of benefit only to those vaccinated.

To clarify the meaning of these observations, a comparison was made of the paralytic attack rate in the unvaccinated segment of the population in 1961 with that observed in 1951–54, prior to use of the vaccine. Fig. 3 reveals a striking uniformity in the difference observed at all age levels. Since use of vaccine varied widely at the different age levels, the unvaccinated at each age level constitute a test group for the amount of virus in circulation. This suggests that less virus was available to which to be exposed and, therefore, for causing disease.

If the assumption is made that the killed-virus vaccine had no effect upon

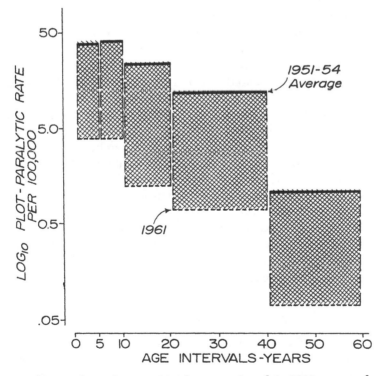

Fig. 3. Paralytic poliomyelitis rates in the unvaccinated in 1961 compared with the average of rates in 1951–54, before vaccine.

virus dissemination and that virus continued to be carried and disseminated by vaccinated individuals as by the unvaccinated before vaccination was introduced into practice, one would have expected the same attack rate among the unvaccinated in 1961 as (compared with the same population) in 1951–54, for example. However, the unvaccinated in 1961 had far less polio than did the unvaccinated in 1951–54. Either the killed-virus vaccine does suppress virus spread, or less virus is present in the population for some other reason. The striking decline in the frequency of recovery of virus from the population at large, and even from sewage in well-vaccinated communities, has provided the reason for the change from merely expecting that the use of a killed-virus vaccine would only prevent paralysis in the individual, to recognizing that the immunologic mechanisms that protect the CNS of the individual also serve to protect the community as well. The mechanism by which this is believed to occur is not only through an effect upon oro-pharyngeal spread, but through a quantitative effect on fecal virus excretion as well.

The foregoing considerations indicate that dissemination of virus is dampened by widespread use of non-infectious vaccine. If we assume that vaccination reduces dissemination of virus to about the same extent as it affects the paralytic rate among those vaccinated, we can estimate the protective effect upon the unvaccinated (through prevention of dissemination of virus) as well as the direct protection afforded those vaccinated. Upon these considerations it is possible to construct a set of curves (Fig. 4) showing relationship between (a) the direct effect of immunization upon those vaccinated (Curve B) and (b) the calculated indirect effect through reduction in the prevention of exposure of the unvaccinated, on the assumption that the vaccinated become ineffective disseminators of virus (Curve C). Curve C, which describes the herd effect, or exposure-protection, is symmetrical because the early effect is that of a small number of vaccinated upon a large number of potential susceptibles and, as immunization progresses, the later effect is that of a large number of vaccinated upon a small number of potential susceptibles. The combined effect directly from immunization (Curve B) and indirectly from the lessened exposure to virus (Curve C) can be calculated and is shown in Curve A. The reciprocal of Curve A is shown as Curve D which describes, as the percentage of effectively immunized individuals is progressively increased, the progressive percentage reduction in attack rate that should occur from a combination of the direct immunization effect upon the vaccinated and the indirect herd effect upon the unvaccinated.

IMMUNIZATION AND VIRUS DISSEMINATION

As the rate of dissemination falls in a given population, one would expect a progressive reduction in the number of foci from which future outbreaks might arise. Thus, new sources of disease would gradually

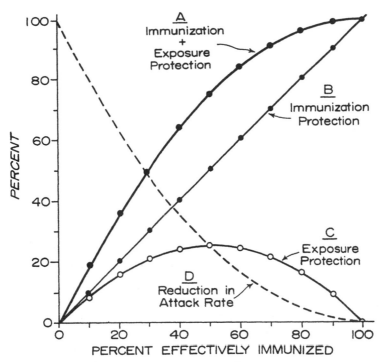

FIG. 4. Relationship between immunization and exposure protection in a given population.

diminish and, if the number of potential disseminators is sufficiently reduced, the virus could reach so low a level of activity as to fall below that required for survival. In Fig. 5 a series of hypothetical lines has been drawn to show what might happen as the number of seedings is reduced. The ratio A/B represents different assumptions for the proportion of latent foci for subsequent establishment of outbreaks in relation to number of virus seedings in the population. It is clear that as the amount of virus seeding is reduced in a given population, the number of latent foci can be reduced to a point where it is less than one for a given unit of population.

It would seem from the foregoing that quantitatively comprehensible laws are operative in the immunologic relationships, both in the individual and in the community; and that extinction is possible for those agents of human disease that exist exclusively in man as the reservoir, and for which either hygienic or immunologic measures, or both, can be applied for interrupting the chain of transmission. For agents transmitted primarily by fecal excreta, as is typhoid, hygienic measures alone are effective. When hygienic measures fail or are inapplicable, then immunization is required. In the case of polio, improvements in hygiene appear to have increased the amount of disease. One interpretation is that non-fecal modes of dissemination have thereby become relatively more important. Observation of the effects of vaccination on preventing spread of virus in the United States and in other countries,

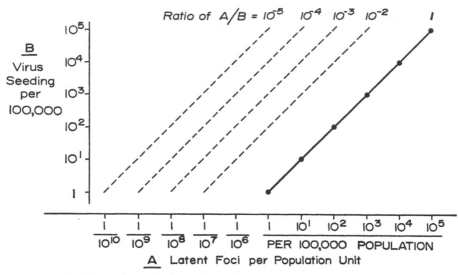

FIG. 5. Hypothetical relationship between virus seeding and latent foci.

where killed-virus vaccine has been employed, has provided the opportunity to alter the view that has prevailed in some quarters that a killed-virus vaccine for polio cannot be expected to affect spread of virus in the community, and that this can be accomplished only by means of a live-virus vaccine.

ARTIFICIAL CONTROL BY IMMUNIZATION

In part, this discussion of the mechanism of the immunity induced by a non-infectious viral antigen has, by implication, been related to the question of the functional equivalence of immunity induced by non-infectious antigens, and that induced by naturally occurring or attenuated virus. Experience with the killed-virus vaccine has indicated that vaccination of about 80–85 per cent of the most susceptible age groups effectively suppresses the occurrence of outbreaks in a community. It has been suggested that about the same proportion would be required to be treated for control of polio through use of live-virus vaccine. Thus, a killed-virus vaccine appears, in this light, to be functionally equivalent to a live-virus vaccine. The killed-virus vaccine principle, in addition, provides the further advantage for simultaneous vaccination against many diseases, by incorporation of many antigens together, and without subjecting the individual or the community to the potentially harmful effects of introduction or maintenance of infectious molecules in the human population.

The possibility of producing large quantities of viral antigens in fertilized eggs, in cultures of animal tissues, and in continuously propagating mammalian cells, affords the opportunity for preparing sufficient quantities of antigenic materials from viruses that propagate in such systems. The availability of techniques that may serve this purpose has altered the previously dominant orientation, which was one of necessity, in which it was expected that a virus would have to multiply in the host for it to be immunized, because it was not heretofore practicable to prepare viral antigens in sufficient quantities for the critical mass necessary for an effective immunizing dose. For the purpose of destroying infectivity, there is the possibility of removing rather than destroying the infectious nucleic acid; there is the further possibility of separating the immunizing antigen in a pure form for combination with other purified antigens, for simultaneous immunization against as many viral antigens as can be compatibly combined.

The fundamental point of view in this discussion is that humoral antibody is one of the essential elements in the immunity mechanism for diseases such as polio and influenza. In both it appears that the immune response is influenced by quantitatively controllable factors where the effects observed are the result of molecular interactions in which the number of molecules of immune substance elaborated in the host is determined by the quantity of immunizing material introduced. The effective antigenic material that induces the formation of antibody appears to be viral protein, and in some instances viral carbohydrate, whether such antigens derive from active infection or from the injection of non-infectious antigens.

Time will not permit more than a glimpse at another example to illustrate other factors that are operative in the immune mechanism of virus diseases.

VIRUS EXTINCTION

It is clear that the smallpox virus can be eliminated from large population groups and for sufficiently long periods to suggest extinction. In such groups there is as yet no evidence of latency, or of the emergence of smallpox virus from whatever may have been its original source of origin. The continued absence of smallpox virus in such groups is not necessarily due to continued immunization which, as a general practice, has been abandoned in some countries. Nor is this due to solid individual immunity in the populations where vaccination practices continue. This is evidenced by cases occurring from exposure to imported cases. This points to the practicable possibility that a well-planned immunization program can bring about extinction of smallpox even without immunizing the entire population and without indefinitely continuing immunization.

However, there is a price that would have to be paid for such an effect, worthwhile and desirable as this may be. I refer here to the relatively rare individuals who are so constituted genetically as to have a defect in the immunological mechanism whereby the host rids itself of vaccinia virus and establishes subsequent immunity. Attention has been drawn to these unusual instances by Kempe who has illuminated two independent systems in the immunity mechanism elicited by vaccinia virus. One is the formation of cell-free or humoral antibody, associated with the gamma globulin fraction of serum protein, and the other is cell-bound antibody of the delayed hypersensitivity type. Essentially, humoral antibody prevents spread of extracellular virus and cell-bound antibody appears to serve the function of clearing away intracellular virus which may otherwise establish a lesion analogous to a tumor with fatal outcome.

In view of these unusual occurrences, there are some who suggest the development of a non-infectious vaccine for this disease, feeling that small-pox immunization will have to be continued for some time, even in areas now free, because of their expectation that eradication programs in other parts of the world will be long in coming.

In concluding these remarks on smallpox, it might be pointed out that the relatively complex chemical constitution of the vaccinia virus, as compared to the smaller poliovirus, for example, may afford opportunity to study the significance of cell-free and cell-bound antibody that seem to be operative in the immune mechanism for this virus. Evidence for other viruses suggests that similar dual mechanisms, involving cell-free and cell-bound antibody are also operative, but there is insufficient time to elaborate upon this now.

CONCLUDING COMMENT

The indications are that certain viruses may, in due course, become extinct, as smallpox virus has disappeared from large population groups. This prospect opens wide vistas for investigation and creates challenges that could be of far-reaching significance with respect to diseases of man and animals. It is for this reason that the question of the nature of the mechanisms of immunity to virus diseases takes on a special meaning.

When we find ourselves thinking about the possibility of the extinction of a virus and the meaning of this in evolutionary and philosophical terms, we begin to wonder about "tampering with nature" and the consequence to man of his deciding which species of life should be exterminated and which should be allowed to survive. It is as if survival will be for the varieties that fit the scheme of man—and how can man know the consequences of his schemes until they have evolved? Nevertheless, it should be evident that the problem of a virus disease for man would disappear if the causative agent was exterminated. Our knowledge of the disease and the agent would then become academic. Man would then have one less active concern, but some new concern will then challenge his ingenuity.

MECHANISMS OF IMMUNITY IN BACTERIAL INFECTIONS

A. A. MILES

The Lister Institute of Preventive Medicine
London, England

I PROPOSE in this communication to adopt as a working hypothesis that there are two episodes of decisive importance in the course of acute infections. The first is the primary lodgement of the infecting microbe, where some of the invaders are destroyed and where the remainder initiate progressive infection (Miles *et al.*, 1957). The second is the episode when, starting from one·or a few of the invaders, there arises the clone of microbes which will eventually grow into the population of parasites that characterize the full-blown, and perhaps lethal, infection. The second episode is perhaps the more important of the two, for suppression of the clone at this point would abort the infection. The reality of the second episode is based on Meynell's biometrical analyses of the dosage-response in acute infections, and his experimental demonstration of the killing by a *monotypical* salmonella bacteraemia of mice that have been infected with mixtures of types (Meynell, 1957a , b; Meynell & Stocker, 1957). In some instances, especially with infection by highly virulent microbes, the two episodes may coincide, the finally infecting clone arising directly from the primary lodgement; in others, the second episode may take place at the site of some metastatic infection, by microbes that have spread from the primary lodgement. I also adopt the hypothesis that the tissue events of both decisive episodes are of the same kind, differing only in the degree to which the various defensive mechanisms are displayed. It follows that resistance to infection should be expressible in terms of the reactions at the tissue site where these episodes occur; modified, of course, by the response of the whole animal to the injury of infection, and by infective episodes at other sites in the body, which, though not themselves decisive in the crucial sense, may nevertheless accelerate or delay the consequences of the decisive episode.

At this site the invader is subjected both inside and outside the tissue cells to antimicrobial factors; and those factors may or may not act with the help of specific antibody. This distinction of intra- and extracellular factors is to some extent arbitrary, because all factors presumably come from cells, and some, like lysozyme, are known to be in effective concentrations, for example, both inside the phagocytes (see, for example, Brumfitt and Glynn, 1961) and in the plasma. The protective role of specific antibody in immunity is unquestioned, though in many instances we do not know which of the many antigens of a microbe are protective, or exactly how protective antibodies work. But it is fairly clear that antibody *per se* has little effect on the viability or metabolism of microbes with which it combines. It is effective in defence either because it neutralizes toxins, or because it makes the microbe susceptible to non-specific defence factors like complement or the phagocyte; and this action may be exquisitely specific, dependent on complementariness with a single one of many antigenic components at the microbial surface (e.g., Adler, 1953). We may then properly consider antibody as accessory to the more fundamental non-specific defence mechanisms and concentrate on these.

It is nevertheless important sometimes to know whether non-specific factors are microbicidal in the absence of antibody. Unfortunately the multiplicity of environmental antigens, either microbial or with structure related to microbial antigens, and the readiness of the animal, from its perinatal days onwards, to indulge in embarrassingly effective displays of immunological competence, make it difficult to deny the participation of traces of specific antibody in what appears to be a non-specific effect. The difficulty, however, is hypothetical, and justifiably countered by the pragmatic assumption that if specificity is not demonstrable, an effect is non-specific until someone proves it to be otherwise.

The non-specific mechanisms to which antibody is an accessory are far from simple. I have neither the time nor the competence to discuss them in full. Much of the subject is enshrined in many excellent reviews and symposia of recent years (e.g., McLeod & Cluff, 1959; Symposium on Bacterial Endotoxins, 1961). Some consistence is now emerging, but the general impression is of a vast archipelago of isolated island facts, which, we must hope, will appear as a coherent continent when we have drained off the waters of ignorance between the islands. Some of these islands are quite large and even have theoretical features by which we can recognize them. And among them, after setting aside all the undoubtedly important considerations of epidemiology, genetics, nutrition, endocrinology and the like, there is a solid body of detailed work on phagocytosis and on serum and tissue factors on the one hand, and, on the other hand, many observations on procedures which either stimulate or depress non-specific resistance in the whole animal.

In some respects the behaviour of the phagocyte parallels that of the whole animal. It makes adaptive responses to the microbe, and when dealing with bacteria of differing virulence discriminates between them much as the animal itself does. The response of the granulocytes includes mobilization of substances like phagocytin (Hirsch & Cohn, 1960), lysozyme and leukin; and the monocytes of immune animals have an increased resistance that is independent of orthodox antibody (e.g., Elberg, 1960; Mackaness, 1962). Other tissue factors include plakins, lysozymes, histones and other basic proteins, polypeptides (Skarnes & Watson, 1957); and, besides complement (whose action is still far from fully understood), the serum factors include bactericidins, the properdins, immunoconglutinins (Coombs *et al.*, 1962), the endotoxin-destroying component (Landy, 1960), and various non-specific opsonins; the list is by no means complete. We should note, as one bar to generalization, that some of these factors and defensive responses are not so much non-specific, as less specific than, say, antibody; thus the bactericidins attack little but certain *Bacillus* spp., phagocytin largely gram-negative and leukins largely gram-positive bacteria; and we should note also that animal species vary greatly in the amount and efficacy of the factors they contain.

It is evident too that these factors and responses are enhanced by procedures like the injection of enterobacterial vaccines or endotoxins, and by infection. But the implication of a substance or a response as significant in immunity still largely depends on the parallelism of its manifestation, or its rise and fall, with resistance of the animal as a whole—a notorious field for indulgence in the fallacy of *post hoc ergo propter hoc*. Taking a broad view, the analysis of non-specific immunity has been very haphazard, and a synthesis in the field is almost impossible. It is easy enough, let us say, to assume that the key to recovery from an infection is intra-phagocytic destruction of the invader. But nature doesn't oblige by introducing the microbe directly to the phagocyte. In natural infection the unit, as it were, of response is not that of parasite to phagocyte, but of parasite to tissue. When the tissue is extravascular, as in the skin, the only representative of the frankly phagocytic cell, whether microphage or a member of the lymphocyte-macrophage system, may be an occasional histiocyte, requiring 2–3 hours stimulation to become phagocytic. There are many possible events between the primary lodgement of the invader and its encounter with a phagocyte. That encounter is generally believed to take place when, as a result of a vascular response to microbial injury, the bactericidal forces of the plasma and white cells are mobilized at the site of infection.

The relation of the primarily infected tissue site to the defences I have sketched is summarized in Fig. 1. The scheme is oversimplified, but serves to illustrate the dependence of the adaptive response of the animal on factors that may be considered, for our purpose, accessory to the events at the primary lodgement of the invader.

Let us look at some instances of immunity at the site of primary lodgement. The reaction at a restricted tissue site is readily observed in the skin of guinea-pigs, where on intracutaneous injection a large variety of pathogens will induce skin-lesions whose diameter at maturity is proportional to log. dose of the organisms (Miles *et al.*, 1957), thus making possible accurate numerical measures of differences in resistance between two sites in the same animal, or between batches of animals. A biological system of this kind approximates well to the condition of natural primary lodgements. Moreover, not only does it permit a large number of comparative estimates of resistance to a variety of pathogens in each of the animals tested; but, if the analogy of primary lodgement with secondary metastatic

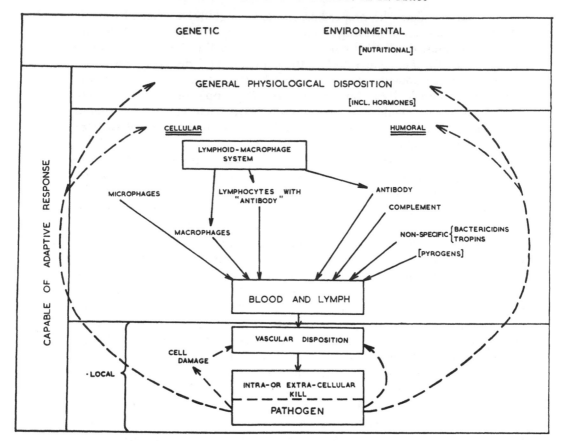

FIG. 1. The main factors determining the outcome of the host-parasite relationship established at the site of primary lodgement of a pathogenic microbe in the tissues of an animal.

lodgements in hitherto uninfected tissue is accepted, the results for a primary lodgement will also be valid for the decisive clonal episode of Meynell. My colleague Ann Brimacombe and I (unpublished) have worked mainly with a general infection by a Group C *Strep. pyogenes* (strains D181 and CN771). Using samples drawn from a control and an infected population of similar animals at varying times during the course of the disease, we tested the skin resistance to infection by the streptococcus itself, and by two other bacteria, *Ps. aeruginosa* (*Ps. pyocyanea*) and *C. ovis*. It is important to note that neither of the last two bacilli had any discoverable antigenic relation to each other or to the infecting streptococcus.

Fig. 2 summarizes the changes, in terms of the resistance of normal controls, taking place during bacteraemia with strain D181. Within four hours of intravenous injection of about one LD40 of the living streptococcus, skin-resistance to all three test organisms rises. Resistance to the streptococcus is maximum in 7 days, declines sharply during the next 2 days, and is much

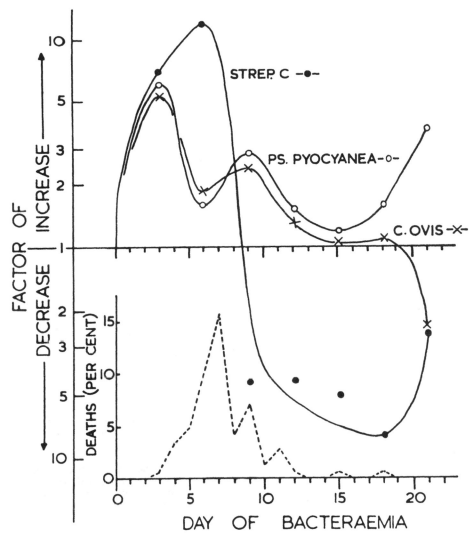

Fig. 2. The time-course of resistance to local infections of the skin by *Strep. pyogenes* Group C, *Ps. aeruginosa* (*pyocyanea*), and *Corynebacterium ovis*, in guinea-pigs infected systemically with *Strep. pyogenes* Group C (strain CN771); of the inflammatory reaction to dead cocci of strain CN771; and of the fatality rate in the batch of 70 guinea-pigs systemically infected for the experiment.

The pathogenicity of the three bacteria was titrated in 3–6 bacteraemic animals and in 3 normal animals. Increase or decrease in resistance of the bacteraemic animals is expressed as the factor by which pathogenicity of the bacteria was, respectively, decreased or increased, in comparison with their pathogenicity in the controls.

less than that in the controls for the next 12 days. The increased resistance to the other two—surely non-specific—undergoes a decline and rise to a second peak at 10 days, and then declines to normal, with a late rise for *Ps. aeruginosa* and decrease for *C. ovis*. Simultaneous skin tests with

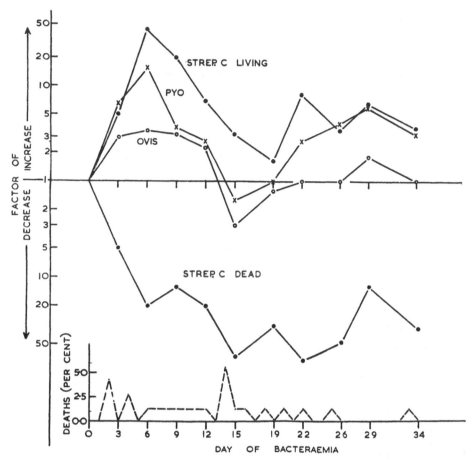

FIG. 3. The time-course of resistance to local infections of the skin by *Strep. pyogenes* Group C, *Ps. aeruginosa* (*pyocyanea*), and *C. ovis*, in guinea-pigs infected systemically with *Strep. pyogenes* Group C (strain D181); and of the fatality rate in the batch of 140 guinea-pigs systemically infected for the experiment. Resistance expressed as in Fig. 2.

dead pathogens made it clear that the reversal of the streptococcal effect is due to the acquisition of substantial delayed hypersensitivity to the coccus—but not to the two bacilli—just after the period when the bacteraemia was at its height, and the incidence of death was highest. After 20–30 days, all the survivors had virtually recovered from the infection.

In some ways the related Strain CN771 behaved differently (Fig. 3). Deaths occurred sporadically throughout 30 days, and animals surviving the severe bacteraemic phase at 5–10 days died later with large abscesses in joints and mediastinum. As with infection by D181, there is a substantial initial rise of resistance to all three organisms, declining to about normal at about the 12th day, and rising, with respect to the coccus and *Ps. aeruginosa*, at the end of 21 days. In other tests with CN771, the late resistance to the coccus was maintained at 10–20 times that of the controls, even in animals within 2 days of the death due to massive internal abscess formation. Infection by this coccus was clearly better than infection by D181 as a stimulant of skin resistance, since resistance was substantial in the face of the equally substantial delayed allergy, as indicated by the exaggerated inflammatory reaction to dead streptococci; an allergy which, arising very early at the 3rd day, persisted to the end, and which, by analogy with the D181 infections, probably contributed to the exacerbation of coccal infection in otherwise resistant skin.

The sequence of events in both types of bacteraemia was confirmed in other experiments. Of the later phases we have no explanation, except that for the possible deleterious effect of delayed hypersensitivity. The initial phase of raised resistance, however, was common to all tests, and applied not only to all three test organisms, but also to pathogens like *Staph. aureus*, *E. coli, Pr. vulgaris, Bord. pertussis,* and *L. monocytogenes.* A similar rise of non-specific resistance occurred in guinea-pigs during the first five days of a fatal systemic infection with the *Ps. aeruginosa.* The time-course and magnitude of this early phase are indeed reminiscent of the non-specific

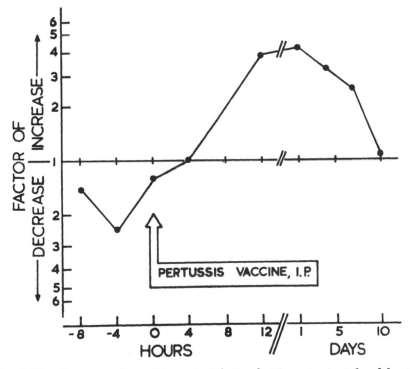

FIG. 4. The changes in skin resistance to infection by *B. pertussis*, induced by intra-peritoneal injection of *B. pertussis* vaccine. Resistance expressed as in Fig. 2.

immunity to general infections induced in mice by enterobacterial vaccines and endotoxins (see Whitby *et al.* 1961); and we confirmed the similarity by testing these stimulants in the guinea-pig skin system. Typhoid vaccine and pertussis vaccine in these conditions produced very similar time-courses of resistance to many of our test organisms; as, for example, in Fig. 4, which summarizes the skin resistance to *B. pertussis* induced by intraperitoneal pertussis vaccine. But stimuli of this kind were by no means consistent in their effect. Thus (Table 1) the streptococcal bacteraemia increased skin resistance to *Pr. vulgaris*, but the two vaccines depressed it; and hyper-thermia induced by holding the animals at 37° for the first four hours after skin injections, to imitate the fever and blood leucocytosis of the bac-teraemia, actually depressed resistance to *C. ovis*.

TABLE 1

Skin infection by	Factor of increase of skin resistance induced by			
	Strep. C Bacteraemia	Hyper-thermia	Pertussis vaccine	Typhoid vaccine
Strep. C	15.0	5.0	10.0	2.0
Staph. aureus	4.5	0.3	nt	nt
C. ovis	5.0	0.3	5.0	12.0
E. coli	10.0	2.0	nt	nt
Ps. aeruginosa	4.0	5.0	2.0	5.0
Pr. vulgaris	5.0	0.2	0.1	0.1

nt = not tested.

Properdin titres we did not attempt to measure, taking the positive response to *C. ovis* and the coccus as being incompatible with a properdin effect. Since the two organisms were insusceptible to fresh guinea-pig serum, we assumed they were so to properdin (if indeed there is such a substance).

In view of the demonstration that fractions of *Staph. aureus* have some of the *in vivo* effects of enterobacterial endotoxin, it is quite possible that the living streptococcus has an endotoxin-like effect—and may therefore, as has been suggested for endotoxin, have mobilized antibody (see Stetson, 1961) and stimulated the reticulo-endothelial system (R.E.S.) (Biozzi *et al.*, 1955). As regards antibody, we have at no time in this period found evidence of frank antibody; and to assume the mobilization of pre-existing antibodies appropriate for the eight different organisms to which we have shown the skin becoming resistant during streptococcal bacteraemia, and, moreover, to a degree that in each case usually induces a 5–20 fold increase in resistance, seems to us at the moment overstretching the notion that specific antibodies are at the bottom of all such manifestations. Stimulation of microphages or of the R.E.S., or of both, is a more plausible explanation; but not a particularly relevant one. The phagocytes lining the circulation are, of course, not directly involved; but neither is a comparable stimulation of R.E. cells in infected tissues, or of those arriving there as a result of inflammation, in question, for the following reasons.

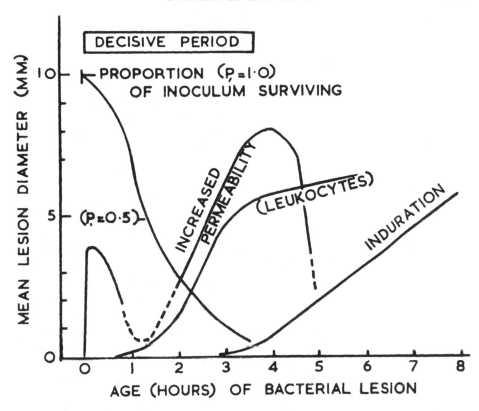

FIG. 5. The time relations of the decisive period of early bacterial infections to the main inflammatory phase of the infection, as indicated by exudation and emigration of leucocytes into the lesion. Characteristic of a number of bacterial pathogens, including *Strep. pyogenes*, *Ps. aeruginosa*, and *C. ovis*. The curve P is an estimate of the rate at which the inoculum is made ineffective by the early tissue defences.

The size of lesions arising from these primary lodgements is determined, as we have shown in a number of ways, by defences that act mainly within the first two hours of the infection. By the time the infection is three hours old, it is insusceptible to procedures that increase resistance, such as bacteraemia, pertussis vaccines, or hyperthermia. That is to say, the 2–3 hour decisive period applies both to normal tissue and to tissues whose resistance is in some way enhanced by the bacteraemia. Nevertheless, as Fig. 5 indicates, during that decisive period, no gross inflammation has taken place; exudation and the diapedesis of leucocytes, and the mobilization of tissue histiocytes—all the orthodox consequences of infective inflammation that are supposed to mobilize the blood defences—occur after the outcome of the skin infection has been decided (Burke & Miles, 1958). It follows that if there *are* cells which are stimulated locally by bacteraemia or endotoxins to greater antimicrobial efforts, they are certainly not microphages or macrophages.

We are left with the conclusion that the local early kill, of which resistance is the manifestation, depends either on soluble antimicrobial substances from plasma present in the intercellular fluid of the skin, or on microbicidal powers, inherent or induced, in the tissue cells themselves. Intercellular fluid certainly contains the plasma constituents; but as far as the early decisive period of infection is concerned we are inclined to doubt the efficacy of any antimicrobial substances present for that reason, since the artificial stimulation of purely liquid exudation into the infected areas at most raises their resistance twofold, whereas we are seeking the reason for increases of the order of tenfold or more. We are, then, left with the non-phagocytic tissue cells themselves. That tissue cells themselves are capable of defence is evident from the reports of the phagocytic and sometimes bactericidal action of such diverse systems as tissue cultures of HeLa cells, monkey kidney, uterine mucosa, foetal skin (Shepard, 1955; Furness, 1958; Richardson, 1959). It would, moreover, be an extraordinary virus preparation whose particle count consistently equalled its plaque count in the wide variety of tissue cultures employed in virology; in other words, all kinds of tissue have the potentiality of inactivating viruses. Again, the peculiarities of organ immunity in various infections cannot all be due to the peculiarities of the anatomical configuration of the organs or their content of orthodox phagocytes; some of them are probably expressions of the antimicrobial action peculiar to the constituent tissue cells. Here, then, is the lead towards a reconciliation of this discrepancy in tissue between the inflammatory response to injury, with its supposed concomitant augmentation of local antimicrobial factors, and the effective kill that occurs in the preinflammatory stage of infection.

I should perhaps express regret that my own contribution to the immunology of bacterial infection should add one more island to the complicated archipelago that symbolizes the subject. I don't even know that it is a true island, or will prove to be the back of an irrelevant migrant whale that happens to show above water. Nevertheless, I think the facts suggest that it would be well to question the notion that the decisive cellular defences are exclusively in the hands of professional phagocytes, union members trained in the doctrines of Metchnikov and Aschoff. We should look at the possible contribution of the non-union amateurs; because these cells after all constitute the ranks from which the professionals, phylogenetically speaking, were recruited.

To do so is not in any way to diminish the importance to immunity of the phagocytes and the humoral factors with which so much investigation has been concerned; but it is to suggest that these systems may exemplify *in excelsis*, as it were, the antimicrobial capacities of the tissues as a whole, and that the non-phagocytic cells may prove to be one of the mainstays of non-specific resistance, both to the primary lodgement of the invader and to all the secondary, metastatic events that determine the course of an infective disease.

REFERENCES

Adler, F. L. 1953. Studies on the bactericidal reaction. II. Inhibition by antibody, and antibody requirements of the reaction. J. Immunol. 70: 79–88.

Biozzi, G., B. Benacerraf and B. N. Halpern. 1955. The effect of *Salm. typhi* and its endotoxin on the phagocytic activity of the reticulo-endothelial system in mice. Brit. J. Exptl. Path. 36: 226–235.

Brumfitt, W., and A. A. Glynn. 1961. Intracellular killing of *Micrococcus lysodeikticus* by macrophages and polymorphonuclear leucocytes: A comparative study. Brit. J. Exptl. Path. 42: 408–423.

Burke, J. F., and A. A. Miles. 1958. The sequence of vascular events in early infective inflammation. J. Pathol. Bacteriol. 76: 1–19.

Coombs, R. A., Annie M. Coombs and D. C. Ingram. 1961. The serology of conglutination and its relation to disease. Blackwell Scientific Publications, Oxford.

Elberg, S. S. 1960. Cellular immunity. Bacteriol. Rev. 24: 67–95.

Furness, G. 1958. Interaction between *Salmonella typhimurium* and phagocytic cells in cell culture. J. Infect. Dis. 103: 272–277.

Hirsch, J. G., and Z. A. Cohn. 1960. Degranulation of polymorphonuclear leucocytes following phagocytosis of microorganisms. J. Exptl. Med. 112: 1005–1014.

Landy, M. 1960. Inactivation of endotoxin by humoral systems. Ann. N.Y. Acad. Sci. 88: 1273–1277.

Mackaness, G. B. 1962. Cellular resistance to infection. J. Exptl. Med. 116: 381–400.

MacLeod, C. M., and L. E. Cluff (editors). 1960. Non-specific resistance to infection. Bacteriol. Rev. 24: 1–200.

Meynell, G. G. 1957. Inherently low precision of infectivity titrations using a quantal response. Biometrics 13: 149–163.

Meynell, G. G. 1957. The applicability of the hypothesis of independent action to fatal infections in mice given *Salmonella typhimurium* by mouth. J. Gen. Microbiol. 16: 396–404.

Meynell, G. G., and B. A. D. Stocker. 1957. Some hypotheses on the aetiology of fatal infections in partially resistant hosts and their application to mice challenged with *Salmonella paratyphi* B or *Salmonella typhimurium* by intraperitoneal injection. J. Gen. Microbiol. 16: 38–58.

Miles, A. A., E. M. Miles and J. Burke. 1957. The value and duration of defence reactions of the skin to the primary lodgement of bacteria. Brit. J. Explt. Path. 38: 79–96.

Richardson, M. 1959. Parasitization *in vitro* of bovine cells by *Brucella abortus*. J. Bacteriol. 78: 769–777.

Shepard, C. C. 1955. Phagocytosis by HeLa cells and their susceptibility to infection by human tubercule bacilli. Proc. Soc. Exptl. Biol. N.Y. 90: 392–396.

Skarnes, R. C., and D. W. Watson. 1957. Antimicrobial factors of normal tissues and fluids. Bacteriol. Rev. 21: 273–294.

Stetson, C. A. 1961. Symposium on bacterial endotoxins. IV. Immunological aspects of the host reaction to endotoxins. Bacteriol. Rev. 25: 457–458.

Symposium on Bacterial Endotoxins. 1961. Bacteriol. Rev. 25: 427–458.

Whitby, J. L., J. G. Michael, M. W. Woods and M. Landy. 1961. Symposium on bacterial endotoxins. II. Possible mechanisms whereby endotoxins evoke increased non-specific resistance to infection. Bacteriol. Rev. 25: 437–446.

MECHANISMS OF IMMUNITY IN INFECTIONS ASSOCIATED WITH EXOTOXINS

NIELS K. JERNE*

*World Health Organization
Geneva, Switzerland*

THERE CAN BE NO DOUBT that the subject assigned to me in this session is easier to deal with than the two preceding ones. The species of pathogenic micro-organisms that produce exotoxins are much fewer than those that don't, and immunity most often depends on a single dominating factor.

PROPERTIES OF EXOTOXINS

Exotoxins are proteins that are secreted by bacterial cells into the surrounding medium during normal growth. They are extremely toxic to mammals and they are antigenic. This generally accepted description excludes the cholera and plague toxins, as well as Shiga neurotoxin and pertussis toxin, which are liberated only after autolysis of the bacterial cells, or can be obtained by extraction from the organisms. It also excludes such low molecular substances as histamine and tryptamine, and bacterial exoenzymes of low toxicity such as hyaluronidase and deoxyribonuclease. If, furthermore, we exclude toxic products, such as tuberculin, which possess little toxicity for a normal animal but may be highly toxic to a sensitized animal, we are left with the true exotoxins, the main ones being: diphtheria toxin, tetanus and botulinus toxin, the toxins of the clostridia that cause gas gangrene, and the toxins of staphylococcus and streptococcus.

Though grouped together according to these restrictive criteria, the exotoxins present a great variety of very characteristic features to which I shall devote a few sentences.

Diphtheria toxin is lethal and dermonecrotic. It will kill a guinea-pig in a dose of about one-tenth of a microgram. It attacks many different types of somatic cells. Pappenheimer (1955) has presented evidence for regarding diphtheria toxin as the protein moiety of cytochrome B produced by the diphtheria organisms in an iron-deficient medium; its toxic action would consist of interference with cytochrome activity in mammalian cells. Strauss (1959, 1960) has recently demonstrated that diphtheria toxin can, within two hours after addition to the medium, inhibit protein synthesis in HeLa cells while the cells continue to synthesize RNA and DNA. All pathogenic

---

*Present address: Department of Microbiology, School of Medicine, University of Pittsburgh, Pittsburgh 13, Pennsylvania, U.S.A.

diphtheria strains seem to elaborate the same toxin. The same applies to a certain extent to tetanus, though culture filtrates containing tetanus toxin must have different toxic components since Llewellyn Smith (1942/43) has shown that different filtrates can differ with respect to the relative doses that are lethal for different species of laboratory animals. As for *Clostridium botulinum*, there are a number of different types of this organism each of which produces an antigenetically distinct toxin. Both tetanus toxin and botulinus toxins are neurotoxic, but the receptor sites at which they attack the motor nervous system are different. These two toxins are the most toxic substances known. Though they are proteins, they will kill a mouse or a guinea-pig in a quantity below 0.001 μg. This lethal dose is more than a thousand times smaller than that of any low molecular weight substance known in pharmacology, such as hydrocyanic acid or the alkaloid aconitin.

Among the clostridia responsible for gas gangrene, the less important ones are *Clostridium septicum* and *Clostridium histolyticum*, the various strains of which all seem to elaborate the same toxin. This is in contrast to the clinically far more important *Clostridium welchii* and *Clostridium oedematiens*, both of which occur in many types that produce a great multiplicity of toxins. The most common and important one of these, and also the best studied, is *Clostridium welchii* alpha-toxin. This exotoxin is dermonecrotic and haemolytic, it can kill a mouse in a dose of less than one-tenth of a microgram, and it has been shown to be an enzyme which hydrolyzes lecithin when activated by calcium or magnesium ions.

Finally, we come to the various exotoxins elaborated by *Streptococcus* and *Staphylococcus*. Pathogenic staphylococci, particularly, produce a number of toxins; the one best studied is probably staphylococcus alpha-toxin which is lethal, haemolytic, and dermonecrotic. Its lethal dose appears to be somewhat less than that of the alpha-toxin of *Clostridium welchii*, but this is difficult to assess because these toxins have not yet been purified sufficiently, and also because toxicity varies in different mammalian species.

ANTITOXIN IMMUNITY

The mechanism of immunity against infections by the bacteria that produce this heterogeneous variety of exotoxins is usually the early development of an appropriate antitoxin. This does not mean that an infection can be dealt with successfully if antitoxin becomes available only after the infection has advanced to a certain point: at that time, either the toxin may already have initiated an irreversible lethal action, or the infected tissues may have become modified to such an extent that antitoxin can no longer reach the focus. A necessary and sufficient safeguard will have been provided if an adequate quantity of one specific antitoxin is present in the blood prior to the onset of the infection. This would be another factor linking these diverse infections into one group.

Unfortunately, we have to recognize the exceptions provided by the staphylococcus and the streptococcus. Whereas, for example, a *Clostridium welchii* infection is associated with the production of a large variety of toxins, the infection will not get under way—as was shown by Evans (1945)— if only alpha-antitoxin is present in the host from the onset and in a sufficient quantity. Staphylococcus infections, on the other hand, which also lead to the production of a large variety of toxins, cannot be prevented by the presence of one antitoxin, at least not with alpha-antitoxin. It still remains to be seen whether any of the other toxins developed by the staphylococcus, such as the leucocidins, play such a major role that an anti-leucocidin might be decisive for immunity. It would appear that the pathogenic properties of staphylococcus and streptococcus are not solely dependent on their production of exotoxins. They therefore fall outside the main group, in being organisms that *per se* present such other problems to the antibacterial defence mechanisms of the host as were discussed earlier by Professor Miles. I am glad to have an excuse for leaving the staphylococci aside, in that the problem of their virulence is the subject of a separate symposium at this Congress.

Apart from the cocci then, the remaining group of organisms producing exotoxins can be characterized by the fact that the presence of a sufficient blood concentration of a single antitoxin confers immunity upon the infected host. That is to say, none of these organisms themselves would present serious problems to ordinary antibacterial defence were not the toxins they secrete so powerful that the host will succumb unless they are neutralized promptly.

From the point of view of the bacteria causing these infections—diphtheria, tetanus, and the other clostridia—this would seem to be an unsatisfactory situation because it does not permit them to multiply extensively or for a long time. If they are permitted to multiply to even a limited extent, their toxins will kill the host they live in, and if the host has antitoxic immunity they will not be permitted to multiply at all.

It does not seem much of an advantage to, for example, tetanus bacilli to be able to secrete a toxin which destroys the nervous system of their host far away from the site of infection, thereby killing the animal in which they have started to grow. One might even suspect, on these grounds, that this group of infections associated with exotoxins are accidental curiosities of nature which lie outside the main stream of evolution in the cold war (and some times hot war) between micro-organisms and mammals, and which generally leads to their co-existence. MacLennan (1962) made a similar remark in his admirable monograph on clostridial infections. I shall quote the following paragraph: "To the clinician, the importance of *Clostridium welchii* rests on its quite fortuitous ability to produce soluble agents capable of poisoning and destroying animal cells. And I would like to emphasise the word *fortuitous.* So far as I am aware the clostridia are primarily and essentially saprophytes, whose toxins are quite incidental and quite as unimportant to their economy as morphine to the poppy plant or digitalis to the foxglove. Yet it is these toxins that determine their pathogenicity."

With respect to diphtheria, one could imagine that the capacity of producing a powerful toxin which destroys cells in the immediate vicinity of
the infection site and thus adds to invasiveness, might be a property that
had been selectively favoured in the evolution of the diphtheria bacterium.
But, in diphtheria, the feeling that we are dealing with an accident of nature
is supported by the finding that the causative bacteria are really perfectly
innocent saprophytes which are normally allowed a limited and peaceful
co-existence with us, until the bacteria themselves get infected by a bacteriophage that forces them to make diphtheria toxin as long as they harbour
this phage or prophage, and thus to become the dreaded cause of a disease
that does not really benefit the survival of the diphtheria species.

From the point of view of the host, the fact that his ordinary bacterial
defence mechanisms are quite capable of dealing with the diphtheria and
clostridial organisms themselves leaves in each case the clear-cut single
problem of dealing with a toxin that is very powerful and that is antigenic.
The host, in order to survive, must neutralize this toxin while it is still
present only in a minute amount; and, as a minute amount of toxin can be
neutralized by a minute amount of antitoxin, we arrive at the spectacular
situation where the presence of a small amount of actively developed or
passively administered antitoxin can make the difference between life and
death, a situation which is perhaps unique in immunology and which is the
basis for the success of the toxoids as prophylactic agents.

CELLULAR AND HUMORAL FACTORS IN ACQUIRED RESISTANCE

After a period, during the earlier part of this century, when circulating
antibodies were thought by many to be the key factor in mammalian defence
and immunity to microbial infection, opinion during the past twenty years
has swung somewhat away from this confidence in antibodies. There is
increasing evidence to suggest that, in some infections, serum antibodies are
not the most important cause of acquired resistance, and it is even possible
that serum antibodies may be harmful to the host in some cases. It has been
shown, for example, that circulating antibodies do not seem to be of any
use in protection against tuberculosis, and that hypo-gammaglobulinaemic
children, who are incapable of producing classical circulating antibodies,
can deal effectively with and develop immunity to measles, vaccinia, etc.
Emphasis is now laid on the study of alternative types of immune response,
such as the development of delayed hypersensitivity, as major factors in
immunity. A recent theory, proposed by Karush and Eisen (1962) attempts
to explain delayed hypersensitivity on the basis of the presence in the
circulation of normally undetectable concentrations of a particular type of
antibody. Several workers have a tendency to disregard the antibodies that
are released by immunologically competent cells and to focus their attention
on these cells themselves as the more important factor in immunity.

The most clear-cut and unassailable defence for the importance of antibodies is provided by the typical infections associated with exotoxins in

which the dominating mechanism of immunity is the production of a single neutralizing antitoxin. Adequate immunization with toxoids would eliminate diphtheria, tetanus, and most clostridial infections from any country by providing everybody with neutralizing antitoxins. A remaining task would be the development of a reliable method for preparing *Clostridium welchii* alpha-toxoid, as it has proved difficult to destroy the toxic properties of this toxin while retaining effective antigenicity. This appears to be the most urgent problem in this field at present.

Here I might stop, were it not that the equation of the mechanism of immunity with the formation of a specific antitoxin does not basically explain anything. What would have to be explained is the mechanism of how this formation of antitoxin comes about. This is easier said than done, or rather, it is easier done than explained, since all of us produce antibodies but none of us knows how. What everybody knows is that there are so-called "immunologically competent cells" in the body that can display their synthetic potentialities, and release specific antibodies, after an appropriate antigenic stimulus. But these words do not get us very far, and here we have the crux of the whole matter, the solution of which would lift immunology out of its descriptive verbosity and up to a level such as was reached in a shorter time by virology.

In regulating its formation of antibodies, it seems obvious that the system of immunologically competent cells obeys what I have called the "Axiom of Burnet": the cells will exert a selection among the potential antigens that present themselves, and refuse to be stimulated by such antigens as are components of the host organism itself (Burnet, 1959). It also seems likely that these cells will obey general laws of protein synthesis by producing antibody molecules as instructed by the RNA templates at their ribosomes. The proposal that the antigen itself acts as a secondary template, determining the final folding of a polypeptide chain into the proper tertiary structure of a specific antibody molecule, does not answer the recognition problem of how the cells manage to discriminate between the body's own antigens, which have to be left alone, and foreign antigens, which are a proper stimulus. Before the cells can act at all, the antigen must be recognized as such, and it appears to me that if it is to recognize a foreign antigenic determinant as a legitimate stimulant of antibody formation, the immunological system must have at its disposal structures that closely resemble antibody combining sites, since these can do exactly what is needed, namely, recognize an antigenic determinant. If follows that structures, similar to the specific combining sites of antibody molecules, must already be present before an antigen can act as a stimulus and, therefore, that these structures can be made by cells without antigenic assistance. The so-called template theories of antibody formation, or instructive theories, which have so long been accepted uncritically, are unnecessary if the Axiom of Burnet is correct and this reasoning would lead us rather to one of the selective theories, either intracellular selection as proposed by Szilard (1960), or cellular selection as proposed by Burnet (1959), or extracellular selection as I proposed seven years ago (Jerne, 1955, 1960).

The problem of the mechanism of immunity in infections associated with exotoxins is the problem of immunity which reduces in the most clear-cut way to the problem of antibody formation.

SUMMARY

Exotoxins are highly toxic antigenic proteins that are secreted by certain bacteria during normal growth. It might seem accidental that this property has turned certain members of a large class of saprophytes into highly dangerous infective agents.

With the exception of staphylococcal and streptococcal infections, immunity in infections associated with exotoxins is, in each case, dependent on the presence of a single antitoxin. This accounts for the success of toxoids in prophylaxis against diphtheria and clostridial infections. The remaining urgent task is the reliable preparation of an effective *Clostridium welchii* alpha-toxoid.

The problem of the mechanism of immunity in these infections reduces to the problem of the mechanism of the formation of circulating antibody.

REFERENCES

Burnet, F. M.   1959.   The clonal selection theory of acquired immunity. Cambridge University Press.

Evans, D. G.   1945.   Treatment with antitoxin of experimental gas gangrene produced in guinea pigs by (a) *Cl. welchii*; (b) *Cl. septicum*; and (c) *Cl. oedematiens*. Brit. J. Exptl. Pathol. 26: 104.

Jerne, N. K.   1955.   The natural selection theory of antibody formation. Proc. Nat. Acad. Sci. (U.S.) 41: 849–857.

Jerne, N. K.   1960.   Immunological speculations. Ann. Rev. Microbiol. 14: 341–358.

Karush, F., and H. N. Eisen.   1962.   A theory of delayed hypersensitivity. Science 136: 1032–1039.

MacLennan, J. D.   1962.   The histotoxic clostridial infections of man. Bacteriol. Rev. 26: 177–276.

Pappenheimer, A. M., Jr.   1955.   The pathogenesis of diphtheria. In Mechanisms of microbial pathogenicity, 5th Symp. Soc. Gen. Microbiol., pp. 40–56. Cambridge University Press.

Smith, M. Llewellyn. 1942/43.   Note on the complexity of tetanus toxins. Bull. Health Org., L.o.N. 10: 104–112.

Strauss, N., and E. D. Hendee.   1959.   The effect of diphtheria toxin on the metabolism of HeLa cells. J. Exptl. Med. 109: 145.

Strauss, N.   1960.   The effect of diphtheria toxin on the metabolism of HeLa cells. II. Effect of nucleic acid metabolism. J. Exptl. Med. 112: 351–359.

Szilard, L.   1960.   The control of the formation of specific proteins in bacteria and animal cells; The molecular basis of antibody formation. Proc. Nat. Acad. Sci. (U.S.) 46: 277–292; 293–302.

SYMPOSIUM VIII

INTERFERENCE AND INTERFERON

Chairman: A. W. DOWNIE

ALICK ISAACS

Interferon and Virus Infection

D. BLAŠKOVIČ

Interference Phenomena against Arthropod-borne Viruses

JOHN P. FOX

Interference Phenomena Observed in the Field

CHAIRMAN'S REMARKS

A. W. DOWNIE

Department of Bacteriology
The University, Liverpool, England

SINCE HOSKINS first clearly described the interfering effect of a non-lethal yellow fever virus injected into a monkey at the same time as, or soon after, a highly virulent strain, a great many instances of virus interference have been studied. In attempts to analyse the phenomenon much experimental work has been carried out in simpler systems than the intact animal—for example, in the chick embryo or its membranes and more recently in tissue cultures. Cross interference has been demonstrated between many different viruses in different animal hosts or cell systems.

At first, living viruses were used to demonstrate the interference effect but it was soon found that inactivated viruses, and especially viruses inactivated by ultraviolet light, could produce interference with infection by a living virus introduced subsequently. A few years ago it was shown by Dr. Isaacs and his colleagues that in at least certain systems the interference was mediated by an apparently non-viral protein which he designated "Interferon." This seems to be produced by tissue cells of various kinds under the influence of living or inactivated virus, and recent studies suggest that, in concentrations which have little effect on cell metabolism, it acts within cells to interfere with the synthesis of viral nucleic acids. It is uncertain whether all types of viral interference are caused by Interferon-like substances—perhaps this is unlikely—but the biological significance of Interferon may be very great. It has been suggested that the production of Interferon may be important in relation to virus virulence and in limiting spread of, and recovery from, virus infection. Recent work has further suggested that the balance between the host and virus which determines chronic or latent infection may be determined by the production of Interferon by virus-infected cells.

However I will leave Dr. Isaacs and subsequent speakers to discuss these extremely interesting possibilities.

INTERFERON AND VIRUS INFECTION

ALICK ISAACS

National Institute for Medical Research
London, England

THE PHENOMENON of virus interference is well recognized among plant, bacterial, and animal viruses but it is only among the last that it has been possible to explain many examples of this phenomenon, at least, as being the result of production of interferon by the infected cell. It seems that the cell reacts to infection by producing an antivirus substance, interferon, which helps the cell to recover from the first virus infection and also protects it from superinfection by a second virus. The production of interferon was studied first in cells of the chick chorio-allantoic membrane treated with an inactivated influenza virus and then superinfected, usually with live influenza virus. Later the production of interferon has been observed in a variety of vertebrate cells infected with animal viruses of many different kinds. Some of the cells which have been shown to produce interferon and some of the viruses shown to initiate its production are listed below.

Animals whose cells have been shown to produce interferon	*Viruses shown to induce the production of interferon*
Chicken, duck, mouse, rat, guinea-pig, rabbit, ferret, dog, pig, sheep, cow, monkey, Man	Numerous arborviruses, polio viruses, numerous myxoviruses, para-influenza viruses, measles, vaccinia, herpes, Rous, polyoma

From this it seems a reasonable conclusion that interferon production is a general response of vertebrate cells to virus infection.

PROPERTIES AND MODE OF ACTION OF INTERFERON

Chick interferon is a protein of molecular weight 63,000 and with an isoelectric point of 4.5 (Burke, 1961). Interferons prepared from different animal species show minor biological and physico-chemical differences, particularly in regard to their species specificity of antiviral action and their stability to heat. However, so far as is known, cells of one animal species produce the same interferon in response to infection with different viruses. Chick interferon has not been found to be antigenic, but recently it was shown that mouse interferon injected into guinea-pigs over a period of some months produced a low-titred antibody (Paucker & Cantell, 1962).

Interferon is active against a wide range of different viruses and it has been known for some time that its action was intracellular and that it blocked an early stage of virus growth. It is most active when given before cells are infected but still inhibits virus growth when given after the infection is two hours under way (Wagner, 1961). It has now been shown to inhibit the replication of virus nucleic acid (De Somer et al., 1962), and this can apparently occur without significant inhibition of the synthesis of the normal cellular nucleic acids, since it is possible to inhibit virus growth without affecting cell division significantly (Baron & Isaacs, 1962). There is some indirect evidence to suggest that interferon may act by inhibiting an oxidative process that supplies energy for viral synthesis. Viruses vary in their requirement of oxygen for virus growth and those with the highest oxygen requirement were found to be the most sensitive to the antiviral action of interferon (Isaacs, Porterfield & Baron, 1961). With larger doses of interferon, cell division is greatly inhibited, but returns to its normal rate once the interferon is removed (Paucker, Cantell & Henle, 1962).

INTERFERON AS A FACTOR IN RECOVERY FROM VIRUS INFECTIONS

Cellular, as distinct from humoral, factors have received increasing attention recently with reference to the process of recovery from virus infection. An early observation was that interferon was liberated rapidly from cells so that its concentration in the surrounding medium was much higher than its concentration within cells (Isaacs & Lindenmann, 1957). This suggested the possibility that it might play a defensive role in virus infection of a cell population.

The studies of Ho and Enders (1959) and Henle et al. (1959) on chronic virus infections of cells in vitro showed that interferon was formed in these cultures and might account for the self-limiting nature of the infections. Further evidence for this conclusion comes from the work of Glasgow and Habel (1962) who found that chronic virus infection of mouse cells in vitro could be cured, maintained, or proceed to cell destruction, simply by a change in the concentration of interferon in the medium. In passing, it is interesting to wonder whether the course of persistent virus infections which are known to occur in man, for example herpes simplex infection, as well as those which are suspected, could be governed by the interferon mechanism. In the chick embryo, Baron and Isaacs (1961) found that the ability to resist the lethal action of a number of viruses developed at the same time as the embryo acquired a functioning interferon mechanism. Here too it is interesting to observe that the effect of virus infections by rubella and vaccinia viruses, occurring during pregnancy, on the developing human embryo is in line with what would be expected if the interferon mechanism played a role. These findings would favour the conclusion that interferon plays an important role in cellular resistance to virus infections.

When we come to consider virus infections of adult vertebrates, humoral and cellular factors both play a role in the processes of recovery. However, there is evidence from the observation of some patients with hypo-gamma-globulinaemia and from the study of animals whose antibody production has been blocked experimentally, that normal recovery from virus infection can occur without significant production of antibody. There is indirect evidence that interferon may play an important role in recovery from virus infections in animals, since two factors that inhibit the action of interferon, increased oxygenation and cortisone, have both been found to produce an adverse effect on virus infections in animals.

Certain lines of tumour cells (Ho & Enders, 1959; Chany, 1961) produce interferon but are very insensitive to its antiviral action. The cells of very young embryos produce low yields of interferon and are very insensitive to its antiviral action (Isaacs & Baron, 1960). This raises the question of the role of the interferon mechanism in the normal cell. It is possible that it plays a role in controlling the rate of nucleic acid synthesis or cell division in the normal cell, and that the relative insensitivity of certain tumour cells and embryonic cells to its antiviral action is a reflection of their rapid rate of growth.

VIRUS VIRULENCE

Virus virulence is a complex virus property which must depend on many different factors. Fenner and Cairns (1959) give a number of examples which show the complexity of this property, and the work of Burnet (1959), Fenner and Comber (1958), and Fraser (1959) on genetic recombinants provides evidence of the multigenic origin of virus virulence. However, little progress has been made in identifying the factors on which virus virulence depends.

Enders (1960) drew attention to the fact that an avirulent strain of measles virus stimulated cells to produce higher yields of interferon than a virulent strain. Enders speculated that this observation might contain a new clue to the problem of virus virulence and De Maeyer and Enders (1963) have since reported that five avirulent strains of polioviruses produced more interferon than did four more virulent strains.

Dr. Ruiz-Gomez and I became interested in this problem in an indirect way. We were interested in the suggestion made by Lwoff and Lwoff (1960) that fever might play an important role in recovery from virus infections. The possibility was considered that the inhibitory effect on virus growth of raising the temperature might operate by favouring either the production or the action of interferon. This question was investigated by studying first the optimal temperature at which a number of different viruses were able to produce plaques in chick embryo cells. This was found to vary between 32° and 42° for different viruses. The optimal temperature for producing interferon was found to be higher than the optimal temperature for virus growth for all the strains investigated. This would therefore be in line with the suggestion that the beneficial effect of fever in virus infections might act by favouring the production of interferon.

It is known from work with polioviruses and poxviruses that a high optimal temperature for virus growth is frequently associated with virus virulence. It became of interest, therefore, to see whether any relationship could be found between the optimal temperature for virus growth, the production of interferon, and the sensitivity to the antiviral action of interferon of this group of viruses. A good correspondence was found between the optimal temperature for virus growth and the sensitivity to interferon, those viruses with a high optimal temperature proving to be much less sensitive to the antiviral action of interferon than viruses with a low optimal temperature. It is more difficult to compare accurately the production of interferon by different viruses than to compare their relative sensitivity to the antiviral action of interferon. Nevertheless, in general, viruses with a low optimal temperature for virus growth were found to give higher yields of interferon than those with a high optimal growth temperature (Ruiz-Gomez & Isaacs, 1963). In general, too, those viruses with a high optimal temperature were found to be virulent in the chick embryo thus supporting Enders' suggestion that the interferon mechanism might afford a clue to the nature of virus virulence. On this hypothesis a virulent virus would be able to avoid one of the normal cellular defence mechanisms. This could occur if the virulent virus were either insensitive to the antiviral action of interferon, or did not stimulate the cells to produce good yields of interferon, or both together.

More convincing evidence of an association of this kind comes from studies of mutants with altered virulence derived from a single virus strain. Wagner (1962) found that a mutant of vesicular stomatitis virus with reduced virulence for mice was more sensitive to the antiviral action of interferon when tested in L cells than the virulent variant; it also seemed to induce the cells to produce slightly more interferon than the virulent variant. Essentially similar results were found by Finter (personal communication) for variants of Semliki Forest virus showing different degrees of adaptation to calf kidney cells. However, we were unable to find much difference in either sensitivity to interferon or the production of interferon between the virulent strain of Newcastle disease virus and the B1 variant of this virus which is less virulent for the chick embryo. On the other hand, it was found that the standard virulent strain of Newcastle disease virus which produces very low yields of interferon in chick cells behaves quite differently in human thyroid cells. In these cells this virus grows very poorly but produces very high yields of interferon. This would suggest that interferon production resembles virus virulence in not being an intrinsic property of particular virus particles but an expression of the interaction between the virus and particular cells.

Virus virulence is obviously a complex problem but these results would suggest that one factor in virus virulence may be the ability of a virus to avoid a normal cellular defence, namely the production of interferon. This could occur if a virus is insensitive to the antiviral action of interferon or if it stimulates cells to give very low yields of interferon. There is also some evidence to suggest that virulent viruses may actually inhibit the production of interferon (Ruiz-Gomez, Rotem & Isaacs, 1963), an observation that recalls the phenomenon of inverse interference described by Lindenmann (1960).

INTERFERON AS A POTENTIAL ANTIVIRAL AGENT IN MAN

The difficulty in finding antiviral substances that could be of practical use in treating virus infections has been that until relatively recently it seemed that any substance that would inhibit the synthesis of viral nucleic acid or protein would also inhibit the synthesis of normal cellular nucleic acid or protein and would therefore prove to be toxic. However, the independence of viral and certain normal cellular synthetic processes is becoming more evident. Thus Franklin and Baltimore (1962) have found that actinomycin D inhibits the synthesis of cellular RNA without inhibiting the production of Mengo (an RNA-containing) virus. Present evidence would suggest that interferon has the reverse effect, i.e. that it inhibits the synthesis of viral nucleic acid at doses which do not inhibit the synthesis of normal cellular nucleic acids. Its broad antiviral spectrum of activity, low toxicity, low antigenicity, and the fact that it normally plays a role in recovery from virus infections suggest that it might prove useful in treating virus infections in man.

These considerations prompted the Medical Research Council in Britain to set up a collaboration with the pharmaceutical industry to see whether interferon could be used to protect against virus infections in man. As a first step, a batch of interferon prepared in monkey kidney tissue was tested to see whether it would inhibit the development of primary vaccination in man. This experiment was chosen because interferon was known to be effective in similar experiments in animals and because an effective experiment in man would give us some idea of which dosage of interferon to aim at in future clinical trials. Volunteers who had not been vaccinated before were given two injections, one of interferon and one of a control fluid, both materials having been supplied in coded form so that the experiment was run as a blind trial. The volunteers were then vaccinated at both sites and the number of takes was observed. The results are shown in Table 1.

TABLE 1

	Control > interferon	Interferon > control	No difference
No. of volunteers with single take	24	1	—
No. of volunteers with double take	8	0	5
TOTAL = 38 volunteers			

A highly significant degree of protection by interferon was found (Scientific Committee on Interferon, 1962). On this basis we are now testing similar preparations of interferon for their ability to prevent the development of common colds, and if this proves successful, to treat established colds. Another trial is being carried out to see whether interferon will have a beneficial effect in treating herpetic infections of the eye. Some preliminary evidence (Jones *et al.*, 1962) suggests that it has a beneficial effect in vaccinial infections of the eye.

FUTURE RESEARCH

During the past five years there have been many interesting findings in this field but many important questions remain to be answered. Confining ourselves to biological questions, we should like to know whether interferon production is a relatively recent event in evolution or whether similar substances are produced during virus infections of bacterial, plant, and insect cells. Another interesting question is the role of interferon in the normal cell. It seems likely that interferon plays some regulating role in the normal cell and that its production in high titre by the virus-infected cell represents an adaptive response that has developed in cells in the course of evolution. Its role in the normal cell then becomes a matter of great interest. A third question of interest is its detailed mode of action: is it directed specifically at the synthesis of virus nucleic acids or does it act indirectly by blocking some oxidative process that supplies the energy for viral synthesis? Finally, a most important question which could have both theoretical and practical interest is what is the exact nature of the stimulus that makes cells produce interferon? Protein synthesis is thought of today in terms of messenger RNA carrying its special code, and viruses are able to bring to cells their full complement of messenger. Perhaps the cell has some means of recognizing what Robert Browning described as "a dusk mis-featured messenger" and responds to foreign nucleic acids by producing interferon. But if the cell does have this special mechanism for excluding unwanted foreign nucleic acids, one wonders whether it might not observe, as Lewis Carroll observed in *Through the Looking Glass*, "He's an Anglo-Saxon Messenger, and those are Anglo-Saxon attitudes."

REFERENCES

Baron, S., and A. Isaacs. 1961. Mechanism of recovery from viral infection in the chick embryo. Nature *191*: 97–98.

Baron, S., and A. Isaacs. 1962. Absence of interferon in lungs from fatal cases of influenza. Brit. Med. J. *i*: 18–20.

Burke, D. C. 1961. The purification of interferon. Biochem. J. *78*: 556–564.

Burnet, F. M. 1959. Virus genetics. Brit. Med. Bull. *15*: 177–180.

Chany, C. 1961. An interferon-like inhibitor of viral multiplication from malignant cells (the viral autoinhibition phenomenon). Virology *13*: 485–492.

De Maeyer, E., and J. F. Enders. 1962. Personal communication.

De Somer, P., A. Prinzie, P. Denys, Jr., and E. Schonne. 1962. Mechanism of action of interferon. I. Relationship with viral ribonucleic acid. Virology 16: 63–70.

Enders, J. F. 1960. A consideration of the mechanisms of resistance to viral infection based on recent studies of the agents of measles and poliomyelitis. Trans. Coll. Phys. Philadelphia 28: 68–79.

Fenner, F., and J. F. Cairns. 1959. Variation in virulence in relation to adaptation to new hosts. In The Viruses, 3: 225–249. Academic Press, London-New York.

Fenner, F., and B. M. Comben. 1958. Genetic studies with mammalian poxviruses. I. Demonstration of recombination between two strains of vaccinia virus. Virology 5: 530–548.

Franklin, R. M., and D. Baltimore. 1962. Patterns of macromolecular synthesis in normal and virus-infected mammalian cells. Cold Spring Harbor Symp. on Quant. Biol. 27: 175–198.

Fraser, K. B. 1959. Features of the MEL X NWS Recombination Systems in influenza A virus. IV. Increments of virulence during successive cycles of double infection with two strains of influenza A virus. Virology 9: 202–214.

Glasgow, L. A., and K. Habel. 1962. The role of interferon in vaccinia virus infection of mouse embryo tissue culture. J. Exptl. Med. 115: 503–512.

Henle, W., G. Henle, F. Deinhardt, and V. V. Bergs. 1959. Studies on persistent infections of tissue cultures. IV. Evidence for the production of an interferon in MCN cells by myxoviruses. J. Exptl. Med. 110: 525–541.

Ho, M., and J. F. Enders. 1959. An inhibitor of viral activity appearing in infected cell cultures. Proc. Nat. Acad. Sci. (U.S.) 45: 385–389.

Isaacs, A., and S. Baron. 1960. Antiviral action of interferon in embryonic cells. Lancet ii: 946–947.

Isaacs, A., and J. Lindenmann. 1957. Virus interference. I. The interferon. Proc. Roy. Soc. B147, 258–267.

Isaacs, A., J. S. Porterfield, and S. Baron. 1961. The influence of oxygenation on virus growth. II. Effect on the antiviral action of interferon. Virology 14: 450–455.

Jones, B., J. E. K. Galbraith, and M. K. Al-Husaini. 1962. Vaccinial keratitis treated with interferon. Lancet i: 875–879.

Lindenmann, J. 1960. Interferon und inverse Interferenz. Zeitschr. f. Hyg. 146: 287–309.

Lwoff, A., and M. Lwoff. 1960. Sur les facteurs du développement viral et leur rôle dans l'évolution de l'infection. Ann. Inst. Past. 98: 173–203.

Paucker, K., and K. Cantell. 1962. Neutralization of interferon by specific antibody. Virology 18: 145–146.

Paucker, K., K. Cantell, and W. Henle. 1962. Quantitative studies on viral interference in suspended L cells. III. Effect of interfering viruses and interferon on the growth rate of cells. Virology 17: 324–334.

Ruiz-Gomez, J., and A. Isaacs. 1963. Interferon production by different viruses. Virology 19: 8–12.

Ruiz-Gomez, J., Z. Rotem, and A. Isaacs. 1963. Optimal temperature for growth and sensitivity to interferon among different viruses. Virology 19 (in press).

Scientific Committee on Interferon. 1962. Effect of interferon on vaccination in volunteers. Lancet i: 873–875.

Wagner, R. R. 1961. Biological studies of interferon. I. Suppression of cellular infection with Eastern equine encephalomyelitis virus. Virology 13: 323–337.

Wagner, R. R. 1962. Cold Spring Harbor Symp. on Quant. Biol. 27: 349.

INTERFERENCE PHENOMENA AGAINST ARTHROPOD-BORNE VIRUSES

D. BLAŠKOVIČ*

Institute of Virology
Czechoslovak Academy of Sciences
Bratislava

INFECTION with the arthropod-borne viruses (arboviruses) served as the first experimental model for the study of interference phenomena with animal viruses. The neurotropic variant of yellow fever virus, the so-called French strain, inoculated into rhesus monkeys along with, or not later than thirty hours after, the viscerotropic Asibi strain of the same virus, protected the animals from death due to the viscerotropic strain (Hoskins, 1935). The same neurotropic variant of yellow fever virus also protected mice against Rift Valley fever virus as well as against the virulent Asibi strain of yellow fever virus.

Conditions under which interference phenomena appear, as well as the basic mechanisms involved, cannot be explained by experiments in laboratory animals. The living organism is too complex a system and is influenced by a variety of factors hard to control. Our knowledge of the mechanisms of interference phenomena has been improved during recent years thanks to the wide use of more simple systems: chick embryos and mainly tissue cultures. The results obtained with these systems have improved our knowledge of interference phenomena induced by and against arboviruses.

It may be said that interference phenomena induced by, as well as against, arboviruses cannot be considered basically different from interference phenomena in other animal viruses. Despite this fact, there is some reason to pay special attention to arboviruses as a model for the study of interference: (*a*) Various arboviruses cause non-lethal infections of different cell cultures, thus providing a suitable interfering virus. (*b*) Some arboviruses have been shown to be very sensitive to the action of interferon and therefore very suitable as indicators of the interference phenomenon. They have therefore been widely used as challenge viruses for the assay of interference induced by heterologous viruses.

INTERFERENCE AGAINST ARBORVIRUSES INDUCED BY HETEROLOGOUS VIRUS

Reviews on virus interference (Henle, 1950; Schlesinger, 1959) contain many data on interference induced by heterologous viruses against different

*This paper was prepared in collaboration with Dr. J. Vilček, whose contribution is deeply appreciated.

arboviruses. Systems in which interference against arboviruses could be induced by various kinds of active or inactivated heterologous viruses, before the discovery of interferon as the effective principle of interference (Isaacs & Lindenmann, 1957), are listed in Table 1.

TABLE 1

Interference against arboviruses induced by heterologous viruses

Interfering virus	Challenge virus	Host system	References
Influenza A	WEE	mouse	Vilches and Hirst, 1947
		chick embryo	Bang, 1949
		mouse	Hirst, 1950
			Schlesinger, 1951
		tissue cultures	Taylor, 1953
	SLE	mouse	Vilches and Hirst, 1947
	Bwamba		
	West Nile	tissue cultures	Lennette and Koprowski, 1945
Influenza A, inactivated	WEE	chick embryo	Henle and Henle, 1945
		mouse	Vilches and Hirst, 1947
Influenza B			
Swine influenza	EEE	chick embryo	Bang, 1949
NDV	WEE	mouse	Vilches and Hirst, 1947
Mouse encephalomyelitis (Theiler)	SLE		Schlesinger et al., 1943, 1944
Columbia SK and MM	WEE	tissue cultures	Huang, 1943

It can be seen that interference phenomena against arboviruses had been studied in all available experimental models: in animals, chick embryos, and tissue cultures. Various hypotheses were advanced to explain interference. Interestingly enough, the altered metabolism of cells caused by the interfering virus had been often emphasized. The inhibition of multiplication of the challenge virus, and eventually the protection of the animal against challenge, had usually been interpreted as a process occurring inside the cell, after the penetration of the challenge virus into it (Henle, 1950; Isaacs & Edney, 1950).

TABLE 2

Activity of interferon against arborviruses

| Origin of interferon | | Activity of interferon | | References |
Inducing virus	Source	Challenge virus	Host system	
Influenza A, inactivated	chick embryo cell cultures	West Nile	chick embryo cell cultures	Isaacs and Westwood, 1959a
Influenza A, inactivated	chick embryo cell cultures	Yellow fever WEE West Nile Bunyamwera	chick embryo cell cultures	Porterfield, 1959
Poliomyelitis, type 2, live	human kidney cell cultures	Sindbis	human amnion cell cultures	Ho and Enders, 1959
Influenza A, live	chick embryo (allantoic fluid)	EEE	chick embryo cell cultures	Wagner, 1960
Influenza A, live	mouse embryo cell cultures, mouse lung (suspension)	Bunyamwera	mice	Hitchcock and Isaacs, 1960

The discovery of interferon (Isaacs & Lindenmann, 1957), and the subsequent isolation from various systems of inhibitors having the properties of interferon, led to the testing of the effect of these substances against different arborviruses. The high degree of sensitivity to various interferon-type inhibitors of arborviruses such as those belonging to Group A (Casals, 1957), including the equine encephalomyelitis and the Sindbis viruses, can be shown clearly even from this heterogenous material. This indicates that the mechanism of action of all these substances must be related (Table 2).

TABLE 3

Interference phenomena induced by arborviruses

Interfering virus	Challenge virus	Host system	References
Yellow fever	Yellow fever (viscerotropic)	monkey	Hoskins, 1935
	Rift Valley fever	mouse	Findlay and MacCallum, 1937
	Vaccinia		Lépine et al., 1947
	West Nile	tissue cultures	Lennette and Koprowski, 1945
	VEE		
	Influenza A		
	Dengue	man	Schlesinger et al., 1956; Sabin, 1952
WEE	EEE	mouse, guinea pig	Schlesinger et al., 1943, 1944
	Vesicular stoma-titis		
EEE	NDV	chick embryo	Bang, 1949
SLE	WEE	tissue cultures	Huang, 1943
	NDV		
	WEE	chick embryo	Duffy, 1944
		rat	Duffy et al., 1952a; Jordan and Duffy, 1952
JBE	WEE		Duffy et al., 1952b
	Poliomyelitis	tissue cultures	Mason and Woodie, 1955
West Nile	VEE		Lennette and Koprowski, 1945
Dengue	Yellow fever	man	Schlesinger et al., 1956
		mosquito	Sabin, 1952

INTERFERENCE PHENOMENA INDUCED BY ARBORVIRUSES

Besides the first interference phenomena described with yellow fever virus (Hoskins, 1935; Findlay & MacCallum, 1937), Henle (1950) and Schlesinger (1959) refer to many other arboviruses capable of inducing interference phenomena in different systems, including animals as well as tissue cultures (Table 3). Despite the relatively great number of systems in which interference had been established, it is difficult to draw any general conclusions or to distinguish any basic mechanism of interference from this material.

Several authors studied the interference phenomena induced by tick-borne encephalitis virus in tissue culture. This virus is very suitable for interference studies because, as with some other members of the Group B arborviruses, its multiplication in tissue cultures of different origin does not lead to the destruction of the host cells and the cells become resistant to superinfection with various heterologous viruses. This phenomenon was observed in several types of primary cell cultures with various challenge viruses: bovine embryo kidney cells are rendered resistant to Newcastle disease and fowl plague viruses; pig, feline, rabbit, and guinea-pig cells to Newcastle disease virus (Morimoto, 1960); sheep kidney cells to Japanese B encephalitis virus (Gaidamovich & Titova, 1961); human embryo and monkey

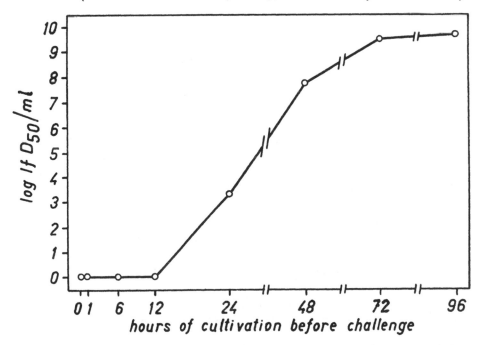

Fig. 1. Dynamics of the establishment of interference by tick-borne encephalitis virus against Western equine encephalomyelitis virus in chick embryo cells. IfD_{50}—50 per cent interference dose of tick-borne encephalitis virus; 0 on the ordinate means $\leqslant 2.5$ log IfD_{50}/ml.

kidney cells to poliovirus (Altstein *et al.*, 1962); and chick embryo cells to Western equine encephalomyelitis virus (Vilček, 1960a).

The time required for the establishment of interference depends on the dose. The dynamics of the appearance of interference against Western equine encephalomyelitis virus in chick embryo cells inoculated with tenfold serial dilutions of tick-borne encephalitis virus and challenged at different times is shown in Fig. 1. It will be shown later that the interference in this system is the result of interferon formation.

It seems that the resistance induced by interference cannot be overcome by even massive doses of the challenge virus. This is certainly true for at least some systems (Morimoto, 1960; Vilček, 1962b; Altstein *et al.*, 1962).

INTERFERON AS MEDIATOR OF THE INTERFERENCE INDUCED BY ARBORVIRUSES

Three different types of cell–virus interaction resulting in interferon formation can be distinguished: (*a*) formation of interferon after contact of the cell with inactivated virus, which is not capable of inducing the reproduction of complete virus or of forming sub-units of virus; (*b*) formation of interferon after interaction of the cell with live virus which multiplies only poorly in the given system, or does not lead to production of infective virus, but eventually can lead to the formation of some kind of incomplete virus; (*c*) formation of interferon after the inoculation of sensitive cells with live virus followed by the complete cycle of virus multiplication.

So far there is no definite evidence for the formation of interferon by members of the arborvirus group after inactivation.

An example of the second type of interferon formation, in relatively insusceptible cells, is its formation by cells of the stable line of human amnion cells inoculated with large doses of Sindbis virus (Gresser & Enders, 1962).

More examples can be given of the third type of interferon formation, i.e., its formation during multiplication of different arborviruses in fully susceptible cells. Interferon formation has been demonstrated with Mayaro (Henderson & Taylor, 1961), with West Nile (Vilček, 1962b), with Sindbis (Ho, 1961) viruses in chick embryo cells; and with O'nyong-nyong (Hitchcock & Porterfield, 1961) and West Nile (Vainio *et al.*, 1961) viruses in mouse brains. Almost twenty years ago Lennette and Koprowski (1945) probably observed interferon formation with the 17 D strain of yellow fever virus multiplying in tissue culture, but no special interest was shown in this phenomenon at that time.

Formation of interferon induced by the interfering virus represents the only known mechanism by which interference can be established by arborviruses.

A different mechanism is suggested by Henderson and Taylor (1961) for the early interference induced with large doses of Mayaro virus against Sindbis virus in cultures of chick embryo cells. An interferon-type inhibitor could not be demonstrated in the culture fluid although at the time multiplication of the Sindbis virus was suppressed, and later on formation of an inhibitor was observed. It is questionable, however, whether an interferon-like inhibitor can be excluded even if its presence could not be shown at the time of challenge. Interferon could be present in concentrations too low to be demonstrated but sufficient to cause some degree of inhibition, or it could be formed shortly after challenge. The latter possibility is important since interferon can suppress virus multiplication even if given after the virus penetrates the cell (Wagner, 1961).

The formation and properties of an interferon from chick embryo cells infected with Central European tick-borne encephalitis virus were thoroughly studied in the Institute of Virology of the Czechoslovak Academy of Sciences. Judged from the dynamics and conditions of interferon formation in the system studied, this substance is responsible for the establishment of interference between tick-borne encephalitis and Western equine encephalomyelitis viruses (Vilček, 1960b).

The presence of interferon in the chick embryo cell cultures is assayed and titrated according to the ability of twofold diluted heated fluids to inhibit completely the cytopathic effect of Western equine encephalo-myelitis virus (Vilček, 1961).

CONDITIONS LEADING TO INTERFERON FORMATION WITH TICK-BORNE ENCEPHALITIS VIRUS IN CHICK EMBRYO CELLS

The dynamics of release of interferon into the medium of chick embryo cell cultures depends on the infective dose of tick-borne encephalitis virus inoculated. When infected with higher doses such as one or more infective

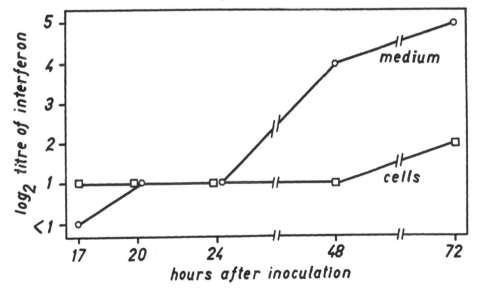

FIG. 2. Dynamics of the appearance of interferon in the medium and cell homogenate of chick embryo cell cultures inoculated with a multiplicity of 10 LD_{50} of tick-borne encephalitis virus per cell.

doses per cell the first detectable interferon appears in the culture medium between the 12th and 24th hour after inoculation, with lower doses of virus between the 24th and 48th hour and sometimes, when the inoculum contained very little infective virus, only after the second day of cultivation. Interferon formation in this system is thus in good accord with interference against Western equine encephalomyelitis virus.

Although relatively high concentrations of interferon are found in the fluid phase of inoculated cultures very little inhibitor can be shown in the homogenate of cells from the same culture (Fig. 2).

Experiments were also designed to show whether interferon formation in the system under study represents only a side product of the synthesis of infective virus by the host cells, or whether, as with influenza virus, certain other myxoviruses, and vaccinia virus, interferon formation can be induced with inactivated virus incapable of self-replication.

We were never able to show interferon formation in cultures which were inoculated with large doses of virus inactivated by mild treatments with ultraviolet irradiation or heating at 37 or 56 C, if the treatment used completely destroyed the infectivity of the virus. If, however, a small part of the population of virus escaped destruction, multiplication of virus to high titres, as well as formation of interferon, occurred. Interferon could then be shown only after 2–3 days of cultivation, as when cultures were inoculated with high dilutions of active virus.

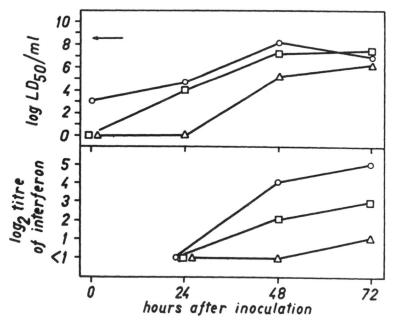

FIG. 3. Multiplication of virus and formation of interferon in chick embryo cells inoculated with tick-borne encephalitis virus kept for different times, at 37 C. Inoculated with virus kept for 72 (○), 96 (□), or 120 (△) hours at 37 C. Arrow indicates the titre of virus inoculated, before inactivation.

The multiplication of virus and formation of interferon took place in chick embryo cells inoculated with suspensions of tick-borne encephalitis virus kept for 3, 4, and 5 days at 37 C (Fig. 3). However, no multiplication of virus and no formation of interferon was found with suspensions kept at 37 C longer than 5 days.

We were thus unable to show interferon formation with tick-borne encephalitis virus without infection of the cell and our present concept of interferon formation in the system studied is that the cell produces virus and interferon simultaneously. This situation is similar to at least two other systems: with poliomyelitis virus (Ho & Enders, 1959) and with Mayaro virus (Henderson & Taylor, 1961). The ability or inability of particular viruses to induce interferon formation without reproduction of the virus is probably conditioned by the structure of the virus particle, presumably by the structure of the virus nucleic acid.

PROPERTIES OF INTERFERON FROM TICK-BORNE ENCEPHALITIS VIRUS-INFECTED CHICK EMBRYO CELLS

Interferon from tick-borne encephalitis virus-infected chick embryo cells shows the same basic physical and chemical properties and the very same basic mode of action as interferon produced by inactivated or live influenza virus, and as other interferon-like substances (Žemla & Vilček, 1961a; Vilček, 1962a). It is notable that the activity of this interferon is not influenced by heating for 1 hour at 75 C. This high degree of thermostability is not shared by all interferon-type inhibitors. Interferon from chick embryo cells infected with tick-borne encephalitis virus can be concentrated and partially purified by precipitation with cold acetone (Žemla & Vilček, 1961b), and attempts to purify it further and to estimate its molecular weight have so far been unsuccessful.

Different techniques were used to study the inhibition of multiplication of various viruses by this interferon. A lack of viral specificity but, on the other hand, a high degree of tissue species specificity was found (Vilček & Rada, 1962; Vilček, 1962a). Western and Eastern encephalomyelitis viruses and the New Jersey N.J.M. strain of vesicular stomatitis virus were the most sensitive of the viruses so far studied to the action of this interferon. Pretreatment of chick embryo cells with interferon inhibited infection by intact Eastern encephalomyelitis virus to the same degree as by infective ribonucleic acid isolated from this virus (Mayer et al., 1961, 1962). These results (similarly to those of Grossberg & Holland, 1961, Ho, 1961, and De Somer et al., 1962) demonstrate that interferon acts after the penetration of the virus nucleic acid into the cell. If interferon was removed from the cultures before inoculation with virus or isolated ribonucleic acid, there was a marked prolongation of the latent period before virus multiplication (Fig. 4). These data indicate that infective ribonucleic acid can penetrate into cells which had been rendered resistant to infection by the action of interferon, and can persist in such cells in an active state. Infective ribonucleic acid can possibly pass at cell division to daughter cells which are still capable of reproducing virus. It is also possible that a cell rendered resistant by the action of interferon can revert to its original sensitivity.

These considerations bring us to the question of the mechanism of action of interferon. We shall not treat this problem in detail, since Dr. Isaacs, who is much more competent in this field, has already considered it in the preceding paper. Let us just mention briefly some observations.

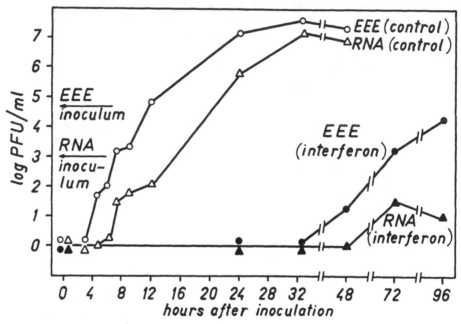

FIG. 4. Multiplication of virus after the inoculation of interferon-pretreated chick embryo cells with Eastern equine encephalomyelitis virus and its isolated ribonucleic acid. 0 on the ordinate means < 1.2 PFU (plaque-forming units)/ml.

Žemla and Schramek (1962a) followed the effect of interferon from tick-borne encephalitis virus-infected cells on the multiplication of Western equine encephalomyelitis virus in chick embryo cells cultivated anaerobically. They were able to show that under anaerobic conditions the multiplication of virus is inhibited by interferon approximately to the same degree as in cultures kept under usual aerobic conditions. The same authors (Žemla & Schramek, 1962b) studied the metabolic effects of interferon on chick embryo cells and showed a greater oxygen uptake and an enhanced aerobic glycolysis in media which do not contain interferon and are not exerting any inhibitory activity on virus multiplication. These results possibly indicate that the observed uncoupling effect of interferon on oxydative phosphorylation (Isaacs *et al.*, 1961a, b) does not necessarily represent the key mechanism of the action of interferon (interferons) against all viruses.

MANIFESTATIONS OF INTERFERENCE PHENOMENA OF ARBORVIRUSES
IN STABLE CELL LINES

The inoculation of some viruses into cultures of stable cell lines can result, in addition to interference, in a biologically important phenomenon which is characterized by continuous release of virus. Such persistently infected cells, carrying the virus over a great, often unlimited number of passages, were studied intensively in recent years, using different viruses, cells, and various conditions of cultivation (Ginsberg, 1958).

L cells (Earle, 1943) persistently infected with Western equine encephalomyelitis virus were studied by Chambers (1957) and Lockart (1960). Autointerference, presumably induced by thermally inactivated virus, is supposed to be responsible for the initiation and maintenance of the carrier state in these cultures, but the formation of an interferon-type inhibitor is also considered (Lockart, 1960). The latter possibility is consistent with the observation that L cells are susceptible to the action of interferon from mouse brain (Vainio et al., 1961).

Persistently infected cultures can be easily obtained from HeLa, Detroit-6, HEp-2, KB, human amnion, and cynomolgus monkey heart cell lines inoculated with both low or high doses of tick-borne encephalitis virus (Mayer, 1962a, b). These persistently infected cells are resistant to super-infection with low doses of poliovirus, they multiply at a lower rate, show altered metabolic activities, and release small quantities of an interferon-like substance. However, the activity of this interferon-type inhibitor can be demonstrated only in primary cultures of human amnion cells, not in the stable cell lines in which interferon is produced. Thus it remains to be elucidated to what degree the interferon-like inhibitor participates in the mechanism leading to the establishment of persistent infection with tick-borne encephalitis virus in stable cell lines.

That the production of interferon can influence substantially the outcome of infection in tissue culture has been recently clearly demonstrated by Gresser and Enders (1962). Stable line human amnion cells are relatively insusceptible to infection with Sindbis virus, but readily produce interferon when inoculated with this virus. Primary human amnion cells are highly susceptible to Sindbis virus and regularly succumb to this virus. If mixed cultures of stable and primary human amnion cells were prepared and inoculated with Sindbis virus, interferon formation by the former cells eventually protected the latter cells from the cytopathic effect of the virus.

It seems therefore very likely that interferon formation can be the cause of the natural resistance of cells to infection, as well as of the initiation and maintenance of a persistent infection. At least four factors are of importance: the ability of virus to induce interferon formation, its sensitivity to the action of interferon, the readiness of the cell to form interferon, and its ability to be rendered resistant by the action of interferon.

PRACTICAL IMPLICATIONS OF INTERFERENCE PHENOMENA OF ARBORVIRUSES

Assay of Non-Cytopathic Viruses

Inoculation of mice is the usual method of isolating and detecting arborviruses. Various kinds of tissue cultures as well as many different techniques of cultivation were tested, and progress has been achieved in producing a cytopathic effect and/or plaque formation with some arborviruses that originally did not do so, but the mouse inoculation test still remains the method of choice for the assay of most arborviruses.

The possibility of using the resistance of tissue culture cells to super-infection with a cytopathogenic virus for the assay of a non-cytopathogenic virus was considered a long time ago by Huang (1943), but this work had not been followed up until recently. Chu Kuan-fu (1959) proposed the use of Western equine encephalitis virus for the detection of Japanese B encephalitis virus in cultures of chick embryo cells. He noticed that if explants of chick embryo tissue had been in contact with Japanese B encephalitis virus, the cells which grew out from this explant were resistant to the cytopathic action of Western equine encephalomyelitis virus. However, the system of plasma-clot cultures proposed by Chu Kuan-fu is rather troublesome. Much simpler are monolayer cultures. Different cells and different challenge viruses were used for the quantitative assay of tick-borne encephalitis virus and antibodies against this virus by interference techniques (Vilček, 1960a; Morimoto, 1960; Gaidamovich & Titova, 1961; Altstein *et al.*, 1962). The sensitivity of these methods was shown to be no better than that of the mouse inoculation test.

The possibility of using interference techniques for the detection of other arborviruses remains to be tested, but there seems to be no reason why such techniques could not be employed with other viruses that multiply without causing cytopathic effect.

Suppression of Arborvirus Infections in Living Organisms by Interferon

The use of interferon for influencing favourably the course of infection with arborviruses has so far been experimental (Hitchcock & Isaacs, 1960); some experiments were quoted earlier. The results were encouraging as are the observations indicating that interferon produced in rabbit kidney cells can suppress local lesions caused by vaccinia virus in rabbits (Isaacs & Westwood, 1959b; Cantell & Tomilla, 1960) and that interferon produced in their own bodies can, under particular conditions, influence the course of experimental influenza infection in mice (Isaacs & Hitchcock, 1960; Link *et al.*, 1961). These findings led to the use of interferon for suppressing the local lesions caused by vaccinia virus in man (Scientific Committee on Interferon, 1962; Jones *et al.*, 1962).

The results obtained encourage further experiments. The possibility of influencing favourably the' course of infection, as well as of revealing the conditions leading to the initiation of hidden and latent infections in organisms is the most important aim of the study of interference phenomena.

REFERENCES

Altstein, A. D., V. A. Kazantseva, and G. A. Shirman. 1962. Interference between tick-borne encephalitis and poliomyelitis viruses in tissue culture. I. Resistance of tick-borne encephalitis virus-infected cells to the cytopathic effect of poliovirus. Acta Virol. 6: 421–427.

Bang, F. B. 1949. Cell blockade in Newcastle disease of chickens and chicken embryos. J. Exptl. Med. 89: 141–154.

Cantell, K., and V. Tomilla. 1960. Effect of interferon on experimental vaccinia and herpes-simplex virus infections in rabbits' eyes. Lancet ii: 682–684.

Casals, J. 1957. The arthropod-borne group of animal viruses. Trans. N.Y. Acad. Sci., Ser. 2, 19: 219–235.

Chambers, V. C. 1957. The prolonged persistence of Western equine encephalomyelitis virus in cultures of strain L cells. Virology 3: 62–75.

Chu Kuan-fu. 1959. Application of the interference phenomenon in tissue culture for the detection of Japanese B encephalitis virus. Acta Virol. 3: 82–88.

De Somer, P., A. Prinzie, P. Denys, Jr., and E. Schonne. 1962. Mechanism of action of interferon. I. Relationship with viral ribonucleic acid. Virology 16: 63–70.

Duffy, C. E. 1944. Interference between St. Louis encephalitis virus and equine encephalomyelitis virus (western type) in the chick embryo. Science 99: 517–518.

Duffy, C. E., R. T. Jordan, and H. M. Meyer. 1952a. Effect of multiple inoculations on interference between St. Louis encephalitis virus and equine encephalomyelitis virus. Proc. Soc. Exptl. Biol. Med. 80: 279–281.

Duffy, C. E., G. C. Pehrson, and P. N. Morgan. 1952b. Interference between Japanese B encephalitis virus and Western equine encephalomyelitis virus in the rat. Proc. Soc. Exptl. Biol. Med. 81: 154–157.

Earle, W. R. 1943. Production of malignancy in vitro. IV. The mouse fibroblast cultures and changes seen in living cells. J. Nat. Cancer Inst. 4: 165–212.

Findlay, G. M., and F. O. MacCallum. 1937. An interference phenomenon in relation to yellow fever and other viruses. J. Path. Bact. 44: 405–424.

Gaidamovich, S. Ya., and N. G. Titova. 1961. Interference between tick-borne and Japanese B encephalitis viruses in sheep embryo kidney epithelial tissue cultures. Acta Virol. 5: 386.

Ginsberg, H. S. 1958. The significance of the viral carrier state in tissue culture systems. Progr. Med. Virol. 1: 36–58.

Gresser, I., and J. F. Enders. 1962. Alteration of cellular resistance to Sindbis virus in mixed cultures of human cells attributable to interferon. Virology 16: 428–435.

Grossberg, S. E., and J. J. Holland. 1961. Interferon effect on virus production in virus-susceptible and insusceptible cells. Fed. Proc. 20: 442.

Henderson, J. R., and R. M. Taylor. 1961. Studies on mechanisms of arthropod-borne virus interference in tissue culture. Virology 13: 477–484.

Henle, W. 1950. Interference phenomena between animal viruses: A review. J. Immunol. 64: 203–236.

Henle, W., and G. Henle. 1945. Interference between inactive and active viruses of influenza. III. Cross-interference between various related and unrelated viruses. Amer. J. Med. Sci. 210: 362–369.

Hirst, G. K. 1950. The relationship of the receptors of a new strain of virus to those of the mumps-NDV-influenza groups. J. Exptl. Med. 91: 177–184.

Hitchcock, G., and A. Isaacs. 1960. Protection of mice against the lethal action of an encephalitis virus. Brit. Med. J. *ii*: 1268–1270.

Hitchcock, G., and J. Porterfield. 1961. The production of interferon in brains of mice infected with an arthropod-borne virus. Virology *13*: 363–365.

Ho, M. 1961. Inhibition of the infectivity of poliovirus ribonucleic acid by an interferon. Proc. Soc. Exptl. Biol. Med. *107*: 639–644.

Ho, M., and J. F. Enders. 1959. Further studies on an inhibitor of viral activity appearing in infected cell cultures and its role in chronic viral infections. Virology *9*: 446–477.

Hoskins, M. 1935. A protective action of neurotropic against viscerotropic yellow fever virus in Macaccus rhesus. Amer. J. Trop. Med. *15*: 675–680.

Huang, C. H. 1943. Titration of St. Louis encephalitis virus and Jungenblut-Sanders mouse virus in tissue culture. Proc. Soc. Exptl. Biol. Med. *54*: 158–160.

Isaacs, A., and M. Edney. 1950. Interference between inactive and active influenza viruses in the chick embryo. I. Quantitative aspects of interference. Austral. J. Exptl. Biol. Med. Sci. *28*: 219–230.

Isaacs, A., and G. Hitchcock. 1960. Role of interferon in recovery from virus infections. Lancet *ii*: 69–71.

Isaacs, A., and J. Lindenmann. 1957. Virus interference. I. The interferon. Proc. Royal Soc. B*147*: 258–267.

Isaacs, A., H. G. Klemperer, and G. Hitchcock. 1961a. Studies on the mechanism of action of interferon. Virology *13*: 191–199.

Isaacs, A., J. S. Porterfield, and S. Baron. 1961b. The influence of oxygenation on virus growth. II. Effect on the antiviral action of interferon. Virology *14*: 450–455.

Isaacs, A., and M. A. Westwood. 1959a. Duration of protective action of interferon against infection with West Nile virus. Nature *184*: 1232–33.

Isaacs, A., and M. A. Westwood. 1959b. Inhibition by interferon of the growth of vaccinia virus in the rabbit skin. Lancet *ii*: 324–325.

Jones, B. R., J. E. K. Galbraith, and M. K. Al-Hussaini. 1962. Vaccinial keratitis treated with interferon. Lancet *i*: 875–879.

Jordan, R. T., and C. E. Duffy. 1952. Interference between St. Louis encephalitis virus and western equine encephalomyelitis virus along a neuronal pathway. J. Inf. Dis. *91*: 165–172.

Lennette, E. H., and H. Koprowski. 1945. Interference between viruses in tissue culture. J. Exptl. Med. *83*: 195–219.

Lépine, P., J. C. Levaditi, and V. Sautter. 1947. Essais d'association des souches neurotropes du virus amaril et du virus vaccinal. Bull. Soc. Path. exot. *40*: 340–343.

Link, F., D. Blaškovič, and J. Raus. 1961. Pathogenesis of influenza infection following inoculation of small doses of adapted virus. I. Dynamics of multiplication of an adapted influenza virus strain in mouse lungs. Acta Virol. *5*: 373–378.

Lockart, R. Z., Jr. 1960. The production and maintenance of a virus carrier state: The possible role of homologous interference. Virology *10*: 198–210.

Mason, H. C., and J. Woodie. 1955. Inhibition of poliomyelitis virus by Japanese B encephalitis (JBE) virus in HeLa tissue culture. Fed. Proc. *14*: 471.

Mayer, V. 1962a. "Partial" cytopathic effect of tick-borne encephalitis virus—a consequence of persistent infection of stable cell lines. Acta Virol. *6*: 92.

Mayer, V. 1962b. Interactions of mammalian cells with tick-borne encephalitis virus. II. Persisting infection of cells. Acta Virol. *6*: 317–326.

Mayer, V., F. Sokol, and J. Vilček. 1961. Effect of interferon on the infection with eastern equine encephalomyelitis (EEE) virus and its ribonucleic acid (RNA). Acta Virol. 5: 264.

Mayer, V., F. Sokol, and J. Vilček. 1962. Infection of interferon-treated cells with eastern equine encephalomyelitis virus and its ribonucleic acid. Virology 16: 359–362.

Morimoto, T. 1960. Interference of Russian spring summer encephalitis with Newcastle disease virus in cell culture of bovine embryonic kidney. Virus (Kyoto) 10: 316–329.

Porterfield, J. S. 1959. A simple plaque inhibition test for antiviral agents: Application to assay of interferon. Lancet ii: 326–327.

Sabin, A. B. 1952. Dengue. In Viral and rickettsial infections of man, ed. T. M. Rivers, pp. 556–568. Lippincott, New York.

Schlesinger, R. W. 1959. Interference between animal viruses. In The Viruses, 3: 157–194. Academic Press, London-New York.

Schlesinger, R. W. 1951. Studies on interference between influenza and equine encephalomyelitis viruses. Arch. ges. Virusforsch. 4: 501–517.

Schlesinger, R. W., P. K. Olitsky, and I. M. Morgan. 1943. Observation on acquired cellular resistance to equine encephalomyelitis virus. Proc. Soc. Exptl. Biol. Med. 54: 272–273.

Schlesinger, R. W., P. K. Olitsky, and I. M. Morgan. 1944. Induced resistance of the central nervous system to experimental infection of equine encephalitis virus. III. Abortive infection with western virus and subsequent interference with the action of heterologous viruses. J. Exptl. Med. 80: 197–211.

Schlesinger, R. W., I. Gordon, J. W. Frankel, J. W. Winter, P. K. Patterson, and W. R. Dorrance. 1956. Clinical and serological response of man to immunization with attenuated dengue and yellow fever viruses. J. Immunol. 77: 352–364.

Scientific Committee on Interference. 1962. Effect of interferon on vaccination in volunteers. Lancet i: 873–874.

Taylor, C. E. 1953. Interference between influenza and equine encephalitis viruses in tissue culture. J. Immunol. 71: 125–133.

Vainio, T., R. Gwatkin, and H. Koprowski. 1961. Production of interferon by brains of genetically resistant and susceptible mice infected with West Nile virus. Virology 14: 385–387.

Vilček, J. 1960a. Interference between tick-borne encephalitis and Western equine encephalomyelitis viruses in chick embryo tissue cultures. Acta Virol. 4: 308–310.

Vilček, J. 1960b. An interferon-like substance released from tick-borne encephalitis virus-infected chick embryo fibroblast cells. Nature 187: 73–74.

Vilček, J. 1961. Studies on an interferon from tick-borne encephalitis virus-infected cells (IF). I. Appearance of IF in infected chick embryo cell cultures. Acta Virol. 5: 278–282.

Vilček, J. 1962a. Studies on interferon from tick-borne encephalitis virus-infected cells (IF). IV. Comparison of IF with interferon from influenza virus-infected cells. Acta Virol. 6: 144–150.

Vilček, J. 1962b. Interferon from tick-borne encephalitis virus-infected cells. Biological Works, Slovak Acad. Sci., Bratislava (in Slovak).

Vilček, J., and B. Rada. 1962. Studies on an interferon from tick-borne encephalitis virus-infected cells (IF). III. Antiviral action of IF. Acta Virol. 6: 9–16.

Vilches, A., and G. E. Hirst. 1947. Interference between neurotropic and other unrelated viruses. J. Immunol. 57: 125–140.

Wagner, R. R. 1960. Viral interference: Some considerations of basic mechanisms and their potential relationship to host resistance. Bacteriol. Rev. 24: 151–166.

Wagner, R. R. 1961. Biological studies of interferon. I. Suppression of cellular infection with Eastern equine encephalomyelitis virus. Virology *13*: 323–337.

Žemla, J., and J. Vilček. 1961a. Studies on an interferon from tick-borne encephalitis virus-infected cells (IF). II. Physical and chemical properties of IF. Acta Virol. *5*: 367–372.

Žemla, J., and J. Vilček. 1961b. Concentration and partial purification of an interferon. Acta Virol. *5*: 129.

Žemla, J., and Š. Schramek. 1962a. The action of interferon under anaerobic conditions. Virology *16*: 204–205.

Žemla, J., and Š. Schramek. 1962b. Notes on the effect of interferon on the metabolism of chick embryo cells. Acta Virol. *6*: 275–277.

INTERFERENCE PHENOMENA OBSERVED IN THE FIELD*

JOHN P. FOX

Division of Epidemiology
Public Health Research Institute of the City of New York, Inc.
New York, U.S.A.

INTERFERENCE generally has been viewed as the dominance of one virus over one or more other viruses competing for cellular sites of multiplication which, in the intact host, may be localized in certain tissues or be disseminated widely in the whole organism. Such dominance may result in prevention, inhibition, or complete suppression of infection with the dominated viruses. Systematic study of the mechanisms involved, most notably interferon, has led to important additional concepts of the nature of interference phenomena. Although such systematic study has been of laboratory nature, interference phenomena obviously can and do occur under field conditions. I shall consider here some of the available evidence for this and attempt to assess the influence of interference on the occurrence and course of viral infection and disease in man.

A first step is to define, in the light of existing theory (1, 2), the types of interference phenomena that may occur under field conditions. In general, these may derive from competition between naturally occurring (wild) viruses, between wild and vaccine viruses, or between two or more vaccine viruses, particularly when competition is for the same cellular sites of multiplication. Although that virus first established usually will dominate, its domination is transient and may decrease in authority as infection subsides. The fact that inactivated or even incomplete virus (1) can induce interference suggests that non-multiplying viral vaccines may afford brief protection against heterotypic viral infection. Finally, we must also consider the possible roles of interferon, already largely suggested by Dr. Isaacs. Not only may interferon be employed as an agent for the prophylaxis or treatment of viral infections, but that produced *in vivo* in response to infection may play an important role in the termination of infection (3). Also, naturally occurring interferon, transported in the blood, may mediate interference between viruses which multiply in widely separated tissue sites such as the lung and the central nervous system (4).

Let us also recall that competition between viruses does not always result in interference. Henle (1) has cited numerous instances of dual infections

*Previously unpublished observations described in this review are based on work supported by Grant A1-03340 funded by the National Institute for Allergy and Infectious Diseases, United States Public Health Service, Bethesda, Maryland.

observed in the laboratory, and I shall cite additional observations in man. Indeed, as occurs with group A Coxsackie (C) and polioviruses (5, 6), a dual infection may result in enhancement of disease, the very reverse of interference.

Finally, definitive demonstration of interference under field conditions is most difficult. The occurrence or non-occurrence of infection and disease are determined by a host of variables which hardly need be enumerated here. Hence, the rigorous demonstration of interference requires strictly comparable observations of the occurrence and course of infections in the presence and in the absence of conditions favoring interference. This requirement is rarely fulfilled by data describing entirely naturally occurring infection and disease.

COMPLETELY NATURAL PHENOMENA

Characteristic disease has been, until the present decade, the only widely available indicator of specific viral infection. Since few viruses produce pathognomonic disease, opportunities for demonstrating interference solely on the basis of disease have been limited. Measles, mumps, and chicken pox should provide examples since they often occur concurrently in the same population segment. However, in open populations the real frequency of dual disease is not known and the expected frequency cannot be estimated because reliable morbidity data do not exist. The nearly concurrent evolution in one child of measles and mumps or chicken pox is seen occasionally in Bellevue Hospital, for example, particularly in children from shelters experiencing concurrent outbreaks (7). While study of such institutional episodes might well be rewarding, I have not encountered relevant reports.

The possible epidemiologic importance of interference as reflected by characteristic disease has intrigued many workers but especially Frederiksen. Following Sabin's report (8) that dengue interferes with yellow fever in monkeys and possibly in mosquitoes, Frederiksen (9) undertook an historical review of their occurrence and concluded that they do not coexist freely. He also drew Dalldorf's attention (10) to the fact that poliomyelitis or Bornholm's disease but never both were epidemic in Denmark in eighteen of twenty-five consecutive years. More recently Frederiksen (11) has noted the inverse relation between influenza A and B in the United States during the period 1948–60, a pattern which now extends to include the 1961–62 season. Since these viruses are not related immunologically but do share season and mode of transmission, he feels strongly that interference may be the determining factor.

Because clinical manifestations are typically non-specific, study of the occurrence of respiratory disease is relevant to interference only when diagnostic laboratory data are obtained. Stille *et al.* (12) determined by sero-diagnosis the frequencies with which adenoviruses (72 per cent), influenza A (3 per cent) and influenza B (6 per cent) were associated with

826 respiratory illnesses among naval recruits in 1958–60. They demonstrated triple infections in 5 and dual infections in 48 illnesses, whereas the calculated expected frequencies were 1 and 52, respectively. Including the triple infections, influenza A and B occurred together 6 times versus 1.4 expected, and a review of relevant published data indicated that, when influenza A coincided in time and place with influenza B or C, dual infections occurred as often as expected. However, more naval recruits with multiple infections required hospitalization than expected. The findings of Stille et al. suggest that, contrary to Frederiksen's belief, infections with influenza A, B, and C and other unrelated respiratory viruses occur independently and that, when mixed infections occur, enhancement of illness rather than a sparing effect may result. However, interference among respiratory viruses may occur on occasion. McClelland et al. (13), in describing an outbreak caused by respiratory syncytial (RS) virus, comment that waves of specific infection commonly do not alter the seasonal pattern of respiratory illness, possibly because a particular virus such as RS gains temporary dominance owing to interference.

Well-documented data regarding enterovirus disease and infections have become most abundant in recent years and have provided quite divergent observations in respect to the interrelation of C viruses and polioviruses. The first group A strains were recovered in 1948 from two children with paralytic disease attributable in retrospect to type 1 poliovirus (P1) (14). Shortly thereafter Melnick et al. (15) found, in studying 47 patients paralyzed in the 1949 outbreak in Easton, Pa., that 64 per cent were shedding group A viruses chiefly (A1) although P1 virus was recovered from 75 per cent. These data suggest that, rather than interfere, C viruses of group A may enhance disease response to poliovirus infection.

With C viruses of group B, a different pattern emerges. Dalldorf (10, 16), in addition to noting the reluctance of Bornholm's disease or pleurodynia and poliomyelitis to be epidemic in the same year, cites evidence suggesting that the substantial occurrence of group B infections is typically associated with a delayed peak in the seasonal occurrence of paralytic poliomyelitis. Recently, Domok and Molnar (17) studied a Hungarian nursery in which a case of paralytic disease had occurred. Although both B2 and P1 viruses were present, only the latter which predominated initially was observed to spread. These data together do suggest some degree of mutual exclusion between polio and C viruses of group B. However, viruses of these two groups can infect one person concurrently, a fact supported by a partial check of my own Louisiana data which reveals 5 such coincidences among 12 dual enterovirus infections in healthy persons.

The inferences as to the interrelation of polio and C viruses drawn from field observations receive substantial support from experimental studies in mice and monkeys (5, 6, 18). Whereas group B viruses appear to exert a sparing effect, group A viruses, if active, tend to enhance the poliovirus disease.

With respect to the poliovirus group itself, Dalldorf (10) suggests that the common tendency for one type to predominate during epidemics is an expression of mutual antagonism or interference. This suggestion, however, is open to serious question. A single poliovirus is but one of many similar enteroviruses, several of which commonly circulate concurrently in any given community, and there seems little reason to expect a special order of antagonism within the small poliovirus group. In our study of the natural occurrence of poliovirus infections in Louisiana (19, 20, 21) we concluded that the predominant type in any given year apparently was determined largely by deficiency in homotypic immunity among children under four years of age.

Epidemiologic studies of enterovirus excretion rather than disease provide additional opportunities to observe naturally occurring interference. Gelfand (22), noting the frequent concurrent multiplicity of enteroviruses and their sharing of season and mode of transmission, suggested that in high risk groups the chances of dual infection should be good. Reviewing isolations from 4,500 specimens collected from 115 young Louisiana children during 1954–56, he noted that of the 610 virus positive specimens (14 per cent), only 3 were shown to contain two viruses as compared with 90 expected. He drew no conclusions because he recognized important technical difficulties in detecting a second virus. First, 128 specimens contained viruses not then identifiable, an unknown proportion of which may have represented dual infections including at least one virus for which typing antiserum was not available (23). Secondly, not only may a second virus have been present in lesser amount or been less adaptable to monkey kidney (MK) cell cultures, but its propagation may have been suppressed non-specifically by antibody to MK cells in the rabbit antisera used to restrain the virus first detected (24, 25). I may add also that the estimated expectancy of dual isolations depended on independence of the individual specimens, an assumption not justified since each child contributed repeated specimens.

In brief summary, available data for completely natural infections include a number of situations in which interference may have operated. They also include definite examples of the failure of interference as illustrated by the demonstration of numerous individual instances of concurrent multiple infections, in some of which there may have been enhancement of disease rather than the sparing associated with interference.

INTERFERENCE IN RELATION TO VIRAL VACCINES

While non-multiplying viral vaccines presumably could stimulate interferon production, demonstrable effect probably would require repeated inoculations which, among accepted vaccine regimens, are given only in Pasteur Treatment. Available relevant data derive only from observations with new-type rabies vaccines in which minor illnesses among vaccine and placebo groups did not differ significantly (26). Also possibly analogous is the undocumented effectiveness of repeated bi-weekly use of vaccinia to combat recurrent herpes.

Live virus vaccines induce infection of appreciable duration which might well prevent or modify the course of disease due to heterotypic viruses. Extensive placebo-controlled trials with special attention to immediately occurring illness have been conducted with various vaccines including yellow fever (17D strain) (27), typhus (strain E of *R. prowazeki*) (28), and Enders' measles vaccine (with gamma globulin) (29). In each instance the vaccinated groups experienced an excess of disease which on statistical grounds was clearly attributable to the vaccine and which served to obscure any possible interference with disease due to heterotypic agents. Immunizing infections with yellow fever vaccine, furthermore, certainly did not always interfere with serum hepatitis virus which was present in many lots of vaccine (30).

Somewhat more specific efforts have been made to determine the influence of live poliovirus vaccines on heterotypic disease. Monotypic P2 vaccine was employed in Singapore and in Hull, England, to combat outbreaks of P1 disease. Published data relate only to Singapore (25, 31) where vaccine was given over a 7-week period to 198,000 children. A week-by-week analysis (32) indicates that vaccinees experienced 8 cases in the first 8 days as compared with 10 expected and only 5 thereafter whereas 39 would have been expected. While no vaccinated cases developed in the 9–19 day interval when, it is suggested, interference should be most evident, the reduced occurrence after day 19 must be attributed in part at least to cross-immunity between P1 and P2 viruses.

On May 5 and 6, 1962, the Health Insurance Plan of Greater New York (HIP) offered Sabin P1 vaccine to its members. Dr. Lila Elveback and I exploited this occasion by ascertaining the recorded frequencies of illness of undetermined but possibly viral causation during each week in May among 4,200 vaccinated and 5,500 unvaccinated children under nine years of age served by two large HIP medical groups (Montefiore and East Nassau). As some measure of normal difference in usage of medical services by the vaccinated and unvaccinated groups, we also determined the recorded frequencies of non-viral illnesses attended and other services rendered. Our findings can be stated very briefly. First, as expected, vaccinated children generally sought more medical care than the unvaccinated. Second, vaccination did not obviously depress the occurrence of "possibly viral" illness. Finally, vaccinated children in the week after feeding experienced a slight excess of respiratory illness, possibly attributable to the vaccine.

We turn now to evidence relating to infection rather than disease and begin with competition between vaccine strains of poliovirus. Among the Lederle strains P3 is dominant (33), whereas P2 is the most aggressive of the Sabin strains (34). The dominance of the Sabin P2 strain is well illustrated by Shirman (35) who fed monotypic vaccines in the order types

1, 2, and 3 with one-week intervals. Not only did P2 usually prevent subsequent infection with P3, but it often suppressed already established P1 infections. Although Horstmann *et al.* (36) observed excellent response to both P2 and P3 when fed as a divalent vaccine, all available evidence indicates that a single feeding of trivalent vaccine cannot be relied upon for satisfactory immunization of triple negative individuals.

The importance of the prevention of immunizing infection with vaccine polioviruses by wild enteroviruses may have been overemphasized. While pre-existing enterovirus infections have been reported to block up to 50 per cent of vaccine strain infections (37, 38), this is not the usual experience. In community groups in Louisiana P3 vaccine infected 17 of 20 (85 per cent) children with a pre-existing infection as compared with 81 of 93 (87 per cent) with no other infection detected (39). In Cleveland pre-existing ECHO (E) type 14 infection prevented P1 vaccine infection in only 1 of 10 nursery infants, and another began shedding both viruses simultaneously (40). Drozdof and Shirman (41) fed P1 vaccine to a group of young children in Estonia, many of whom were already excreting wild P2 virus. In general, P1 infection took over when the fecal titer of P2 was low but was blocked if the P2 titer was 10^4 per gram or higher. Low P2 titers were assumed to reflect infections that had just begun or were past their peak. Thus, existing evidence would suggest that, except when unusually prevalent, wild enteroviruses will not interfere greatly with vaccination. Further, Sabin *et al.* (42) have demonstrated that satisfactory immunization can be achieved in areas of high enterovirus prevalence by mass feeding of two doses of trivalent vaccine.

Limitation of spread of vaccine polioviruses by wild enteroviruses represents another facet of interest. As discussed elsewhere (39), a number of factors exert a significant influence on the spread of Sabin vaccine strains. Hence, estimation of limitation of spread can be attempted only under carefully controlled conditions. In the Cleveland nursery episode of 1960 a high prevalence of E14 virus did not prevent spread of the P1 vaccine strain to 20 or 30 contacts (40). Perhaps more relevant are data from studies of vaccine spread in households and in communities in Louisiana (39). In the household studies, vaccine was fed to a single susceptible family member and the spread to other members was observed. Patterns in individual households could be found to illustrate both spread and failure of spread in the presence of a wild virus. In the aggregate, among 56 families studied, slightly more spread occurred among susceptible child contacts harboring a wild virus in the week after vaccination (32 per cent) than among those apparently free of other infection (26 per cent). In the community studies, all children in 25 families received P3 vaccine and in 26 control families all received a placebo. Fecal specimens were collected twice weekly for 11 weeks from both groups. Review of the original data reveals that, of 96 placebo-fed children, 71 excreted a wild virus at some time and 30 (42 per cent) of these also shed the P3 vaccine strain; in contrast, only 3 (12 per cent) P3 infections were detected among the remaining 25 children. These data, thus, indicate that the same children tended to acquire both vaccine and wild virus infections. Since these children also were characterized by young age, immunologic susceptibility and poor personal hygiene apparently exerted more influence on virus spread than did interference. The only possible indication of interference observed was the frequent abrupt replacement of one virus, wild or vaccine, by another in serially collected specimens.

Finally, vaccine polioviruses do influence infection with wild viruses. Not only may the vaccine virus replace an established wild virus but it also affords brief protection against new wild virus infections. Thus, in the Louisiana communities (39) during the first two weeks after feeding, wild viruses invaded 7 placebo families but only 1 of those fed vaccine. Similarly, in Singapore (25) examinations within four weeks of vaccination revealed wild viruses in 12.9 per cent of 464 controls but in only 3.6 per cent of 469 vaccinated children. Finally, as shown in Toluca, Mexico (42), and in Hungary (43), really mass vaccination temporarily displaces wild viruses in the community at large.

PHENOMENA BASED ON INTERFERON

I already have reviewed the negative evidence for transient protection against heterotypic disease which might result from interferon produced *in vivo* after administration of viral vaccines. Indeed, limited efforts so far made to demonstrate interferon production in man have been unsuccessful. These include the study of lung material from 11 fatal cases of influenzal pneumonia (44) and of nasal secretions from common colds (45). However, Gresser (46) does report interferon production *in vitro* by freshly collected human leucocytes stimulated by measles or Sendai viruses.

If theory as suggested by Isaacs (3) and by Horsfall (47) be accepted, the most common natural phenomenon dependent on interferon is recovery from viral infection. Distinctly more controversial is the suggestion (48) that the developing ability of embryos to produce and respond to interferon explains why maternal rubella induces congenital defects only in the first trimester.

Finally, there is the exciting possibility that interferon derived from non-host sources can be used in preventing or treating infection. The preliminary data regarding prevention of vaccinia takes (49) and treatment of vaccinial keratitis (50) are highly encouraging. Hopefully, we shall hear much more about this in the future.

DISCUSSION AND SUMMARY

I have tried in the foregoing to anticipate the manifestations of interference that may both occur and be susceptible to detection under field conditions and to present selected observations which provide some measure of the influence of interference on human infection and disease.

I have ignored at least two types of well-studied phenomena. High multiplicity of infection (47, 51) or an infecting inoculum overburdened with non-infective virus (1) may result in limited development of infection or "auto interference." This phenomenon probably does not occur naturally but does suggest that excessive doses of live virus vaccines should be avoided. In rhesus monkeys, for example, viremia and antibody response were inversely proportional to the dose of yellow fever vaccine given (52). A second phenomenon is persistent infection which, *in vitro*, seems to depend on interferon (2). Although persistent infections with viruses and rickettsiae *in vivo* are well known, their dependence on interference is not yet clear.

The most certainly demonstrated results of competition between naturally occurring viruses illustrate failure of interference. Multiple infections definitely occur, sometimes with the frequency expected in the absence of interference, and may result in enhancement of disease rather than the sparing associated with interference. Although the completely natural occurrence of interference must be conceded, its conclusive demonstration is virtually impossible, and I personally doubt that it is a factor of major epidemiologic importance. As Henle (1) has emphasized, the occurrence of interference in the laboratory depends on rather exacting conditions which, one may surmise, do not always pertain in the field. Furthermore, when they do, the resulting resistance is short lived and, if periodic re-exposure to a second virus be postulated, immunologic susceptibility must be the dominant factor.

The foregoing conclusion is supported by the frequent concurrent presence and spread of multiple, potentially competing viruses in human populations. It is further supported by statistical theory. My colleague, Dr. Elveback, has explored the influence of interference on the basis of simple models of concurrent outbreaks in closed populations in which one infection was postulated to afford during its full course complete resistance to heterotypic infection (53). In the extreme and presumably rare case, well-established virus A could temporarily so reduce the number susceptible to virus B that, if introduced during this short period, the latter would be unable to spread. However, under any conditions permitting virus B to become established, the effects of interference would be minor. As an example, an 8-week outbreak might be prolonged to 10 or 11 weeks and the total cases reduced by from 2 to 5 per cent.

Interference is potentially more important to live virus vaccines. Although vaccine infections may induce transient protection against heterotypic wild viruses, prevention of immunization because of wild viruses is of greater concern. This concern, however, probably has been overly stressed in relation to poliovirus vaccines at least. More important in this case is interference between vaccine strains which prohibits reliance on administration of a single dose of trivalent vaccine.

Despite my devaluation of the importance of interference to the natural occurrence of human infection and disease, knowledge of interference has potentially great implications for the future. These are largely spelled out at present in the name interferon. However, interference also provides a tool for the assay and study of viruses such as rubella (54) whose presence can be detected only indirectly.

REFERENCES

1. Henle, W. 1950. Interference phenomena between animal viruses: A review. J. Immunol. *64*: 203–236.
2. Wagner, R. R. 1960. Viral interference: Some considerations of basic mechanisms and their potential relationship to host resistance. Bacteriol. Rev. *24*: 151–166.
3. Isaacs, A., and G. Hitchcock. 1960. Role of interferon in recovery from virus infections. Lancet, July 9: 69–71.
4. Hitchcock, G., and A. Isaacs. 1960. Protection of mice against the lethal action of an encephalitis virus. Brit. Med. J. *2*: 1268–1270.
5. Dalldorf, G., and H. Weigand. 1958. Poliomyelitis as a complex infection. J. Exptl. Med. *108*: 605–616.
6. Stanley, N. F. 1952. Attempts to demonstrate interference between Coxsackie and poliomyelitic viruses in mice and monkeys. Proc. Soc. Exptl. Biol. Med. *81*: 430–433.
7. Krugman, S. Personal communication.
8. Sabin, A. B. 1952. Research on dengue during World War II. Am. J. Trop. Med. Hyg. *1*: 30–50.
9. Frederiksen, H. 1955. Historical evidence for interference between dengue and yellow fever. Am. J. Trop. Med. Hyg. *4*: 483–491.
10. Dalldorf, G. 1961. A great experiment. Yale J. Biol. Med. *34* (3,4): 234–238.
11. Frederiksen, H. 1961. Epidemiological significance of the interference phenomenon. Am. J. Trop. Med. Hyg. *10*(2): 271–272.
12. Stille, W. T., W. Pierce, and Y. E. Crawford. 1961. Multiple infections in acute respiratory illness. I. Severity of illness of naval recruits and independence of infectious agents. J. Inf. Dis. *109*: 158–165.
13. McClelland, L., M. R. Hilleman, V. V. Hamparian, A. Ketler, C. M. Reilly, D. Cornfeld, and J. Stokes, Jr. 1961. Studies of acute respiratory illnesses caused by respiratory syncytial virus. II. Epidemiology and assessment of importance. New Eng. J. Med. *264*: 1169–1175.
14. Dalldorf, G. 1952. From *Clostridium welchii* to the Coxsackie viruses: Changing microbiology. J. Mt. Sinai Hosp. *19*: 396–410.
15. Melnick, J. L., A. S. Kaplan, E. Zabin, G. Contreras, and N. W. Larkum. 1951. An epidemic of paralytic poliomyelitis characterized by dual infections with poliomyelitis and Coxsackie viruses. J. Exptl. Med. *94*(6): 471–492.
16. Dalldorf, G., and R. Albrecht. 1955. Chronologic association of poliomyelitis and Coxsackie virus infections. Proc. Nat. Acad. Sci. (U.S.) *41*: 978–982.
17. Domok, I., and E. Molnar. 1961. Enterovirus studies in connection with the 1959 poliomyelitis epidemic in Hungary. Acta Microbiol. *8*(2): 189–203.
18. Dalldorf, G. 1951. The sparing effect of Coxsackie virus infection on experimental poliomyelitis. J. Exptl. Med. *94*(1): 65–71.
19. Fox, J. P., H. M. Gelfand, D. R. LeBlanc, and D. P. Conwell. 1957. Studies

on the development of natural immunity to poliomyelitis in Louisiana. I. Overall plan, methods and observations as to patterns of sero-immunity in the study group. Am. J. Hyg. 65: 344–366.

20. Gelfand, H. M., D. R. LeBlanc, J. P. Fox, and D. P. Conwell. 1957. Studies on the development of natural immunity to poliomyelitis in Louisiana. II. Description and analysis of episodes of infection observed in study group households. Am. J. Hyg. 65: 367–385.

21. Potash, L., H. Gelfand, and J. P. Fox. 1960. Studies on the development of natural immunity to poliomyelitis in Louisiana. VI. The incidence of polio-virus infections during 1958 as an indication of the effect of Salk type vaccine on virus dissemination. Am. J. Hyg. 71(3): 418–426.

22. Gelfand, H. M. 1961. The occurrence in nature of the Coxsackie and ECHO viruses. Progr. Med. Virol. 3: 193–244.

23. Gelfand, H. M. 1959. The incidence of certain endemic enteric virus infections in southern Louisiana. South. Med. J. 52 (7): 819–827.

24. Habel, K. 1958. The effect of anticellular sera on virus multiplication in tissue culture. Virology 5: 7–29.

25. Hale, J. H., L. H. Lee, and P. S. Gardner. 1961. Interference patterns encountered when using attenuated poliovirus vaccines. Brit. Med. J. Sept. 16: 728–732.

26. Schwab, M. P., J. P. Fox, D. P. Conwell, and T. A. Robinson. 1954. Avianized rabies virus vaccination in man. Bull. Wld. Health Org. 10: 823–835.

27. Fox, J. P., E. H. Lennette, C. Manso, and J. R. S. Aguiar. 1942. Encephalitis in man following vaccination with 17D yellow fever virus. Am. J. Hyg. 36: 117–142.

28. Fox, J. P., J. A. Montoya, M. E. Jordan, and M. Espinosa. 1955. Immunization of man against epidemic typhus by infection with avirulent *Rickettsiae prowazeki* (Strain E). III. The serologic response and occurrence of post-vaccination reactions in groups of vaccinated under field conditions in Peru. Am. J. Hyg. 61: 183–196.

29. Stokes, J., Jr., R. Weibel, R. Halenda, C. M. Reilly, and M. R. Hilleman. 1962. Enders' live measles-virus vaccine with human immune globulin. Am. J. Dis. Child. 103: 366–372.

30. Fox, J. P., C. Manso, H. A. Penna, and M. Para. 1942. Observations of the occurrence of icterus in Brazil following vaccination against yellow fever. Am. J. Hyg. 36: 68–116.

31. Hale, J. H., M. Doraisingham, L. H. Lee, K. Kanagaratnam, K. W. Leong, and E. S. Monteiro. 1959. Large-scale use of Sabin type 2 attenuated poliovirus vaccine in Singapore during a type 1 poliomyelitis epidemic. Brit. Med. J. 5137: 1541–1549.

32. Knowelden, J., J. H. Hale, P. S. Gardner, and L. H. Lee. 1961. Measurement of the protective effect of attenuated poliovirus vaccine. Brit. Med. J. i: 1418–1420.

33. Cox, H. R., V. J. Cabasso, F. S. Markham, M. J. Moses, A. W. Moyer, M. Roca-Garcia, and J. M. Ruegsegger. 1959. Immunological response to trivalent oral poliomyelitis vaccine. Brit. Med. J. ii: 591–597.

34. Sabin, A. B. 1957. Properties and behavior of orally administered attenuated poliovirus vaccine. J. Am. Med. Assoc. 164: 1216–1223.

35. Shirman, G. A. 1961. Interaction of viruses in the intestinal tract of man. II. Interference between poliovirus vaccine strains. Acta Virologica 5(6): 359–366.

36. Horstmann, D. M., J. R. Paul, M. Godenne-McCrea, R. H. Green, E. M. Opton, A. I. Holtz, and J. C. Niederman. 1961. Immunization of preschool

children with oral poliovirus vaccine (Sabin). J. Am. Med. Assoc. *178*: 693–701.

37. Benyesh-Melnick, M., J. L. Melnick, and M. R. Alvarez. 1959. Poliomyelitis infection rate among Mexican children fed attenuated poliovirus vaccines. *In* Live poliovirus vaccines, PASB Pub. 44, pp. 272–285.

38. Ramos-Alvarez, M., F. G. Santos, L. R. Rivera, O. Mayes, L. Bustamante, S. Martin-Sosa, and A. G. Duran. 1960. Use of Sabin's live poliovirus vaccine in Mexico. Bol. med. Hosp. infant. (Mex.) *1*(3): 170–179.

39. Fox, J. P., H. M. Gelfand, D. R. LeBlanc, L. Potash, D. I. Clemmer, and D. Lapenta. 1960. The spread of vaccine strains of poliovirus in the household and in the community in southern Louisiana. *In* Poliomyelitis: Papers and discussions presented at the 5th Intl. Poliomyelitis Cong., Copenhagen, Denmark, pp. 368–383.

40. Ingram, V. G., M. L. Lepow, R. J. Warren, and F. C. Robbins. 1962. Behavior of Sabin type 1 attenuated poliovirus in an infant population infected with ECHO 14 virus. Pediatrics *29*(2): 174–180.

41. Drozdov, S. G., and G. A. Shirman. 1961. Interaction of viruses in the intestinal tract of man. I. Interference between wild and vaccine poliovirus strains. Acta Virol. *5*(4): 210–219.

42. Sabin, A. B., M. Ramos-Alvarez, J. Alvarez-Amezquita, W. Pelon, R. H. Michaels, I. Spigland, M. A. Koch, J. M. Barnes, and J. S. Rhim. 1960. Live, orally given poliovirus vaccine: Effects of rapid mass immunization on population under conditions of massive enteric infection with other viruses. J. Am. Med. Assoc. *173*: 1521–1526.

43. Domok, I., E. Molnar, and A. Jancso. 1961. Virus excretion after mass vaccination with attenuated polioviruses in Hungary. Brit. Med. J. *i*: 1410–1417.

44. Baron, S., and A. Isaacs. 1962. Absence of interferon in lungs from fatal cases of influenza. Lancet *i*: 18–20.

45. Tyrrell, D. A. J. 1962. Personal communication.

46. Gresser, I. 1961. Production of interferon by suspensions of human leucocytes. Proc. Soc. Exptl. Biol. Med. *108*: 799–803.

47. Horsfall, F. L., Jr. 1961. Factors contributing to recovery from viral diseases. Can. Med. Assoc. J. *84*: 1221–1226.

48. Isaacs, A., and Baron, S. 1960. Antiviral action of interferon in embryonic cells. Lancet, Oct. 29: 946–947.

49. A Report to the Medical Research Council from the Scientific Committee on Interferon. Effect of interferon on vaccination in volunteers. 1962. Lancet *i*: 873–875.

50. Jones, B. R., J. E. K. Galbraith, and M. K. Al-Hussaini. 1962. Vaccinial keratitis treated with interferon. Lancet *i*: 875–878.

51. Wagner, R. R., and A. H. Levy. 1960. Interferon as a chemical intermediary in viral interference. Ann. N.Y. Acad. Sci. *88*(5): 1308–1318.

52. Fox, J. P., and H. A. Penna. 1943. Behavior of 17D yellow fever virus in Rhesus monkeys: Relation to substrain, dose and neural or extraneural inoculation. Am. J. Hyg. *38*: 152–172.

53. Elveback, L. To be published.

54. Parkman, P. D., M. S. Artenstein, J. McCown, and E. L. Buescher. 1962. Characteristics of an agent recovered from recruits with rubella. Fed. Proc. *21*: 466.

SYMPOSIUM IX

DEMONSTRATION OF VIRUSES IN NEOPLASIA

Chairman: A. B. SABIN

FRANK L. HORSFALL

Role of Infectious Agents in the Pathogenesis of Neoplasia

W. BERNHARD

Les Problèmes de la mise en évidence de virus oncogènes
au microscope électronique

GEORGE KLEIN

Genetic Aspects of the Relationship Between Viruses and Tumors

CHAIRMAN'S REMARKS

A. B. SABIN

The Children's Hospital Research Foundation
University of Cincinnati
Cincinnati, Ohio, U.S.A.

ONE OF THE MOST INTRIGUING QUESTIONS in microbiology and medical science today is whether or not human cancers are caused by viruses. Up to the present time, there is no evidence that any human cancer is caused by a virus. There are, however, at least three important reasons for pursuing the viral hypothesis of human cancer: the first is that several *spontaneously occurring* cancers of lower animals have been shown to be caused by viruses and it seems unlikely that human beings would be an exception; the second is that two viruses which are harmless under natural conditions and which are not known to be the cause of any spontaneous tumors—the polyoma virus of mice and the vacuolating virus of rhesus monkeys—can under very special experimental conditions produce cancers after injection in certain newborn or very young animals; and the third reason is that two "human" adenoviruses not known to be associated with any particular disease have in recent months also been shown to produce cancers after injection in newborn hamsters. We are faced with the intriguing enigma that the viruses that have been proved to be the cause of naturally occurring mammalian cancers, like the mammary carcinoma and the leukemias of mice, are highly species-specific and thus far have resisted all attempts at identification by tissue culture methods, so that the procedures by which they have been discovered cannot be used in the study of human cancer. On the other hand, the experimentally oncogenic viruses which are most readily detected by tissue culture methods, like the polyoma virus of mice and the vacuolating virus of monkeys, are not known to cause any naturally occurring tumors, and when the polyoma virus has been isolated from spontaneous mouse cancers, the tumors actually had another cause, as, for example, the Gross leukemia virus. Moreover, the experimental studies with polyoma virus have shown that a virus can cause a cancer and then seemingly disappear from the subsequent generations of malignant cells.

We are therefore faced with great dilemmas in our attempts to demonstrate the role of viruses in human cancer. This is the reason that the title of our symposium is: "Demonstration of Viruses in Neoplasia." We are fortunate that Drs. Horsfall, Bernhard, and Klein, who are well known for their synthetic as well as analytic capabilities, have consented critically to evaluate and synthesize our present knowledge about viruses in neoplasia and thereby provide some indication of the possible approaches to studies on the role of viruses in human cancer.

ROLE OF INFECTIOUS AGENTS IN THE PATHOGENESIS OF NEOPLASIA

FRANK L. HORSFALL, JR.

Sloan-Kettering Institute for Cancer Research
New York, New York, U.S.A.

THIS COMMUNICATION was to have been prepared and presented by the late Dr. Jerome T. Syverton. His sudden and untimely death in January, 1961, at the early age of 53 made this commendable plan of the program committee impossible of fulfilment. It is both an honor and a privilege to have been invited to develop the subject that was assigned to my friend of many years before his tragic death. I have been happy to accept this invitation because of my admiration for the vigor, enthusiasm and imagination with which Dr. Syverton approached the numerous problems which aroused his curiosity, because of my wish to offer tribute to the memory of an outstanding and original investigator and also because from numerous discussions with him through the years I am confident that our views on the subject that now confronts us were not dissimilar in any significant way.

Although the title of this communication makes it feasible to consider the role of all types of infectious agents in the pathogenesis of neoplasia, this symposium is aimed primarily at a broad consideration of the relation of one variety of such agents to tumors. In consequence, I shall confine my comments to the smallest of known infectious agents, the viruses, and the infective chemical components that can be separated from them, the viral nucleic acids. At the outset it needs to be pointed out that it may be desirable for purposes of analogy and illustration to draw on findings broadly scattered throughout the viral field and to consider as possibly related to the problems before us facts which have been established with certain viruses that are not known to have any direct relation to the neoplastic alteration. So too as regards the nucleic acids and their biological activities which, although designated as infective when the substances are derived from viral particles, are not commonly referred to in this manner when transformation of bacterial characters is under consideration. And yet these formally similar activities, as well as those ascribed to the nucleic acids of temperate phages, may each have some usefulness for purposes of analogy and illustration in clarifying the role of viruses, as it is seen at present, in the pathogenesis of neoplasia.

It has been a long time since 1911 and the first unequivocal demonstration (1) that a solid tumor could be induced by an infectious agent, now generally designated Rous sarcoma virus. As Rous himself indicated recently in an unpublished lecture, the state of the art bearing on the understanding of neoplasia was not ready for this pioneering discovery at the time it was made. Cancer was a disease of unknown cause and therefore, by definition, the tumors induced by the chicken sarcoma agent could not be cancers. It was generally held and almost universally believed that cancer could not be, and in fact was not, in any way related to an infectious process. On grounds which are now even more difficult to understand, the agent was not generally accepted as a virus until many years had passed, despite the fact that Rous had demonstrated clearly that cell-free filtrates retained the capacity to induce typical sarcomas (2). Thus, the discovery that a virus could induce the various cell alterations that lead to the development of a malignant neoplasm represented a wholly new concept of the etiology of cancer which was opposed vigorously by many and considered as a serious possibility by only a very few.

From 1911 through 1914, Rous and his associates published a number of now classical papers "on the causation by filterable agents of . . . chicken tumors" (3). Not only the original sarcoma, but also an osteo chondro-sarcoma and a sarcoma of intracanalicular pattern, were shown to be inducible by such agents. Transmission to the developing chicken embryo, even with cell-free filtrates, was demonstrated and so it was shown for the first time that a virus could be propagated in this useful immature host (4). Developing, newborn or suckling animals were not employed widely in the study of virus-induced tumors until more than twenty-five years had passed; not until the milk agent of mice had been discovered by the late Dr. John J. Bittner (5) and the first leukemia virus of mice had been found by Gross (6). Rous (7) showed that there were two kinds of resistance to the fowl tumors, one of which was directed against the preformed and implanted tumor cells as such, while the other was directed against the filterable agent itself. In addition, and how modern this now seems, he showed that ultraviolet light rapidly killed the cells of the transplantable sarcoma without affecting the filterable etiological agent significantly (7). Studies of the agents that induced three histologically distinct types of fowl sarcomas revealed that these viruses were of about the same size and possessed similar properties (3). Thus was discovered a new group of viruses which induce in fowl malignant neoplasms of diverse character and the beginning of the long pursuit of the relation of viruses to cancer was at hand.

Some well-known investigators who have devoted themselves to the study of sarcomas of chickens and the Rous sarcoma virus have indicated that it is not easy to ask questions to which at least part of the answers were not already available as a result of the extensive and penetrating early investigations of Rous and his associates.

As has happened so often when a new and quite unexpected concept emerges, a long incubation period followed this pioneering work. Relatively little further study was directed toward the first cancer-inducing viruses for almost two decades although Andrewes (8) and a few other pioneers kept the small flame of interest burning. In the book on *Filterable Viruses* (9), edited by the late Dr. Thomas M. Rivers, which appeared in 1928, there are only a few references to the Rous sarcoma virus. Most extensive among these are the brief comments of Carrel concerning the alterations induced in macrophages in culture by the virus. Because latent or dormant viruses and their activation by non-specific stimuli, such as the injection of normal tissue suspensions or certain chemicals, were not then recognized, the production of tumors by such means and the finding that they contained the Rous virus served more to confuse than to clarify the problem.

The discoveries by Shope (10) of the fibroma virus of rabbits in 1932 and of the papilloma virus (11) in 1933 served to bring the incubation period to an end and it was soon accepted widely that viruses could in fact induce true tumors, even though benign, in a mammalian host. Although early experiments on the transmission of human warts by cell-free filtrates had been confirmed (12) in 1919, little attention or interest was aroused by these reports.

Only one year after the discovery of the Shope papilloma virus, Rous and Beard (13) reported that carcinomatous changes sometimes developed in papillomas induced by this agent. Moreover, they presented evidence that this mammalian tumor was an "autonomous new growth, purposeless, parasitic, and, on occasion, progressive" (14). In 1935, they described the progression to cancer of virus-induced rabbit papillomas which had been under observation for more than six months (15). Such cancers became markedly anaplastic, metastases were frequent and the tumors were transplantable ultimately to suckling rabbits (16). It was concluded that "the virus that gives rise to the rabbit papillomas must be looked upon as the primary cause of the cancers developing therefrom" (15).

In experiments with chemical carcinogens, such as methylcholanthrene and tar, Rous and his co-workers showed that the chemical agents acted to accelerate the development of the malignant alterations initiated by the virus (17). In fact, long-continued tarring of the skin led, on intravenous injection of the virus, to the development of primary cancers which were malignant from the first (18). The late Dr. Francisco Duran-Reynals ultimately carried the enhancement of viral effects by chemical compounds much further and demonstrated that certain classical virulent viruses, such as fowl pox, could be associated with the development of tumors under these special conditions (19).

With the transplantable cancer, which had originated eight years previously from a virus papilloma in a domestic rabbit, 22 successive transfers during a period of 3½ years continued to show evidence of viral antigen as indicated by the development of active immunity to and antibodies against the Shope virus (20). As is now well known, such evidence for the presence of the agent could not be obtained after the 46th serial transplant although there was no discernible change in the character of the cancer (20). As

Shope (21) has stated: "the carcinoma has run through a complete cycle from virus-induced papilloma to carcinoma that is apparently virus-induced, and finally on to carcinoma with which no recognizable virus can be identified. It has thus come to resemble the classical malignant tumors in that it now no longer gives any recognizable sign of the nature of its actuating cause." It should be emphasized that this is neither unique nor any longer surprising. Syverton and his associates (22) showed that cancers deriving from virus-induced papillomas in wild cottontail rabbits also fail to yield evidence of the presence of the intact infective agent. As Shope (23) has stressed recently, tumors induced by Rous sarcoma virus in turkeys, polyoma virus in hamsters or papilloma virus in domestic rabbits all fail to yield infective viral particles in the usual tests. These findings are analogous to those with bacteria which have been altered by temperate phages. Infective phage particles or even phage antigens cannot be demonstrated directly until the prophage is activated by non-specific stimuli and viral reproduction is initiated. In this connection, the recent demonstration by Ito and Evans (24) that infective viral DNA can be obtained from rabbit papillomas devoid of viral infectivity is of special interest.

From 1936 to the present time, new information about cancer-inducing viruses has become available at a progressively increasing rate until now some thirty different viruses capable of initiating the development of cancer have been reported (25). Among the outstanding accomplishments during these sixteen years were the discovery of the milk agent of mice by Bittner (5) in 1936, the identification of certain viruses of the avian leukosis complex by Hall and his associates (26) in 1941, and the discovery of the first leukemia virus of mice by Gross (6) in 1951. During the last five years discoveries in this field have tumbled one over another with the demonstration of several other leukemia viruses of mice by Friend (27) in 1957 and Moloney (28) in 1960, the identification of polyoma virus by Stewart and her associates (29) in 1957, and the recent indications that simian virus 40 of monkeys (30) as well as adenovirus (31), type 12 and possibly type 18, can induce tumors in hamsters. The very recent finding (32) that SV40 can induce changes in human cells in culture may be of considerable importance. The tumor-inducing capacity of DNA separated from polyoma virus was demonstrated in 1959 by di Mayorca and his co-workers (33), and that from Shope papilloma virus in 1961 by Ito (34). This year, the tumor-inducing capacity of RNA separated from erythroblastosis virus was reported by Lacour and Harel (35), and that from a mouse leukemia virus by Moloney (36). Friend and her associates (37) have recently discovered a new virus capable of inducing lymphomas in mice.

There appears now to be wide agreement that the following facts have been demonstrated beyond any reasonable doubt. Certain viruses can initiate the cancerous alteration in animal cells growing separately from the intact host and therefore, except for their genetic composition, wholly removed from host influences. It appears, however, that such changes in cultured cells have not yet been demonstrated decisively with either radiation or chemical compounds, the other major categories of factors that are believed to be capable of inducing cancer. Many viruses can incite the development of a number of different types of cancer, either as solid tumors or as diffuse forms in various animal species which include amphibian, avian and numerous mammalian hosts. Some viruses induce cancers most readily when inoculated into newborn or very young animals. Others can induce cancers even when they are introduced into adult animals. One virus, avian lymphomatosis, can be transmitted through the eggs of infected but normal-appearing hens and can lead to neoplastic disease when the chicks mature. Another virus, the Bittner agent, is transmitted through the milk of infected but normal-appearing mice and can induce cancer in breeding female offspring. Several viruses are capable of initiating the development of several forms of cancer in the same host species and one, polyoma, can induce as many as twenty different varieties of cancer in mice.

There are, in biochemical terms, only two kinds of cancer-inducing viruses: those with nucleic acid cores of the RNA type and those with such cores of the DNA type. RNA-containing viruses include, apparently, all of the avian sarcoma-leukosis agents and several of the mouse leukemia agents. As was stated earlier, two viruses in the RNA group have been found recently to yield infective nucleic acids capable of initiating the development of tumors. DNA-containing viruses include Shope papilloma and polyoma, both of which have yielded infective nucleic acids capable of inciting the development of tumors in the intact animal host.

The cancer-inducing viruses are closely comparable to many other members of the large family of viruses as regards their size, form, composition and growth cycle. At present, there does not seem to be any valid basis for thinking of them as a distinct and separate group. Most of these agents have been shown to be capable of initiating infections which do not lead to the development of cancer. With the exception of the avian leukosis agents, it appears that natural infection with a virus potentially capable of inducing tumors does not commonly result in the development of cancer. The investigator himself appears to play an important role in this field and can markedly increase the probability that a given virus will induce cancer by establishing highly artificial experimental conditions.

Certain of these viruses produce specific immune reactions in their hosts, but several, particularly the mouse milk agent and some of the mouse leukemia viruses, are very poor antigens. The Friend leukemia virus has been shown to yield a viral vaccine that is moderately effective in preventing the development of leukemia in mice when the same agent is inoculated (38). Much additional work remains to be done on vaccines of this kind and on immune reactions to tumors.

Tumor-inducing viruses, like the other agents in this large family, are the smallest of known infective agents, with dimensions which are best expressed in Angstrom units. They represent the smallest biological entities which possess the major attributes of living matter including, most importantly, a genetic apparatus that guides and controls their heritable characters. In terms of present knowledge, viruses, whether inducing cell necrosis or proliferation, whether virulent or oncogenic, may be considered as vehicles for the trasmission of infective nucleic acid; to be specialized organelles for the introduction of new genetic material into host cells (39).

This concept places viruses as a group in a unique category unlike that of any other infective agents. Their properties are not strictly comparable to those of other biological phenomena in which the transfer of genetic material from one cell to another is well known, as in the case of fertilization of ova by sperm, transformation of bacterial characters by deoxyribonucleic acid, or transduction of bacterial properties by phage. Viruses appear to represent natural mutational factors, which, while having no life of their own when separate from cells, lead host cells, once they have gained entry, to make new materials and to manifest properties which normally such cells would not have. Among the large number of alterations that viruses can induce in host cells those that do not kill the cells but persist and endure are of most interest.

Cell necrosis or suicide resulting from the processes that lead to viral reproduction is a common phenomenon and serves to provide an explanation for many of the features of the classical viral diseases such as yellow fever, poliomyelitis and the numerous encephalitides. But this would be a dead-end phenomenon if the virus were incapable of finding other susceptible host cells in which to initiate still further destructive cycles. Through death of the host or recovery, about the mechanism of which there is still much to be learned (40), the infective process ultimately ceases to be of consequence and an equilibrium between host and virus may develop which, in the surviving host, often leads to specific immunity to reinfection.

With the tumor-inducing viruses, as too with temperate phages, a very different relationship between altered host cell and inciting agent appears commonly to develop. This is especially evident with the DNA-containing viruses, which have been most exhaustively studied, and appears to be characterized in the majority of host cells by disappearance of the virus as an intact infective agent and the emergence of new properties on the part of the host cell (41). The alterations in the properties of the cells, which may take many different forms, tend not to lead to their destruction as with the virulent viruses, and the daughter cells which are produced on growth and division faithfully show the same new features as the altered parent cells. There appears to be a provocative analogy between the effects of some temperate phages on their bacterial hosts and the effects of certain tumor-inducing viruses on animal cells. In both instances the altered host cells produce more cells with like properties without the need for any further infection by the inciting virus. In contrast to the single-cycle potentially dead-end relationship between virulent viruses and host cells in which continuation of the process is dependent on successive infection of new host cells at each reproductive cycle, a persistent and enduring relationship between viral components and host cells appears to be established which is not dependent on further infection and is perpetuated, as in the case of classical mutations, by cell division.

With the virulent viruses, those which induce the many well-known acute viral diseases, a single effective association between one viral particle and one host cell can in theory lead ultimately to the destruction of innumerable host cells through infection of other host cells by new virus particles in an expanding series. This is, of course, the basis on which the plaque technique for counting infective viral particles was developed with phages and later adapted by Dulbecco (42) for the same purpose to several animal viruses. In sharp contrast, with certain tumor-inducing viruses as with temperate phages, a single effective association between one viral particle and one host cell can in theory lead ultimately to the production of innumerable host cells with new properties simply by the usual process of cell growth and division. Under laboratory conditions, such altered cells may retain their new properties indefinitely and on continuous cultivation constantly produce new cells of the same kind. Like cancer cells which arise from undetermined causes, those which result from the effects of certain viruses also continue to produce daughter cells with neoplastic features on cultivation. As with classical mutations these new properties appear to be heritable from parent cells to daughter cells. If the animal host does not possess effective means for reacting to and disposing of such altered cells and they reproduce in sufficient number, a tumor containing them may develop. If it is uncontrolled in growth and invasive, such a tumor is designated as malignant and may lead ultimately to the destruction of the host organism.

As a concluding comment, it seems appropriate to emphasize that the discovery of cancer-inducing viruses in animals has not been a simple task. To accumulate decisive and convincing evidence of their relation to the development of cancers has been still more difficult. Although such agents have not yet been shown to be associated with the initiation of cancer in man, it will be surprising indeed if closely similar tumors are found ultimately to have dissimilar incitants merely because they arise in different mammalian hosts.

REFERENCES

1. Rous, P. 1911. A sarcoma of the fowl transmissible by an agent separable from the tumor cell. J. Exptl. Med. *13*: 397–411.
2. Rous, P. 1911. Transmission of a malignant new growth by means of a cell-free filtrate. J. Am. Med. Assoc. *56*: 198.
3. Rous, P., and J. B. Murphy. 1914. On the causation by filterable agents of three distinct chicken tumors. J. Exptl. Med. *19*: 52–69.

4. Rous, P., and J. B. Murphy. 1911. Tumor implantations in the developing embryo: Experiments with a transmissible sarcoma of the fowl. J. Am. Med. Assoc. *56*: 741–742.
5. Bittner, J. J. 1936. Some possible effects of nursing on the mammary gland tumor incidence in mice. Science *84*: 162.
6. Gross, L. 1951. "Spontaneous" leukemia developing in C3H mice following inoculation, in infancy, with Ak-leukemic extracts, or Ak-embryos. Proc. Soc. Exptl. Biol. Med. *76*: 27–32.
7. Rous, P. 1913. Resistance to a tumor-producing agent as distinct from resistance to the implanted tumor cells: Observations with a sarcoma of the fowl. J. Exptl. Med. *18*: 416–427.
8. Andrewes, C. H. 1932. Some properties of immune sera active against fowl-tumor viruses. J. Path. Bact. *35*: 243–249.
9. Rivers, T. M. (ed.). 1928. Filterable viruses. Williams and Wilkins, Baltimore.
10. Shope, R. E. 1932. A filterable virus causing tumor-like condition in rabbits and its relationship to virus myxomatosum. J. Exptl. Med. *56*: 803–822.
11. Shope, R. E. 1933. Infectious papillomatosis of rabbits. J. Exptl. Med. *58*: 607–624.
12. Wile, U. J., and L. Kingery. 1919. The etiology of common warts: Their production in the second generation. J. Am. Med. Assoc., *73*: 970–973.
13. Rous, P., and J. W. Beard. 1934. Carcinomatous changes in virus-induced papillomas of the skin of the rabbit. Proc. Soc. Exptl. Biol. Med. *32*: 578–580.
14. Rous, P., and J. W. Beard. 1934. A virus-induced mammalian growth with the characters of a tumor (the Shope rabbit papilloma). III. Further characters of the growth: General discussion. J. Exptl. Med. *60*: 741–766.
15. Rous, P., and J. W. Beard. 1935. The progression to carcinoma of virus-induced rabbit papillomas (Shope). J. Exptl. Med. *62*: 523–548.
16. Smith, W. E., J. G. Kidd and P. Rous. 1952. Experiments on the cause of the rabbit carcinomas derived from virus-induced papillomas. I. Propagation of several of the cancers in sucklings, with etiological tests. J. Exptl. Med. *95*: 299–318.
17. Rous, P., and W. F. Friedwald. 1944. The effect of chemical carcinogens on virus-induced rabbit papillomas. J. Exptl. Med. *79*: 511–538.
18. Kidd, J. G., and P. Rous. 1938. The carcinogenic effect of a papilloma virus on the tarred skin of rabbits. II. Major factors determining the phenomenon: The manifold effects of tarring. J. Exptl. Med. *68*: 529–562.
19. Duran-Reynals, F. 1956. Realities and hypotheses of viral infection as a cause of cancer. Rev. can. de Biol. *14*: 411–428.
20. Rous, P., J. G. Kidd and W. E. Smith. 1952. Experiments on the cause of the rabbit carcinomas derived from virus-induced papillomas. II. Loss by the Vx2 carcinoma of the power to immunize hosts against the papilloma virus. J. Exptl. Med. *96*: 159–174.
21. Shope, R. E. Personal communication.
22. Syverton, J. T., H. E. Dascomb, E. B. Wells, J. Koomen, Jr., and G. P. Berry. 1950. The virus-induced papilloma-to-carcinoma sequence. II. Carcinomas in the natural host, the cottontail rabbit. Cancer Res. *10*: 440–444.
23. Shope, R. E. 1962. Are animal tumor viruses always virus-like? J. Gen. Physiol. *45*: 143–154.
24. Ito. Y., and C. A. Evans. 1961. Induction of tumors in domestic rabbits with nucleic acid preparations from partially purified Shope papilloma virus

and from extracts of papillomas of domestic and cottontail rabbits. J. Exptl. Med. *114*: 485–500.

25. Gross, L. 1961. Oncogenic viruses. Pergamon Press, New York.
26. Hall, W. J., C. W. Bean and M. Pollard. 1941. Transmission of fowl leucosis through chick embryos and young chicks. Am. J. Vet. Res. *2*: 272–279.
27. Friend, C. 1957. Cell-free transmission in adult Swiss mice of a disease having the character of a leukemia. J. Exptl. Med. *105*: 307–318.
28. Moloney, J. B. 1960. Biological studies on a lymphoid leukemia virus extracted from sarcoma 37. I. Origin and introductory investigations. J. Nat. Cancer Inst. *24*: 933–951.
29. Stewart, S. E., B. E. Eddy, A. M. Gochenour, N. G. Borgese and G. E. Grubbs. 1957. The induction of neoplasms with a substance released from mouse tumors by tissue culture. Virology *3*: 380–400.
30. Eddy, B. E. 1962. Tumor induction by a virus from monkey kidney. *In* Perspectives in virology, vol. III. Burgess Press, Minneapolis.
31. Trentin, J. J., Y. Yabe and G. Taylor. 1962. Tumor induction in hamsters by human adenovirus. Proc. Am. Assoc. Cancer Res. *3*: 369.
32. Shein, H. M., and J. F. Enders. 1962. Transformation induced by simian virus 40 in human renal cell cultures. I. Morphology and growth characteristics. Proc. Nat. Acad. Sci. (U.S.) *48*: 1164–1172.
33. di Mayorca, G. A., B. E. Eddy, S. E. Stewart, W. S. Hunter, C. Friend and A. Bendich. 1959. Isolation of infectious deoxyribonucleic acid from SE polyoma-infected tissue cultures. Proc. Nat. Acad. Sci. (U.S.) *45*: 1805–1808.
34. Ito, Y. 1960. A tumor-producing factor extracted by phenol from papillomatous tissue (Shope) of cottontail rabbits. Virology *12*: 596–601.
35. Lacour, F., and J. Harel. 1962. Lésions néoplasiques provoquées chez le poulet par l'acide ribonucléique extrait de tissus leucémiques (erythroblastose aviaire). Compt. rend. des séances de l'Acad. des Sci. *254*: 4231–4232.
36. Moloney, J. B. 1962. Presented at VIII International Cancer Congress, Moscow, U.S.S.R.
37. Friend, C., E. de Harven and J. Haddad. 1962. Presented at VIII International Cancer Congress, Moscow, U.S.S.R.
38. Friend, C. 1959. Immunological relationships of a filterable agent causing leukemia in adult mice. J. Exptl. Med. *109*: 217–228.
39. Horsfall, F. L., Jr. 1960. Viral infection and viral disease in man. Proc. Mayo Clin. *35*: 269–282.
40. Horsfall, F. L., Jr. 1961. Factors contributing to recovery from viral diseases. Can. Med. Assoc. J. *84*: 1221–1226.
41. Dulbecco, R., and M. Vogt. 1960. Significance of continued virus production in tissue cultures rendered neoplastic by polyoma virus. Proc. Nat. Acad. Sci. (U.S.) *46*: 1617–1623.
42. Dulbecco, R. 1952. Production of plaques in monolayer tissue cultures by single particles of an animal virus. Proc. Nat. Acad. Sci. (U.S.) *38*: 747–752.

LES PROBLÈMES DE LA MISE EN ÉVIDENCE DE VIRUS ONCOGÈNES AU MICROSCOPE ÉLECTRONIQUE

W. BERNHARD

Institut de Recherches sur le Cancer
Villejuif, Seine, France

LE DESTIN de la théorie virale du cancer est étrange. Enoncée au début du siècle par Borrel, microbiologiste pastorien, elle ne fut ensuite défendue que par quelques rares pathologistes et biologistes contre l'opinion de la grande majorité des bactériologistes et virologistes. Depuis peu d'années les tumeurs à virus sont à nouveau travaillées avec le plus grand succès par des chercheurs issus de la Microbiologie. Les recherches expérimentales de la dernière décennie ont permis d'établir un grand nombre de faits nouveaux. Elles ont même apporté quelques découvertes qui ont réussi à convaincre leurs plus critiques adversaires du bien-fondé des idées de quelques chercheurs solitaires. Il existe au moins une trentaine de tumeurs à virus connues chez l'animal et il serait étonnant que l'Homme, seul, échappât totalement à l'action de ces agents alors que l'on trouve des virus oncogènes chez de nombreuses espèces, des poissons jusqu'aux singes. *Mais pourquoi n'a-t-il pas été possible jusqu'ici de prouver indiscutablement l'origine virale au moins de certaines tumeurs ou leucémies humaines ?*

Afin de pouvoir répondre à cette question, nous passerons d'abord brièvement en revue les méthodes biologiques employées pour la mise en évidence d'agents oncogènes chez l'animal avant d'insister plus particulièrement sur le rôle joué par la microscopie électronique. Puis, nous essayerons d'évaluer les chances d'une détection éventuelle de virus oncogènes chez l'Homme. Enfin, nous évoquerons brièvement le problème de la carcinogénèse virale, qui nous semble dominer à l'heure actuelle la virologie du cancer et intéresse, au plus haut point, le microscopiste électronicien.

I. LA DÉTECTION DE VIRUS CANCÉRIGÈNES CHEZ L'ANIMAL

(a) Le rôle des souches pures

On ne saurait trop souligner l'importance de la génétique dans les découvertes de virus cancérigènes chez l'animal et, plus particulièrement, chez la souris. L'histoire de la mise en évidence du facteur lacté par Bittner chez des souris A et C3H en fournit l'exemple le plus célèbre. Comment aurait-on pu purifier cet agent sans l'incidence très élevée de tumeurs dans une souche donnée, et l'identifier au microscope électronique si l'on avait dû se baser sur des tumeurs mammaires spontanées de souris génétiquement impures et sans données épidémiologiques précises ? Un deuxième exemple est la découverte par Ludwik Gross en 1951 de la transmissibilité par filtrat de la leucémie de souris. Elle ne fut possible que grâce à l'emploi de souches à incidence leucémique élevée, AK et C58, qui furent les donneurs de virus, les souches C3H et C57 étant les receveuses particulièrement susceptibles à l'agent leucémique. Enfin, il ne faut pas oublier que la découverte du virus du Polyome est intimement liée à celle du virus leucémique de Gross (1953). La mise en évidence de tous ces agents aurait été impensable sans ce travail de sélection génétique préalable.

(b) L'utilisation des animaux nouveau-nés

Duran-Reynals (1942) avait déjà observé que le passage du virus de Rous aux canards n'était possible que s'il employait des cannetons après l'éclosion. Ludwik Gross (1951) a pu montrer la filtrabilité de la leucémie de souris grâce à l'injection de filtrats leucémiques à des souriceaux âgés de quelques heures. Tous les autres travaux sur des virus oncogènes consécutifs à ceux de Ludwik Gross se basent ainsi sur l'emploi d'animaux nouveau-nés ou très jeunes avec un système de défense immunitaire absent ou faible, et donc particulièrement sensibles à l'action d'agents oncogènes. C'est grâce aux passages répétés des virus leucémiques sur des souriceaux que leur virulence fut augmentée et leur étude au microscope électronique ne devint fructueuse qu'après cette étape.

(c) Le rôle de la culture de tissu

La microscopie électronique a bénéficié depuis environ une demi-douzaine d'années de l'emploi de cette technique en virologie du cancer. La culture *in vitro* du virus de Rous selon la technique proposée par Rubin (1957), Rubin et Temin (1958) a permis l'étude du cycle évolutif de cet agent (Haguenau et coll., 1960). La culture du fibrome de Shope (Febvre, et coll., 1957), des virus myélo- et erythroblastiques (Bonar et coll., 1959; Heine et coll., 1961; Beard, 1962) a également éclairci beaucoup de problèmes concernant la formation de ces particules virales. La culture *in vitro* du virus du polyome de la souris (Stewart et coll., 1958), et du virus SV40 du singe découvert par Sweet et Hilleman (1960) furent particulièrement riches de conséquences pour la microscopie électronique. La recherche directe de ces agents dans les tumeurs qu'ils induisent aurait été à peu près sans espoir. Il fallait d'abord les démasquer dans un système cellulaire susceptible où ils apparaissent alors en énorme quantité. Il y a encore quelques années, on opposait l'action cytostimulante des virus cancérigènes au pouvoir cytolytique de certains virus classiques. Les travaux de Stewart et coll. (1958, 1959), puis de l'école de Toronto (voir Ham et coll., 1961), établissant que suivant le système choisi, le même virus oncogène peut être soit cytostimulant, soit cytolytique (« incorporé » ou « non incorporé », selon Dulbecco (1961)), fut une véritable révélation pour les cancérologues.

Une découverte importante sur laquelle nous reviendrons plus loin, est la transformation *in vitro* de cellules embryonnaires normales en cellules malignes par l'action du virus du polyome, réussie pour la première fois par Vogt et Dulbecco (1960), puis confirmée par les travaux de Sachs (1961) et de ses collaborateurs, Stoker (1961) et Negroni (1961). Voici des cellules tumorales dont la malignité a été induite *in vitro* par un virus qui lui-même disparaît ensuite totalement sans laisser de traces, tout au moins de traces décelables avec nos méthodes actuelles (Dulbecco, 1961). Des résultats semblables ont été rapportés sur la transformation de fibroblastes de poulet en cellules sarcomateuses par le virus de Rous (Prince, 1960). Ces observations ont une valeur théorique considérable dans la recherche sur l'origine virale des tumeurs humaines et pourraient expliquer l'échec enregistré ici par la microscopie électronique.

(d) L'utilisation du hamster pour révéler l'action cancérigène d'un virus

Il n'y a que fort peu de temps que le hamster est utilisé dans le domaine de la virologie du cancer. L'étude d'Eddy et coll. (1958) avait déjà prouvé qu'il était facile d'induire des tumeurs diverses chez cet animal par le virus du polyome de la souris. Plus récemment, le hamster fut à nouveau utilisé pour révéler l'action cancérigène de virus provenant d'espèces éloignées. Le virus vacuolisant SV40, virus latent chez le macaque, y provoque des sarcomes très malins (Eddy et coll. 1961; Girardi et coll. 1962) et l'adénovirus type 12 de l'Homme y déclenche la croissance rapide de tumeurs malignes, également sarcomateuses, quelques semaines après l'infection (Trentin et coll. 1962). Ce système détecteur si sensible va donc intéresser tous ceux et notamment les microscopistes électroniciens, qui s'efforcent de révéler des virus oncogènes éventuels dans des tissus humains.

(e) Le rôle de la microscopie électronique

Nous insisterons plus longuement sur l'emploi de cet instrument dans la détection de virus oncogènes. Le moment semble propice pour définir plus exactement le rôle de cette technique en virologie du cancer. Son importance a été soit surestimée, soit sous-estimée dans le passé et il est donc nécessaire de connaître les avantages et les limites de la seule méthode permettant la mise en évidence directe de virus oncogènes. *Il ne saurait être question de dissocier les faits ainsi acquis de leur contexte biologique. Bien au contraire, la microscopie électronique ne peut donner le maximum de renseignements que si elle est intégrée dans l'expérimentation cancérologique.* Que ceux qui jugent les contributions morphologiques négligeables en virologie consultent la revue d'Oberling et Guérin sur les virus oncogènes parue en 1954. Il y a huit ans seulement, ces auteurs étaient encore obligés de défendre sur des pages entières leur point de vue, peu partagé à ce moment-là, selon lequel les virus oncogènes seraient des virus véritables et non des plasmagènes ou autres particules hypothétiques d'origine endogène. Il y a peu de temps enfin, Peyton Rous (1959) a dû élever vigoureusement la voix contre la théorie de la mutation somatique qui, par l'esprit fataliste qui l'inspire, a fait tant de mal en cancérologie expérimentale.

La mise en évidence au microscope électronique de la presque totalité des virus oncogènes connus a contribué d'une manière décisive à démontrer qu'il n'existe pas de barrière entre virus classiques et virus cancérigènes et que ces agents ont une morphologie si caractéristique qu'il est impossible de les confondre avec des structures cellulaires normales. La microscopie électronique a ainsi créé une base morphologique solide pour l'expérimentation biologique qui était d'autant plus nécessaire que les recherches s'attaquent de plus en plus aux systèmes cellulaires plutôt qu'à l'organisme, et nécessitent ainsi une connaissance approfondie des ultrastructures allant jusqu'à l'échelle moléculaire. Des mises au point sur ce sujet ont déjà été publiées à plusieurs reprises (Bernhard, 1960, 1963; Amano, 1961; Dmochowski, 1960), voir aussi le livre de Dalton et Haguenau (1962). Nous n'insisterons donc pas sur l'anatomie ultrastructurale des différentes particules ni sur la grande variété de leurs cycles évolutifs. Mais de ces recherches entreprises dans de nombreux laboratoires on peut dégager certains problèmes susceptibles de nous intéresser plus particulièrement ici.

1. *Quelle est la fréquence des particules virales visibles dans des tumeurs d'origine virale connue ?* La réponse varie suivant la tumeur étudiée mais dans la plupart des cas, cette recherche s'avère longue et difficile. Les difficultés sont d'abord inhérentes à la méthode employée dans tous les laboratoires : celles des coupes ultrafines. Une coupe ultrafine ne montre qu'une partie infime de la masse cellulaire, et par conséquent, nous avons peu de chances de tomber sur des virus si ceux-ci ne sont pas répartis d'une manière homogène, par plusieurs milliers, dans toute la cellule. D'autre part, on connaît depuis longtemps de nombreux exemples de tumeurs à virus qui ne libèrent que fort peu de particules virales ou cessent même totalement d'en produire : Sarcome de Rous (Rous & Murphy, 1914; Bryan et coll., 1955); Polyome (Rowe et coll., 1960; Habel & Silverberg, 1960). Le cas classique est celui d'une tumeur dérivée du papillome de Shope qui peut totalement cesser la production de virus infectieux, et plus tard, même de l'antigène viral (Kidd & Rous, 1940; Rous et coll., 1952). Les examens de ces tissus tumoraux au microscope électronique restent négatifs. Shope (1962) a récemment insisté sur ce fait en prenant comme principal exemple le papillome de Shope bénin dans lequel il est impossible de mettre en évidence des virus complets ou des antigènes viraux dans la couche proliférative de la tumeur. Les particules détectables apparaissent seulement dans la couche kérato-hyaline biologiquement morte (Noyes & Mellors, 1957). Cet auteur conclut que dans certaines tumeurs, bénignes ou malignes, dont l'origine virale est sûre, l'agent qui entretient la croissance tumorale n'est plus « virus-like », c'est-à-dire, peut perdre son caractère physique de virus complet. Or, si ces agents ne subsistent que sous forme d'acide nucléique

intimement lié aux structures cellulaires de l'hôte, comment sera-t-il possible d'en trouver la trace morphologique ?

Rien ne prouve que nous ne nous trouvons pas dans une situation semblable quand nous examinons — sans résultat — des tumeurs humaines. Même dans des tumeurs expérimentales qui restent constamment filtrables, comme les lymphomes des souris AK et C58, et dans la leucémie de Friend, on ne peut mettre en évidence des particules que dans la moitié des cas environ (Bernhard & Guérin, 1958; de Harven, 1962). Inversement, il existe des tumeurs mammaires chez des souris biologiquement « sans » facteur lait où l'on trouve des particules virales du type B (Bernhard et coll., 1955), dont l'identification avec le virus de Bittner semble prouvée (Moore et coll., 1959). Dans des tissus adénomateux prénéoplasiques de souris considérées comme dépourvues du facteur lacté, de Ome et ses collaborateurs, ont pu également montrer des particules virales. De Ome (1962) en conclut que ces particules visibles au microscope électronique ne seraient pas directement responsables des tumeurs mammaires de la souris, mais cette interprétation ne nous semble pas la seule possible.

Il faut à ce sujet rappeler l'étude de Benedetti (1957) sur la présence de nombreuses particules virales dans des embryons de poulets normaux. Cette observation nous troubla beaucoup à l'époque puisque nous utilisions ces tissus comme contrôles pour une étude sur l'érythroblastose et le Sarcome de Rous du poulet où nous venions de mettre en évidence exactement le même type morphologique de particules. On aurait pu conclure à la non-spécificité des particules présentes dans les tissus tumoraux, mais nous pensions déjà que le virus présent dans les contrôles serait un agent étroitement lié aux virus oncogènes du poulet, pouvant devenir oncogène à son tour, comme par exemple celui de la lymphomatose. Le travail de Friesen et Rubin (1961) en culture de tissu sur le virus RIF vient d'y ajouter un important argument.

Le cas idéal pour la détection de virus oncogènes au microscope électronique se présente seulement quand on peut cultiver l'agent *in vitro*, c'est-à-dire lorsque les cellules en culture possèdent un nombre beaucoup plus élevé de particules que les tumeurs. Dans les tumeurs spontanées autres que celles qui apparaissent avec une fréquence très élevée dans une souche pure (par exemple les tumeurs mammaires de la souris), il est par contre très difficile de découvrir des virus même si ces tumeurs sont d'origine virale.

2. *Est-il possible de déceler des lésions cellulaires induites par la présence d'un virus latent ?* Nous avons observé de temps à autre des lésions nucléaires dans des cellules tumorales, particulièrement dans des cellules hodgkiniennes ou dans des lymphosarcomes humains, qui ressemblent beaucoup à celles signalées à maintes reprises dans des infections virales classiques (Leplus et coll., 1961). Ces lésions sont caractérisées par l'apparition dans le nucleoplasme d'un ou de plusieurs corps denses. De plus, on peut voir des nucléoles anormaux présentant au contact du nucléolonema des

amas d'une substance granulaire. Des altérations semblables ont été obser-vées dans le molluscum contagiosum, le sarcome de Rous, la varicelle, l'ectromélie, l'infection par le virus EMC et surtout dans des phases précoces du cycle évolutif des virus du polyome et du SV40 (Granboulan et coll., 1963). Il n'est pas possible à l'heure actuelle de dire s'il s'agit là d'une simple analogie morphologique de lésions ayant une cause différente ou si, au contraire, les aspects anormaux des noyaux dans certaines tumeurs humaines, dont l'origine virale peut paraître probable, sont effectivement liés à une infection virale latente en rapport avec le processus tumoral, mais sans production de particules virales complètes. Les recherches de virus dans des tissus tumoraux de l'Homme ont été si décevantes jusqu'ici qu'il est nécessaire de tenir compte des moindres signes cytologiques soupçonnés de traduire une phase du cycle évolutif d'un virus hypothétique. Mais d'une part, ces signes n'ont été observés que rarement, d'autre part les processus de nécrobiose, très fréquents dans des tumeurs à croissance rapide, pour-raient éventuellement provoquer des altérations semblables dans la trame fine du nucleoplasme. Nous devons nous imposer une extrême prudence dans l'interprétation de ces phénomènes et nous garder d'en tirer des conclusions hâtives qui ne manqueraient pas de discréditer une méthode indispensable dans les recherches sur des tumeurs d'étiologie inconnue.

3. *Peut-on mettre en évidence des virus non oncogènes dans des tumeurs* ? Cette question a été posée à maintes reprises par tous les virolo-gistes qui savent que les virus se multiplient plus facilement dans des cellules dédifférenciées, et par conséquent dans les tissus cancéreux ana-plasiques qui peuvent offrir un terrain idéal pour toutes sortes de virus latents. Nous rappelons ici les travaux d'Alice Moore (1960) qui a utilisé des virus oncolytiques dans une tentative thérapeutique. Huebner (1962) et ses collaborateurs ont isolé des adénovirus à partir de tumeurs de la souris. Ainsi l'objection principale que l'on faisait aux microscopistes électroniciens était la présence possible, dans des tumeurs, de virus non-oncogènes ayant une morphologie semblable à celle des virus oncogènes. Mais au fur et à mesure que l'on progressait dans l'identification morphologique des virus en général, on s'apercevait que le danger de confondre des agents spéci-fiques et non spécifiques était relativement faible. On peut même prétendre que, dans la majorité des cas, la microscopie électronique a d'emblée pu identifier l'agent effectivement responsable de la croissance tumorale. A deux reprises seulement, on a photographié des virus n'ayant probablement aucun rapport avec la tumeur en question. Ce fut un réovirus de la souris, vu par Selby et coll. (1954), avant l'identification biologique de celui-ci, dans des cellules ascitiques d'Ehrlich. Puis, Bernhard et Granboulan (1961) ont trouvé dans des cellules d'un lymphosarcome de la souris l'agent thymique dé-crit par Rowe et Capps (1961). N'est-il-pas étonnant que des virus si répandus dans beaucoup d'élevages comme ceux de la chorioméningite lymphocytaire (LCM), et de l'ectromélie n'aient jamais été signalés dans des tumeurs de

la souris ? Nous avons depuis lors adopté la règle que, si des particules virales sont fréquemment associées à un tissu tumoral donné, il y a une très forte chance pour qu'elles représentent un virus du groupe oncogène plutôt qu'un virus latent non spécifique ; mais il est évident que seule l'expérimentation biologique sera susceptible de trancher cette question.

Toutefois, depuis l'importante observation faite par Trentin et collaborateurs sur le pouvoir cancérigène de l'adénovirus type 12 (1962) il sera difficile d'exclure qu'un virus du type classique et considéré jusqu'ici comme non-oncogène ne puisse être rendu responsable du déclenchement d'une croissance tumorale. Toutes les données classiques paraissent ainsi bouleversées. Dès lors, qui oserait encore affirmer qu'un adénovirus banal trouvé *par hasard* dans une tumeur n'a aucun rapport avec le processus cancéreux ? Qui s'aventurerait aujourd'hui à dire que l'action cancérigène ne restera liée qu'au type 12 de l'Adénovirus ? Tout dépendra du système détecteur choisi. Le morphologiste devra se borner à décrire le virus qui se trouve dans un tissu donné sans lui attribuer trop vite une étiquette. Il est ainsi amené à évaluer les chances qui lui restent pour détecter de nouveaux virus cancérigènes spécifiques d'une manière peu optimiste.

II. LES NOMBREUSES DIFFICULTÉS SUPPLÉMENTAIRES DE LA DÉTECTION DE VIRUS CANCÉRIGÈNES CHEZ L'HOMME

Comme le souligne Ludwik Gross (1961), l'un des plus grands obstacles d'une étude épidémiologique du cancer humain est le fait que nos observations renferment une période de vie toujours beaucoup trop courte, une à deux générations, plus rarement trois. Or, si l'on admet qu'un virus hypothétique suit la transmission verticale plutôt qu'horizontale, c'est-à-dire qu'il peut passer d'une génération à l'autre sans toutefois se manifester cliniquement dans chaque individu porteur, il sera toujours impossible de dresser une image épidémiologique comparable, même de loin, à ce qui a été fait chez l'animal. En cherchant un virus oncogène dans des tumeurs humaines variées on s'expose à des difficultés comparables à celles que l'on aurait rencontrées si l'on avait voulu détecter le virus de Bittner d'emblée chez des souris sauvages. L'existence du facteur lacté y a, en effet, été démontrée, mais seulement après une vingtaine d'années de recherches approfondies sur des souris C3H et d'autres lignées pures (Andervont & Dunn, 1956). Sans cette base de comparaison sûre, la découverte d'un virus mammotrope et oncogène chez la souris sauvage aurait été certainement vouée à l'échec.

L'expérimentation cancérologique chez l'Homme n'est possible que dans une mesure très limitée. Que l'on se rappelle le rôle que jouent actuellement les souriceaux et hamsters nouveau-nés dans le démasquage de virus oncogènes chez l'animal. Quel *système de détection* pouvons nous alors choisir pour l'Homme ? A en juger d'après les très nombreux résultats négatifs enregistrés par beaucoup de chercheurs qui, suivant les premiers résultats spectaculaires de Grace et coll. (1960) injectent des extraits de tumeurs humaines variées à des souriceaux nouveau-nés, il n'y a qu'une chance assez faible de révéler de cette manière des agents cancérigènes chez l'Homme. Toolan (1960) a pu isoler à partir de tissus cancéreux humains un virus de très petite taille après injection de filtrats à des hamsters (H₁ virus). Toutefois, ce virus semble être identique au K-virus du rat, et il n'a pas été possible jusqu'ici de prouver que cet agent, qui induit un mongolisme chez cet animal, ait une action cancérigène. La recherche de virus dans des tumeurs humaines par des *moyens immunologiques* peut être particulièrement difficile, sinon impossible, puisque nous savons que des tumeurs déclenchées chez l'animal peuvent perdre entièrement l'antigène viral. C'est, comme nous l'avons vu, le cas de certaines tumeurs dérivées du papillome de Shope et du polyome. Habel (1962) a montré que certaines tumeurs, où l'on ne décèle plus le virus du polyome qui les a déclenchées, contiennent un nouvel antigène différent de l'antigène viral. Si l'on peut démontrer que certaines tumeurs humaines ont acquis un nouvel antigène, comment prouvera-t-on que celui-ci est lié au passage d'un virus oncogène ?

Quant à la *culture de tissu*, depuis la mise en évidence du polyome, elle est quotidiennement employée dans un grand nombre de laboratoires pour détecter un effet cytopathogène provoqué éventuellement par des agents — cancérigènes ou non — présents dans des extraits de tumeurs humaines. Les quelques résultats publiés à ce sujet par Stewart et Irwin (1960) sont certes intéressants, mais n'ont pas eu de suite. Pouvons-nous d'ailleurs être sûrs qu'avec un système cellulaire choisi au hasard, un virus X provoquera nécessairement des lésions cellulaires, ou, s'il passe dans le surnageant, donnera obligatoirement des tumeurs chez la souris et le hamster ? Le cas du virus H₁ de Toolan (1960) peut servir de mise en garde.

Quant à la *microscopie électronique*, plusieurs résultats positifs ont été signalés pour des tumeurs humaines. Il ne fait pas de doute que Braunsteiner et coll. (1959) ont pu montrer quelques particules de type viral au contact de cellules leucémiques humaines. Dmochowski et coll. (1959) ont photographié quelques rares particules virales dans des ganglions lymphatiques de malades atteints de leucémies et de maladie de Hodgkin. Plus récemment, Sorensen (1961) a pu démontrer la présence de particules de type viral dans des vacuoles de cellules plasmocytaires d'une maladie de Kahler. Ces dernières images sont particulièrement impressionnantes. Que penser de ces observations qui sont restées rarissimes par rapport au grand nombre d'examens au microscope électronique de cellules tumorales humaines ? Il va de soi que ces travaux ne nous apportent aucune certitude sur la nature réelle de ces particules dont le caractère viral paraît probable, mais n'est pas absolument certain. L'interprétation d'images semblables doit donc être faite avec la plus grande prudence. Cependant, il ne faut pas non plus rejeter d'emblée des observations que l'on pourra interpréter seulement si l'on peut lier une activité biologique quelconque à la présence de ces particules.

III. L'IMPORTANCE DES RECHERCHES SUR LA CARCINOGÉNÈSE VIRALE IN VITRO

Après la découverte de Trentin et collaborateurs (1962), la recherche sur la cause virale possible de tumeurs humaines peut s'orienter selon une voie toute différente de celle choisie jusqu'ici. Si hier un microscopiste électronicien avait montré des adénovirus dans un ganglion leucémique, on aurait jugé cette observation banale ; dès lors, nous devons nous demander dans quelles conditions un virus considéré comme non-oncogène est susceptible de déclencher une croissance maligne. Plus le système que nous étudierons sera simple, plus nous aurons la chance de comprendre le mécanisme de la malignité. Après la transformation probablement maligne effectuée *in vitro* par le virus SV40 sur des cellules humaines (Koprowski et coll., 1962) on fera sans doute des tentatives pour transformer des cellules humaines *in vitro* par des adénovirus et d'autres virus humains. Si de tels essais devaient être couronnés de succès, nous pourrions alors espérer un éclaircissement rapide du phénomène de la carcinogénèse virale en général, et du déclenchement de la croissance tumorale chez l'Homme en particulier. Cependant, l'analyse des processus intimes qui se jouent à l'échelle moléculaire ne pourra se faire que si elle est basée sur l'emploi simultané des techniques les plus récentes de la biologie cellulaire et si le généticien, le biochimiste, le virologiste, l'immunologiste et le microscopiste électronicien arrivent à travailler ensemble en étroite collaboration. Quand nous connaîtrons aussi bien les phénomènes intracellulaires de la multiplication de virus cancérigènes que nous connaissons actuellement les mécanismes de l'infection des bactéries par les phages, nous aurons résolu l'essentiel du problème du cancer, à savoir la transformation maligne. A juste titre, Luria (1960), Dulbecco (1960) et Lwoff (1960) ont proposé aux cancérologues de s'inspirer du modèle bactérie-phage pour l'analyse de la cellule animale infectée par un virus oncogène. Il ne peut s'agir d'une analogie, mais plutôt d'un exemple méthodologique. Les travaux de Dulbecco et de ses collaborateurs illustrent parmi d'autres combien cette voie est fertile. La théorie virale aura surtout contribué à réduire ce problème à sa base la plus simple, donc la plus accessible à l'étude, *la cellule*. C'est là, à nos yeux, la véritable signification et le mérite historique de cette théorie. Où en serions-nous en génétique humaine, si les grandes lois de la génétique n'avaient pas été analysées d'abord chez Pisum ou chez Drosophila ?

Quand nous aurons à revenir plus tard à l'organisme, nous rencontrerons à nouveau les mêmes difficultés expérimentales qui nous semblent insurmontables aujourd'hui, mais qui se présenteront alors sous un angle entièrement nouveau. L'ubiquité de virus latents chez l'animal et chez l'Homme n'a plus besoin d'être prouvée. Le tout est de savoir ce que ces agents sont capables de faire au niveau des centres régulateurs de la vie cellulaire. L'ère de la détection de virus spécifiquement oncogènes n'est certes pas close, mais on peut prévoir que c'est l'étude de la cancérisation *in vitro* par ces agents qui attirera de plus en plus l'intérêt des chercheurs, car jamais auparavant ils n'ont pu utiliser des systèmes expérimentaux aussi nettement définis sur le plan génétique, biochimique et morphologique, entraînant une transformation maligne contrôlable en si peu de temps. La complexité du phénomène cancéreux reste énorme à l'échelle de l'organisme. Elle est très grande à l'échelle des tissus. Au niveau cellulaire cette complexité est considérablement réduite et devenue accessible à une analyse rationnelle dans laquelle le microscopiste électronicien peut et doit jouer son rôle.

REMERCIEMENTS

Nous tenons à remercier le Prof. agr. P. Tournier pour les suggestions qu'il nous a prodiguées lors de la rédaction de ce manuscrit. La Mutuelle Générale de l'Education Nationale nous a accordé son appui financier.

REFERENCES

Amano, S. 1961. Host-virus interrelationships in cancerogenesis as observed under the electron microscope. *In* Progress in experimental tumor research, *2*: 36–66. S. Karger, Basel.

Andervont, H. B., and T. B. Dunn. 1956. Studies on the mammary tumor agent carried by wild house mice. Acta Un. int. Cancr. *12*: 530–543.

Beard, J. W. 1962. Etiologic aspects of the avian leukemias. *In* Progress in Hematology, *3*: 105–135. Grune & Stratton.

Benedetti, E. L. 1957. Présence de corpuscules identiques à ceux du virus de l'érythroblastose aviaire chez l'embryon du poulet et des poussins normaux. Bull. Cancer *44*: 473–482.

Bernhard, W. 1960. The detection and study of tumor viruses with the electron microscope. Cancer Res. *20*: 712–727.

Bernhard, W. 1963. Some problems of fine structure in tumor cells. *In* Progress in experimental tumor research, *3*: 1–34. S. Karger, Basel.

Bernhard, W., and M. Guerin. 1958. Présence de particules d'aspect virusal dans les tissus tumoraux de souris atteintes de leucémie spontanée. Compt. rend. Acad. Sci. Paris *247*: 1802–1805.

Bernhard, W., and N. Granboulan. 1961. Morphology of oncogenic and non-oncogenic mouse viruses. *In* Ciba Foundation Symposium on tumour viruses of murine origin, ed. Wolstenholme and O'Connor, pp. 6–49.

Bernhard, W., M. Guerin and C. Oberling. 1955. Mise en évidence de corpuscules d'aspect virusal dans différentes souches de cancers mammaires de la souris. Acta Un. int. Cancr. *12*: 544–557.

Bonar, R. A., D. F. Parsons, G. S. Beaudreau, G. Becker and J. W. Beard. 1959. Ultrastructure of avian myeloblasts in tissue culture. J. Nat. Cancer Inst. *23*: 199–210.

Braunsteiner, H., K. Fellinger und F. Pakesch. 1959. Ueber die Anwesenheit virusähnlicher Einschlüsse in menschlichen leukämischen Geweben. Wiener Ztschr. f. inn. Med. *40*: 384–388.

Bryan, W. R., D. Calnan and J. B. Moloney. 1955. Biological studies on the Rous sarcoma virus. III. The recovery of virus from experimental tumors in relation to initiating dose. J. Nat. Cancer Inst. *16*: 317–335.

Dalton, A. J., and F. Haguenau (eds.). 1962. Tumors induced by viruses: Ultrastructural studies. Academic Press.

De Ome, K. B. 1962. The mouse mammary tumor virus. Fed. Proc. *21*: 15–18.

Dmochowski, L. 1960. Viruses and tumors in the light of electron microscope studies: A review. Cancer Res. *20*: 977–1015.

Dmochowski, L., C. E. Grey, J. A. Sykes, C. C. Shullenberger and C. D. Howe. 1959. Studies on submicroscopic structure of human leukemic tissues. Acta Un. int. Cancr. *15*: 768–778.

Dulbecco, R. A. 1960. A consideration of virus-host relationship in virus-induced neoplasia at the cellular level. Cancer Res. *20*: 751–761.

Dulbecco, R. A. 1961. Viral carcinogenesis. Cancer Res. *21*: 975–980.

Duran-Reynals, F. 1942. The reciprocal infection of ducks and chickens with tumor-inducing viruses. Cancer Res. *2*: 343–369.

Eddy, B. E., G. S. Borman, W. H. Berkeley and R. D. Young. 1961. Tumors induced in hamsters by injection of Rhesus monkey kidney cell extracts. Proc. Soc. Exptl. Biol. Med. *107*: 191–197.

Eddy, B. E., S. E. Stewart, R. Young and G. B. Mider. 1958. Neoplasms in hamsters induced by mouse tumor agent passed in tissue culture. J. Nat. Cancer Inst. *20*: 747–761.

Febvre, H. L., J. Harel et J. Arnoult. 1957. Observation, pendant la phase muette du développement intracellulaire du virus du fibrome de Shope, de corps d'inclusion diffus, sans virus corpusculaires, correspondant avec la présence d'un antigène soluble. Bull. Cancer *44*: 92–105.

Friesen, B., and H. Rubin. 1961. Some physicochemical and immunological properties of an avian leucosis virus (RIF). Virology *15*: 387–396.

Girardi, A. J., B. H. Sweet, V. B. Hotnick and M. R. Hilleman. 1962. Development of tumors in hamsters inoculated in the neonatal period with vacuolating virus SV$_{40}$. Proc. Soc. Exptl. Biol. Med. *109*: 649–660.

Grace, J. T., E. A. Mirand, D. T. Mount and R. Metzgar. 1960. Oncogenic properties of extracts of human tumors. Proc. Amer. Assoc. Cancer Res. *3*: 115.

Granboulan, N., P. Tournier, R. Wicker and W. Bernhard. 1963. An electron microscope study of the development of SV$_{40}$ virus. J. Cell. Biol. *17*: 423–441.

Gross, L. 1951. "Spontaneous" leukemia developing in C3H mice following inoculation, in infancy, with Ak-leukemic extracts, or Ak-embryos. Proc. Soc. Exptl. Biol. Med. *76*: 27–32.

Gross, L. 1953. A filterable agent, recovered from Ak-leukemic extracts, causing salivary gland carcinomas in C3H mice. Proc. Soc. Exptl. Biol. Med. *83*: 414–421.

Gross, L. 1961. Oncogenic viruses. Pergamon Press, New York.

Habel, K. 1962. Immunological determinants of polyoma virus oncogenesis. J. Exptl. Med. *115*: 181–193.

Habel, K., and R. J. Silverberg. 1960. Relationship of polyoma virus and tumor in vivo. Virology *12*: 463–476.

Haguenau, F., H. L. Febvre and J. Arnoult. 1960. Ultrastructural morphology of Rous sarcoma grown in vitro. *In* Perspectives in virology, vol. II, ed. M. Pollard, pp. 160–173. Burgess Press, Minneapolis.

Ham, H. W., E. A. McCulloch, L. Siminovitch, A. F. Howatson and A. A. Axelrad. 1961. The process of viral carcinogenesis in the hamster kidney with the polyoma virus. *In* Ciba Foundation Symposium, pp. 284–301.

Harven, E. de. 1962. Ultrastructural studies on three different types of mouse leukemia: A review. *In* Tumors induced by viruses, ed. A. J. Dalton and F. Haguenau. Academic Press, New York.

Heine, U., G. S. Beaudreau, C. Becker, D. Beard and J. W. Beard. 1961. Virus of avian erythroblastosis. VII. Ultrastructure of erythroblasts from the chicken and from tissue culture. J. Nat. Cancer Inst. *26*: 359–388.

Huebner, R. J. 1962. Communication personnelle.

Kidd, J. G., and P. Rous. 1940. A transplantable rabbit carcinoma originating in a virus-induced papilloma and containing the virus in masked or altered form. J. Exptl. Med. *71*: 813–837.

Koprowski, H., J. A. Ponten, F. Jensen, R. G. Ravdin, P. Moorhead and E. Saksela. 1962. Transformation of cultures of human tissue infected with simian virus 40. J. Cell. Comp. Physiol. *59*: 281–292.

Leplus, R., J. Debray, J. Pinet et W. Bernhard. 1961. Lésions nucléaires décélées au microscope électronique dans des cellules de "lymphomes malins" chez l'homme. Compt. rend. Acad. Sci. Paris. *253*: 2788–2790.

Luria, S. E. 1960. Viruses, cancer cells, and the genetic concept of virus infection. Cancer Res. *20*: 677–688.

Lwoff, A. 1960. Tumor viruses and the cancer problem: A summation of the conference. Cancer Res. *20*: 820–829.

Moore, D. H., E. Y. Lasfargues, M. R. Murray, C. D. Haagensen, and E. C. Pollard. 1959. Correlation of physical and biological properties of mouse mammary tumor agent. J. Biophys. Biochem. Cytol. *5*: 85–92.

Moore, A. E. 1960. The oncolytic viruses. *In* Progress in experimental tumor research, ed. Homburger, *1*: 411–439. S. Karger, Basel.

Negroni, G. 1961. The properties of Mill Hill Polyoma Virus (MHP). *In* Ciba Foundation Symposium on tumour viruses of murine origin, ed. Wolstenholme and O'Connor, pp. 332–364. London.

Noyes, W. F., and R. C. Mellors. 1957. Fluorescent antibody detection of the antigens of the Shope papilloma virus in papillomas of the wild and domestic rabbit. J. Exptl. Med. *106*: 555–562.

Oberling, C., and M. Guerin. 1954. The role of viruses in the production of cancer. *In* Advances in cancer research, *2*: 353–423. Academic Press. New York.

Prince, A. M. 1960. Quantitative studies on Rous sarcoma virus. VI. Clonal analysis of in vitro infection. Virology *11*: 400–424.

Rous, P. 1959. Surmise and fact on the nature of cancer. Nature *183*: 1357–1361.

Rous, P., J. G. Kidd and W. E. Smith. 1952. Experiments on the cause of the rabbit carcinomas derived from virus-induced papillomas. II. Loss by the Vx2 carcinoma of the power to immunize hosts against the papilloma virus. J. Exptl. Med. *96*: 159–174.

Rous, P., and J. B. Murphy. 1914. On the causation by filterable agents of three distinct chicken tumors. J. Exptl. Med. *19*: 52–69.

Rowe, W. P., and W. I. Capps. 1961. A new mouse virus causing necrosis of the thymus in newborn mice. J. Exptl. Med. *113*: 831–844.

Rowe, W. P., J. W. Hartley, J. D. Estes and R. J. Huebner. 1960. Growth curves of polyoma virus in mice and hamsters. *In* National Cancer Institute, Monograph 4, Symposia tumor viruses, pp. 189–209.

Rubin, H. 1957. The production of virus by Rous sarcoma cells. Ann. N.Y. Acad. Sci. *68*: 459–472.

Rubin, H., and H. M. Temin. 1958. Infection with the Rous sarcoma virus in vitro. Fed. Proc. *17*: 994–1003.

Sachs, L. 1961. The "in vitro" analysis of malignancy induced by polyoma virus. *In* Ciba Foundation Symposium on tumour viruses of murine origin, ed. Wolstenholme and O'Connor, pp. 380–409. London.

Selby, C. C., C. E. Grey, S. Lichtenberg, C. Friend, A. E. Moore and J. J. Biesele. 1954. Submicroscopic cytoplasmic particles occasionally found in the Ehrlich mouse ascites tumor. Cancer Res. *14*: 790–794.

Shope, R. E. 1962. Are animal tumor viruses always virus-like? J. Gen. Physiol. 45: 143–154.

Sorensen, G. D. 1961. Electron microscopic observations of viral particles within myeloma cells of man. Exptl. Cell Res. 25: 219–221.

Stewart, S. E., B. E. Eddy and N. Borghese. 1958. Neoplasms in mice inoculated with a tumor agent carried in tissue culture. J. Nat. Cancer Inst. 20: 1223–1244.

Stewart, S. E., B. E. Eddy, M. F. Stanton and S. L. Lee. 1959. Tissue culture plaques of SE Polyoma virus. Proc. Am. Assoc. Cancer Res. 3: 67.

Stewart, S. E., and M. L. Irwin. 1960. Cellular proliferation in primary tissue cultures induced with a substance derived from cell-free concentrates from human neoplastic material. Cancer Res. 20: 766–767.

Stoker, M. 1961. Studies on transformation by polyoma virus in vitro. In Ciba Foundation Symposium on tumour viruses of murine origin, ed. Wolstenholme and O'Connor, pp. 365–379. London.

Sweet, B. H., and M. R. Hilleman. 1960. The vacuolating virus, S.V.$_{40}$. Proc. Soc. Exptl. Biol. Med. 105: 420–427.

Toolan, H. W. 1960. Experimental production of mongoloid hamsters. Science 131: 1446–1448.

Trentin, J. J., Y. Yabe and G. Taylor. 1962. Tumor induction in hamsters by human adenovirus. Proc. Am. Assoc. Cancer Res. 3: 369.

Vogt, M., and R. Dulbecco. 1960. Virus-cell interaction with a tumor-producing virus. Proc. Nat. Acad. Sci. (U.S.) 46: 365–370.

GENETIC ASPECTS OF THE RELATIONSHIP BETWEEN VIRUSES AND TUMORS

GEORGE KLEIN

Institute for Tumor Biology
Karolinska Institutet Medical School
Stockholm, Sweden

GENETICAL CONSIDERATIONS enter into discussions regarding the relationship between viruses and tumors essentially at three main levels. The first concerns the relations between the oncogenic virus and its target cell; the second, the interaction between the virus and its animal host; and the third, the relationship between the virus-induced tumor cell and the host. It may be convenient to subdivide the present discussion into three corresponding sections and to focus on some cases where natural genetic variation or virus-induced genetic changes appear to play an important role in influencing the properties of the system.

I. VIRUS-CELL RELATIONSHIPS

Information concerning the relationship between oncogenic viruses and their host cells is still fragmentary and difficult to obtain, but it is at least possible to formulate some questions which appear to be relevant. The following will be discussed: (*a*) Does the cellular change occurring during virus-induced neoplastic transformation involve the level of structurally coded genetic information or is it localized to other levels, such as regulating mechanisms and gene expression? (*b*) Do neoplastic cells of established, originally virus-induced tumors contain information contributed by the viral genome, and if so, is this a necessary and sufficient prerequisite for their neoplastic properties? (*c*) Concurrently with the neoplastic transformation, do oncogenic viruses induce other phenotypic changes in their target cells than those that are obviously related to their neoplastic properties? (*d*) Is the tendency of a cell to undergo neoplastic transformation influenced by its genetic constitution?

(*a*) Genetics and Virus-induced Neoplastic Transformation at the Cellular Level.

Before the intracellular level at which an oncogenic virus may modify the target cell can be discussed for a given system, it is necessary to raise the question in each case whether the virus acts directly on the cells that turn neoplastic, or, alternatively, affects the host organism in some indirect fashion. In the latter case, the virus merely increases the probability of a neoplastic transformation which does not exclusively depend on the virus. Indirect actions of this type occur very probably in a number of virus-tumor systems. To this category belong the "conditioning" or "promoting" effects of viral infections which have been postulated as the most probable explanations of several well-documented cases of oncogenesis (17). It appears that tumor viruses may play a number of different roles: they may initiate the neoplastic process; they may promote the development of a tumor that has been initiated by other agents; or they can contribute to the progression of established tumors towards more independent forms (37). This can be true even for a single host-tumor system. It has been shown (53) that the Shope papilloma virus can act as an initiator, inducing papillomas that become malignant at a later stage; or as a promotor when introduced into methyl-cholanthrene-treated skin; and, finally, as a "transforming" influence when acting on tar-induced papillomas which it may change into carcinomas. A similar multiplicity of action mechanism has also been shown for some chemical carcinogens, within the same animal species but with regard to different target tissues; the action of urethane is a case in point (6).

Because of this diversity of possible action mechanisms, it is always necessary to prove a direct interaction between a virus and a neoplastic cell product within a given system before a discussion of the intracellular level of viral oncogenesis can be meaningful. The most clear-cut demonstration of direct action has come from studies on the Rous agent and the polyoma virus.

In the case of the Rous agent (and other fowl tumor viruses), the transformation of normal cells into fully established tumor cells is rapid and almost immediate. Moreover, the cellular change leads to an exact reproduction of the tumor type from which the agent has been derived. This appears to be true even with regard to the particular degree and type of differentiation which characterized the original source. Thus, the virus appears to direct the recipient cells into new and sometimes very unusual pathways of differentiation (15). This, together with the absence of recognizable intermediate steps during the conversion process, is already suggestive of direct action. The development of in vitro assay procedures, cloning techniques, and the demonstration of a direct proportionality between the number of "infective centers," consisting of morphologically altered, presumably malignant cells, and the dose of infective virus has yielded more decisive evidence on this point (56).

The neoplastic conversion induced by the polyoma virus has been studied both in vitro and in vivo in several different species, particularly the hamster and the mouse. Exposure of normal hamster cell suspensions to the virus, followed by cloning and determination of the number of normal and morphologically changed, presumably neoplastic, colonies has led Stoker (68) to conclude that the change is induced by the direct action of the virus. This conclusion was based mainly on the direct relationship between

virus dose and the yield of transformed colonies, the absence of any cytopathogenic effect in the hamster system, and the fact that the transformed
colonies developed without delay.

For the systems where a direct oncogenic action of the virus is well
established, the question may be raised whether the cellular change involves
the genetic level, that is, structurally coded information (and this includes
both DNA and RNA) or some other level. As alternative possibilities, one
may consider situations where abnormal states of differentiation "arise from
alterations of gene-repression mechanisms due to changes in state of episomes, including latent viruses" (38).

While these questions can be stated rather clearly, they cannot be
answered with any degree of certainty at the present state of our knowledge.
They are closely related to the more general problems concerning genetic
versus epigenetic changes in somatic cells of higher organisms (43). A
meaningful approach will only become possible after methods have been
developed for the genetic analysis of somatic cells. Among possible
approaches towards such an analysis, the demonstrated occurrence of
cellular fusion has received increasing attention recently. The experiments
of Barski *et al.* (3, 4) and of Sorieul and Ephrussi (65) have shown that it
is possible to hybridize different established cell lines in tissue culture. It
was also found that identity of origin was not a prerequisite for fusion. It is
apparently also feasible to obtain fusion of virus-induced tumor cells with
cells of other types. In the cell lines where it has been shown to occur,
fusion is not a very rare event and, fortunately enough, the fused cells show
a selective advantage in competition with their parental strains. No regular
segregation has yet been found, but accidental losses of chromosomes do
occur, allowing at least some degree of segregation. Such losses seem to take
place more frequently when the number of chromosomes is high.

If cell fusion can be shown to be a regular occurrence in combinations of
several different, representative cell lines, tumor cells of different origin
and derivation may be mated with each other and with normal cells and
it will be possible to decide whether the neoplastic properties of tumor cells
of various kinds are dominant or recessive. If they turn out to be recessive,
genetic losses will have to be considered and the question will also arise
whether the fused product of two neoplastic cells induced in different ways
may give rise to "wild type," that is, normal cells. Such experiments have
not yet been performed but the tools seem to be available now.

Among other possibilities for genetic analysis it appears that the phenomenon of somatic crossing over, which has been found so useful for genetic
mapping in the experiments of Pontecorvo on Aspergillus (45), may possibly
occur in mammalian cells (31). If further substantiated, this may open the
way for genetic mapping. Genetic analysis of this type or of other types,
such as transformation by DNA or transduction by viruses, is a necessary
requirement for the understanding not only of the neoplastic transformation
but also of differentiation. One of the first questions to be decided concerns

the problem whether all somatic tissue cells of higher organisms contain the same genetic information in agreement with classical genetic dogma, or not. Developmental changes may be imprinted at the genetic level and genetic models of differentiation have been constructed (for ref. see 31), but it is more customary to regard them as epigenetic in nature, affecting the expression of genetic information rather than the structural code itself.

An answer to these questions is a prerequisite for a meaningful attack on the cellular genetics of neoplastic transformation, whether this is induced by viruses or by other means. This is in line with Luria's generalization (38) that the study of virus infection at the cellular level is a branch of cellular genetics. He also points out (37) that the cellular changes which have to be considered to explain the neoplastic cellular transformation encompass the same range of mechanisms that must be considered in connection with normal tissue differentiation, namely gene mutations, chromosomal rearrangements, mutations in non-chromosomal genetic determinants, or alterations in self-maintaining steady-state mechanisms regulated by metabolic feedback.

(b) *Possible Role of the Virus Genome in the Determination of the Neoplastic Phenotype.*

The question whether genetic information contributed by the oncogenic virus is a necessary condition for the maintenance of the neoplastic character of the target cell or, alternatively, whether the virus merely triggers a permanent cellular change that is self-perpetuating in the absence of the virus, has been the subject of much debate. Conclusive evidence is not available on this point for any single system. More refined methods of genetic and biochemical analysis still have to be applied to the study of this question. Only circumstantial evidence can be discussed now and even this is scarce. One case in point is represented by polyoma-induced tumors in mice and in hamsters. In both species, established virus-induced tumors release little virus or none at all, and single cell clones of non-releasing cells could be established. These resisted numerous attempts to induce virus release by treatments which are known to induce phage maturation in lysogenic bacteria (12, 20, 74, 75, 76). Neoplastic cells, transformed by the polyoma virus *in vitro* or *in vivo*, are regarded by Dulbecco and Vogt (12) as intrinsically non-virus releasers. This fact, taken together with the demonstrated resistance of *in vitro* transformed lines against the cytopathogenic effect of live polyoma virus, has led Vogt and Dulbecco (75) to conclude that the virus is probably integrated into the cellular genome, in analogy with the integration of the prophage in lysogenic bacteria. They modified this view later, however, when it was shown (22) that most *in vivo* induced tumors are fully susceptible to the cytopathogenic effect of superinfecting polyoma virus and the resistance of *in vitro* transformed cultures is therefore an epiphenomenon, probably due to the fact that large amounts of virus are present during transformation and resistant cells are therefore being selected for continuously. In agreement with this view, it was also found that cell populations that have been selected for resistance against polyoma superinfection *in vitro* tend to become sensitive during serial isotransplantation *in vivo* while they maintain their neoplastic properties unchanged (21).

The recognition of the fact that neither resistance against superinfection nor the ability to release virus are essential qualities of the neoplastic cells now seems to stimulate the view that the virus genome is not integrated with the tumor cells at all. This is not a necessary or even a plausible conclusion, however. The original parallel with lysogeny and the more recent opposite view are both based on rather superficial analogies with bacterial systems; while stimulating, such analogies should not be taken too literally as far as details are concerned. The fact that infectious virus is **not being released** spontaneously or after various treatments by no means proves that parts of the virus genome may not be present in the cells. Even in bacterial systems, incomplete phages may become integrated with the genome of the recipient bacterium and the incorporation of a complete phage genome seems to be an extreme situation, by no means the general rule. In transduction, where host genes and phage genes are carried together in the same particle, it has not been proven in any single case that the entire genome of the phage is incorporated into a transducing particle (38). It is conceivable that only parts of the virus genome, those responsible for the neoplastic transformation, are incorporated selectively into the genome of the recipient cell. These would not be necessarily inducible. When the transducing phage P1 is carrying genetic markers of the host bacteria, all intermediates can be found between almost fully competent phages that can make almost normal phage particles and transducing elements that give no indication of having received any phage genes at all, being unable even to produce immunity. The last type could be, according to Luria, a chromosomal cell fragment, without any phage genes or, more probably, it may still include some phage genes which make it capable of multiplying in the transduced cells. Thus, absence of immunity against superinfection and failure to release mature virus particles are not safe criteria which could prove the absence of genetic material contributed by the virus even in bacterial systems; they are still less useful when the many unknowns and the increased complexity of higher cells have to be faced.

Among other things, virus-induced tumor cells and lysogenic bacteria are completely different with regard to their natural history. Under natural conditions, lysogenic bacteria carrying a prophage must have a selective advantage over corresponding non-lysogenic forms when both are exposed to the homologous phage. This advantage may explain why lysogenic systems have become established so readily during evolution. In such systems immunity would have a positive survival value, in the same way as in mouse embryo tissue cultures exposed to the polyoma virus, where in the presence of large quantities of mature virus particles, resistant cell lines become established, concurrently with the neoplastic transformation. Tumor induction by polyoma virus *in vivo* occurs under quite different circumstances, however. By the time tumors appear *in vivo*, the serum of their host contains a high titer of antiviral antibodies and extracellular virus is readily neutralized. Resistance against superinfection could hardly have a positive survival value for tumor cells under such circumstances. The resistant forms appear to be at selective disadvantage when competing with sensitive cells in the absence of large quantities of extracellular virus: as mentioned above, cell lines made resistant *in vitro* tend to become sensitive when passaged *in vivo*.

It follows from these considerations that there is no reason to postulate exact and detailed analogies between the bacterial and the neoplastic cell systems and that the absence of resistance to superinfection in the latter is by no means useful as a criterion by which to exclude the possible integration of at least parts of the viral genome into some self-replicating template system—whether chromosomal or episomal—of the host cell.

Are there any *positive* indications of such an integration? The most suggestive evidence concerns the antigenicity of polyoma-induced tumors in mice (18, 19, 62, 61) and probably also in hamsters (19, 2). Animals previously exposed to the polyoma virus were found to be resistant against small, cellular isografts from established polyoma tumors while the same grafts grew regularly in untreated controls. In addition to the virus, homografts of serially transplanted polyoma tumor lines which no longer released virus were also found capable of inducing transplantation resistance against genetically compatible polyoma tumor isografts. Since there appeared to be complete cross-reaction between different polyoma-induced tumors in the latter type of experiment (61, 19), the most probable interpretation was that tumors induced by the polyoma virus in mice contained a new, cellular antigen which appeared to be common for this whole etiological group of neoplasms. With a few occasional exceptions of doubtful significance, the same antigen seemed to be absent from tumors that arose spontaneously in polyoma-free colonies or were induced by chemical carcinogens or by other tumor viruses. Humoral serum antibodies against the polyoma-tumor antigen could not be demonstrated with certainty while lymph node cells of presensitized animals did show a certain neutralizing effect, indicating that the rejection mechanism may be akin to a straightforward homograft response. Sensitization to the tumor antigen would then be responsible for the resistance of adult mice against the oncogenic action of polyoma virus. It is not known whether there is any relationship between the new cellular antigen and any viral antigen; the cellular antigen must be different from those viral antigens that induce the formation of antibodies inhibiting viral hemagglutination, however, since such antibodies cannot be demonstrated in isograft-resistant animals, previously exposed to polyoma-tumor homografts. Antiviral antibodies of the HI-type are neither necessary nor sufficient for the rejection response. While the cellular antigen appears to be the same in polyoma tumors induced in different inbred mouse strains, it seems to be different in mouse and in hamster tumors.

Tumor-specific antigens, critically distinguishable from isoantigenic differences caused by genetical divergence between the original and the recipient hosts, have now been demonstrated to exist in several other host-tumor systems, with no known virus etiology (35, 34, 44, 47, 48). In comparison with these, the antigenicity of polyoma tumors has some unique features. The differences concern such details as the presence or absence of cross-reaction between different tumors induced by the same agent, and the permanence and stability of the antigenicity. Most if not all sarcomas induced by methylcholanthrene are characterized by individually distinct antigenicity and different tumors do not cross-react, even though they have been induced by the same dose of methylcholanthrene in the same tissue of the same genotype (35, 44, 32). This is in sharp contrast with the extensive and apparently general cross-reaction of polyoma tumors within a given species. Another possible difference is indicated by unpublished findings of Sjögren in our laboratory who applied continuous, protracted selection pressure against antigenic polyoma tumor cells by propagating several lines in presensitized, relatively resistant mice through 15–42 transfer generations. While this type of negative selection against cells containing isoantigens can lead to the emergence of antigenically deficient cell variants in other systems (23, 29), this was not the case here and all tested tumors maintained their antigenicity undiminished. This stability was also in contrast to the individually distinct, tumor-specific antigens of methylcholan-threne-induced sarcomas which were occasionally lost or diminished (48, 32).

The stability of the polyoma tumor antigen indicates that it may be an expression of an indispensable cellular characteristic, an obligatory requirement for their neoplastic properties or for their viability. While this cannot be taken to prove that the viral genome or parts of it are carried in some integrated form by the cells, this appears as the most probable explanation. The alternative possibility, that the virus has made the cells neoplastic and antigenic at the same time but does not participate in the maintenance of these conditions, is less likely, since populations of neoplastic cells are known to be very plastic and usually yield to selection pressure by throwing off variants that do not contain antigens which have become unsuitable for their growth in a given host type. Even if it is assumed that the virus induces the same change in all transformed recipient cells and the antigenicity is just another expression of the same neoplastic cellular phenotype, it is difficult to imagine that this phenotype could not be modified further in the course of continued serial transfer and of tumor progression and that no dissociation would be possible between antigenicity and neoplastic character whenever the former becomes a burden in the preimmunized host. It seems more plausible that the virus genome does exist in some integrated form in the host cell and actually maintains the neoplastic phenotype and the antigenicity as well, whether these are different expressions of the same cellular property or not. This picture would correspond to bacterial conversion (38) where the integration of a converting phage into the genome of the recipient cell is both necessary and sufficient for the induction and the maintenance of a new cellular property, such as a surface antigen. The antigen-determining phage genes seem to control the production of enzymes that catalyse specific steps in the biosynthesis of complex polysaccharides present on the surface of the host Salmonella cells. Since non-converting phage mutants, as well as mutants determining altered forms of the antigens, have been isolated, it might be rewarding to look for variant forms of the polyoma virus which may determine antigenic specificities differing from the currently known form. It is of particular interest that in bacterial conversion systems, prophage mutations to defectiveness do not affect antigen production. It is thus easy to postulate a form of integration in line with what has been said above where parts of the viral genome would be incorporated into the cellular genome but the system would still not be inducible and it would be impossible to obtain complete virus particles.

The possible antigenicity of other virus-induced tumor cells is less well known. In the mouse, lymphomas induced by the Gross virus have been found antigenic in isologous hosts, even though their antigenicity was weaker than that of polyoma tumors (64, 33). This system is particularly convenient to study because, in contrast with other tumor systems, the lymphoma cells are susceptible to the cytotoxic action of the serum of resistant, isologous recipients whose resistance was built up either by small subliminal isografts or by homografts of other leukemias induced by Gross virus. Different lymphomas induced by the Gross virus showed extensive cross-reaction with each other, both in transplantation and in cytotoxic tests. The cross-reaction was not complete in the latter series of tests, however, and it remains to be seen whether the antigenic overlapping was only partial or, alternatively, whether the different individual tumors varied with regard to their sensitivity to the same cytotoxic isoantibody. Whichever is the case, the tumor-specific antigen or antigens of the Gross lymphomas appeared to be quite different from the common antigen present in polyoma tumors in the preliminary tests carried out so far (33).

Recently, Sachs has suggested (58) that a lymphoma induced by the Moloney virus may contain a tumor-specific antigen. Other systems where there are strong indications that new cellular antigens, foreign to the host, may develop concurrently with viral induction of tumors include the Rous sarcoma (55) and the Shope papilloma (14). In both cases antigenicity of this type is probably responsible for the regression of established primary tumors.

With regard to the Rous sarcoma system, a close integration of the virus and the cell genomes has been postulated by a number of investigators (70, 50, 57) although this has not been definitely proven in any case so far. Part of the evidence concerning the Rous virus which is relevant in this connection will be discussed under the next heading (c).

Another interesting situation is represented by the papilloma induced by

Shope virus in wild, cottontail rabbits. It has been shown (39) that virus protein is only synthesized in differentiating, keratinizing cells, but not in the proliferating epidermal cells derived from the basal cell layer. The latter cells presumably contain the viral genome in some naked, replicating, but probably non-infectious form (37). Another relevant aspect of the Shope papilloma system concerns its behavior in different types of hosts. While virus can be isolated regularly from the papillomas induced in wild cottontail rabbits, in domestic rabbits the same virus induces papillomas of similar structure which permit the isolation of only a little or no infectious virus. This was again interpreted to indicate a qualitative change in the nature of the virus. This view was criticized by Beard (5), however, in whose opinion findings of this type reflect the small quantity of virus present in the tumors rather than any qualitative change.

If the domestic rabbit papillomas are protected from mechanical injuries, they regularly give rise to very malignant cancers which do not yield infectious virus at all. Serological data indicate that the virus persists in these tumors in a masked, non-infectious form. The blood of domestic rabbits with a papilloma or a carcinoma derived from it contains antibodies that neutralize the virus and fix complement. The virus antigen could not be eliminated by grafting the cancers through animals hyperimmunized against the virus. In one serially transplanted line, the Vx2 carcinoma, the antigenicity was only lost after eight years of serial transplantation (28, 54). This extremely prolonged maintenance of a virus-determined characteristic is, again, in line with the postulated integration of the viral genome, consisting of DNA, with the cellular genome.

The work with the papilloma virus has been recently reviewed by Shope (60). He presents the hypothesis that the virus can exist in the papillomas it has induced in two different forms: one, the complete mature virus, composed of nucleic acid and protein; and the other, immature virus, composed of naked viral nucleic acid without protein. The function of the mature papilloma virus would be to initiate tumor formation and that of the immature virus to maintain neoplasia. In the non-infective domestic rabbit papilloma, the viral nucleic acid and protein would not combine to form mature infective virus and neoplasia would be maintained by the activity of the viral nucleic acid alone. Experimental support for this concept has been obtained by Ito and Evans, who were able to isolate infective viral DNA from non-infectious domestic rabbit papilloma (26).

(c) Other New Phenotypic Characteristics in Virus-induced Tumor Cells.

The discussion under this heading can be subdivided into two parts: the first concerns the question whether an oncogenic virus induces its target cell to change its phenotype in other respects than what is obviously related to its neoplastic behavior; and the second, closely related to the discussion immediately above, whether different virus mutants can be isolated that are distinguishable by phenotypic differences among their respective neoplastic cell products. The importance of the first question has been emphasized particularly by Luria (37). He stressed that the amount of genetic information in several tumor viruses must be quite limited, since they are very small. For this reason, he postulated that any change in the growth pattern of a cell exposed to oncogenic virus must depend on only one or a few virus-controlled reactions. He continued: "In view of the limited amount of genetic information available in a virus, whenever a specific biochemical activity appears in a virus-induced tumor, it becomes important to decide whether this is directly controlled by viral genes, because any such new function has a significant chance of being *the key* function in the tumoral transformation." He quotes the case of arginase that has been shown (51) to be present in high concentration in the cells of rabbit papillomas induced by Shope virus and in the previously mentioned cancers which originate from them and which are presumably still carrying the viral genome, perhaps in a defective form. Tumor-bearing animals contain a precipitin in their blood serum, not present in controls, which reacts with the tumor arginase. Furthermore, the amino acid composition of the tumor arginase seems to differ from that of normal rabbit liver arginase, which is in agreement with the view that its amino acid sequence is dictated by the DNA template of the virus itself (52).

Other cases of this type include the specific new antigens of virus-induced tumors discussed under the preceding heading and the various unusual and abnormal products of cell differentiation induced by the fowl sarcoma viruses, where each virus imposes upon the recipient cell the exact type and specificity of differentiation characterizing the tumor from which it has been derived (15). In the opinion of Foulds, it is not possible to account for the individualities of all the diverse forms by assuming a different normal cell of origin for each of them. He believes that the cell of origin imposes limits on what kind of tumor *can* develop, but within these limits the virus and not the cell of origin determines what particular kind of tumor *does* develop. While imposing a particular degree and type of differentiation, the agents may direct the cells into a pattern of differentiation which, aside from the neoplastic change, they only follow under very exceptional circumstances.

Other changes of the cellular phenotype occurring in connection with the neoplastic transformation which are more probably related to the neoplastic character of the cells themselves include the decrease in contact inhibition observed after neoplastic transformation of normal cells *in vitro* by the Rous agent (56) and by the polyoma virus (75, 12), respectively. Since the change in contact inhibition is believed to be related to the invasiveness of tumor cells (1), this is perhaps just another expression of the neoplastic change.

The other area, concerning the question of viral mutations as related to cellular phenotype, has not been explored to any significant extent with the exception of the recent interesting work of Temin (69, 70, 71). After having worked out a technique to collect virus selectively from single isolated foci of transformed cells, induced by exposing normal chick fibroblasts to the Rous virus, he could separate three different virus variants that induced characteristically different types of colonies. The different colony types bred true during serial passage. The host cell also played a role in determining the cellular change, since the same virus line produced different effects on different kinds of fibroblasts but the type of change induced was a genetically determined character of the virus line. When cells already transformed by a given virus variant were exposed to superinfection with one of the other two variants, they either continued to release virus of the original type, or changed and went on to release virus of the superinfecting type, or continued to release both the original and the superinfecting types together. The cells that released both virus types could morphologically correspond to either one of them; thus cellular morphology could be controlled by the original or by the superinfecting virus type as well and there was no dominance relationship between them. In certain cell clones the ability to release both virus types was inherited during many cell generations. Temin concluded that the Rous virus is inherited from cell generation to cell generation in a stable way, and that in cells which contained both virus genomes one could reproduce without being expressed in cellular morphology. Furthermore, it appeared that a cell can sometimes lose the virus type it originally contained when superinfected with another type. In his most recent work, Temin found indications (71) that superinfection with one type could actually induce the production of the original virus type which was not released previously by the colony in question. This is so far a unique observation in the field of tumor viruses. Work of this type is of great potential significance since, as mentioned previously, many authors assume that the Rous virus genome is in some way integrated with Rous sarcoma cells, even if the latter do not release virus at all. The findings of Temin suggest that the virus genome participates directly in the control of the cellular phenotype and its mutations can lead to changes at the cellular level. Another important conclusion that Temin could draw from his work on mixed infection with two different virus variants was based on the observation that in the superinfection experiments the original virus was replaced by the superinfecting virus, in the majority of cases, indicating that the number of inherited copies of the original virus was very small at the time of superinfection. The fact that some cells continued to release both types of virus through prolonged periods of time was interpreted to mean that there was some special mechanism in the cell for the transmission of the virus equally to the daughter cells, or this stability would not be expected.

(d) *Influence of Target Cell Genetics on Their Tendency to Undergo a Neoplastic Transformation.*

With many tumor viruses, the genetic constitution of the host plays an important role in influencing the probability that the virus will induce a given tumor. The genetic factors involved may operate at a number of different levels. Some of them influence the host, its immune response to the virus, its endocrine environment, etc. In addition to these, there are well-documented cases to show that genetic factors may influence the tendency of the target tissue cells themselves to undergo a given neoplastic transformation after exposure to a certain carcinogenic agent. This has been shown to be the case for a number of nonviral carcinogens and for some viruses as well (for review, see 24). As a rule, the experiments in question were based on the knowledge that F_1 hybrid animals produced by the crossing of two different inbred strains accept tissues grafted to them from *both* parental hosts. Normal target tissues of two different parental strains, one susceptible and the other insusceptible to a given carcinogenic influence, were grafted to a common F_1 hybrid recipient. The hybrid host was subsequently exposed to the carcinogenic agent. The incidence of tumors was often found to be higher in the tissue derived from the susceptible parent than in the tissue of the resistant strain. Since both target tissues were present in the same host, the genetic difference influencing their susceptibility must be assumed to be localized at the tissue level itself. This does not imply that the tissue level is the only level where genetically determined host factors act—in fact, there is much evidence to the contrary—but there is no doubt that this is one of the important modes of action. This is true for several well-documented cases of carcinogenesis by chemical substances, hormones and viruses. As far as viruses are concerned, the work of Prehn (46) has shown that, with the mammary tumor agent, genetic susceptibility influences tumor formation directly at the tissue level. The site of gene action has also been localized to the target tissue, that is, the thymus, in the case of experimental lymphoma induction by various means, including a viral agent (40). Strain differences have also been found with regard to the sensitivity of different tissues to the polyoma virus (9, 63) but it is not yet known whether the genetic factors involved operate directly at the cell response level or indirectly at the immune response level. The peculiar absence of salivary gland tumors in the A strain (63) is probably due to factors operating at the tissue level; these might be genetic and/or developmental.

Developmental factors have been shown to be important in other cases. This was to be expected, since there are clear-cut cases with non-oncogenic viruses, such as the influenza virus, where it has been shown that the host cell may become, through differentiation, incapable of fulfilling some of the virus-dictated orders so that no complete virus can be made (16). With the tumor viruses, the previously mentioned example of the Shope papilloma in cottontail rabbits, where mature virus can be found in the keratinizing but not in the proliferating cells, shows, as pointed out by Luria (37), that cellular differentiation and formation of viral protein are closely inter-related and both of them are incompatible with a rapid cell proliferation. Furthermore, the developmental state of the recipient cells is important not only from the point of view of virus maturation but also with regard to the oncogenic response of the recipient tissue. The work of Dawe (9) with organ cultures of salivary glands exposed to polyoma virus shows that there is a trend from the youngest to the oldest tissue towards an increasingly active proliferative response, while there was a trend in the opposite direction with respect to the cytolytic response. There may be a parallel between this and the hemorrhagic versus proliferative response of the chicken-Rous virus system (13). The state of differentiation has also been shown to be of importance in determining the susceptibility of the lymphoid cells of the thymus to leukemogenic viruses (27).

II. VIRUS-HOST RELATIONSHIPS

This is a rather extensive field since genetic variation of the virus and of the recipient host are of importance as well. In addition, possible host-induced modification of the virus may also play a role. Several reviews of recent date are available, particularly with regard to the behavior of the fowl tumor viruses, and no attempt will be made to review them here in a comprehensive way. Only a few points will be emphasized, particularly with regard to the mouse.

The known mouse tumor viruses differ greatly with regard to their antigenicity within the species. For instance, the polyoma virus is strongly antigenic and induces the formation of high titers of neutralizing and hemagglutination-inhibiting antibodies within a comparatively short time after inoculation. The lymphoma viruses of Gross and of Moloney and the mammary tumor agent have not been shown to be antigenic in the mouse. The Friend virus is possibly antigenic, but if so, its antigenicity seems to be weaker than that of polyoma. The antigenicity of the different viruses in their home species may be correlated with their host specificity. The polyoma virus induces tumors exclusively in newborn mice or in adults that have received a high dose of total body irradiation prior to virus inoculation (10). On the other hand, with none of the leukemia agents is host susceptibility to the virus restricted exclusively to newborn animals. Originally, the Gross virus was rather restricted and induced lymphomas only in newborn or a few days old animals of certain specific strains. After selective animal passage, its virulence has increased considerably, however, and the susceptible age includes now even young adults of certain strains. The range of susceptible strains has also become wider. Nevertheless, the Gross virus is still highly strain-specific and the same is true for the Friend virus. Other agents like the milk factor are still somewhat restricted in their host range but not to the same degree. Still others like polyoma and the Moloney virus do not seem to be restricted at all (with one exception which will be mentioned below).

The resistance of a certain strain to a given virus is not necessarily due to an immunological reaction of the host against the virus; many other levels are conceivable and genetic or developmental differences influencing the tendency of host tissues to undergo a neoplastic transformation, as discussed above, represent some other alternatives. From the genetic point of view, the best analysed case is represented by the role of the milk agent in the induction of mammary cancers in mice. It has been firmly established that, in addition to the virus, a certain hormonal influence and the genetic constitution of the host also play important roles in increasing or decreasing the probability of mammary tumor development (8). The miscellaneous complex of multiple genetic factors has now been resolved into at least three subcategories. Certain genetic determinants influence the tendency of the mammary tissue itself to undergo the neoplastic transformation; these have been mentioned previously. Others influence the hormonal environment ("inherited hormonal influence") and make it more or less favorable for tumor development (8). Still others control the multiplication of the virus itself; these appear to be particularly relevant for the present discussion. In a series of beautiful experiments, Heston et al. have shown (25) that the agent carried by the susceptible C3H strain is eliminated rapidly if a sufficient part of the genetic background is replaced by the genome of the resistant C57BL strain by serial backcrossing. After the agent disappeared, it did not reappear again when C3H chromatin was re-introduced. This indicated that the introduction of the C57BL chromatin really eliminated the agent rather than changed it to a latent or inactive form. The early elimination of the agent in the C57BL to C3H backcrosses suggested that probably only few genes controlled the agent and perhaps there was only a single pair (25, 24).

The elimination of the mammary tumor agent on the C57BL background is of interest for several reasons. Although there is no evidence to indicate that the mammary tumor agent is antigenic in mice and that its elimination is caused by an immunological reaction of the host, there is no decisive evidence against it either. Heston tends to believe that the agent is lost by simple dilution, not being able to reproduce on the C57BL genetic background, but it is difficult to distinguish between this possibility and a host reaction that is not detectable by available methods. The position of the C57BL strain as a good immunological reactor has been documented in different types of experiments. It has a uniquely high titer of natural agglutinins against sheep red cells and shows a strong immune response against heterologous red cells (66, 11). With regard to the natural antibodies, the difference between C57BL and C3H has been shown to be due, at least in part, to genetic factors (67). Furthermore, C57BL is a low tumor strain and, unless irradiated, it is notorious for showing considerable resistance against most, if not all, known tumor viruses. It is completely resistant against the strain-specific Gross and Friend viruses, and it shows a certain relative resistance against the polyoma virus (9), and the Moloney virus (41). The latter two are highly pathogenic for all other mouse strains tested. C57BL is also characterized by a strong homograft reaction. While a number of inbred mouse strains do not show the weakest form of homograft reaction, the rejection of male skin by genetically compatible, isologous females, C57BL is characterized by perhaps the most regular response. Its reactivity is determined by genetic factors, probably by either one of two dominant genes (30). The C57BL strain also reacts strongly against the highly pathogenic ectromelia virus (59) and its reactivity is, again, determined genetically and is probably due to one, or, possibly, one of two (30) alternative dominant autosomal factors. The exceptionally good immunological reactivity of the C57BL strain may be related to the known fact that it is difficult, if not impossible to induce immunological tolerance to homografts in newborn C57BL mice (7), probably because immunological reactivity develops earlier in this strain than in several other strains (42).

On the basis of data available at present, it cannot be decided whether the relative resistance of the C57BL strain against known tumor viruses is due to its high immunological reactivity, or to some other cause, such as differences with regard to the development or relative proportion of virus susceptible cells. Whichever the case may be, the fact remains that this is a case of genetically determined differences in susceptibility to oncogenic viruses. It will be an important task for future research to break down this phenomenon into its component parts and to differentiate between immunological and other phenomena as well as to analyse the genetic determination mechanisms involved.

Other cases where a genetic analysis of tumor virus resistance has been initiated include the Rous virus system. Lines of inbred chickens have been produced that are resistant against or susceptible to the virus (72). The data obtained from appropriate crosses indicate that the susceptibility to the intracerebral inoculation of Rous sarcoma virus is dominant to resistance—a situation which is apparently the inverse of what has been said above about the immunological reactivity of C57BL mice—and is dependent for expression upon a single pair of autosomal genes. Similar conclusions were reached earlier by Prince (49) who used other lines of animals. The inbred lines of chicken used in the work of Waters *et al.* (72) have also been employed for studies on resistance to erythroblastosis (73). A relatively simple type of inheritance seemed to be involved in this case too, apparently depending for complete expression on only one pair of autosomal dominant genes (73).

III. CELL-HOST RELATIONSHIPS

This section can be made quite brief for two reasons: very little is known and what is known has already been considered to some extent above (particularly in I (*b*)). Some aspects nevertheless deserve special emphasis. As discussed above, it has been shown that polyoma-induced mouse tumors (18, 19, 62, 61), polyoma tumors of the hamster (19, 2), lymphomas induced by the Gross virus (33, 64), and, probably, lymphomas induced by the Moloney virus (58) contain new cellular antigens, not necessarily identical with any virus antigen. They seem to be capable of inducing, under appropriate circumstances, the formation of humoral antibodies and/ or a homograft type of response after grafting to genetically compatible, isologous hosts and presumably also in the primary host. Strong indications have been obtained that the same may be true for Rous sarcoma cells (55) and for Shope papilloma cells (14). In all these systems, the evidence seems to be critical in excluding possible sources of error arising from isoantigenic donor-host differences in genetically heterogeneous animal material and in proving the genuine tumor specificity of the phenomena observed. This may have important theoretical and practical implications. The polyoma tumor antigen seems to be common for all tumors induced by this virus in a given species. It appears probable (19) that the resistance of adult mice to the oncogenic activity of the virus is due to the comparatively strong antigenicity of the neoplastic cells which are formed under the influence of the virus. A reaction akin to the homograft response would then prevent their growth into gross neoplasms in immunologically mature animals. On the other hand, when newborn mice are injected with the virus, normal cells would change to neoplastic before the host response had time to mature and at least some of them would be able to emerge successfully from the race between neoplastic cell proliferation and the maturation of the host response. As an alternative, tolerance has been considered to explain the behavior of the newborn, but this is difficult to maintain, since mice that have received the virus as newborn are *not* tolerant against the tumor antigen, as judged by their resistance to small isografts of established polyoma tumors (62). It is nevertheless possible, however, that a certain tolerance can be induced by the inoculation of X-irradiated tumor cells into newborn mice of at least certain strains (19).

Many interesting problems regarding the role of host defence in the development of virus-induced tumors arise from these observations and they all merit further investigation. It seems particularly important to examine very closely why mice inoculated with polyoma when newborn can resist grafts of living, genetically compatible, polyoma tumor cells as adults but are nevertheless unable to prevent the outgrowth of their own primary tumors. One possibility is that the reaction against the tumor antigen is too slow in developing and remains weak in the situation where only occasional foci of a few neoplastic cells are present in the body and these are at their natural tissue site, sheltered by ordinary tissue barriers. A sudden graft of a large cell number from established tumors at a less natural location may represent a stronger antigenic stimulus and induce what would essentially correspond to a "second set response." For this reason, very small cell numbers transformed *in situ* could "sneak through" the immunological recognition mechanism until it is too late; medium size inocula grafted from established tumors to unnatural sites would induce resistance; and grafts of larger size would break through the resistance barrier. So far, this is in agreement with available facts. It may also be recalled that established, vascularized, slightly antigenic grafts are known to be less vulnerable to a homograft reaction than new grafts. The above explanation could be proved if it could be shown that mice inoculated with the virus as newborn develop no or fewer tumors if they are given an antigenic inoculum from an established polyoma tumor at adult age which they successfully resist.

Problems of this type, with suitable modifications, arise in other cases where tumors have been shown to be antigenic for genetically compatible hosts. In particular, sarcomas induced by methylcholanthrene have been considered from this aspect and considerable discussion has arisen as to whether it is necessary to postulate a depression of the immune reponse during carcinogenesis in order to explain the outgrowth of antigenically foreign cell clones, or whether it is sufficient to attribute the findings to the delicate time balance between the growth of the neoplastic cells and the delay in the host response. At present, experimental findings can be quoted in support of both concepts and the situation is equivocal (cp. 36).

Already the antigenic systems known at present allow the conclusion that there is a clear-cut difference with regard to the "strength" of tumor antigenicity. While polyoma tumors in mice are strongly antigenic, lymphomas induced by the Gross virus are only weakly so. This may explain the difference in their behavior in newborn as compared to adult mice: polyoma is exclusively pathogenic for newborn; the Gross virus is preferentially but not exclusively so.

The possible prophylactic significance of virus-tumor antigenicity is obvious. In cases where there is a common, strong antigen, specific vaccination may be an efficient preventive measure. Conversely, when dealing with individually distinct antigens in systems like the methylcholanthrene-induced sarcomas, non-specific bolstering of the immunological response of the host by, for example, BCG treatment may be useful and it has actually been applied with some success (44) with methylcholanthrene-induced sarcomas, with the probably virus-induced, "spontaneous" lymphomas of the AK strain, and with milk agent induced, mammary carcinomas as well. Even though their frequency was not reduced, the appearance of the tumors was delayed in all systems. The immunological nature of these phenomena still remains to be proved, but the findings appear promising.

ACKNOWLEDGMENT

The work of the author and his collaborators quoted in this paper has been supported by the Swedish Cancer Society and by grant C-4747 from the National Cancer Institute, U.S. Public Health Service.

REFERENCES

1. Abercrombie, M. 1958. *In* Symposium on the chemical basis of development, ed. W. D. McElroy and B. Glass, pp. 318–328. Johns Hopkins University Press.

2. Atanasiu, P., G. Orth et P. Dragonas. 1962. Resistance antitumorale specifique tardive chez le hamster immunisé peu après la naissance avec le virus du polyome. Comp. rend. Acad. Sci. Paris *254*: 2250–2252.

3. Barski, G. 1961. Clones cellulaires "hybrides" isolés à partir de cultures cellulaires mixtes. Compt. rend. Acad. Sci. Paris *253*: 1186–1188.

4. Barski, G., S. Sorieul et F. Cornefert. 1960. Production dans des cultures in vitro de deux souches cellulaires en association, de cellules de caractère "hybride". Compte. rend. Acad. Sci. Paris *251*: 1825–1827.

5. Beard, J. W. 1956. Fallacy of the concept of virus "masking": A review. Cancer Res. *16*: 279–291.

6. Berenblum, I., and N. Trainin. 1960. Possible two-stage mechanism in experimental leukemogenesis. Science *132*: 40–41.

7. Billingham, R. E., and L. Brent. 1957. A simple method for inducing tolerance of skin homografts in mice. Transplantation Bull. *4*: 67–71.

8. Bittner, J. J. 1958. Genetic concepts in mammary cancer in mice. Ann. N.Y. Acad. Sci. *71*: 943–975.

9. Dawe, C. J. 1960. Cell sensitivity and specificity of response to polyoma virus. *In* Monograph *4*, National Cancer Institute, pp. 67–128.

10. Dawe, C. J., L. W. Law and T. B. Dunn. 1959. Studies of parotid tumor agent in cultures of leukemic tissues of mice. J. Nat. Cancer Inst. *23*: 717–797.

11. Davidsohn, I., and K. Stern. 1954. Heterohemoantibodies in inbred strains of mice. II. Immune agglutinins and hemolysins for sheep and for chicken red cells. J. Immunol. *72*: 216–223.

12. Dulbecco, R., and M. Vogt. 1960. Significance of continued virus production in tissue cultures rendered neoplastic by polyoma virus. Proc. Nat. Acad. Sci. U.S. *46*: 1617–1623.

13. Duran-Reynals, F., and R. M. Thomas. 1940. Hemorrhagic disease occurring in chicks inoculated with Rous and Fujinami viruses. Yale J. Biol. Med. *13*: 77–98.

14. Evans, C. A., R. S. Weiser and Y. Ito. 1962. Antiviral and antitumor immunologic mechanisms operative in the Shope papilloma-carcinoma system. Cold Spring Harbor Symp. Quant. Biol. *27*: 453–462.

15. Foulds, L. 1958. Neoplastic development. *In* Symposium on the chemical basis of development, ed. W. D. McElroy and B. Glass, pp. 680–700. Johns Hopkins University Press.

16. Fulton, F., and A. Isaacs. 1953. Influenza virus multiplication in the chick chorioallantoic membrane. J. Gen. Microbiol. *9*: 119–131.

17. Furth, J., and D. Metcalf. 1958. An appraisal of tumor-virus problems. J. Chron. Dis. *8*: 88–112.

18. Habel, K. 1961. Resistance of polyoma virus immune animals to transplanted polyoma tumors. Proc. Soc. Exp. Biol. Med. *106*: 722–725.

19. Habel, K. 1962. Immunological determinants of polyoma virus oncogenesis. J. Exptl. Med. *115*: 181–193.

20. Habel, K., and R. J. Silverberg. 1960. Relationship of polyoma virus and tumor in vivo. Virology *12*: 463–476.

21. Hellström, I., K. E. Hellström and H. O. Sjögren. 1962. Further studies on superinfection of polyoma-induced mouse tumors with polyoma virus in vitro. Virology *16*: 282–300.

22. Hellström, I., K. E. Hellström, H. O. Sjögren and G. Klein. 1960. Superinfection of polyoma-induced mouse tumors with polyoma virus in vitro. Exptl. Cell Res. *21*: 255–259.

23. Hellström, K. E. 1960. Studies on isoantigenic variation in mouse lymphomas. J. Nat. Cancer Inst. *25*: 237–269.

24. Heston, W. E., 1959. Site of gene action and carcinogenesis. *In* Genetics and cancer, ed. R. W. Cumley, pp. 226–240. University of Texas Press, Austin.

25. Heston, W. E., M. K. Deringer and T. B. Dunn. 1956. Further studies on the relationship between the genotype and the mammary tumor agent in mice. J. Nat. Cancer Inst. *16*: 1309–1334.

26. Ito, Y., and C. A. Evans. 1961. Induction of tumors in domestic rabbits with nucleic acid preparations from partially purified Shope papilloma virus and from extracts of papillomas of domestic and cottontail rabbits. J. Exptl. Med. *114*: 485–500.

27. Kaplan, H. S. 1961. The role of cell differentiation as a determinant of susceptibility to virus carcinogenesis. Cancer Res. *21*: 981–983.

28. Kidd, J. G. 1942. The enduring partnership of a neoplastic virus and carcinoma cells. J. Exptl. Med. *75*: 7–70.

29. Klein, E., G. Klein and K. E. Hellström. 1960. Further studies on isoantigenic variation in mouse carcinomas and sarcomas. J. Nat. Cancer Inst. *25*: 271–294.

30. Klein, E., and O. Linder. 1961. Factorial analysis of the reactivity of C57BL females against isologous male skin grafts. Transplantation Bull. *27*: 457–459.

31. Klein, G. 1963. Somatic cell genetics. *In* Methodology in mammalian genetics, ed. W. J. Burdette, pp. 407–468. Holden-Day, San Francisco.

32. Klein, G., and E. Klein. 1962. Antigenic properties of other experimental tumors. Cold Spring Harbor Symp. Quant. Biol. *27*: 463–470.

33. Klein, G., H. O. Sjögren and E. Klein. 1962. Demonstration of host resistance against isotransplantation of lymphomas induced by the Gross agent. Cancer Res. *22*: 955–961.

34. Klein, G., H. O. Sjögren and E. Klein. 1962. Demonstration of host resistance against sarcomas induced by implantation of cellophane films in isologous (syngeneic) recipients. Cancer Res. *23*: 84–92.

35. Klein, G., H. O. Sjögren, E. Klein and K. E. Hellström. 1960. Demonstration of resistance against methylcholanthrene induced sarcomas in the primary autochthonous host. Cancer Res. *20*: 1561–1572.

36. Linder, O. E. A. 1962. Survival of skin homografts in methylcholanthrene-treated mice and in mice with spontaneous mammary cancers. Cancer Res. *22*: 380–383.

37. Luria, S. E. 1960. Viruses, cancer cells, and the genetic concept of virus infection. Cancer Res. *20*: 677–688.

38. Luria, S. E. 1962. Bacteriophage genes and bacterial functions. Science *136*: 685–692.

39. Mellors, R. C. 1958. Viruses, genes and cancer. Fed. Proc. *17*: 714–723.

40. Miller, J. F. A. P. 1961. Etiology and pathogenesis of mouse leukemia. Adv. Cancer Res. *6*: 291–368.

41. Moloney, J. B. 1960. Biological studies on a lymphoid leukemia virus extracted from sarcoma 37. I. Origin and introductory investigations. J. Nat. Cancer Inst. *24*: 933–951.

42. Möller, G. 1961. Studies on the development of the isoantigens of the H-2 system in newborn mice. J. Immunol. *86*: 56–68.

43. Nanney, D. L. 1958. Epigenetic control systems. Proc. Nat. Acad. Sci. (U.S.) *44*: 712–717.

44. Old, L. J., E. A. Boyse, D. A. Clarke and E. A. Carswell. 1962. Antigenic properties of chemically-induced tumors. Ann. N.Y. Acad. Sci. *101*, Art. 1: 80–106.

45. Pontecorvo, G. 1958. Trends in genetic analysis, pp. 1–145. Columbia University Press, New York.
46. Prehn, R. T. 1953. Tumors and hyperplastic nodules in transplanted mammary glands. J. Nat. Cancer Inst. *13*: 859–871.
47. Prehn, R. T. 1960. Tumor-specific immunity to transplanted dibenz(a,h)-anthracene-induced sarcomas. Cancer Res. *20*: 1614–1617.
48. Prehn, R. T., and J. M. Main. 1957. Immunity to methylcholanthrene-induced sarcomas. J. Nat. Cancer Inst. *18*: 769–778.
49. Prince, A. M. 1958. Quantitative studies on Rous sarcoma virus. II. Mechanism of resistance of chick embryos to chorio-allantoic inoculation of Rous sarcoma virus. J. Nat. Cancer Inst. *20*: 845–850.
50. Prince, A. M. 1960. Quantitative studies on Rous sarcoma virus. VI. Clonal analysis of in vitro infections. Virology *11*: 400–424.
51. Rogers, S. 1959. Induction of arginase in rabbit epithelium by the Shope rabbit papilloma virus. Nature *183*: 1815–1816.
52. Rogers, S. 1960. Concerning the nature of the induction of arginase by the Shope papilloma virus. Fed. Proc. *19*: 401.
53. Rogers, S., J. G. Kidd, and P. Rous. 1960. Relationships of the Shope papilloma virus to the cancers it determines in domestic rabbits. Acta Un. int. Cancr. *16*: 129–130.
54. Rous, P., J. G. Kidd, and W. E. Smith. 1952. Experiments on the cause of the rabbit carcinomas derived from virus-induced papillomas. II. Loss by the Vx2 carcinoma of the power to immunize hosts against the papilloma virus. J. Exptl. Med. *96*: 159–174.
55. Rubin, H. 1962. The immunological basis for non-infective Rous sarcomas. Cold Spring Harbor Symp. Quant. Biol. *27*: 441–452.
56. Rubin, H., and H. M. Temin. 1958. Infection with the Rous sarcoma virus in vitro. Fed. Proc. *17*: 994–1003.
57. Rubin, H., and H. M. Temin. 1959. A radiological study of cell-virus interaction in the Rous sarcoma. Virology *7*: 75–91.
58. Sachs, L. 1962. Transplantability of an X-ray induced and a virus induced leukemia in isologous mice inoculated with a leukemia virus. J. Nat. Cancer Inst. *29*: 759–764.
59. Schell, K. 1960. Studies on the innate resistance of mice to infection with mouse pox. II. Route of inoculation and resistance; and some observations on the inheritance of resistance. Austral. J. Exptl. Biol. Med. Sci. *38*: 289–299.
60. Shope, R. E. 1962. Are animal tumor viruses always virus-like? J. Gen. Phys. *45*: 143–154.
61. Sjögren, H. O. 1961. Further studies on the induced resistance against isotransplantation of polyoma tumors. Virology *15*: 214–219.
62. Sjögren, H. O., I. Hellström, and G. Klein. 1961. Transplantation of polyoma virus-induced tumors in mice. Cancer Res. *21*: 329–337.
63. Sjögren, H. O., and N. Ringertz. 1962. Histopathology and transplantability of polyoma-induced tumors in strain A/Sn and three coisogenic resistant (IR) substrains. J. Nat. Cancer Inst. *28*: 859–895.
64. Slettenmark, B., and E. Klein. 1962. Cytotoxic and neutralization tests with serum and lymph node cells of isologous mice with induced resistance against Gross lymphomas. Cancer Res. *122*: 947–954.
65. Sorieul, S., and B. Ephrussi. 1961. Karyological demonstration of hybridization of mammalian cells in vitro. Nature *190*: 653–654.
66. Stern, K., and I. Davidsohn. 1954. Heterohemoantibodies in inbred strains of mice. I. Natural agglutinins for sheep and chicken red cells. J. Immunol. *72*: 209–215.

67. Stern, K., K. S. Brown, and I. Davidsohn. 1956. On the inheritance of natural anti-sheep agglutinins of inbred strains. Genetics *41*: 517–527.
68. Stoker, M. 1962. Studies on transformation by polyoma virus in vitro. *In* Ciba Foundation Symposium on tumor viruses of murine origin, ed. Wolstenholme and O'Connor, pp. 365–379. London.
69. Temin, H. M. 1960. The control of cellular morphology in embryonic cells infected with Rous sarcoma virus in vitro. Virology *10*: 182–197.
70. Temin, H. M. 1961. Mixed infection with two types of Rous sarcoma virus. Virology *13*: 158–163.
71. Temin, H. M. 1962. Separation of morphological conversion and virus production in Rous sarcoma virus infection. Cold Spring Harbor Symp. Quant. Biol. *27*: 407–414.
72. Waters, N. F., and B. R. Burmester. 1961. Mode of inheritance of resistance to Rous sarcoma virus in chickens. J. Nat. Cancer Inst. *27*: 655–661.
73. Waters, N. F., B. R. Burmester, and W. G. Walter. 1958. Genetics of experimentally induced erythroblastosis in chickens. J. Nat. Cancer Inst. *20*: 1245–1256.
74. Winocour, E., and L. Sachs. 1961. Cell-virus interactions with the polyoma virus. II. Studies on the nature of the interaction in tumor cells. Virology *13*: 207–226, 1961.
75. Vogt., M., and R. Dulbecco. 1960. Virus-cell interaction with a tumor-producing virus. Proc. Nat. Acad. Sci. (U.S.) *46*: 365–370.
76. Vogt, M., and R. Dulbecco. 1962. Studies on cells rendered neoplastic by polyoma virus: The problem of the presence of virus-related materials. Virology *16*: 41–51.

SYMPOSIUM X

PLEUROPNEUMONIA-LIKE ORGANISMS AS AGENTS OF HUMAN AND ANIMAL DISEASES

Chairman: HARRY E. MORTON

E. KLIENEBERGER-NOBEL

Some Current Trends in the Field of PPLO

L. DIENES

Comparative Morphology of L Forms and PPLO

PAUL F. SMITH

The Role of Sterols in the Growth and Physiology of
Pleuropneumonia-like Organisms

SHMUEL RAZIN

Structure, Composition and Properties of the PPLO Cell Envelope

P. PLACKETT, S. H. BUTTERY and G. S. COTTEW

Carbohydrates of Some *Mycoplasma* Strains

CHAIRMAN'S REMARKS

HARRY E. MORTON

Department of Microbiology
University of Pennsylvania
Philadelphia, U.S.A.

A SYMPOSIUM on the pleuropneumonia-like organisms (PPLO) is timely because of the increased interest in these organisms and the new developments which are constantly occurring in this area. To illustrate the rapid change which may occur in our knowledge about PPLO it needs only to be pointed out that since this symposium was organized much has appeared to indicate that the Eaton virus, the cause of some forms of primary atypical pneumonia, may be certain strains of PPLO. It used to be the belief that PPLO were quite host specific. Indeed some strains of PPLO become established only within certain organs or tissues in their specific host species. With more sensitive means of strain differentiation it now appears that some strains of PPLO are capable of parasitizing more than one animal species. This means that we must learn something about PPLO regardless of their source.

Having the distinction of being the smallest cells capable of being grown on artificial media makes PPLO challenging subjects for studying cellular physiology. It has been shown that the metabolism of PPLO differs from that of nearly all other organisms. One of the aims of this symposium is to elucidate some of the areas in which these micro-organisms differ from all others. At the same time it is hoped that data will be presented which indicate the role these organisms play as the connecting link between the submicroscopic form of life and the more highly organized bacteria.

SOME CURRENT TRENDS IN THE FIELD OF PPLO

E. KLIENEBERGER-NOBEL

The Lister Institute, London, England

VARIOUS KINDS of PPLO have been found in rats, mice, dogs, cattle, sheep, goats, man and, as recent researches have shown, in poultry and swine. Isolations have yielded not only different types, but also, as would be expected, aberrations from the apparently well-defined types. For example, my collaborator, Dr. Lemcke (1961) isolated an organism from the nose of a rat which was identical neither with the typical rat lung strains nor with the typical rat polyarthritis strain. This strain, R38, was, however, a rat pathogen. It produced abscesses in the animals when inoculated subcutaneously. The abscesses regressed within four to six weeks. The organism was isolated from the spleen or the enlarged axillary or inguinal lymph nodes in some of the experimental rats, showing that the infection could be systemic. In this respect R38 resembled the polyarthritis strains, but was less virulent and never produced a high serum titre; the highest observed was 320. Complement fixation tests (C.F.T.) showed that R38 was related to a typical polyarthritis strain but the latter contained antigens not possessed by R38. This fact may account for the difference in virulence between the two strains.

The more strains we examine and the better our diagnostic methods, the more we will come across strains that differ from so-called type strains. The results of a recent detailed examination in Australia (J. R. Hudson, personal communication, 1962) of goat strains collected from various countries illustrates this very well. It is therefore of paramount importance that strains which have been isolated from pathological conditions and described in the literature should be preserved so that various isolates can be compared. Above all, we should be cautious and conservative in giving names to single organisms before sufficient information has been collected.

I am not familiar with the PPLO situation in swine. Work in this field has been carried out for years at Cambridge (Whittlestone, 1957), and more publications will probably appear soon.

Extensive studies on the human strains have been carried out in my laboratory (Card, 1959). It is generally recognized that the mouth and throat strains are non-pathogenic and belong to a particular type. More than 80 of a large number of strains from human genitals have been investigated by C.F.T. and found to be more or less identical antigenically. We have formed the opinion that this particular antigenic type is the pathogen often responsible for non-gonococcal urethritis and other pathological conditions. This so-called "human genital PPLO type 1" is not the only organism of the group which has been isolated from genitalia. In America but not in the United Kingdom another type represented by the "Campo strain" has been cultivated on various occasions. We collected the available cultures of this so-called "human genital type 2" organism, compared them with all the other organisms available and found them to be indistinguishable from our rat polyarthritis PPLO. There is no reason why such organisms should not live on human genitalia as saprophytes; not long ago we found a mouse lung strain in this location. These findings support the view that there is only one human genital organism of pathological significance.

Another organism, designated "G" type, occurring in man has been isolated by Ruiter and Wentholt (1953) on several occasions from the genital mucosa in gangrenous lesions containing a fusospirillary flora. "G" type strains are distinct from other human organisms, but their pathogenic significance is doubtful. I have been trying to give a brief review of the strains found, and at the same time to demonstrate the difficulty of the typing. The necessity of identifying unknown PPLO cannot be overestimated. This may entail a lot of expert work as cultural and serological methods have to be employed and the new isolate has to be compared with a number of known types.

Great interest has been aroused lately by the discovery of a new type in man and its apparent association with disease. I am of course speaking of the Eaton agent. I do not want to describe any of the work carried out in this field because all that has been done in our laboratory is the cultural and serological examination of Hayflick's strain from primary atypical pneumonia. We have been able to grow this strain well; it produces typical colonies with dark centres and lighter peripheries and they grow to a reasonable size. Dr. Lemcke was able to produce an antigen from cultures in liquid media which reacted with convalescent but not acute phase serum from patients with primary atypical pneumonia.

I have mentioned most of the types that have been discovered so far, except the poultry organisms. As you know the organism causing chronic respiratory disease (C.R.D.) in chickens and sinusitis in turkeys was discovered by Nelson (1935), who not only described it but also proved its pathogenicity. The coccobacilliform body strains can certainly be distinguished from ordinary PPLO and from the saprophytic ones found in chickens. I do not consider them to be *Mycoplasmas* proper; they might be classified under *Mycoplasmatales* but not under *Mycoplasmataceae*. I should like to propose the genus name of *"Nelsonia"* for these organisms.

We know particularly from the electron micrographs that very small granular elements are produced in PPLO. The question of their viability arises. It can be shown by ultra-filtration experiments that they are viable and often occur in large numbers. Elford was the first to develop filters in which pore diameter could be precisely determined. In 1931 he showed that the cultures of pleuropneumonia bovis and agalactia of sheep and goats contained viable particles 125–175 mμ in diameter. I have myself carried out a number of ultra-filtrations and confirmed Elford's findings. The results depend largely on the state of the culture, the organism used, and the techniques employed. Only a few organisms have been examined, and in this field much remains to be done. Density-gradient centrifugation is a promising new method for isolation of the various elements of a PPLO culture. It is effective because PPLO cells differ in density as well as in size, and sediment accordingly. Morowitz and Tourtelotte (1962), using this method, found that young cultures contain mainly large cells and old ones mainly the minimal reproductive units. I have never found the very small elements in coccobacilliform body strains, the pathogens which cause coryza in chickens. The average diameter of coryza-elements is 0.25 μ (250 mμ). This is one of the reasons why I think they should be distinguished from *Mycoplasma* proper.

I should like to mention that I found in filtration experiments that the smallest elements of well-adapted L form strains were larger as well as less numerous than those of PPLO.

From the medical point of view the most important problems are those of the pathogenicity and epidemiology of PPLO. Of course the veterinarians, who have studied pleuropneumonia bovis and agalactia of sheep and goats in the field and in the laboratory for decades, have collected a large amount of information. Those who are working on diseases of man and of domestic and small laboratory animals can learn a great deal from their reports. The epizootics of pleuropneumonia and agalactia usually affect a large number of individuals. The infected ones do not always develop the disease. It is well known that agalactia as a rule does not break out until the females are under the stress of lambing or kidding and in the lactation period, though they may have been infected months previously while grazing in a contaminated place. Pleuropneumonia cannot easily be transmitted from one animal to another. Yet in northern Australia and in Africa, where the disease is enzootic, whole herds may succumb to it when they are driven over large areas of country in unfavourable weather conditions to find new pastures. These examples show that the presence of the organism is not enough to produce disease and that other factors are involved. This applies also to other PPLO diseases. Bronchopneumonia of rats eventually affects all the stock animals. The suckling rats and the young animals have the organism in their nasopharynx, receiving the infection from their mothers; yet they are quite healthy. Under stress, however, the lungs may become invaded and the disease may take an acute and fatal course. Usually the lungs become diseased when the rats age and then the disease takes a chronic course. A very quick and striking way of producing bronchopneumonia in young rats was discovered by my collaborator Cheng who tied off one bronchus in young rats which had no PPLO in their lungs. In the ligated lobe in which stagnation had been produced the disease developed within a week; the lobe became hepatized and ten days after the operation big abscesses had formed. An enormous crop of the rat lung PPLO was cultivated from the diseased tissue and the abscesses.

Polyarthritis, another PPLO disease of the rat, can occur as an acute and often also fatal disease. Although it usually is not possible to infect healthy animals with a pure culture of the organism, I have succeeded in producing severe polyarthritis by injecting an emulsion of agar or mammalian cells with the organisms.

An experiment which illustrates that a second factor plays a role was carried out by Mooser (1949). He showed that a particular mouse PPLO injected intraperitoneally into mice soon died and did not harm the animals. When he gave the mice Ectromelia at the same time, this PPLO developed abundantly in the peritoneum producing a large amount of purulent exudate. I also obtained growth of the organism of agalactia in the peritoneum of mice when I injected it together with Ectromelia, and the animals became severely ill. However, when saprophytic strains from soil or sewage were used together with Ectromelia, no such effect was achieved and the saprophytes soon disappeared from the peritoneal cavity.

The antibody response in PPLO infection has been studied in my laboratory by C.F.T. for a number of years. Lemcke (1961) has studied naturally occurring and experimental infections in small laboratory rodents. She examined first bronchiectasis of rats and found that antibody is absent or present only at very low titre in young rats which do not yet have PPLO in their lungs. As the rats age the lungs are invaded and eventually bronchopneumonic lesions develop. The highest titres are found in rats with severe and extended lesions; but they never exceeded 1:320. The reason for the relatively low titres is the strict localization of the lung condition. This is different in rat polyarthritis which is, at a certain stage, a systemic disease, when the organisms can be found in the enlarged spleen, the lymph glands, and the blood. Antibody production is correspondingly high, giving titres of 1:2000 and 1:5000.

In mice also the incidence of lung infection increased with age and the serum titres increased correspondingly. The primary seat of infection is the nasopharynx; but in contrast to the rats not all the mice become infected, and nasal infection is not always followed by lung disease. However, in mice as in rats there was a high correlation between the presence of PPLO, the degree of the disease, and the occurrence of specific antibodies in the blood.

The established relationship between PPLO infection and specific serum titre in rats and mice supports our view of the significance of serum titres against genital PPLO in man. We are of the opinion that antibody against human genital PPLO is indicative of past or present PPLO infection.

The last section of my talk deals with the colony characteristics and morphology of PPLO. I have often been asked to give a definition of PPLO, but this is impossible. We are all familiar with the usual low magnification microscopical appearance of the colonies with their dark centres and lighter peripheries. However, in several publications dots which mean little to the reader have been shown in photographs and described as colonies. These dots may be the first manifestations of PPLO colonies, or they may be artifacts. To convince us that they have isolated PPLO these workers must learn to grow these tiny colonies into proper PPLO colonies. That the "dots" or "spots" can be transferred and multiplied is no proof of their living nature. In 1940 Brown, Swift, and Watson published a paper bearing on PPLO pseudocolonies, and what they wrote then still applies today: "Unless recognized in their various forms the pseudocolonies . . . may be confused with the growth of filterable microorganisms, for not only in their morphology do they mimic colonies of pleuropneumonia-like microorganisms, but by applying the cultural techniques commonly used to propagate these microorganisms in subcultures, the pseudocolonies appear to multiply to a remarkable degree." Even if we succeed in obtaining characteristic colonies a diagnosis may be premature. We have also to grow them on liquid media and to examine their growth in the phase and darkfield microscope, in stained preparations, and perhaps in the electron microscope. Only the sum total of these examinations can establish our diagnosis beyond doubt.

My interpretation of the developmental cycle of PPLO is shown in two diagrams published in my recent book. I have been guided by the idea that the development must be similar in both liquid and solid media even if the appearances are widely different. The first diagram illustrates the growth in liquid medium (Plate I). It starts with the minimal reproductive unit, a granule of 125–175 mμ diameter. These granules grow into elements of various shapes, round, oval, or filamentous; they can probably divide and branch at this stage. In the next stage, concentrated and thin parts arise in the cytoplasm and the concentrated areas produce the new minimal reproductive units. These granules may be shed and start the development again as shown under (1) and (2); or they may remain attached to the mother cell and grow out in various ways as shown under (5). On the solid medium (Plate II) the development is similar, but, owing to the plastic nature of the elements which do not possess a rigid cell wall, the single elements spread flatly on the surface and thus grow into discs or sheets of different size and shape. After a period of spreading and dividing, a differentiation into concentrated and thinner areas takes place, as in the liquid medium, and minimal reproductive units are formed within the mother cells. These may grow again if enough nutrient is present. Spreading, simple division, production of minimal reproductive units, and their further development can occur simultaneously in one culture, thus producing a complex picture.

It may be seen from electron micrographs, recently produced in collaboration with Dr. R. C. Valentine (National Institute for Medical Research,

PLATES I and II. Developmental cycle of PPLO: Plate I in liquid media, Plate II on solid media. See text for explanation. Reproduced from Klieneberger-Nobel (1962) by permission of Academic Press.

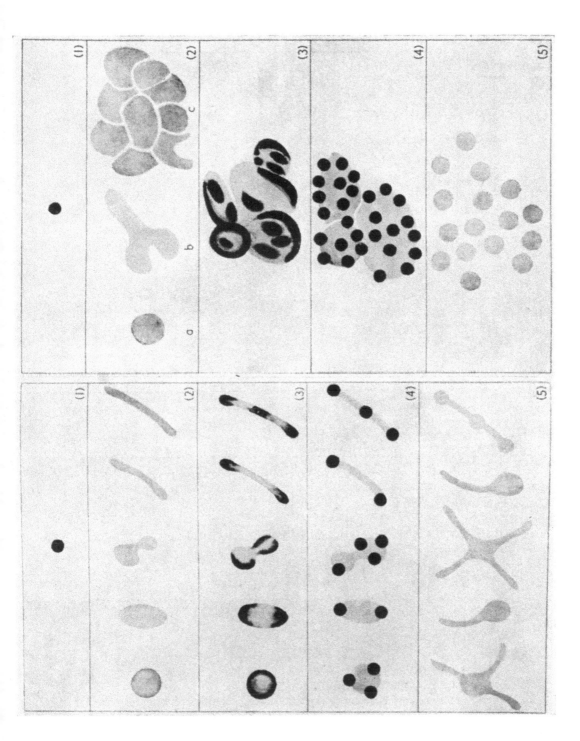

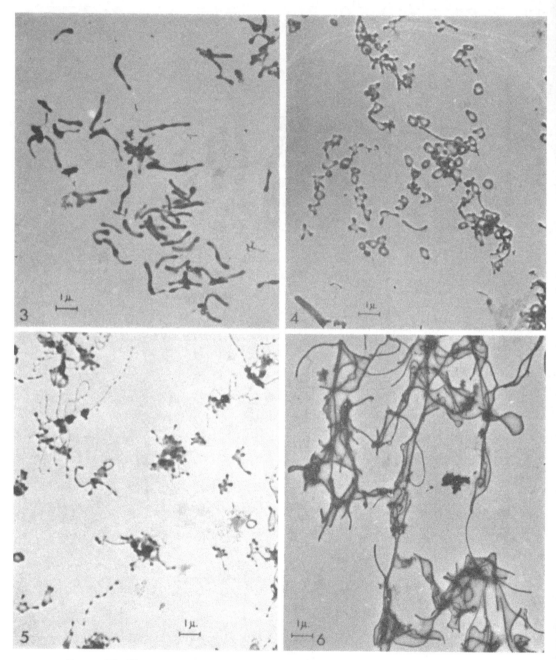

PLATE III. Electron micrographs of PPLO's. Fig. 3, caprine pleuropneumonia; Fig. 4, agalactia; Fig. 5, rat lung organism; Fig. 6, unidentified organism from tissue cultures.

London), that many of the structures are much too small for proper resolution by the light microscope (Plate III). The cultures were grown in liquid media and the suspensions for the electron micrographs prepared according to the method of Rodwell and Abbot (1961). A carbon supporting-film and a Siemens U M 100 electron microscope were used. In an overnight culture of caprine pleuropneumonia filaments of varying thickness can be seen, some with swellings and some with cytoplasm of varying density (Fig. 3 of Plate III). In the organism of agalactia (Fig. 4 of Plate III) there are some filaments and many cells (vesicles) showing a concentration of material round the periphery. In some the characteristic granules have formed which have grown out into elongated forms. Very interesting pictures have been obtained of the rat lung organism (Fig. 5 of Plate III). Filaments of an extraordinary fineness are produced and develop into rows of granules. There are also bigger forms which produce the granules at the periphery. The last organism of which E.M.'s have been prepared was isolated by Hayflick from tissue cultures (Fig. 6 of Plate III). It is not the human genital type which has been found in HeLa cell cultures and so far we have been unable to identify it with any other culture in our collection. It produces exceptionally long filaments interspersed with some vesicular forms that show concentration contours.

Ultrathin sections of PPLO give information about the cell components. They have not taught us much about the life cycle. Of course, when ultrathin sections are made, fixation should be carried out with caution. Osmic acid does not seem to be a good fixative, nor is formaldehyde unless used in a hypertonic solution. So far the ultrathin sections have given us valuable information on the envelope of the elements. We shall doubtless learn more about their cytoplasmic and nuclear content in the future. By means of the method we have employed and by means of negative staining we should be able to learn a good deal more about the developmental cycle in liquid media if all the organisms available are examined and conditions of growth, in particular the time of incubation, are varied.

REFERENCES

Bridré, J., and A. Donatien. 1923. Le microbe de l'agalaxie contagieuse et sa culture *in vitro*. C. R. Acad. Sci., Paris *187*: 262.

Brown, T. M., H. F. Swift, and R. F. Watson. 1940. Pseudo-colonies simulating those of pleuropneumonia-like microorganisms. J. Bacteriol. *40*: 857.

Card, D. H. 1959. PPLO of human genital origin: Serological classification of strains and antibody distribution in man. Brit. J. Vener. Diseases *35*: 27.

Chu, H. P., and W. I. B. Beveridge. 1954. Chronic balanoposthitis in dogs associated with pleuropneumonia-like organisms. Symp. sur les uretrites non gonococciques, Monaco.

Cordy, D. R., H. E. Adler, and R. Yamamoto. 1955. A pathogenic pleuropneumonia-like organism from goats. Cornell. Vet. *45*: 50.

Edward, D. G.ff. 1940. The occurrence in normal mice of pleuropneumonia-like organisms capable of producing pneumonia. J. Pathol. Bacteriol. *50*: 409.

Klieneberger, E., and D. B. Steabben. 1937. On a pleuropneumonia-like organism in lung lesions of rats with notes on the clinical, and pathological features of the underlying condition. J. Hyg. Camb. *37*: 143.

Klieneberger-Nobel, E. 1959. Pleuropneumonia-like organisms in genital infections. Brit. Med. J. *i*: 19.

Klieneberger-Nobel, E. 1962. Pleuropneumonia-like organisms (PPLO) Mycoplasmataceae. Academic Press, London and New York.

Laidlaw, P. P., and W. J. Elford. 1936. A new group of filterable organisms, Proc. Roy. Soc. B*120*: 292.

Lemcke, R. M. 1961. Association of PPLO infection and antibody response in rats and mice. J. Hyg. Camb. *59*: 401.

Lemcke, R. M., and G. W. Czonka. 1962. Antibodies against pleuropneumonialike organisms in patients with salpingitis. Brit. J. Ven. Diseases *38*: 212.

Mooser, H. 1949. Die Mobilisation von *Musculomyces* durch das Virus der Ektromelie. Experientia *5*: 364.

Morowitz, H. J., and Tourtelotte. 1962. The smallest living cells. Scient. Amer. *206*(3): 117.

Nelson, J. B. 1935. Coccobacilliform bodies associated with an infectious fowl coryza. Science *82*: 43.

Nocard, E., and E. R. Roux, avec la colloration de M. M. Borrel. 1898. Salimbeni et Dujardin-Beaumetz. Le microbe de la péripneumonie. Ann. Inst. Pasteur *12*: 240.

Ruiter, M., and H. M. M. Wentholt. 1953. Incidence, significance and bacteriological features of pleuropneumonia-like organisms in a number of pathological conditions of the human genito-urinary tract. Acta derm. venereol. Stockh. *33*: 130.

Sabin, A. B. 1938. Identification of the filtrable, transmissible neurolytic agent isolated from toxoplasma-infected tissues. Science *88*: 575.

Seiffert, G. 1937. Ueber das Vorkommen filtrabler Mikroorganismen in der Natur und ihre Züchtbarkeit. Zbl. Bakt. I, Abt. Orig. *139*: 337.

Shoetensack, H. M. 1934. Pure cultivation of the filtrable virus isolated from canine distemper. Kitasato Arch. *11*: 277.

Whittlestone, P. 1957. Some respiratory diseases of pigs. Vet. Rec. *69*: 1354.

COMPARATIVE MORPHOLOGY OF L FORMS AND PPLO *

L. DIENES

*Departments of Bacteriology and Medicine
Massachusetts General Hospital
and
Robert W. Lovett Memorial Foundation
for the Study of Crippling Diseases
Harvard Medical School
Boston, Mass., U.S.A.*

PLEUROPNEUMONIA-LIKE ORGANISMS (PPLO) are morphologically one of the best characterized groups of micro-organisms. Their fragility, their variable size and shape and the structure of their colonies allow identification without difficulty. However, a similar form of growth, usually designated as the L form, may be found under special conditions in almost every species of bacteria. The similarities between PPLO and L forms are generally recognized, as is the fact that, with experience, the two can be distinguished. My impression is that the similarities between the two groups involve essential properties such as structure and reproductive processes. Dissimilarities are in less important properties such as size, growth requirements and greater or lesser tendency to autolysis. Such differences may be the result of the fact that PPLO are well-established organisms in nature and adapted to live in this form, whereas L forms, as we know them, are artificial products of the laboratory.

The study of the morphology of these organisms has been and still is confused by the use of inadequate techniques. These organisms are easily distorted and destroyed and the conditions of culture influence greatly their size and shape. A special technique is necessary to see the individual organisms with the light microscope. The difficulties in the use of the electron microscope, especially with the L forms, are far from being solved. The simple technique of staining the agar cultures *in situ*, as used in our laboratory (Madoff, 1960), is probably most appropriate to obtain the basic information concerning their morphology and reproductive processes and to check the results obtained by more complicated techniques. The observations to which I shall refer and the photographs illustrating them were obtained with this simple technique.

Two basic properties distinguish the L forms from regular bacteria. The first is the absence of a rigid cell wall. The second is multiplication in the

*A large part of the work on which this report is based was supported by a grant from the National Institute of Arthritis and Metabolic Diseases, U.S. Public Health Service, Bethesda, Maryland, U.S.A. This is publication No. 332 of the Robert W. Lovett Memorial Foundation for the study of Crippling Disease.

form of soft granules considerably smaller than bacteria, at least during certain periods in the development of the culture. These properties have been observed always to be associated with two others: the tendency of the small granules to grow into an agar medium leading to a characteristic structure of the colonies, and the tendency of the organisms to enlarge and to grow to large bodies, "giant forms," sometimes more than 20 μ in diameter. It is possible that the two latter-mentioned properties are the consequence of the former ones. These properties define a morphologically well-characterized group and the name of L forms should be applied only when these properties are present. Transitional forms between the bacteria and their L forms have not been observed. Bacteria may grow into large bodies and the cultures may be extremely pleomorphic, but multiplication proceeds in more or less regular bacterial forms and the colonies retain the structure of bacterial colonies. The young colonies usually consist of regular bacteria. Transformation to L forms occurs when growth starts in the form of soft granules. This is always connected with the appearance of the other properties of L forms and it is the dividing line between bacterial and L forms.

L type cultures obtained from different bacteria and possessing these basic characteristics vary considerably in appearance, in growth requirements, in metabolic activities, in susceptibility to phages and also in the tendency to resume bacterial form. It is important that L forms obtained from a single bacterial strain may present considerable differences persisting in cultivation, including differences in the cell wall. I do not agree with Klieneberger that stability, meaning the loss of the ability to resume the regular bacterial structure, should be included in the definition of L forms.

The absence of a rigid cell wall in L forms is indicated by their physical

---

PLATE I

FIG. 1. A broth culture after 3 hours incubation transferred to agar. The fusion of two segments of the short filaments and the development of large bodies at the site of fusion is apparent. X 1600. Unstained.

FIG. 2. Broth culture after 16 hours. All bacteria developed to large bodies. Stained with safranin. X 2000.

FIG. 3. The chromatin granules in the large bodies. X 3000.

FIG. 4. One large body, after incubation overnight on agar, greatly increased in size and filled with chromatin granules. X 3000.

FIG. 5. Two large bodies on agar returning to the regular bacillary forms. X 2000.

FIG. 6. The earliest growth of L form from a large body. X 3000.

FIG. 7. The earliest growth of the granules of L forms from a large body of *H. influenzae*. The large body is not in sharp focus and is faintly visible between the groups of granules. X 2350.

FIG. 8. Growth of the granules of L forms from Proteus after 2½ hours incubation in agar pour plate. X 2350.

FIG. 9. Same as Fig. 7, after 4 hours incubation. One large body has grown to a very large size. X 2350.

FIG. 10. Well-developed L colony of Salmonella. X 30.

FIG. 11. Well-developed colony of a human urethral PPLO. X 900.

FIG. 12. Large bodies full of small granules at the periphery of a *B. prodigiosus* L colony. X 2100.

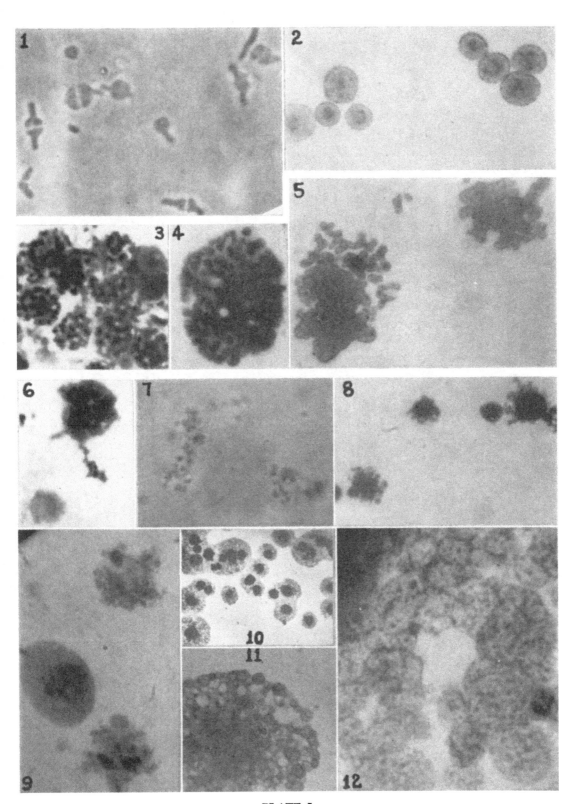

PLATE I

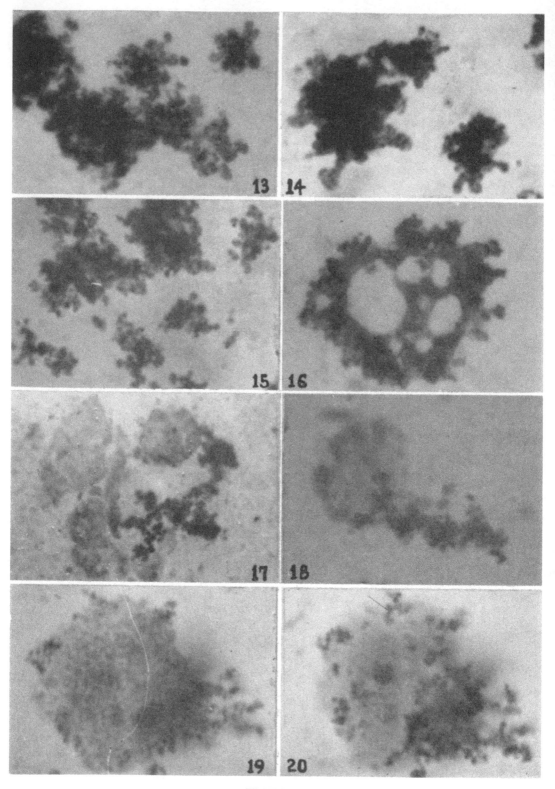

PLATE II

properties, by their fragility and by their ease of deformation. Examinations of thin sections with the electron microscope also indicate a considerably thinned cell wall. Several antigens and chemical components responsible for the rigidity of the cell wall of bacteria are absent in the L forms, but some constituents may also be absent which are not connected with the cell wall.

The L forms are often produced by direct injury to the cell wall. Such injury is also the cause of the pleomorphism of bacteria. The first effect of the weakening of the cell wall is growth of bacillary forms into long filaments. A further change is their growth into spherical or flat large bodies. The L forms always develop after the bacteria have grown into large bodies either directly from the large bodies or from the granules left after their disintegration. This observation is of great interest for the understanding of the nature of L forms and also of the large bodies. Nevertheless, it leads only to confusion to regard the large bodies growing from bacteria as L forms. Large bodies often cannot be induced to grow, and when they do they usually reproduce regular bacteria and not the small granules of the L forms. The large bodies are part of the pleomorphism of bacteria. The L forms derive from a further alteration of the large bodies and their properties are different from those of pleomorphic bacteria.

In a few cases it has been possible to follow step by step the development of large bodies from bacteria and to observe their structure, their reproductive processes and the growth of L forms from them. Most information has been obtained with a strain of *Bacteroides* (Dienes & Smith, 1944). This bacterium produced L forms spontaneously and no penicillin was used in the experiments. The bacillus grew on agar in the form of short rods. Growth started in similar form in broth, but after a few hours the bacilli grew into short filaments. These started to divide but the division was not completed, the segments fused together, and at the point of fusion large bodies developed (Figs. 1, 2). For two to three hours the developing large bodies, when transferred to fresh media, divided into a group of bacteria

PLATE II

Fig. 13. Six-hour growth on agar of a human urethral PPLO. Notice the size of the organisms and the presence of very small organisms in the periphery of some colonies. X 2400.

Fig. 14. Twelve-hour-old colonies on agar of another human urethral strain. X 3000.

Figs. 15–18. L forms of a Group A beta hemolytic streptococcus. 15: Six-hour growth on agar, X 2500; 16: A large body transplanted is vacuolized and the periphery grows into granules, X 2400; 17: Initial growth on the plate inoculated with the streptococcus consisting of large bodies and growth of small granules, X 2200; 18: Small granules grow into the agar from a transferred large body, X 2400.

Fig. 19. A large body of a human urethral PPLO transferred to fresh medium grows on the surface to a very large size. It is full of small granules and similar granules grow into the medium. X 2300.

Fig. 20. This photograph shows the same large body, putting the focus of the microscope below the surface. Granules start to grow at different sites from the large body. X 2300.

that retained the fusiform shape of the developing large bodies. This indicates that the large bodies were not produced from the bacteria by a physical process, for instance imbibition of water, and that they were not giant single organisms but that they were produced by the growing units of bacteria, multiplying without separation, inside a common envelope (Figs. 3–4).

For the next twelve hours all large bodies developed to bacteria when they were transferred either to fresh broth or to agar (Fig. 5). Later, an increasing number either did not develop at all or developed into L colonies on transfer to agar (Fig. 6). The organisms growing inside the large body gradually lost the ability to develop the regular cell wall, but after being transferred to fresh agar medium a few continued to grow as L forms. These L forms do not derive from the bacteria simply by weakening of the cell wall and continuing to grow without it, but appear to be the result of a special growth process inside the large bodies. The structure of the large bodies and the growth of bacteria and L forms from them, observed in this case, have also been observed in other species (Fig. 7). In most cases, however, the consecutive steps of the derivation of L forms from bacteria cannot be seen so clearly.

The tendency to return to bacterial form varies to a large extent in L forms. It is remarkable that in all cases in which the origin of bacteria has been observed they developed from the large bodies of the culture. The small granules never resumed directly the usual bacterial structure. There is a type of L culture, which I designated at 3B, in which some of the large bodies start to resume bacterial form immediately after elimination of penicillin. But in this case too the initial multiplication starting from bacteria is in the form of small granules. In most instances the L cultures do not contain any organism which immediately resumes bacterial form under appropriate conditions. Re-transformation into bacteria occurs only very rarely after a period of growth in the L form, from one among many millions of growing organisms. In some cases re-transformation occurs only in broth, not on agar media, and in some cases it has never been observed. The tendency to return to bacterial form is often lost after long cultivation, apparently as a consequence of aging. It does not seem to be justified to base a principal distinction on this loss between "stable" and "unstable" L forms. First of all, it is often not possible to tell whether or not this tendency is completely lost. Reappearance of bacteria in the L form is one of their most interesting properties and there is no reason to believe that its loss indicates the elimination of transitory forms in the cultures.

The growth of bacteria to large bodies suggests a natural process. The large bodies have been known since the early days of bacteriology. In some groups of bacteria, for example in *Neisseria*, in *Hemophilus*, in *Bacteroides*, and in *Streptobacillus moniliformis*, it is not uncommon that after some growth the cultures are transformed either partly or *in toto* into large bodies (Dienes & Weinberger, 1951). As long as intact large bodies are present, transfers will usually grow, and the development of bacteria from the large bodies has been observed repeatedly. The reason that this is not generally known is that the large bodies are very fragile and in the usual smear preparations are not recognized. Large bodies can be seen in the natural habitat of bacteria, such as in feces or on the mucous membranes. Large bodies were studied often in highly artificial conditions; however, it is more important that these artificial conditions are often not necessary for their development and that the large bodies seem to play some role in the life of bacteria.

In contrast to the large bodies, the L forms consisting in the growth of small granules from the large bodies, as we observe them in the laboratory, may be entirely artificial products. Most suggestive in this respect is the role which the agar plays in their growth. Their development from bacteria was observed only on agar media and not on other solid media or in broth. The physical conditions provided by the agar have as much importance as the nutrients for their growth. This suggests that the small granules are able to grow in agar because the agar substitutes for some of the conditions present in the large bodies and necessary for their growth.

Although the L forms may be artificial products, their similarity to PPLO and to some of the large viruses gives great interest to them. The impression of most investigators interested in these organisms is that the PPLO derived at some time from L forms, became stabilized, and have continued to live in this form.

The question arises: Do PPLO derive from bacteria at present? No direct evidence for this has been found to date, and most of the claims made for it are poorly supported. However, there are observations which suggest that the weakening of the cell wall may play a part in the adaptation of parasitic bacteria to the host. It seems to me of great importance that bacteria often show signs of the weakening of cell walls in pathologic processes. It was mentioned previously that various bacteria have the tendency to grow to large bodies and produce L forms spontaneously. This occurs usually for a short period following their isolation from infectious processes. In one case of peritonitis there was evidence suggesting that *Bacteroides* multiplied in the L form in phagocytic cells (Dienes & Smith, 1944). Such observations suggest that bacteria may adapt themselves to injury to the cell wall and also suggest the way in which bacteria may have taken the form of PPLO and remained permanently in this form. The study of the possible role of L forms in infectious processes needs much clinical material and much time-consuming work, but it is in many respects more promising than to study the variation of bacteria under artificial conditions.

There are observations of other types, the follow-up of which with present methods of electron microscopy and genetics may give important information on the nature of L forms. In some cases large bodies are evidently formed by the fusion of two segments of a bacterial filament. Observations with a strain of *Bacteroides* have been mentioned; a similar process can be observed occasionally also in *Salmonella* and *Escherichia* exposed to penicillin (Weinberger, Madoff, & Dienes, 1950). Thus far, no genetic changes have been observed in bacteria recovered from L forms. We have to bear in mind that we are at the very beginning in the study of a complex process.

In order to evaluate the significance of the similarities and differences between PPLO and L forms we have to consider the structure, the whole range of variation of size and shape of the organisms, and their reproductive processes. The structure is similar in the two groups in so far as it is accessible to study at present. The cell envelope, the simplicity of inner structure and the indication of nuclear material as they appear with the electron microscope appear to be similar. Chemical and metabolic studies do not indicate principal differences between the two groups. It seems to me especially significant that the structure and reproductive processes of the large bodies are similar in bacteria, in L forms and in PPLO.

The similarity of the gross and microscopic appearance and structure of the colonies on agar is generally admitted (Figs. 10, 11, 12). The well-developed colonies of L forms can usually be distinguished from PPLO by their larger size and by the larger size of the organisms. Young colonies of both forms may be indistinguishable (Figs. 13, 14, 15, 17). The size and arrangement of granules growing out from the large bodies and invading the agar are similar (Figs. 8, 9, 16, 18, 19, 20). It is apparent in young colonies that they are produced by the growth of small granules and the invasion of the agar occurs by active growth and not by passive transport of the small granules as has been claimed by some authors. Multiplication in large colonies occurs mostly in the center of the colony embedded in the agar, and the streaming of the organisms from there to the surface can be observed in both groups. Colonies with similar structure have not been observed in any other groups of micro-organisms.

The individual organisms vary in size and form in both groups and the distribution of various sizes in the culture is greatly influenced by the physical environment, the nutrients present and the age of the culture. In some of the PPLO cultures small, round or elongated organisms between 0.1 and 0.2 μ are visible with the electron microscope. The viability of these is proven by filtration. Only very few of the organisms are of such small size. The majority of growing organisms are between 0.3 and 1 μ. Organisms several μ in diameter may occur on the surface of the agar and may develop to much larger flat, round or polygonal forms. While young, these large bodies consist of small granules and are viable (Fig. 12, 16, 19, 20). The small forms multiply by division or by extrusion of a thin short filament on the end of which the new granule develops (Turner, 1935; Liebermeister, 1953). The double granules so formed are characteristic to both PPLO and L forms. In a few PPLO strains long filaments develop which may disintegrate into granules or develop swellings from which new filaments grow. In most PPLO strains and in L forms long filaments have not been observed.

The electron microscope indicated organisms in the cultures of L forms as small as in PPLO (Dienes, 1953). According to the available filtration experiments the size of the smallest viable organisms in the L forms is slightly larger than in PPLO. This can hardly be regarded as an important difference between the two groups because the L form is less well adapted to grow in our media, especially in broth. More important than size is the fact that the small organisms are produced in the same way in both groups, either by direct multiplication or by multiplication inside the large bodies.

Comparison of broth cultures of PPLO and L forms is difficult because PPLO produce an even turbidity consisting of small granules, while the L forms produce clumps consisting of large bodies. Multiplication of L forms in broth occurs by the growth of granules inside the large bodies and the development of granules again into large bodies. The different behavior in broth is not a principal difference between PPLO and L forms because similar types of multiplication occur in both groups, and their occurrence is influenced greatly by the physical environment.

The similarities between PPLO and L forms, if studied with appropriate techniques, are as impressive now as they seemed to be when the L forms were first observed.

PLATES

The photographs are intended to give concrete examples of the basic observations to which I have referred. Most of them were made from stained agar preparations: Figs. 7, 10, 11, 12, 19, and 20 from wet and Figs. 8, 9, 13, 14, 15, 16, 17, and 18 from dried preparations. Figs. 2–6 were obtained from preparations made with the agar fixation technique of Klieneberger.

REFERENCES

References to the early literature on L forms can be found in the review article of Dienes, L., and Weinberger, H. J. 1951. Bacteriol. Rev. *15*: 245–288.

The recent literature is well covered by E. Klieneberger-Nobel in her book: Pleuropneumonia-like organisms (PPLO) Mycoplasmataceae. 1962. Academic Press, London and New York.

Dienes, L. 1953. Electron micrographs made from L forms of Proteus and two human strains of Pleuropneumonia-like organisms. J. Bacteriol. *66*: 280–286.

Dienes, L. and W. E. Smith. 1944. The significance of pleomorphism in Bacteroides strains. J. Bacteriol. *48*: 125–153.

Liebermeister, K. 1953. Untersuchungen zur Morphologie der Pleuropneumonia-(PPLO)-Gruppe. Z. Naturforsch. *8b*: 757.

Madoff, S. 1960. Isolation and identification of PPLO. Ann. N.Y. Acad. Sci. 79: 383–392.

Turner, A. W. 1935. A study on the morphology and life cycles of the organisms of pleuropneumonia contagiosa bovum (*Borrelomyces peripneumoniae* nov. gen.) by observation in the living state under dark ground illumination. J. Pathol. Bacteriol. *41*: 1–32.

Weinberger, H. J., S. Madoff, and L. Dienes. 1950. The properties of L forms isolated from Salmonella and the isolation of L forms from Shigella. J. Bacteriol. *59*: 765–775.

THE ROLE OF STEROLS IN THE GROWTH AND PHYSIOLOGY OF PLEUROPNEUMONIA-LIKE ORGANISMS

PAUL F. SMITH

State University of South Dakota
Vermillion, U.S.A.

THE EXISTENCE of two major groups of pleuropneumonia-like organisms (PPLO) based on the presence or absence of a growth requirement for sterol is generally acknowledged. That these organisms alone among the bacteria possess such a requirement has given impetus to a study of the possible function it plays in their vital physiological mechanisms. The absence of a typical bacterial cell wall and their apparent stability in various physical environments have directed interest toward an examination of the cell membranes of these organisms. When these two aspects, lipid function and cell membranes, are viewed together one cannot help but consider PPLO as an exemplary tool for the study of fundamental biochemical phenomena surrounding cell membrane function.

Experimental studies on PPLO conducted over the last decade have yielded enough data to allow the derivation of some postulates concerning their cellular physiology. The subject of my discussion centers on the thesis that the non-saponifiable lipids of PPLO carry out a bifunctional role, i.e., the maintenance of the structural integrity of the cell membrane and as intermediates or carries of substrates and metabolic end-products for transport across cell membranes.

There is a specificity for a given molecular structure. The sterols required for growth, such as cholesterol, cholestanol, β-sitosterol and ergosterol all possess an available -OH group at C-3 and a hydrocarbon side chain (Smith & Lynn, 1958). Compounds lacking the -OH group at C-3 (Δ^4 cholesten-3 one, cholestane, biocholesteryl ether and testosterone) and compounds lacking a hydrocarbon side chain (testosterone, the androstene diols, estradiol and estrone) are inactive. Closer examination reveals that the specificity is even more pronounced since some of the 3-OH compounds with the side chain are also inactive. Further insight into the reasons for this specificity will be afforded in the discussion of function of sterols.

The strains that do not require sterol for growth (Laidlaw B and B-15), are able to synthesize their non-saponifiable lipid (NSL) *de novo* (Smith & Rothblat, 1962) and incorporate C^{14} from acetate-1-C^{14} and mevalonic acid-2-C^{14} into their NSL, whereas strains that require sterols cannot. The ability to synthesize non-saponifiable lipid does not alter the capacity to incorporate sterols in their stead. Indeed, sterols active in support of growth of sterol-requiring strains spare the synthesis of NSL by non-sterol-requiring strains (Smith, 1962).

Awareness of these facts, the molecular specificity of the sterol required for growth, the synthetic capacity of non-sterol-requiring strains and the sparing activity of sterol on synthesis of NSL, will now permit an analysis of the function of NSL in PPLO.

Structural function. The cell or protoplasmic membrane is considered to be a bimolecular layer of lipids separating two layers of adsorbed proteins constituting a double membrane about 70 A in thickness. The envelope surrounding PPLO cells has been shown by Van Iterson and Ruys (1960) to be a double membrane of these dimensions. In essence, then, the external cell covering of PPLO is, morphologically speaking, a protoplasmic membrane. Little is known about the specific chemical composition of this membrane except for the NSL component (Smith & Rothblat, 1960; Rothblat & Smith, 1961; Smith, 1962). After sonic lysis, 69 to 83 per cent of the NSL of the cells is found in the insoluble residue in pigmented cells. The pigment is also largely associated with the residue or membrane fraction. Since PPLO contain 5 to 10 per cent of their dry weight as NSL, NSL must comprise a significant quantity of the membrane. As will be discussed later, the composition of the NSL is rather specific and is dependent upon the metabolic capabilities of the organisms.

PPLO, whether sterol-requiring or not, adsorb certain sterols. This process is not dependent upon any energy-yielding reactions and indeed can occur with heat killed cells. There is a requirement for certain proteins which appear to regulate the uptake of sterol and for some surface active agent which will increase the aqueous solubility of the steroid yet not exhibit pronounced toxicity to the cell (Smith & Boughton, 1960). The surface active agent may also act by altering the permeability of the outer protein layer enabling passage of sterol to the underlying lipid layer. Whether a given compound can be adsorbed or not depends on its molecular structure; Steroids possessing a non-polar side chain are irreversibly adsorbed while those lacking the side chain are not. It would appear that adsorption occurs via the non-polar end of the molecule. The -OH group at C-3 is immaterial to this process. Adsorbed steroid cannot be removed by washing, even with solutions of surface active agents not lysing the cells; it can be removed with lipid solvents.

There is evidence that the site of adsorption is phospholipid in nature. Cells extracted with lipid solvents no longer take up steroid, but cells extracted with acetone, in which phospholipids are not soluble, are not affected. Uptake is inhibited by polyvalent cations, such as UO_2^{++}, La^{++}, and Ba^{++}, which are thought to be bound to phosphate groups of phospholipids.

The uptake of appropriate steroid continues over several hours before completion. Cells grown in optimal levels of sterol exhibit a capacity for

520   x. pplo: *P. F. Smith*

further uptake in the metabolic resting state. None of the sterol adsorbed is degraded and all can be recovered as NSL. This finding is compatible and explainable according to the thesis of Willmer (1961), whereby the packing arrangements of steroid with phospholipid molecules vary with the molar ratios. Thus variation of ratios of sterol to phospholipid from 3:1 to 1:3 are compatible with the integrity of lipid monolayers. Continued incorporation of sterol by resting cells could result in a rearrangement of the molecular packing.

Organisms grown in concentrations of sterol greatly exceeding the optimum exhibit a marked reduction in capacity to adsorb sterol in the resting state. As would be expected, surface active agents, such as digitonin, sodium oleate and lecithin, and saponins in sufficient concentration result in disruption of the lipoprotein membrane with ensuing lysis of the organisms.

Non-sterol-requiring strains grown in the absence of sterol synthesize NSL comprised entirely of carotenoid pigments (Smith, 1963). Two basic molecular structures are detectable in all strains examined. One, found in small quantity, is the hydrocarbon, neurosporene. The other, found in greatest quantity, is a dihydroxy neurosporal. Both appear to occur naturally as the all trans isomers. Although the exact location of the -OH groups on the molecule is not known, most naturally occurring carotenols are oxygenated at positions 3 and 3′. Fig. 1 presents the molecular con-

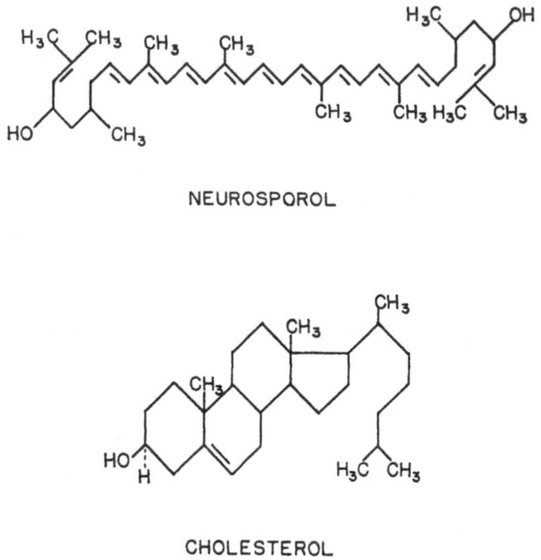

NEUROSPOROL

CHOLESTEROL

FIG. 1. Comparative molecular structures of neurosporol and cholesterol.

figurations of both cholesterol and neurosporol. An analogy can be seen in their structures. Both possess an -OH group at C-3 and both possess a long hydrocarbon segment.

It is proposed that the non-saponifiable lipid of PPLO, be it sterol or carotenol, forms a portion of the bimolecular lipid layer of the cell mem-

brane, being interspersed between phospholipid molecules and held together principally by van der Waal forces between the non-polar segments
of the respective molecules and the repulsion of water by the hydrocarbon
chains. There may also be a bonding between polar groups on the phospholipids and sterol or carotenol but forces between such groups can be
as repulsive as cohesive, according to Willmer (1961). The fact that
steroids incapable of supporting growth are incorporated irreversibly with
the same ease as steroids supporting growth favors binding by non-polar
chains only. It also accounts for the relative side chain specificity of the
molecule. An explanation for the necessity of a polar group, specifically
an OH group, on the molecule, is forthcoming upon examination of the
second proposed function of NSL in PPLO, namely, permeability processes.

Permeability function. As mentioned earlier, only certain 3-OH sterols
support growth. In close scrutiny of the molecular configuration of the 3-OH
sterols with the structures drawn in the preferred chair conformation (Fig.
2), with the radicals attached to C-3 and C-5 denoted as axial or equatorial,

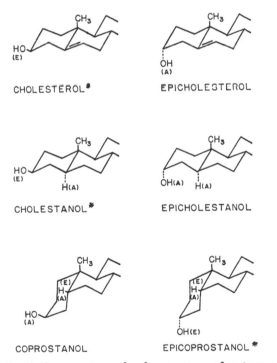

FIG. 2. Comparative molecular structures of various sterols.

a similarity between sterols active in supporting growth can be noted.
Equatorial bonds are defined as those lying in the general plane of the fused
ring while axial bonds lie at right angles to the general plane of the ring.
All sterols capable of supporting growth possess the 3-OH radical in equatorial configuration. Those which are inactive have the 3-OH radical in

axial configuration. This is the only factor governing the specificity of the molecule and it is immaterial whether the 3-OH group is α or β. The configuration of the hydrogen atom at C-5 is of little concern although all active sterols which contain it have it in the axial configuration relative to the A ring. Generally speaking, substituents in the equatorial orientation are more stable and an equatorial hydroxy group is more easily esterified and hydrolyzed chemically or enzymatically because of less steric hindrance. Introduction of a double bond at the 5 position, as in cholesterol, results in a conformation closely resembling cholestanol, i.e., the 3 β-OH is equatorial, rather than a conformation resembling coprostanol in which the 3 β-OH is axial. Apparently the cis or trans relationship of ring A to ring B has little bearing on the effectiveness of the sterol. Whether this configuration has an effect on incorporation is not known as yet. Basically the configurational requirements for uptake are only relatively specific. Hence one must look elsewhere for an explanation of the high degree of configurational specificity of the active sterols. Since specificity is one notable property of enzymes, it was thought that some enzymatic function vital to the organisms is concerned with the non-saponifiable lipids.

Analysis of the non-saponifiable lipids of both sterol- and non-sterol-requiring strains has yielded information compatible with its participation in enzyme reactions (Rothblat & Smith, 1961; Smith, 1963). Non-glucose fermenting, sterol-requiring strains contain unesterified and esterified cholesterol. The volatile fatty acids in ester linkage are predominately butyric and acetic. Glucose-fermenting sterol-requiring strains contain esterified and unesterified cholesterol and cholesteryl β-D glucoside. Glucose-fermenting non-sterol-requiring strains contain neurosporene, esterified and unesterified neurosporol and a neurosporyl glucoside. The volatile fatty acid in ester linkage is acetic only in both glucose-fermenting strains. Obviously to form ester and glycosidic linkage with the sterol or carotenol, the organisms must possess esterases and glycosidases.

An esterase distinct from lipase activity and capable of synthesizing cholesteryl esters of fatty acids and of hydrolytic or thiolytic cleavage of cholesteryl esters has been demonstrated to exist in all strains (Smith, 1959). Like the NSL the site of the esterase is in the insoluable residue (cell membrane) following sonic lysis. No specific information is available yet on the proposed glycosidase. Nevertheless, when resting cells of glucose-fermenting strains are incubated with glucose-C^{14}, labelled cholesteryl glucoside is formed only when the organisms are actively metabolizing glucose. When one relates the groups attached to the sterol or carotenol to the substrate and end-product of metabolism, particularly of glucose-fermenting strains, it can be seen that they are identical. That is, glucose is the initial substrate and can be found in glycosidic linkage with sterol or carotenol, and acetate, the end-product of aerobic glucose metabolism, is the principal fatty acid and sole volatile fatty acid found in ester linkage with sterol or carotenol. The picture is not as clear with non-glucose-fermenting strains but one can speculate that acetate, butyrate or both are metabolic end-products or initial substrates for strains possessing oxidative activity for short-chain fatty acids.

It is proposed tentatively that the sterol or carotenol acting as a carrier in conjunction with the esterase and glycosidase acting as permeases (Cohen & Monod, 1957) function in transport of metabolizable substrate across the cell membrane into the cell and of metabolic end-products out of the cell. Fig. 3 presents the proposed scheme using glucose as an example.

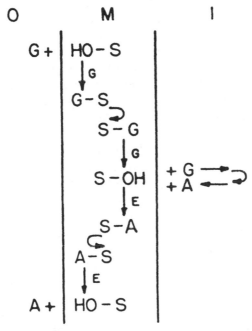

Fig. 3. Schematic pathway of transport across cell membrane of PPLO. O—outside of cell; M—cell membrane; I—interior of cell; G—glucose; S-OH—sterol or carotenol; G—glucosidase; GS—steryl or carotenyl glucoside; A—acetate; E—esterase; S-A—steryl or carotenyl acetate.

External glucose is coupled with cholesterol or neurosporol, the -OH groups of which face the outside of the cell, by the action of a glucosidase (assumed to be present in the membrane), to form cholesteryl or neurosporyl glucoside. The increase in polarity of the sterol molecule as a result of glucosidation would give reason for rotational or translational movements in the membrane causing rearrangement of the molecule making the glucosyl group available to the inside of the cell (Danielli, 1954). In this orientation the glucosidase could cleave the glucosyl group from the glucoside. Such a reaction would be favored, for the enzymatic mechanism for degradation of glucose is present in the cell and would force the glucosidase reaction in the direction of cleavage. The free alcohol would remain in this orientation being prepared to accept the end-product of glucose metabolism, acetate. Following degradation of glucose to acetate inside the cell the acetate would be coupled to the sterol or carotenol by the action of the esterase in the membrane. Esterification results in a decrease in polarity of the molecule. This change in polarity would give reason for another rotational or translational movement in the membrane, this time making the acetyl group available to the outside of the cell. Again the esterase could catalyse cleavage of the ester with the production of the free alcohol and liberation of acetate. The sterol or carotenol would be in the proper orientation to participate in another cycle of transport.

A dihydroxy neurosporol would possess an advantage over cholesterol by virtue of its possessing a polar group at either end of the molecule. These -OH groups could face or lie in the protein layers of the membrane, the central non-polar segment between the phospholipid molecules. The hydroxy group facing the inside of the cell could be esterified while the other facing the exterior of the cell could be linking with glucose. One rotational movement could achieve both transport of glucose into the cell and transport of acetate out of the cell.

Obviously this mechanism is highly theoretical but at present it explains the necessity for a sterol of a highly specific molecular configuration, the presence of free, esterified and glucosidyl derivatives of sterol and carotenol, and the existence of and the cellular location of the NSL and esterase. An extended discussion of the relative fit of this proposed transport mechanism with evidence supporting transport systems proposed for other cells is too time-consuming for this presentation. It can be stated that this proposed mechanism is similar to the enzymatic carrier concept of active transport described by Danielli (1954), Cirillo (1961) and many other investigators. There is no evidence yet to conclude whether this transport is one of facilitated diffusion or an energy-dependent accumulation process. The mechanism proposed above can readily account for the stereospecificity of membrane transport, the Michaelis-Menten relationships found in membrane permeation (Morgan, Post & Park, 1961) and in glucose transport, the proposed carrier complex and the competition among hexoses for the transport system (Wilbrandt, 1961).

References

Cirillo, V. P.   1961.   Sugar transport in microorganisms. Ann. Rev. Microbiol. *15*: 197–218.

Cohen, G. N., and J. Monod.   1957.   Bacterial permeases. Bacteriol. Rev. *21*: 169–194.

Danielli, J. F.   1954.   Morphological and molecular aspects of active transport. Symp. Soc. Exptl. Biol. 8: 502–515.

Morgan, H. E., R. L. Post, and C. R. Park.   1961.   Glucose transport and phosphorylation in the perfused heart of normal and diabetic rats. *In* Membrane transport and metabolism, ed. A. Kleinzeller and A. Kotyk, pp. 423–430. Academic Press, Inc., New York.

Rothblat, G. H., and P. F. Smith. 1961. Nonsaponifiable lipids of representative pleuropneumonia-like organisms. J. Bacteriol. *82*: 479–491.

Smith, P. F. 1959. Cholesterol esterase activity of pleuropneumonia-like organisms. J. Bacteriol. 77: 682–689.

Smith, P. F. 1963. Carotenoids of Mycoplasma. J. Gen. Microbiol. (in press).

Smith, P. F., and J. E. Boughton. 1960. Role of protein and phospholipid in the growth of pleuropneumonia-like organisms. J. Bacteriol. *80*: 851–860.

Smith, P. F., and R. J. Lynn. 1958. Lipid requirements for the growth of pleuropneumonia-like organisms. J. Bacteriol. 76: 264–269.

Smith, P. F., and G. H. Rothblat. 1960. Incorporation of cholesterol by pleuropneumonia-like organisms. J. Bacteriol. *80*: 842–850.

Smith, P. F., and G. H. Rothblat. 1962. Comparison of lipid composition of pleuropneumonia-like and L-type organisms. J. Bacteriol. *83*: 500–506.

Van Iterson, W., and A. C. Ruys. 1960. The fine structure of the Mycoplasmataceae (microorganisms of the pleuropneumonia group = PPLO). I. *Mycoplasma hominis*, *M. fermentans* and *M. salivarium*. J. Ultrastruct. Res. *3*: 282–301.

Wilbrandt, W. 1961. The sugar transport across the red cell membrane. *In* Membrane transport and metabolism, ed. A. Kleinzeller and A. Kotyk, pp. 388–398. Academic Press, New York.

Willmer, E. N. 1961. Steroids and cell surfaces. Biol. Rev. *36*: 368–398.

STRUCTURE, COMPOSITION AND PROPERTIES OF THE PPLO CELL ENVELOPE *

SHMUEL RAZIN

Department of Clinical Microbiology
The Hebrew University–Hadassah Medical School
Jerusalem, Israel

PLASTICITY is a most prominent feature of the pleuropneumonia-like organisms. This characteristic has led to the assumption that PPLO have a peculiar cell envelope and are devoid of rigid walls as found in eubacteria. Yet, until recently, very little was done to elucidate the nature of this peculiar cell envelope. The rapid progress made during the last decade in the study of bacterial membranes has provided both the impetus and the means for investigating the properties of the PPLO cell envelope.

MORPHOLOGICAL STUDIES

Electron microscopic studies of the whole PPLO cells have indicated the absence of a rigid cell wall (Morton et al., 1954; Klieneberger-Nobel & Cuckow, 1955). Recent studies of ultrathin sections showed the PPLO to be limited by an envelope much thinner than that of eubacteria (Freundt, 1960; Sharp, 1960; Edwards & Fogh, 1960; Van Iterson and Ruys, 1960; Ruys & Van Iterson, 1961). Thanks to the elaboration of fixation and staining techniques for electron microscopy a better definition of the structure of the bacterial cell envelopes has become possible. Electron microscopy of ultrathin sections showed various eubacteria to be covered by a cell wall of varying thickness (usually 100–200 A) underneath which lies a plasma membrane, usually 70–80 A thick (Van Iterson, 1961; Koike & Takeya, 1961; Imaeda & Convit, 1962). The plasma membrane was shown to be composed of two electron-opaque layers and a less dense layer in between. This three-layered structure corresponds to the "unit membrane" (Robertson, 1959) which covers cells and organelles of various origin. It is believed to consist of a single bimolecular leaflet of lipid ($\sim$ 35 A thick) bordered by monolayers ($\sim$ 20 A thick) of protein or polysaccharide (Robertson, 1959). Van Iterson and Ruys (1960) and Ruys and Van Iterson (1961) succeeded in obtaining PPLO cell-sections showing very clear cell membranes. These

*This research was supported in part by a grant from the Joint Research Fund of the Hebrew University–Hadassah Medical School.

The help of Mr. M. Argaman throughout this study is gratefully acknowledged.

membranes resembled the plasma membranes of bacteria in their triple-
layered structure and in having a thickness of ~75 A. The morphological
similarity between PPLO and bacterial protoplast membranes was confirmed
in our study, as well. Protoplasts of *Micrococcus lysodeikticus* prepared by
lysozyme digestion (Gilby & Few, 1960a) and cells of *Mycoplasma laidlawii*
were mixed with 2 per cent agar containing 1 M sucrose, fixed and sectioned
according to Van Iterson and Ruys (1960). The sections clearly showed the
striking resemblance between the membranes covering the PPLO and
bacterial protoplasts.

CHEMICAL COMPOSITION

   Kandler and Zehender (1957) and Plackett (1959) were unable to detect
diaminopimelic acid and hexosamines in several PPLO strains. This suggested that PPLO are devoid of the "mucopeptide" polymer, responsible for
the rigidity of bacterial cell walls. We were able to confirm these findings
(Razin & Argaman, 1961) and provide additional evidence for the absence
of the "mucopeptide" polymer, by demonstrating the complete resistance of
PPLO to lysozyme. None of the PPLO strains examined was lysed by
lysozyme, even when several methods suitable for lysis of gram-positive and
gram-negative bacteria were used (Smolelis & Hartsell, 1949; Becker &
Hartsell, 1954; Repaske, 1956; Grula & Hartsell, 1957; Kohn, 1960). The
absence of the "mucopeptide" polymer from PPLO was to be expected
because of the marked plasticity of the cells and their complete resistance to
penicillin.
   Various methods for obtaining isolated PPLO membranes for chemical
analysis were tried out. Lysis by osmotic shock, the method of choice for
isolation of bacterial protoplast membranes, could not be applied, because
PPLO were found to resist this treatment (Razin & Argaman, 1962). Disruption of PPLO cells by sonic or ultrasonic energy resulted in complete
destruction of the delicate cell membranes, as evidenced by electron microscopy. The best method for obtaining isolated cell membranes was found
to be lysis of PPLO suspended in deionized water by alternate freezing and
thawing. Electron microscopy of PPLO suspensions treated in this way
showed them to consist almost entirely of very thin membranes (Fig. 1).
In order to obtain enough membrane material for chemical analysis, the
PPLO were ruptured in the Hughes press. *Mycoplasma laidlawii* was grown
in 10 litre quantities of liquid Edward medium (Razin and Oliver, 1961)
supplemented with 1 per cent Bacto-PPLO serum fraction and 0.75 per cent
glucose. After 16–18 hours of incubation at 37 C the cells were sedimented
by high speed centrifugation and washed once with deionized water. A
thick paste of washed cells was then crushed without abrasives in the
Hughes press, previously cooled to —35 C. The crushed material was diluted
with deionized water and centrifuged at 8,000 g for 20 min. The sediment
was discarded and the highly opalescent supernatant fluid was centrifuged

FIG. 1. Isolated cell membranes of *Mycoplasma laidlawii*.

at 20,000 g for 30 min. The resulting transparent yellow sediment was freeze-dried. Samples taken from the sediment formed at 8,000 g and examined by the electron microscope showed many broken cells, debris, and a few membranes. The sediment formed at 20,000 g consisted almost entirely of cell membranes.

Membranes of *Micrococcus lysodeikticus* protoplasts, prepared according to Gilby, Few and McQuillen (1958), were included in the chemical studies for purposes of comparison. Total nitrogen and phosphorus of the membranes were determined as described by Umbreit *et al.* (1957). Protein was estimated according to Lowry *et al.* (1951). Lipids were extracted by methanol and ether (Gilby, Few and McQuillen, 1958) and evaporated to dryness under vacuum. Cholesterol was determined in the non-saponifiable lipid fraction by the Liebermann-Burchard reaction as outlined by Cook (1958). Total carbohydrate was estimated according to Dubois *et al.* (1956). Nucleic acids were extracted according to Ogur and Rosen (1950); RNA was determined by the method of Drury (1948) and DNA according to Burton (1956).

The results of the chemical analysis of the PPLO and bacterial protoplast

TABLE 1

CHEMICAL ANALYSIS OF CELL MEMBRANES

			mg/100 mg dry weight								
			Lipid			Carbo-hydrate	Nucleic Acids				
	Protein		Total				RNA		DNA		
Organism	Mean	Range	Mean	Range	Choles-terol	Mean	Range	Mean	Range	Mean	Range
Myco-plasma laidlawii	62	55–67	27	25–30	0–3.5	7	7–8	3	2.1–4.7	0.2	0.15–0.50
Protoplasts of *Micro-coccus lyso-deikticus*	52	43–56	25	22–26	0	11	8–13	1	0–2	1.2	1.1–1.4

membranes are summarized in Table 1. Although no more than preliminary and still incomplete, the results show a striking similarity in the chemical composition of the PPLO and bacterial protoplast membranes. Our data for the composition of the protoplast membranes conform well with those obtained by Gilby, Few and McQuillen (1958). The only substantial difference found in this preliminary study between membranes of *M. laidlawii* and those of *M. lysodeikticus* protoplasts was the presence of significant amounts of cholesterol in the former. It must be stressed, however, that the amount of cholesterol found in *M. laidlawii* depended on its concentration in the growth medium (Rothblat & Smith, 1961). Thus, cholesterol could not be detected in *M. laidlawii* grown in a cholesterol-free synthetic medium (Razin & Cohen, unpublished).

Mycoplasma mycoides var. *mycoides* was found to require glycerol, cholesterol and long-chain fatty acids for growth (Rodwell & Abbot, 1961). There are several indications that these compounds are utilized for the biosynthesis of the PPLO cell envelope. Thus, Plackett (1961) brought evidence for the incorporation of glycerol by *M. mycoides* var. *mycoides* into a cardiolipin-like compound resembling the complex phosphatidic acid present in bacterial protoplast membranes (Gilby, Few & McQuillen, 1958; Weibull & Bergström, 1958; Macfarlane, 1961).

SUSCEPTIBILITY TO LYSIS

Valuable information on the properties of the PPLO cell envelope was obtained by testing the susceptibility of PPLO cells to lysis by various physical and chemical agents. For purposes of comparison, lysozyme-produced protoplasts of *Micrococcus lysodeikticus* (Gilby & Few, 1960a), penicillin-induced spheroplasts of *Escherichia coli* (Lederberg, 1956) and the stable L forms of *Streptobacillus moniliformis* were included in this study. Table 2 summarizes some of the results obtained. It may be seen

TABLE 2

Per Cent Lysis of PPLO, Bacterial Protoplasts, Spheroplasts
and L Forms by Various Chemical Agents

Agent	*Myco-plasma laid-lawii*	*Myco-plasma mycoides* var. *capri*	Proto-plasts of *Micro-coccus lyso-deikticus*	Sphero-plasts of *Escheri-chia coli*	L form of *Strepto-bacillus monili-formis*	Intact cells of *Micro-coccus lyso-deikticus*
Sodium lauryl sulphate (5×10^{-4} M)	95	97	95	60	65	5
Cetyltrimethyl-ammonium bromide (5×10^{-5} M)	70	5	90	10	0	0
Sodium taurocholate (0.25%)	83	60	85	40	45	0
n-Propanol (1.68 M)	90	85	90	20	30	0
n-Butanol (0.40 M)	85	80	92	30	55	0
NaOH (0.25 M)	90	90	70	80	40	15
Pancreatic lipase (500 μg/ml)	80	80	60	45	30	0
Digitonin (120 μg/ml)	85	85	0	0	0	0

All experiments were carried out in 1 M sucrose + 0.05 M NaCl solution. Optical density measured at 500 mμ at zero time and after 30 min incubation at room temperature.

$$\text{Per cent lysis} = \frac{\text{OD (time 0)} - \text{OD (time 30)}}{\text{OD (time 0)}} \times 100.$$

from this table that PPLO, like bacterial protoplasts, were very sensitive to lysis by surface active agents, primary alcohols, alkali and pancreatic lipase. The marked sensitivity of PPLO to lysis by these agents provides additional evidence for the lipoprotein nature of their envelope. According to Gilby and Few (1960a), primary alcohols act on the lipid component of the protoplast membrane and cause lysis by disruption of the membrane permeability. Similarly, pancreatic lipase degrades the lipid component of the membrane, causing its structural disintegration (Spiegelman, Aronson & Fitz-James, 1958). The cationic detergent cetyltrimethylammonium bromide combines with the phosphatidic acid present in the membrane, causing lysis by impairing membrane permeability (Gilby & Few, 1960b). The anionic detergent sodium lauryl sulphate acts mainly on the protein component of the membrane, which it dissolves (Gilby & Few, 1960b). Sodium lauryl sulphate caused a marked clearing of PPLO membrane suspensions.

An important difference between PPLO and bacterial protoplasts, spheroplasts and L forms was the sensitivity of the former to lysis by digitonin and saponin (Table 2). Lysis of several PPLO strains by digitonin has already been recorded by Smith and Rothblat (1960). Digitonin apparently causes lysis by combining with the cholesterol present in the PPLO cell envelope. *Mycoplasma laidlawii* grown in a cholesterol-free synthetic medium (Razin & Cohen, unpublished) and found to contain no detectable amounts of cholesterol, was almost completely resistant to lysis by digitonin.

Bacterial spheroplasts and L forms were more resistant to lysis by the chemical agents tested than bacterial protoplasts and PPLO (Table 2). The defective cell walls which still cover the plasma membrane of spheroplasts and L forms (McQuillen, 1960) are apparently responsible for this resistance. However, the spheroplasts and L forms were considerably more sensitive to lysis by the above-mentioned agents than intact bacterial cells.

Another difference between PPLO and bacterial protoplasts was found with respect to lysis by osmotic shock. Whereas protoplasts of M. lysodeikticus underwent almost complete and immediate lysis when transferred from 1 M sucrose to 0.25 M sucrose solution, the PPLO strains were not lysed to any significant degree, even when transferred from the concentrated sucrose solution to deionized water. Resistance of PPLO to osmotic shock has already been indicated by several authors (Smith & Sasaki, 1958; Plackett, 1959; Butler & Knight, 1960). Several hypotheses may be provided to explain this resistance. (a) The very small dimensions and spherical shape of most PPLO cells are factors which reduce the adverse effects of osmotic pressure changes (Mitchell & Moyle, 1956). (b) The PPLO cell envelope might be very elastic and eminently capable of withstanding stretching. The cholesterol present in the cell envelope might contribute to this elasticity, for cholesterol is believed to be interspersed between the phospholipid residues in biological membranes and to stabilize their structure (Ponder, 1961). (c) The PPLO cell may have a low internal osmotic pressure. Various bacteria differ widely with respect to their internal osmotic pressure. Thus gram-positive cocci have osmotic pressures of 20–30 atm (Mitchell & Moyle, 1956), while gram-negative rods such as Escherichia coli or Aerobacter species have internal osmotic pressures of only 4–8 atm (Gebicki & James, 1960; Hugo & Russell, 1960). We have no direct measure of the internal osmotic pressure of PPLO cells. However, indirect evidence for a low internal osmotic pressure in these cells was obtained by freezing and thawing experiments. PPLO suspended in deionized water were sensitive to lysis by alternate freezing and thawing. Addition of low concentrations of sucrose or NaCl protected the cells from lysis. A concentration of 0.25 M sucrose gave complete protection, while 0.12 M sucrose sufficed to protect almost all PPLO cells. The protoplasts of M. lysodeikticus, which have an internal osmotic pressure of about 20–30 atm (Mitchell & Moyle, 1956) were lysed by alternate freezing and thawing even when suspended in 1 M sucrose solution. The protective effect is probably due to the shrinkage of the plastic PPLO cells owing to osmotic dehydration in the hypertonic media (Postgate & Hunter, 1961). The cell envelope of the shrunk cell is likely to offer more resistance to the shearing forces of the ice crystals. If this explanation is correct, then 0.25 M sucrose solution has to be regarded as hypertonic, and 0.12 M sucrose as about isotonic to the PPLO cells. The osmotic pressure of 0.12 M sucrose solution is about 3 atm (Handbook of Chemistry and Physics, 1954–1955). Hence the internal osmotic pressure of PPLO seems to be remarkably low. On the other hand, the requirement of the PPLO for a rather high tonicity of the growth medium (Leach, 1962) seems to contradict the above assumption.

CONCLUSION

The PPLO cells are limited by a membrane of lipoprotein nature. Morphological and chemical studies of this membrane indicate its close resemblance to the plasma membrane of bacteria.

ACKNOWLEDGMENTS

We wish to thank Mrs. E. Friedberg and Mr. M. Wormser for their valuable technical assistance.

REFERENCES

Becker, M. E., and S. E. Hartsell. 1954. Factors affecting bacteriolysis using lysozyme in dual enzyme systems. Arch. Biochem. Biophys. 53: 402–410.

Burton, K. 1956. A study of the conditions and mechanism of the diphenylamine reaction for the colorimetric estimation of deoxyribonucleic acid. Biochem. J. 62: 315–323.

Butler, M., and B. C. J. G. Knight. 1960. The survival of washed suspensions of Mycoplasma. J. Gen. Microbiol. 22: 470–477.

Cook, R. P. 1958. Cholesterol. Academic Press, Inc., New York.

Drury, H. F. 1948. Identification and estimation of pentoses in the presence of glucose. Arch. Biochem. 19: 455–466.

Dubois, M., K. Gilles, K. Hamilton, P. Rebas, and E. Smith. 1956. Determination of carbohydrates by phenol. Anal. Chem. 28: 350.

Edwards, G. A., and J. Fogh. 1960. Fine structure of pleuropneumonia-like organisms in pure culture and in infected tissue culture cells. J. Bacteriol. 79: 267–276.

Freundt, E. A. 1960. Morphology and classification of the PPLO. Ann. N.Y. Acad. Sci. 79: 312–325.

Gebicki, J. M. and A. M. James. 1960. The preparation and properties of spheroplasts of *Aerobacter aerogenes*. J. Gen. Microbiol. 23: 9–18.

Gilby, A. R. and A. V. Few. 1960a. Lysis of protoplasts of *Micrococcus lysodeikticus* by alcohols. J. Gen. Microbiol. 23: 27–33.

Gilby, A. R., and A. V. Few. 1960b. Lysis of protoplasts of *Micrococcus lysodeikticus* by ionic detergents. J. Gen. Microbiol. 23: 19–26.

Gilby, A. R., A. V. Few, and K. McQuillen. 1958. The chemical composition of the protoplast membrane of *Micrococcus lysodeikticus*. Biochim. et Biophys. Acta 29: 21–29.

Grula, E. A. and S. E. Hartsell. 1957. Lysozyme in the bacteriolysis of gram-negative bacteria. I. Morphological changes during use of Nakamura's technique. Can. J. Microbiol. 3: 13–21.

Handbook of Chemistry and Physics. 36th ed., 1954–1955. Editor-in-Chief, C. D. Hodgman. Chemical Rubber Publishing Co. Cleveland, Ohio.

Hugo, W. B., and A. D. Russell. 1960. Quantitative aspects of penicillin action on *Escherichia coli* in hypertonic medium. J. Bacteriol. 80: 436–440.

Imaeda, T., and J. Convit. 1962. Electron microscope study of *Mycobacterium leprae* and its environment in a vesicular leprous lesion. J. Bacteriol. 83: 43–52.

Kandler, O., and C. Zehender. 1957. Ueber das Vorkommen von α, ϵ-Diaminopimelinsäure bei verschiedenen L-Phasentypen von *Proteus vulgaris* und bei den pleuropneumonieähnlichen Organismen. Z. Naturforsch. *12*b: 725–728.

Klieneberger-Nobel, E., and F. W. Cuckow. 1955. A study of organisms of the pleuropneumonia group by electron microscopy. J. Gen. Microbiol. *12*: 95–99.

Kohn, A. 1960. Lysis of frozen and thawed cells of *Escherichia coli* by lysozyme, and their conversion into spheroplasts. J. Bacteriol. *79*: 697–709.

Koike, M., and K. Takeya. 1961. Fine structure of intracytoplasmic organelles of mycobacteria. J. Biophys. Biochem. Cytol. *9*: 597–608.

Leach, R. H. 1962. The osmotic requirements for growth of Mycoplasma. J. Gen. Microbiol. *27*: 345–354.

Lederberg, J. 1956. Bacterial protoplasts induced by penicillin. Proc. Nat. Acad. Sci. (U.S.) *42*: 574–577.

Lowry, O. H., N. J. Rosebrough, A. L. Farr, and R. J. Randall. 1951. Protein measurement with the folin phenol reagent. J. Biol. Chem. *193*: 265–275.

Macfarlane, M. G. 1961. Composition of lipid from protoplast membranes and whole cells of *Micrococcus lysodeikticus*. Biochem. J. *79*: 4p.

McQuillen, K. 1960. Bacterial protoplasts. *In* The bacteria: A treatise on structure and function, ed. I. C. Gunsalus and R. Y. Stanier, *1*: 249. Academic Press, New York.

Mitchell, P., and J. Moyle. 1956. Osmotic function and structure in bacteria. Symp. Soc. Gen. Microbiol. *6*: 150.

Morton, H. E., J. G. Lecce, J. J. Oskay, and N. H. Coy. 1954. Electron microscope studies of pleuropneumonia-like organisms isolated from man and chickens. J. Bacteriol. *68*: 697–717.

Ogur, M., and G. Rosen. 1950. The nucleic acids of plant tissues. I. The extraction and estimation of desoxypentose nucleic acid and pentose nucleic acid. Arch. Biochem. *25*: 262–276.

Plackett, P. 1959. On the probable absence of "mucocomplex" from *Mycoplasma mycoides*. Biochim. et Biophys. Acta *35*: 260–262.

Plackett, P. 1961. A polyglycerophosphate compound from *Mycoplasma mycoides*. Nature *189*: 125–126.

Ponder, E. 1961. The cell membrane and its properties. *In* The cell, ed. J. Brachet and A. E. Mirsky, *2*: 2–84. Academic Press, New York.

Postgate, J. R., and J. R. Hunter. 1961. On the survival of frozen bacteria. J. Gen. Microbiol. *26*: 367–378.

Razin, S., and M. Argaman. 1961. Properties of the Mycoplasma (PPLO) cell envelope. Bull. Res. Council Israel 9E: 121–122.

Razin, S., and M. Argaman. 1962. Susceptibility of Mycoplasma (pleuropneumonia-like organisms) and bacterial protoplasts to lysis by various agents. Nature *193*: 502–503.

Razin, S., and O. Oliver. 1961. Morphogenesis of Mycoplasma and bacterial L-form colonies. J. Gen. Microbiol. *24*: 225–237.

Repaske, R. 1956. Lysis of gram-negative bacteria by lysozyme. Biochim. et Biophys. Acta *22*: 189–191.

Robertson, J. D. 1959. The ultrastructure of cell membranes and their derivatives. Biochem. Soc. Symp. *16*: 3–43.

Rodwell, A. W. and A. Abbot. 1961. The function of glycerol, cholesterol and long-chain fatty acids in the nutrition of *Mycoplasma mycoides*. J. Gen. Microbiol. *25*: 201–214.

Rothblat, G. H., and P. F. Smith. 1961. Nonsaponifiable lipids of representative pleuropneumonia-like organisms. J. Bacteriol. *82*: 479–491.

Ruys, A. C., and W. Van Iterson. 1961. Some characteristics of pathogenic avian PPLO. Antonie van Leeuwenhoek *27*: 129–138.

Sharp, J. T.   1960.   The cell wall of bacterial L-forms and pleuropneumonia-like organisms. Ann. N.Y. Acad. Sci. 79: 344–355.

Smith, P. F., and G. H. Rothblat.   1960.   Incorporation of cholesterol by pleuropneumonia-like organisms. J. Bacteriol. 80: 842–850.

Smith, P. F., and S. Sasaki.   1958.   Stability of pleuropneumonia-like organisms to some physical factors. Appl. Microbiol. 6: 184–189.

Smolelis, A. N., and S. E. Hartsell.   1949.   The determination of lysozyme. J. Bacteriol. 58: 731–736.

Spiegelman, S., A. I. Aronson, and P. C. Fitz-James.   1958.   Isolation and characterization of nuclear bodies from protoplasts of *Bacillus megaterium*. J. Bacteriol. 75: 102–117.

Umbreit, W. W., R. H. Burris, and J. F. Stauffer.   1957.   Manometric techniques, 3rd ed. Burgess Publishing Company, Minneapolis.

Van Iterson, W.   1961.   Some features of a remarkable organelle in *Bacillus subtilis*. J. Biophys. Biochem. Cytol. 9: 183–192.

Van Iterson, W., and A. C. Ruys.   1960.   The fine structure of the Mycoplasmataceae (microorganisms of the pleuropneumonia group = P.P.L.O.). I. *Mycoplasma hominis*, *M. fermentans* and *M. salivarium*. J. Ultrastruct. Res. 3: 282–301.

Weibull, C., and L. Bergström.   1958.   The chemical nature of the cytoplasmic membrane and cell wall of *Bacillus megaterium*, strain M.   Biochim. et Biophys. Acta 30: 340–351.

CARBOHYDRATES OF SOME *MYCOPLASMA* STRAINS

P. PLACKETT*, S. H. BUTTERY and G. S. COTTEW

Division of Animal Health
Animal Health Research Laboratory, C.S.I.R.O.
Parkville, Victoria, Australia

ALTHOUGH SEROLOGICAL TESTS play a large part in studies of the Mycoplasmataceae, little has been done by way of chemical characterization of the antigens. An exception is the work of Kurotchkin (1937) who, twenty-five years ago, reported the isolation of a specific carbohydrate substance from *Mycoplasma mycoides*. Although active in precipitin tests, it did not fix complement with bovine antisera. Large quantities of the substance were shown to be present both in culture supernatants and in the blood of animals in severe cases of the disease. More recently Dafaalla (1957, 1959) achieved the separation of two antigenic fractions from *M. mycoides*. One of these (fraction A), precipitated by 67 per cent ethanol, was probably related to Kurotchkin's carbohydrate. The other (fraction B), extractable from the cells with 67 per cent ethanol, was active in both precipitin and complement fixation tests. Fraction B was found attached to the cells only, whereas fraction A was present also in culture supernatants, in exudates, and in the blood of moribund animals. White (1958) used immunodiffusion tests to demonstrate the presence of three soluble antigens in extracts of *M. mycoides* and in material from lesions and exudates. One or two of these could often be found in sera from dying animals.

M. mycoides cells were fractionated into protein, carbohydrate, and lipid fractions by Yoshida (1961). The lipid fraction contained complement-fixing antigens; the protein and carbohydrate fractions did not.

It is of interest that Knight and Cowan (1961), who prepared a soluble complement-fixing antigen by a modification of Dafaalla's method, found that the product did not fix complement with bovine antisera unless a heat-labile factor, present in normal bovine sera, was added to the system.

We first became interested in the carbohydrate components of the V5 strain of *M. mycoides* as a potential source of error in the determination of the nucleic acids. It was found that the organisms synthesized a galactose polymer of rather unusual properties, amounting to about 10 per cent of the dry weight of the cells. The preparation and some of the properties of the crude galactan have already been reported (Buttery & Plackett, 1960). We

*Dr. Plackett presented this paper on invitation of the Congress Committee. Mr. Buttery to whom an invitation had been extended was unable to attend.

have made further studies of this polysaccharide, and have examined some other Mycoplasma strains for the presence of carbohydrates.

DISTRIBUTION OF SUGARS

The strains examined are listed, together with the sources from which they were obtained, in Table 1.

TABLE 1

DISTRIBUTION OF SUGARS IN *Mycoplasma* STRAINS

Strain	Origin	Received from	Hexose components
Bovine			
V5	pleuropneumonia	Parkville	*Galactose*, glucose
Gladysdale	pleuropneumonia	Parkville	*Galactose*, glucose
3278	pleuropneumonia	N.C.T.C.	*Galactose*, glucose
L2917	arthritis	G. Simmons	Glucose
N29	arthritis	G. Simmons	Glucose
BGL	genital	Lister Inst.	Glucose (galactose, mannose?)
542	nasal	Parkville	Glucose
Goat			
Ca	pleuropneumonia	Lister Inst.	Glucose
HG	pleuropneumonia	Parkville	Glucose
GY	peritonitis	L. Laws	*Galactose*, glucose
OG	polyarthritis	R. Olds	*Galactose*, glucose
Sheep			
JD	lung	Parkville	Glucose
Avian			
M1316	duck, nasal	G. Simmons	Glucose
1252	non-pathogenic	M. Pulsford	Glucose
Tu	fowl	H. P. Chu	(Glucose, galactose, mannose?)
S6	turkey	M. Pulsford	(Glucose?)
Saprophytic			
Laidlaw B	sewage	P. F. Smith	Glucose

Except where sugars were present in traces only (shown in brackets) identifications are based on comparison with authentic sugars on paper chromatograms run in at least three different solvent systems, and upon the spectra observed in the cysteine-sulphuric acid reaction (Dische *et al.*, 1949). Glucose in the presence of galactose was estimated with glucose oxidase (Huggett & Nixon, 1957), all samples containing galactose at the same concentration.

All strains except 542, Tu, and S6 were grown in "BVF-OS" (Turner, Campbell & Dick, 1935). In some experiments this was supplemented with 0.03 M glucose, 0.003 M glycerol and 2×10^{-5} M Na oleate. The growth of *M. mycoides* (V5 strain), whether measured by optical density or by colony count, is much improved by the provision of additional amounts of these nutrients, which are known to be essential (Rodwell, 1960). The initial pH of the supplemented medium was adjusted to 7.9–8.0 with NaOH. The modified medium is unlikely to give better growth of strains which grow poorly in BVF-OS. It does give better growth of other *M. mycoides* strains, the bovine arthritis strains (L2917 and N29), and *M. laidlawii* (Laidlaw B). Strain S6 was grown in the supplemented medium with ox serum replaced by horse serum. Strain BGL was grown in the standard medium but with twice the usual concentration of ox serum. Strains 542 and Tu were grown in the medium described by Provost (1957). After one to six days, depending on the rate of growth, the cultures were harvested by centrifugation.

After washing in cold 0.2 M NaCl, the organisms were examined according to the scheme outlined in Fig. 1. Most of the methods were those used in studies of the V5 strain of *M. mycoides* (Buttery & Plackett, 1960). Samples to be tested for the presence of amino sugars were hydrolysed in 6 N HCl and chromatographed on Dowex 50 (Plackett, 1959).

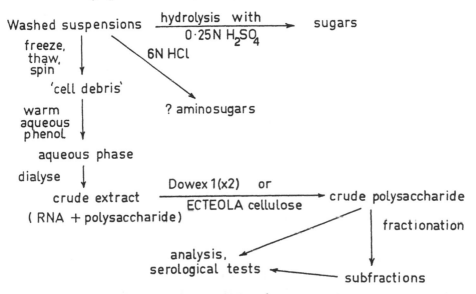

Fig. 1. Examination of *Mycoplasma* suspensions.

From some of the strains we obtained polysaccharides by extraction with phenol. The frozen and thawed cells, buffered to pH 8 with 0.04 M TRIS-HCl, were centrifuged at 26,000 g. The pellet ("cell debris") was resuspended in water and heated with an equal volume of a mixture of phenol and water (6:1,w/w) according to Westphal, Lüderitz and Bister (1952). The aqueous phase obtained by cooling and centrifuging the mixture, and dialysing to remove phenol, will be termed "crude extract." The preliminary freezing and thawing simplified subsequent purification because most of the RNA passed into the supernatant. The remaining RNA, which was extracted from the "cell debris" with polysaccharide, was removed by passing the crude extract through columns of Dowex 1 × 2 (Cl′-form) or of ECTEOLA-cellulose. This operation did not remove or alter any serologically active component detectable in immuno-diffusion tests. The crude polysaccharide obtained in this way contained less than 0.5 per cent of RNA.

It is to be expected that the sugar content of washed suspensions will depend on the physiological age of the culture at the time of harvesting. Fig. 2 shows results obtained with the V5 strain of *M. mycoides*. The amount of carbohydrate recoverable in washed suspensions, per unit volume of

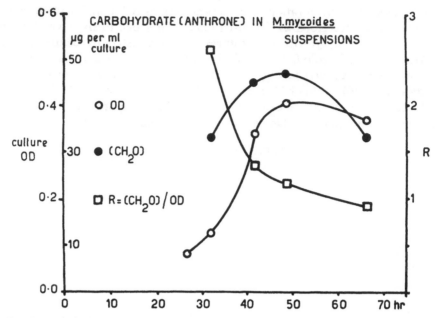

FIG. 2. Carbohydrate content of cells harvested from supplemented BVF-OS medium. Total carbohydrate was determined by the anthrone method (Trevelyan & Harrison, 1952) using galactose as the standard. Optical density was measured in an Evelyn colorimeter with a 660 mμ filter.

culture, passed through a maximum shortly before the maximum optical density was attained. The amount of carbohydrate per unit of optical density declined continuously throughout the period of measurement. A similar but less rapid decline was observed in a parallel experiment with the bovine arthritis strain L2917. These results were not unexpected. Kurotchkin and Benaradsky (1938) found that considerable quantities of polysaccharide were released into the culture medium during growth. In cultures like that shown in Fig. 2, material giving positive precipitin reactions was detected in the supernatant long before the maximum optical density was attained and was released continuously thereafter. This is consistent with the shape of the curves in Fig. 2. The amount of polysaccharide recovered from the supernatant of a culture harvested at the optical density maximum was about three times that present in the cells. It is not known how much of this material was excreted by living organisms and how much was released by lysis of dead ones.

The methods of culturing, harvesting, and extracting the organisms throughout this survey were those found suitable for *M. mycoides* and the bovine arthritis organisms. No systematic study of growth conditions for the other strains was made and it is not known whether the methods used were optimal for the demonstration of polysaccharides in these strains also. Since complex and undefined growth media were used, washing of the organisms was essential and chemical analysis of the supernatants was not practicable.

It is possible that some of the strains found to contain very little carbohydrate produce abundant polysaccharide under different conditions, or that a polysaccharide is produced which is much less firmly bound to the cells than that of *M. mycoides*.

Table 1 shows the distribution of the hexoses in the various strains. Ribose and one or more aldohexoses were found in all of them, although in some instances, shown by brackets in Table 1, only faint traces of hexose were detected on paper chromatograms. No deoxyhexose (methylpentose), heptose, or uronic acid was found in any of the strains. Only L2917, Ca, Tu, and S6 were analysed for hexosamines. Strain Tu yielded a small amount of hexosamine-like material, equivalent to 0.6 μg hexosamine-N per mg total N. Such a small quantity could be due to contamination of the washed organisms with medium constituents. The amounts found in the other strains were even smaller. Earlier studies of saprophytic and murine strains (Kandler & Zehender, 1957), and the V5 strain of *M. mycoides* (Plackett, 1959), showed that these strains probably do not form hexosamines.

The three bovine pleuropneumonia strains, and the strains GY and OG, which were isolated from natural cases of disease (not pleuropneumonia) in goats, are closely related serologically (Hudson & Cottew, 1962). All of them contain large amounts of galactose, together with a little glucose. Analyses of hydrolysates of strains 3278, Gladysdale, and OG with glucose oxidase showed that only 2–4 per cent of the total hexose was glucose. Similar products were obtained from all five strains by the phenol method. Reactions of identity between the main components of these preparations were observed in gel-diffusion tests. To avoid entanglement in taxonomic niceties we shall refer to these five strains as the galactan group. None of the other organisms examined contained more than a trace of galactose or mannose. Neither GY nor OG appears to have any relationship to the goat pleuropneumonia strains Ca or HG, being much more closely akin to *M. mycoides* var. *mycoides*.

The bovine strains L2917 and N29, both of which were isolated from natural cases of arthritis in Australian cattle, contained glucose as the only hexose. They cross-reacted strongly with each other, but not with members of the galactan group, and feebly, if at all, with other strains. They were rich in carbohydrates, and polysaccharides obtained from them will be described in more detail later.

The goat strain Ca contained small amounts of glucose, and the ratio of hexose to pentose was at least ten times smaller than that found for any member of the galactan group or the bovine arthritis strains. Ca is not serologically related to *M. agalactiae* nor to the other goat strain HG. The latter also contains glucose, and although not related to the galactan group, is related, both serologically and culturally, to *M. agalactiae*, which we have not analysed.

Strains Tu, S6, and Laidlaw B did not cross-react with each other, nor with any of the preceding groups, in agglutination or complement fixation tests made with hyperimmune donkey sera. The serological relationships of the remaining strains have not been studied in detail. An M1316 suspension was agglutinated by rabbit antisera to strains JD and 542, and a Tu suspension by rabbit antiserum to 1252, but no significant cross-reactivity was demonstrated between these strains and any of the others. All contained at least traces of glucose, but only in BGL, 542, and Laidlaw B was the hexose content comparable with that of the galactan group and the bovine arthritis strains. BGL and 542 grew poorly in our cultures and no attempt was made to prepare polysaccharides from them. Crude extracts made by the phenol method from the "cell debris" of strains Ca, JD, M1316, 1252, and Laidlaw B contained less than 20 μg of hexose per mg total cell N. Yields from *M. mycoides* and bovine arthritis strains under comparable conditions were at least ten times greater. No serological activity was found in these preparations. The pentose content of extracts from Ca, JD, M1316 and the galactan strains OG and Gladysdale was determined. The amounts found corresponded closely to the RNA content determined by ultraviolet absorbance measurements. It is unlikely that the extracts contained pentosans or pentose phosphate polymers.

These observations do not, of course, imply the absence of carbohydrate antigens from these strains. The amounts of sugar detected, though small enough to discourage chemical studies, may well be of immunological significance. Strain Ca certainly has at least one heat-stable antigen.

SPECIFIC POLYSACCHARIDES

Extraction with warm aqueous phenol (Westphal, Lüderitz & Bister, 1952) is a convenient method for the separation of polysaccharides and RNA from other macromolecular cell constituents. It has been applied with considerable success to the isolation of specific lipopolysaccharides from a wide range of gram-negative bacteria. Although it is probable that these products often contain more than one serologically distinct molecular species (Kabat, 1961), fractionation of material extracted from *Pasteurella pestis* yielded a lipopolysaccharide satisfying rigorous tests of homogeneity (Davies, 1956).

Some results obtained with preparations from the V5 strain of *M. mycoides* and from the bovine arthritis strains are reviewed in this section. Besides giving strong precipitin reactions, the crude polysaccharides could be used to sensitize sheep erythrocytes for indirect haemagglutination (Cottew, 1960), and fixed complement with bovine antisera, provided that a heat-labile factor, present in normal bovine serum, was added to the system (Cottew, 1962). The substances are probably haptens rather than complete antigens. No antibody responses, and no toxic or pyrogenic effects, were observed after injection of the *M. mycoides* galactan into experimental animals.

The physico-chemical properties of the polysaccharides are given in

TABLE 2
PROPERTIES OF *Mycoplasma* POLYSACCHARIDES

	Galactan from *M. mycoides*		Glucan from bovine arthritis organism	
	Crude galactan	Fraction P6e	Crude glucan strain L2917	Fraction Ip strain N29
Reducing sugar (anhydro)	90	92[a]	94[b]	98[b]
Total N	<0.2	0.06	0.12	0.07
Total P	<0.1	0.02	—	0.02
$[\alpha]_D$	−140°	−150°	−9.6°	—
Predominant linkage	-6-O-β-D-galactofurnosyl-1-		-2-O-β-D-glucopyranosyl-1-	

[a]After hydrolysis in 0.1 N H_2SO_4 for 1.5 hr.
[b]After hydrolysis in 0.5 N H_2SO_4 for 18–19 hr.

Table 2. The predominant linkages are assigned on the basis of acid-lability, optical rotation, periodate oxidation data, and the properties of the disaccharides obtained by partial acid hydrolysis (Plackett & Buttery, 1962). We failed to detect glucose in our preparations until it was pointed out to us (we are very grateful to Dr. M. Heidelberger for this information) that an *M. mycoides* antiserum reacted with polysaccharides containing glucose but not galactose, namely, barley glucan and the specific polysaccharide of type II pneumococci. When we re-examined the question, using paper chromatography and glucose oxidase, we found that the crude galactan did indeed contain glucose to the extent of about 1 per cent of the total hexose. The amount varied somewhat between preparations and between subfractions of the same preparation. The glucose linkages were split at a rate consistent with the pyranose configuration. It is interesting to note that Kurotchkin and Benaradsky (1938) reported cross-reactions between *M. mycoides* and pneumococci of types I and II.

Although less complex chemically than the lipopolysaccharides of typical gram-negative bacteria, the preparations were heterogeneous. Ultracentrifugation showed the presence of at least two components, while immunodiffusion experiments with subfractions of the crude polysaccharides showed that at least four serologically distinct components were present and that some, if not all, were polydisperse.

By repeated precipitation from 70 per cent (v/v) ethanol, followed by high-speed centrifugation, the major component of the *M. mycoides* galactan was obtained as a fraction (P6e in Table 2), which was almost homogeneous in gel-diffusion tests with hyperimmune donkey serum. But traces of a minor component were detectable and the material was still polydisperse. The material soluble in 70 per cent ethanol, most of which appeared to differ from the major component of P6e only with respect to molecular weight, was further fractionated with ethanol and n-propanol, and by ultracentrifugation. All subfractions gave at least three lines in gel-diffusion tests. The most soluble fraction (SCc), which was not precipitated by 90 per cent (v/v) n-propanol, was very similar to a preparation of the complement-fixing antigen obtained by Dafaalla's method, in tests with both bovine and donkey sera.

Fraction P6e differed from the crude galactan, and from the material not precipitated by 70 per cent ethanol, in that no turbidity developed during acid hydrolysis, indicating that it contained much less bound lipid. Also, the serological activity of the major component was not destroyed by heating in alkaline solution (e.g., in 0.25 N NaOH at 56° for 30 min), as was that of the minor components.

Moreover, some bovine antisera reacted feebly or not at all with the major component, while reacting strongly with one or more of the minor components. It must be emphasized that these sera were obtained from diseased animals or from animals vaccinated with viable organisms. The hyper-immune donkey sera, which reacted strongly with the major component, were obtained by intravenous injection of killed suspensions.

A phenomenon frequently observed in severe cases of bovine pleuropneu-monia is the "eclipse" of the agglutination reaction by circulating antigen (Turner, 1962b). In such sera, large quantities of a substance serologically identical with the major component, and with material prepared by Kurotch-kin's method, were demonstrable in gel-diffusion tests. In the example shown in Fig. 3 (serum D71), additional components were present, as well as *antibodies* to at least two of the minor components.

The low reactivity of many bovine sera to the major component of the galactan may be explained simply by the copious release of the substance from the organisms during multiplication *in vivo*, leading to partial neu-

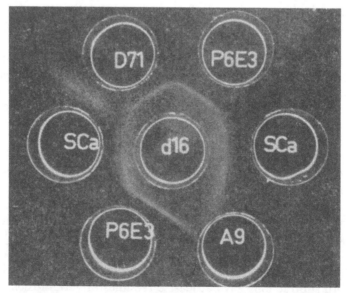

FIG. 3. Immunodiffusion with bovine antisera. 1 per cent agar in 2.5 per cent NaCl. Galactan fractions P6E3 (a subfraction of P6e) and SCa (enriched in minor components) at 0.2 mg/ml. Hyperimmune donkey serum (d16) in central well.

TABLE 3
HAEMAGGLUTINATION TESTS WITH GALACTAN SUBFRACTIONS

Sensitization		Donkey serum 1				Bovine serum 656					
		1:80	160	320	640	1:80	160	320	640	1280	2560
P6e	10 µg/ml	4	4	1	—	—	—	—	—	—	—
	50 µg/ml	4	4	3	1	3	tr	—	—	—	—
SCc	10 µg/ml	4	2	—	—	4	4	4	4	1	—
	50 µg/ml	4	4	4	—	4	4	4	4	1	—

tralization of the corresponding antibodies. The haemagglutination and complement fixation titres of such sera depend primarily on antibodies to determinants not present in the major component and not released from the mycoplasmas in soluble form *in vivo*. Eclipse of the complement-fixation and indirect haemagglutination reactions is certainly rare, although it may occur during severe bacteraemia.

The behaviour of the subfractions in haemagglutination tests was consistent with the results of immunodiffusion. As shown in Table 3, both P6e and SCc could be used to sensitize erythrocytes for indirect haemagglutination by hyperimmune donkey serum, P6e inhibited agglutination of cells sensitized with either fraction. With a bovine serum (656), however, titres with SCc cells were at least eight times higher than those with P6e cells, and P6e did not inhibit the agglutination of SCc cells by this serum.

Although heating with alkali did not affect the activity of the major component as an inhibitor of the indirect haemagglutination reaction of donkey serum, the treated material was no longer able to sensitize erythrocytes for the reaction. This shows that the molecule has some alkali-labile grouping, distinct from the antigenic determinants, which is necessary for attachment to the surface of the red cell. Heating with alkali destroyed both the sensitizing and the inhibitory activity of the minor components irrespective of the serum used.

Indirect evidence suggests that the determinants involved in the indirect haemagglutination reaction with bovine sera, although not shared with the major component, are carbohydrate in nature. The inhibitory activity of the crude galactan was destroyed by reaction with periodate (Table 4) and the rate of inactivation by acid hydrolysis was consistent with the hypothesis that galactofuranoside linkages are important.

TABLE 4
INHIBITION OF HAEMAGGLUTINATION BY
PERIODATE-OXIDIZED GALACTAN

Time (hr)	Periodate consumed*	Minimum inhibitory concentration (µg/ml)
0	0.00	3
0.25	0.07	3
2	0.41	12
4	0.47	33
8	0.63	>100
24	0.85	>100

*moles/mole hexose.

We postulate that the minor components are glycolipid substances and that multivalent aggregates are present in aqueous solution. Splitting of the lipid portion by alkali, which releases fatty acid from the unfractionated galactan, or acid hydrolysis of a furanoside linkage close to the attachment of the lipid moiety, give fragments, carrying the specific groupings, but of relatively low molecular weight. These are of low serological activity, either because they have few determinant groups per molecule, or because the orientation of the groups in the postulated multivalent aggregates (and on the surface of the organisms themselves), confers an additional element of specificity.

Attempts to identify the specific determinant groups of either the major or the minor components have not been successful. The tri- and tetra-saccharide fractions obtained from partly hydrolysed galactan were less active, by a factor of at least 10^3, than the unhydrolysed material as inhibitors of haemagglutination in either bovine or donkey sera. Periodate oxidation of the galactan showed that there were few if any unsubstituted galactofuranose groups at the non-reducing ends of the chains. Thus specificity may be determined by terminal groups of different configuration, or by the secondary structure of the macromolecule. Cross-precipitation and inhibition studies suggest that glucose and galactopyranose residues may be important determinants.

The glucan from the bovine arthritis strain N29 was fractionated with ethanol. The major component (fraction I_p, Table 2) was precipitated three times from 60 per cent (v/v) ethanol. A number of minor components, soluble at higher ethanol concentrations, were present, but could not be separated from each other. Material apparently identical with the main component was detected by gel-diffusion in the serum of an infected bovine. Antibody reacting with one or more minor components was also present.

A 1:2-β-glucan is found also in the culture medium of the crown-gall organism, *Agrobacterium tumefaciens* (Putman, Potter, Hodgson & Hassid, 1950). A sample of crown-gall polysaccharide gave a strong precipitation reaction with antiserum to strain L2917, and was a good inhibitor of the indirect haemagglutination reaction, although it did not sensitize sheep red cells for this reaction. To test the hypothesis that lipid substituents might play some part in the attachment of carbohydrate haptens to erythrocytes, a sample of crown-gall polysaccharide was treated with palmitoyl chloride in the presence of pyridine. The product did in fact sensitize sheep erythrocytes for agglutination by antiserum to strain L2917, although not so efficiently as the *Mycoplasma* glucan.

DISCUSSION

Only a very limited range of sugar types was encountered in this survey. This is consistent with the very restricted biosynthetic ability of the Mycoplasmataceae. The large battery of enzymes needed for the synthesis of the complex heteropolysaccharides present in the walls of typical bacteria, or the capsules of the pneumococci for example, might entail the storage of too much additional genetic information.

While we cannot generalize from two instances, it is remarkable that the two polysaccharides we have found have unusual linkages. Until recently the only polysaccharide known to contain galactofuranose residues was galactocarolose, of *Penicillium charlesii*, in which the linkages are 1:5-β (Haworth, Raistrick & Stacey, 1937; Gorin & Spencer, 1959). Galacto-furanose groups have since been found in a disaccharide isolated from the culture medium of *Betacoccus arabinosaceous* (Bourne *et al.*, 1961), and in the specific polysaccharide of type 34 *Pneumococcus* (Roberts *et al.*, 1962). A number of species of *Agrobacterium* are known to produce glucans in which all, or nearly all, the linkages are 1:2-β- (Putman *et al.*, 1950; Gorin, Spencer and Westlake, 1961), but this is perhaps the least common type of linkage found in glucose polymers.

The mucopeptides of bacterial cell-walls and the capsular polypeptides of some bacteria, which contain a high proportion of D-amino acids, are resistant to many of the commoner proteolytic enzymes and peptidases (Salton, 1961). Perhaps the synthesis of a homopolysaccharide with unusual linkages is one way in which a parasite of very limited metabolic ability may form a structure resistant to the enzymes present in host tissues. Antigen may persist for remarkably long periods in pleuropneumonia autopsy specimens and has been detected by the precipitin reaction even in putrefy-ing material (White, 1958; Turner, 1962a). Most galactosidases probably do not attack galactofuranosides (Wallenfels & Malhotra, 1961), although we have found that a commercial enzyme preparation, prepared from culture filtrates of *Aspergillus niger*, will split the *M. mycoides* galactan. Enzymes splitting β-1,2-glucans may also be uncommon, although Reese, Parrish and Mandels (1961) found inducible β-1,2-glucanases in several species of fungi. We have found that enzyme preparations from *Helix pomatia* and *Stachybotrys atra* will split the glucan of the bovine arthritis organism.

Polysaccharides of unusual structure may have survival value for another reason, namely that there is less chance of encountering cross-reacting antibody in a previously uninfected host. This might be particularly im-portant for organisms which are ill adapted for survival outside the host. We have no idea of the biological function of the polysaccharide. It may be a capsular or slime layer substance, but since most of the carbohydrate remains with the "cell debris" after freezing and thawing, it may also be an integral part of some surface structure. No clear evidence of any capsule can be seen in electron micrographs.

Studies of the sensitization of erythrocytes for indirect haemagglutination reactions may be relevant to the question of how the antigenic determinants are attached to the *Mycoplasma* elements. The surface of a *Mycoplasma* may resemble that of an animal cell more closely than that of a typical bacterium, and glycolipid haptens may be oriented at the surface as proposed by Rapport (1961).

REFERENCES

Bourne, E. J., J. Hartigan, and H. Weigel. 1961. Biosynthesis of α-D-glucopyranosyl D-galactofuranoside and other D-galactose-containing saccharides by *Betacoccus arabinosaceous*. J. Chem. Soc.: 1088–1092.

Buttery, S. H., and P. Plackett. 1960. A specific polysaccaride from *Mycoplasma mycoides*. J. Gen. Microbiol. 23: 357–368.

Cottew, G. S. 1960. Indirect haemagglutination and haemagglutination inhibition with *Mycoplasma mycoides*. Austral. Vet. J. 36: 54–56.

Cottew, G. S. 1962. Enhancement of the complement fixation reaction with a soluble antigen from *Mycoplasma mycoides*. Nature 194: 308.

Dafaalla, E. N. 1957. A study of the antigenic structure of the contagious bovine pleuropneumonia organism. Bull. Epiz. Dis. Africa 5: 135–145.

Dafaalla, E. N. 1959. Some immunological observations on the organism of contagious bovine pleuropneumonia. Proc. XVIth Int. Vet. Congr., Madrid 2: 539–542.

Davies, D. A. L. 1956. A specific polysaccharide of *Pasteurella pestis*. Biochem. J. 63: 105–116.

Dische, Z., L. B. Shettles, and M. Osnos. 1949. New specific color reactions of hexoses and spectrophotometric micromethods for their determination. Arch. Biochem. 22: 169–184.

Gorin, P. A. J., and J. F. T. Spencer. 1959. 5-0-β-D-galactofuranosyl-D-galactose from galactocarolose. Can. J. Chem. 37: 499–502.

Gorin, P. A. J., J. F. T. Spencer, and D. W. S. Westlake. 1961. The structure and resistance to methylation of 1,2-β-glucans from species of agrobacteria. Can. J. Chem. 39: 1067–1073.

Haworth, W. N., H. Raistrick, and M. Stacey. 1937. Polysaccharides synthesised by micro-organisms. III. The molecular structure of galactocarolose produced from glucose by *Penicillium charlesii* G. Smith. Biochem. J. 31: 640–644.

Hudson, J. R. and G. S. Cottew. 1962. Unpublished observations.

Huggett, A. St. G. and D. A. Nixon. 1957. Enzymic determination of blood glucose. Biochem. J. 66: 12P.

Kabat, E. A. 1961. Experimental immunochemistry, 2nd ed., p. 834. C. C. Thomas, Springfield, Illinois.

Kandler, O., and C. Zehender. 1957. Ueber das Vorkommen von α-,ϵ-Diaminopimelinsäure bei verschiedenen L-Phasentypen von *Proteus vulgaris* und bei den pleuropneumonieähnlichen Organismen. Z. Naturforsch. 12b: 725–728.

Knight, G. J., and K. M. Cowan. 1961. Studies on allegedly non-complementfixing immune systems. I. A heat labile serum factor requirement for a bovine antibody complement-fixing system. J. Immunol. 86: 354–360.

Kurotchkin, T. J. 1937. Specific carbohydrate from *Asterococcus mycoides* for serologic tests of bovine pleuropneumonia. Proc. Soc. Exptl. Biol. Med. 37: 21–22.

Kurotchkin, T. J., and C. V. Benaradsky. 1938. Serological diagnosis of bovine pleuropneumonia through the use of the specific carbohydrate of *Asterococcus mycoides*. Chinese Med. J., Suppl. 2: 269–278.

Plackett, P. 1959. On the probable absence of "mucocomplex" from *Mycoplasma mycoides*. Biochim. et Biophys. Acta 35: 260–262.

Plackett, P., and S. H. Buttery. 1962. Unpublished observations.

Provost, A., and R. Queval. 1957. Recherches immunologiques sur la peripneumonie. I. La réaction d'agglutination. Rev. elev. med. vet. pays trop. 10: 357–368.

Putman, E. W., A. L. Potter, R. Hodgson, and W. Z. Hassid. 1950. The structure of crown-gall polysaccharide. J. Am. Chem. Soc. 72: 5024–5026.

Rapport, M. M. 1961. Structure and specificity of the lipid haptens of animal cells. J. Lipid Res. 2: 25–36.

Reese, E. T., F. W. Parrish, and M. Mandels. 1961. β-D-1,2-glucanases in fungi. Can. J. Microbiol. 7: 309–317.

Roberts, W. K., G. J. Buchanan, and J. Baddiley. 1962. Galactofuranose units in the specific substance from type 34 Pneumococcus. Biochem. J. 82: 42P.

Rodwell, A. W. 1960. Nutrition and metabolism of Mycoplasma mycoides var. mycoides. Ann. N.Y. Acad. Sci., 79: 499–507.

Salton, M. R. J. 1961. The anatomy of the bacterial surface. Bact. Rev. 25: 77–99.

Trevelyan, W. E., and J. S. Harrison. 1962. Studies on yeast metabolism. I. Fractionation and microdetermination of cell carbohydrates. Biochem. J. 50: 298–303.

Turner, A. W. 1962a. Detection of Mycoplasma mycoides antigen and antibody by means of precipitin tests, as aids to diagnosis of bovine contagious pleuropneumonia. Austral. Vet. J. 38: 335–337.

Turner, A. W. 1962b. Circulating M. mycoides antigen as a cause of loss of agglutination and complement fixation reactivity during acute pleuropneumonia. Austral. Vet. J. 38: 401–405.

Turner, A. W., A. D. Campbell, and A. T. Dick. 1935. Recent work on pleuropneumonia contagiosa boum in North Queensland. Austral. Vet. J., 11: 63–71.

Wallenfels, K., and O. P. Malhotra. 1961. Galactosidases. Advances in Carbohydrate Chem. 16: 239–298.

Westphal, O., O. Lüderitz and F. Bister. 1952. Ueber die Extraktion von Bakterien mit Phenol/Wasser. Z. Naturforsch. 7b: 148–155.

White, G. 1958. Agar double diffusion precipitation reaction applied to the study of Asterococcus mycoides. Nature 181: 278–279.

Yoshida, T. 1961. Antigenicity of cell components of antigenic variants of contagious bovine pleuropneumonia organisms in serological tests. Nat. Inst. Anim. Health Quart. 1: 199–206.

SYMPOSIUM XI

THE VIRULENCE OF STAPHYLOCOCCI

Chairman: R. E. O. WILLIAMS

R. E. O. WILLIAMS

Ecological Evidence for the Existence of Virulent Strains
of Staphylococci

PHYLLIS M. ROUNTREE

The Origin and Spread of Virulent Staphylococci

KIRSTEN ROSENDAL

Correlation of Virulence of Staphylococci from Patients with
Bacteraemia with Various Laboratory Indices

D. E. ROGERS

The Phagocytosis of Staphylococci

J. B. DERBYSHIRE

Immunization against Staphylococcal Infections

ECOLOGICAL EVIDENCE FOR THE EXISTENCE OF VIRULENT STRAINS OF STAPHYLOCOCCI

R. E. O. WILLIAMS

Wright-Fleming Institute
St. Mary's Hospital Medical School
London, England

THERE ARE FEW more certain ways of provoking an argument than to attempt to define the use of the word "virulent" as applied to microbes. But we can hardly escape some attempt to suggest, at the beginning, what it is we are going to discuss during this symposium. We can best follow Miles (1955) in using the word "pathogenic" to characterize a species or group of organisms the members of which are liable to produce disease. The word "virulent" is then used to describe the capacity of an individual strain of the species to produce disease. Thus when we say that a particular strain of the admittedly pathogenic species *Staphylococcus aureus* is virulent we mean that it, in contradistinction to some other unmentioned strains of the same species, is able to produce disease.

Quite clearly several limitations are needed even at this point, for staphylococci can produce a variety of diseases in different animals—cutaneous or generalized infection in man, mastitis in cattle, pyaemia in sheep and, if given the right circumstances, pyelonephritis in mice. We have to define virulence in terms of the particular challenge that is offered to the staphylococcus.

In this symposium, we propose to discuss virulence from two aspects. First, and briefly, we must review the evidence that there are variations in the ability of different strains of staphylococci. And secondly we must consider what factors may distinguish the more virulent from the less virulent strains.

We can envisage a minimal staphylococcus, which has just those characteristics that are needed for the taxonomists to allow it a place in the species, but none of the extra and taxonomically optional "virulence factors" such as capsule, haemolysins, etc. Can such a minimal staphylococcus produce disease in any circumstances? If not, how many and which of the optional characters have to be added to enable it to produce disease when put into the situation favouring it the most? And with how many more does it have to be endowed to make it a strain with the propensity for producing epidemic disease?

In all studies of virulence factors we have inevitably to rely on laboratory tests, usually with cultures of the microbe, to detect the factor whose relation to virulence we are trying to determine. We should remember the fundamental problem that bacteria do not always produce in artificial culture the same complex of antigens and enzymes that they produce in the animal. There is good evidence of this from antibody studies of patients convalescent from streptococcal infections: nearly all infected patients produce anti-hyaluronidase, though many of the strains isolated from these patients fail to produce detectable hyaluronidase in culture.

METHODS USED FOR RECOGNIZING VIRULENT STRAINS

We may first review the different approaches that have been adopted in studies of virulence. These include attempts to produce experimental infection in animals and man; studies of resistance to phagocytosis; and prospective or retrospective epidemiological studies in man.

Experimental Infection

The ideal method for determining which strains of staphylococci are virulent for man would be to test cultures for their ability to infect man. But quite clearly the situations in which such a test can be contemplated are very few. Elek and Conen (1957) explored the use of intradermal inoculation in man and obtained some valuable information on the minimal infecting dose; while Foster and Hutt (1960), also with human subjects, used inoculation on to the surface of traumatized epidermis. In both cases, however, some of the subjects developed unpleasant infective complications, and neither method is suitable for general use. The staphylococcus enterotoxin has also been tested in humans (e.g., Dolman, 1934) but again the severity of the reaction may be too great for this to be generally acceptable. The veterinarians have an obvious advantage over medical investigators in that experimental infection of their relevant host by the relevant route can be used, and Derbyshire's contribution to this symposium illustrates the results that can be achieved.

Experimental infection of animals has much more often been used to detect factors that are thought to be relevant to virulence for man. But the validity of, for example, intraperitoneal or intravenous challenge of mice as a measure of cutaneous or even blood-stream virulence for man is not by any means self-evident, and it seems clear that no mechanism of virulence inferred from animal experiment ought to be accepted as appropriate for human infections without an explicit test to establish that the correlation holds in man as well as in the animal.

An extension of the technique of experimental infection as a means of recognizing virulence factors is to immunize against specific factors recognized in cultures and to measure the protective effect of this procedure. Again this is more easily achieved in animals than in man, because of the facility of artificial challenge in animals (as in Derbyshire's contribution). However there are possibilities of using the same technique in man, if the immunized subjects can be observed to experience the challenge of natural exposure to infection. Long-term controlled field trials are thus needed, but immunization of pregnant women to protect against possible staphylococcal infection in the puerperium, and immunization of patients with a history of recurrent skin sepsis, seem to offer possible experimental material.

Resistance to Phagocytosis

With the pneumococcus there is good evidence that capsulation is partly resonsible for virulence and that the capsule acts as an antiphagocytic factor. It seems reasonable that resistance to phagocytosis should, generally, be correlated with virulence and that phagocytosis tests should be capable of yielding valuable information on at least one aspect of virulence. However, the isolated phagocytic system, even if the phagocytes are derived from the animal host under study, is very artificial and behaviour of bacteria in such systems may not be related very closely to their behaviour in the whole animal (as was hinted at in the work of Fleck, 1956, on streptococcal infections in mice). Again, confirmatory tests will certainly be needed to demonstrate the clinical relevance of any virulence factors discovered: by analogy with the pneumococcus, artificial immunization might offer a way of obtaining such confirmatory evidence.

Prospective Studies in Man

The nearest available counterpart to the animal experiment, with man as the animal, is the prospective study of the outcome of introduction into human tissues of staphylococci with differing properties. There are a few situations in which this can be observed to happen. For example, small traumatic wounds, if examined bacteriologically soon after infliction, are sometimes found to be contaminated with staphylococci; and some of the cases of clinical sepsis that develop subsequently are attributable to the persistence and multiplication of these contaminants. Williams and Miles (1949) tried to determine the importance of α-haemolysin production by comparing the sepsis rates of wounds contaminated initially with toxigenic staphylococci with those of wounds yielding non-toxigenic strains. More recently using the same principle though in a more indirect way, we compared the wound infection rate in patients who were initially nasal carriers of antibiotic-sensitive or antibiotic-resistant staphylococci (Williams et al., 1959). Rosendal has used the same technique in her study of bacteraemia, which is reported in this symposium.

The essential of this approach is that the strains compared should be known, initially, to have similar opportunities for producing disease, and in this it differs from the next method.

Retrospective Study of Staphylococci from Different Sources

There are numerous reported studies in which the significance of particular "virulence" factors has been assessed by comparing their frequency in strains from various sorts of infective lesion with that in strains from carrier sites, it being assumed that this represents a comparison between pathogenic and non-pathogenic strains. From all we know of the epidemiology of staphylococcal infections it is clear that, as a generalization, this assumption is unjustified. Staphylococci derived from the noses of healthy carriers can without doubt be shown on occasion to produce disease, either in the carrier himself, or in other people to whom his staphylococci are conveyed. Nevertheless many nasal strains certainly are lacking in virulence, so that, for the comparison of carrier and lesion strains to be valid, we need to be able to eliminate from the carrier strains those that can give rise to disease when introduced into suitable sites from those that seem to do so only with difficulty. Studies of phage-type distributions suggest that some approach to this might be possible.

ECOLOGICAL EVIDENCE FOR EXISTENCE OF VIRULENT STRAINS

The application of phage-typing of staphylococci on a wide scale has given us a new understanding of the differing behaviour of different strains of staphylococci and it seems a useful introduction to the rest of the symposium to recall the evidence for the existence of characteristic epidemiological behaviour associated with particular phage types. An analysis of the type distribution of staphylococci sent from various sources to the Staphylococcus Reference Laboratory was published by Williams and Jevons (1961) and provides a general picture, which can now be supplemented with information on later years (kindly made available to me by Dr. M. T. Parker and Dr. M. Patricia Jevons). Information on the staphylococci from particular diseases is also available from special investigations.

Williams and Jevons (1961) analysed the types of 2,381 staphylococci from: (1) healthy nasal carriers, (2) septic lesions such as boils, whitlows and septic lacerations in patients having no immediate connection with hospital, and (3) septic lesions in hospital patients, particularly postoperative wound infections and skin infections in newborn infants. Some of the hospital strains were drawn from recognized "epidemics," here defined as consisting of three or more associated cases; others were so far as was known sporadic cases. The material for the analysis of the hospital staphylococci consisted of staphylococci sent to the Staphylococcus Reference Laboratory for typing and there is inevitably bias in the selection of strains. There must be a predominance of antibiotic-resistant strains and there may be a tendency for epidemics due to notorious types to be studied more intensively than others. For the present purpose, however, it seems that the trends are sufficiently reliable.

Fig. 1 presents a re-analysis of some of the data from the Williams and Jevons report. It is worth comparing the frequency in various sources of a few types.

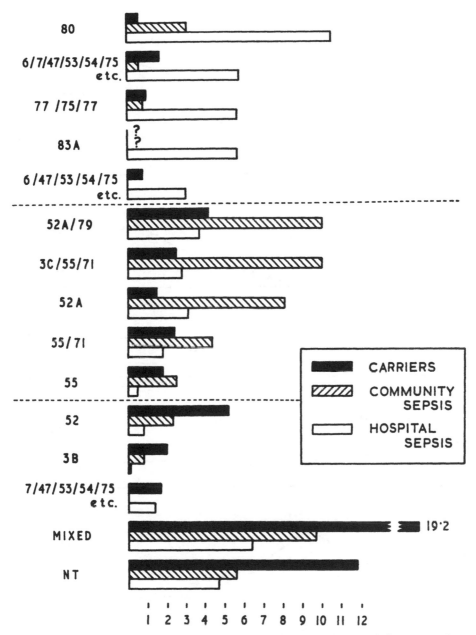

FIG. 1. Percentage frequency of the commonest phage types in staphylococci in three sources (based on Williams and Jevons, 1961).

Hospital Infections

Not unexpectedly 70 per cent of the strains of type 80 (probably almost all 80/81) were from hospital infections. The same was true of several types within phage group III. Certainly a contributory factor in this hospital

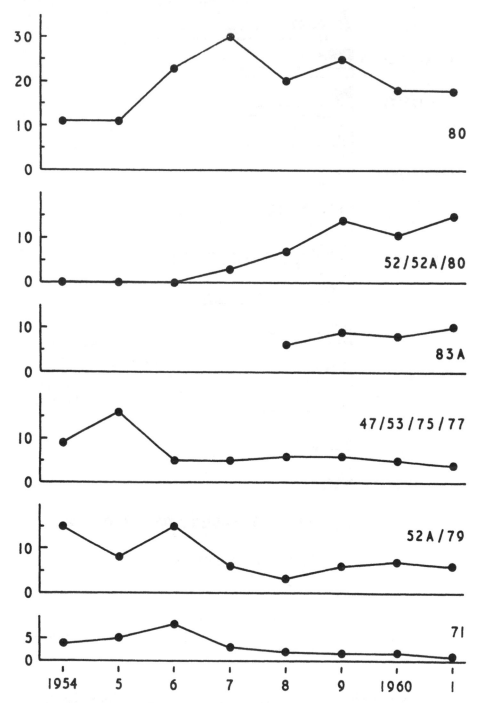

FIG. 2. Percentage frequency of 6 phage types among strains from "epidemics" of hospital infection, 1954–61 (from Williams and Jevons, 1961, and later records kindly supplied by Dr. M. T. Parker and Dr. M. P. Jevons).

spread of a few strains is their capacity to give rise to antibiotic-resistant variants, but the changes in prevalence of a few types recorded during the last few years show that antibiotic resistance is certainly not the only factor.

At present three types appear to account, between them, for some 50 per cent of the epidemics of hospital infection recognized in Britain. The trend of the dominant "epidemic" types recognized in the material examined at Colindale over the last eight years is shown in Fig. 2. There was a decline in the relative predominance of type 47/53/75/77 and 52A/79 after 1955 and 1956, and an increase in 80, 52/52A/80 and, since 1958, 83A. Certainly the first of these (47/53/75/77) commonly had the same antibiotic sensitivity pattern as 80 and 52/52A/80. On the other hand, 83A is commonly more resistant, and this might account for its recent spread. But strains of many other types are equally resistant to antibiotics and yet have not become such widespread epidemic types; isolated epidemics of considerable vigour have been observed with many other types but the frequency of association with epidemics is relatively much less. It seems that some types, and perhaps some strains within other types, are endowed with a special character, which, following Fekety and Bennett (1959), we may call "epidemiological virulence" and which is certainly not understood. Epidemiological virulence appears to be correlated with resistance to mercuric chloride (Moore, 1960) but there is no clue as to the significance of this correlation.

A different example of the varying behaviour of strains of staphylococci in hospital is offered by the observations in a five-year study in a surgical ward (see Shooter et al., 1958; Williams et al., 1959). During the course of this study we observed well over 200 distinguishable phage types of staphylococci among the patients.

There were 27 separate introductions, of a total of 17 different types, each resulting in the colonization of 5 or more patients (Table 1). These introductions differed markedly in the extent to which they were followed simply by nasal colonization, on the one hand, or by septic complications

TABLE 1

RATIO OF LESIONS TO NASAL CARRIERS IN INTRODUCTIONS TO A SURGICAL WARD RESULTING IN INFECTION OF FIVE OR MORE PATIENTS

Ratio: lesions/carriers*	No. of introductions	Types	Mean no. patients per introduction
0–	9	29/52, 3C/55, 6/7/47 etc., 6/53/77, 55/53, 52/80, 52A/79, 79, 52/52A/79/80/7/42E	11.7
0.1–	1	53/77	9.0
0.2–	7	80/81, 80/81, 79, 75/77, 53/77, 6/7/47 etc., 6/42E/47/75	20.7
0.3–	2	6/53/77, 75/77	9.5
0.4–	3	80/81, 83A, 6/7/47 etc.	9.3
0.5–	2	80/81, 53/77	19.5
0.6 and over	3	53, 83A, 52/55	8.0

*The ratio is the number of patients developing staphylococcal lesions to the total number becoming nasal carriers following the introduction of a particular type into the ward.

in wounds, chest or elsewhere on the other. In the table, the introductions have been classed by the ratio of the number of patients with septic lesions to the total with nasal colonization. Thus in 10 introductions only 10 per cent or less of the colonized patients had septic lesions, while in 8 introductions 40 per cent or more had lesions. Yet, with the exception of 2 introductions, the average number of patients infected was not notably different.

Most of the types whose spread resulted in a number of septic lesions are, of course, the hospital epidemic types already discussed. But what deserves comment is the frequent occurrence and quite wide spread of particular types among patients' noses without the production of any septic complication in wound, chest or elsewhere. In most cases these incidents were due to types other than those notoriously responsible for epidemics, though sometimes epidemic types spread without generating any septic lesions.

One cannot draw very firm conclusions from a single survey of this sort, even though it lasted for several years, because the extent to which a staphylococcus, when introduced, spreads within a hospital ward depends to some extent on the "dispersal ability" of the patients infected by it (Noble, 1962). But the results in the table seem to indicate that the factors leading to "communicability" are different from those enabling the staphylococcus to produce disease after invasion and are, in one sense, another aspect of virulence.

Analogous observations have been reported from maternity units. Thus Poole (1960) noted that some of the staphylococci introduced by nurses infected the babies and then continued to spread among the babies even when the introducer had left; other strains infected the babies only when the introducer was still present. Presumably both sorts of staphylococcus had skin virulence for the infants, but only one sort had the power of spreading.

Community Infections

Leaving the hospital strains, there were more surprisingly a number of types whose commonest "source" was septic lesions outside hospital (Fig. 1), and for four types—52A, 52A/79, 3C/55/71 and 42E—the predominance in such lesions was almost as great as that for the notorious epidemic types in hospital. This dominance must be due to some virulence factor other than antibiotic resistance, and, despite the fact that, in individuals, self-infection from the nose is well established, the commonest types in septic lesions are not the commonest types in the nose (see also Miller *et al.*, 1962). In Britain it is even now the case that hospital epidemic staphylococci (like type 80/81) are rare in the community outside hospital, either in lesions or as carrier strains.

The association of type 71 with impetigo (Parker *et al.*, 1955; Parker & Williams, 1961) offers a special example of a staphylococcus type responsible for epidemic infection outside hospital. Again we have no explanation for this association.

The one staphylococcus disease for which we imagine we can "explain" the association with phage type is food poisoning: the fact that some 70 per cent of food poisoning outbreaks are due to strains of phage group III (e.g., Williams & Jevons, 1961) is presumably attributable to widespread diffusion of enterotoxin production among strains of this group.

There are relatively few types that are commonly found in the nose of healthy carriers but rarely found in infective lesions. Types 52 and 3B, the various unclassifiable types, and the untypable strains are, however, in this class. Types 52 and 3B are apparently common but largely non-virulent staphylococci. The unclassifiable and untypable strains are common in carriers but are not so rare as causes of infection.

CONCLUSION

Thus phage typing surveys of staphylococci indicate that there are indeed strains with differing abilities to cause disease, and the extent to which some of these differences are correlated with phage type suggests that they relate to some stable genetic characteristics. The studies also indicate the various facets of the concept of "virulence." There are types which, like type 71, have a particular association with one specific disease. There is a group of types which includes almost all the strains capable of producing enterotoxin. There appear to be strains, if not types, with great powers of communicability but little ability to invade. There are types that can invade the tissues but appear to lack communicability. And, lastly, there are the types which, led by type 80/81, have elevated the staphylococcus to the status of a national problem by their ability both to spread and to invade. The characteristics responsible for these differences are the virulence factors we should like to discover.

REFERENCES

Dolman, C. E. 1934. Ingestion of staphylococcus exotoxin by human volunteers with special reference to staphylococcic food poisoning. J. Infect. Dis. 55: 172–183.

Elek, S. D., and P. E. Conen. 1957. The virulence of *Staphylococcus pyogenes* for man. A study of the problems of wound infection. Brit. J. Exptl. Pathol. 38: 573–586.

Fekety, F. R., and I. L. Bennett, Jr. 1959. The epidemiological virulence of staphylococci. Yale J. Biol. Med. 32: 23–32.

Fleck, D. G. 1956. Mouse protection and enhancement of phagocytosis by antisera to *Streptococcus pyogenes*. Brit. J. Exptl. Pathol. 37: 406–414.

Foster, W. D., and M. S. R. Hutt. 1960. Experimental staphylococcal infections in man. Lancet *ii*: 1373–1376.

Miles, A. A. 1955. The meaning of pathogenicity, 5th Symposium, Society for General Microbiology, pp. 1–16. Cambridge University Press.

Miller, D. L., J. C. McDonald, M. P. Jevons, and R. E. O. Williams. 1962. Staphylococcal disease and nasal carriage in the Royal Air Force. J. Hyg. (Lond.) *60*: 451–465.

Moore, B. 1960. A new screen test and selective medium for the rapid detection of epidemic strains of *Staph. aureus.* Lancet *ii*: 453–458.

Noble, W. C. 1962. The dispersal of staphylococci in hospital wards. J. Clin. Path. *15*: 552–558.

Parker, M. T., and R. E. O. Williams. 1961. Further observations on the bacteriology of impetigo and pemphigus neonatorum. Acta Paediat. Uppsala *50*: 101–112.

Parker, M. T., A. J. H. Tomlinson, and R. E. O. Williams. 1955. Impetigo contagiosa: The association of certain types of *Staphylococcus aureus* and of *streptococcus pyogenes* with superficial skin infections. J. Hyg. (Camb.) *53*: 458–473.

Poole, P. M. 1960. The reinvasion of a maternity unit by *Staphylococcus aureus.* Mon. Bull. Minist. Health Lab. Serv. *19*: 113–123.

Shooter, R. A., M. A. Smith, J. D. Griffiths, Mary E. A. Brown, R. E. O. Williams, Joan E. Rippon, and M. Patricia Jevons. 1958. Spread of staphylococci in a surgical ward. Brit. Med. J. *i*: 607–613.

Williams, R. E. O., and M. Patricia Jevons. 1961. Lysotypen von Staphylococcus aureus verschiedener Herkunft. Zbl. Bakt. *181*: 349–358.

Williams, R. E. O., M. Patricia Jevons, R. A. Shooter, C. J. W. Hunter, J. A. Girling, J. D. Griffiths, and G. W. Taylor. 1959. Nasal staphylococci and sepsis in hospital patients. Brit. Med. J. *ii*: 658–662.

Williams, R. E. O., and A. A. Miles. 1949. Infection and sepsis in industrial wounds of the hand: A bacteriological study of aetiology and prophylaxis. Spec. Rep. Ser. Med. Res. Coun., Lond. No. 266.

THE ORIGIN AND SPREAD OF
VIRULENT STAPHYLOCOCCI

PHYLLIS M. ROUNTREE

Fairfax Institute of Pathology
Royal Prince Alfred Hospital
Sydney, Australia

DURING THE PAST FIFTEEN YEARS, bacteriologists have been observing the rapid course of micro-evolution in the staphyloccoci. Selection of and accumulation of antibiotic-resistant mutants have produced a staphylococcal flora in civilized man which appears to differ markedly from that existing before 1947. Attention has been focussed on the effects of the introduction of certain strains into nurseries for the newborn, on the increased incidence of staphylococcal septicaemia and on the occurrence of epidemics of furunculosis in hospital personnel and in families. Certain strains, notably those typing as 80/81 or of closely related phage patterns, but also other strains, have been implicated frequently in these epidemics and it has become customary to regard the ability to cause epidemics as synonymous with virulence.

Virulence must, however, be considered as a relative character dependent on the relationship between a parasite and its hosts. A micro-organism capable of causing a fatal infection in one species may be completely innocuous for another. Similarly, within a susceptible species, such as man, there will be all gradations of susceptibility up to and including complete immunity to infection.

Man's association with the staphylococcus goes far back into antiquity and possibly to his primate ancestors. This long association has led to a well-adjusted balance in which the parasite's survival and transmission from generation to generation has been assured while the host normally suffers little or no disability. This state of tolerance breaks down from time to time, the bacteria invade the tissues and may, in rare cases, cause the death of the host.

The question then arises as to whether this breakdown in tolerance is due to alterations in the host or in the parasite. In other words, has the parasite become more virulent or has the host become more susceptible?

Virulence may be defined as the capacity of a strain to produce disease in a particular host. Infectivity, on the other hand, involves the transmission of a strain from one host to the next. A strain may be fully virulent for an individual but may lack characters which permit it to be readily transmitted.

Within the framework of these definitions, an epidemic strain could be regarded as one that is both virulent and readily transmissible.

The distinction between virulence and infectivity is not, however, clear cut. Transmissibility may depend on the numbers of organisms available for transmission and these, in turn, may be determined by the type of lesion produced in an individual host. For example: a strain that causes a minimal skin lesion, such as a thrombophlebitis at the site of an intravenous infusion, may invade the blood stream and cause a septicaemic death; the same strain might readily colonize the nose and umbilicus of newborn babies and spread rapidly in a nursery without causing clinical infection. In the first situation it could be regarded as virulent but of low infectivity; in the second as of low virulence but of high infectivity.

Keeping in mind, therefore, the difficulties inherent in this distinction between virulence and infectivity, some aspects of the origin of virulent strains will be discussed and some of the possible factors concerned in their spread will be considered.

THE ORIGIN OF VIRULENT STRAINS

There is no evidence that virulent strains of *Staph. aureus* have not always existed. In 1852, T. Hunt published in the *Lancet* an account of the "furuncloid epidemic" which appeared to break out in "all four quarters of the globe at one and the same time" and which in London reached its peak in the first quarter of 1852. Hunt mentions epidemics of boils in London and other English towns, in France, Austria, the Cape of Good Hope and Philadelphia. Nearer in time, Chickering and Park (1919) described an epidemic of staphylococcal pneumonia associated with the influenza pandemic of 1918–19.

Epidemics of infection in the newborn were reported during the 1940's, by which time methods were available for distinguishing strains. It is of particular interest that, in England, phage type 3A, which was penicillin-sensitive was a common cause of these outbreaks (Allison, 1949; Parker & Kennedy, 1949). This strain has now disappeared as a cause of nursery epidemics while one important feature of strains causing neonatal infections during more recent years has been their penicillin resistance.

The hypothesis that the introduction of antibiotics is the chief factor that has influenced the emergence of the *current* virulent strains has much evidence to support it. In hospital populations which provide opportunities for the spread of infection, the use of penicillin led to the selection of penicillinase-producing strains as the causative organisms in hospital-acquired infections. Resistance to streptomycin and then to tetracycline, to chloramphenicol and to erythromycin were added to these strains following the introduction of these antibiotics. Up to 1953, most of these resistant strains belonged to Phage Group III.

Barbour and Edwards (1953) found that strains of Group III had a higher mutation rate to streptomycin resistance than did those strains of Groups I and II that they tested. It had been suggested that these anti-biotic-resistant strains might be genetically more unstable and therefore of higher adaptability in a changing environment (Barber & Whitehead, 1949).

One character of particular interest in these strains is that, although they colonize the noses of patients and staff in hospitals, infect clean surgical wounds, and cause pneumonia, enterocolitis and septicaemia, they rarely give rise to pathognomic skin lesions such as boils and carbuncles. They have spread outside hospitals to a very limited extent. On the other hand, strains that readily mutate to antibiotic resistance and in addition readily produce skin lesions could be expected to spread freely both within and outside hospitals. Such strains were reported in increasing numbers from 1954 onwards and belong chiefly to phage type 80/81 and related phage patterns.

Their origin is a matter for speculation. They were found almost simul-taneously in Australia (Rountree & Freeman, 1955), Canada (Bynoe, Elder & Comtois, 1956) and the United States (Shaffer, Sylvester, Baldwin and Rheins, 1957) but in Great Britain as a cause of an epidemic only in 1955 (Duthie, 1957). Later it was stated that strains of this phage pattern had been identified in a collection of staphylococci that had been made between 1927 and 1947 (Blair & Carr, 1960). However, only one strain of the specific 80/81 pattern was found in this collection of 276 strains although strains of related patterns were present.

Since type 80/81 strains owe their particular phage pattern to the carriage of a completely defective prophage (Rountree & Asheshov, 1961), it is possible that they were derived from earlier strains (typing as 52/52A/80/81) by lysogenization. Such a change has been reported *in vitro* (Sakurai, Up-dyke, Nahmias & Gerhardt, 1961).

Even if the ancestors of the present type 80/81 strains were these earlier strains, it is apparent either that the earlier strains were lacking in some attribute that permitted them to spread widely or that conditions in hospitals were such that epidemics were unlikely. The latter seems improbable, especially in nurseries for the newborn, yet it was only after the appearance of the present strains that nursery epidemics became a matter for general concern. It seems a reasonable conclusion, therefore, that some time about 1953 penicillin-resistant strains possessing some biologically distinctive characters arose as mutants of previously existing strains.

In general, epidemics of neonatal infection seem to have been the means whereby these strains were seeded into the population outside hospitals. Their introduction into families was followed by the spread of clinical infection in the family (Hurst & Grossman, 1960) in contrast to the paucity of lesions produced when other strains were brought home from hospitals. In Australia by 1958 infection was so widespread that 58 per cent of boils, carbuncles and styes occuring in the general population were due to this strain (Johnson *et al.*, 1960) and there was usually no history of any recent contact with a hospital.

In contrast to these 80/81 strains, the multiple resistant strains of Group III, so characteristic of surgical infection in hospitals, have been rarely found in people with no recent hospital experience. This would seem to indicate that the Group III strains are readily transmissible *only* in hospitals and to hosts particularly susceptible to infection.

It may be concluded therefore that the epidemiological success of certain strains depends on (1) their genetic lability which permits them to adapt to the antibiotic-laden environment of the modern hospital, and (2) their possession of certain characters that allow ready transmissibility to new hosts.

FACTORS INFLUENCING TRANSMISSIBILITY

The factors that influence transmissibility are certainly complex and may well interact with each other. Some of possible significance, both inside and outside hospitals, will now be discussed separately.

1. *The Numbers of Organisms Disseminated from the Host*

The extent and nature of the lesions produced by the virulent strain will determine the numbers of cocci available for transmission to a new host. The ability to initiate lesions is necessarily of importance in this regard (but will be discussed by other speakers).

Certain clinical conditions are associated with widespread contamination of the patient's surroundings. Hare and Cooke (1961) found that contamination of the bodies, bedding and general environment of persons with skin infections and staphylococcal pneumonia and enterocolitis was higher than that found in patients with post-operative wound infection. Similarly, Rountree and Beard (1962) observed that the blankets of patients with staphylococcal pneumonia were heavily contaminated with organisms identical with those in the patient's respiratory tract.

Nasal carriers are also known to contaminate their environment, although usually to a more limited extent. However, Eichenwald *et al.* (1961) found that, in a nursery, babies whose noses were colonized with type 80/81 staphylococci contaminated their surroundings heavily only when a virus infection of the respiratory tract was superimposed.

The numbers of patients having a simultaneous respiratory tract infection with a virus and staphylococci will normally be few at any given time and such people cannot be regarded as the chief source from which epidemic staphylococci are dispersed. Because infected surgical wounds are covered with a dressing there has been a tendency to regard them as insignificant reservoirs of infection. Colebrook (1950), however, pointed out that dispersal of organisms can be heavy while dressings are being removed.

The larger the area infected, the greater the numbers of cocci available for dispersal. The load from a patient with septicaemia may be negligible compared with that of a burned patient infected with the same strain.

Persistence of infection in an individual, exemplified by the person who has frequent crops of boils, and characteristic of type 80/81 infections, could provide significant numbers of organisms for dissemination to new hosts over a long period.

2. *Survival of Staphylococci outside the Body*

Since infected persons and carriers contaminate their environment, this poses the following questions: (1) For how long after being shed from the body, are these organisms viable and capable of infecting new hosts? (2) Are there differential survival rates for different strains?

Lidwell and Lowbury (1950) examined the death rates at various relative humidities of *Staph. aureus* present in samples of dust collected in three hospitals. K, the death rate per day, varied from 0.030 in a dry atmosphere to 0.53 at 84 per cent relative humidity. Maltman, Orr and Hinton (1960) studied the death of the Wood 46 strain dried on glass. After six days storage at room temperature, the viable count was reduced by 90 per cent. After three days, the virulence of the strain for mice by the intramuscular, intracerebral and intravenous routes was markedly reduced (Hinton *et al.*, 1960). These workers therefore suggested that staphylococci shed from the body and surviving in the environment have suffered "sub-lethal damage which is associated with an overall decrease in infective potential."

The Wood 46 strain was isolated more than thirty years ago and its behaviour may not be representative of more recent epidemic strains. This question of the viability of dried staphylococci has therefore been examined further using a system that attempts to simulate conditions in the hospital ward or home. The behaviour of 37 strains belonging to a variety of phage types and isolated from epidemic and non-epidemic situations was compared.

Measured doses of staphylococci in the log phase of growth in broth were deposited on squares of cotton lint and allowed to dry at room temperature in a cupboard. The numbers of viable organisms were counted at intervals and the death rate per day calculated. The temperature of storage varied from 66 to 70 F and the relative humidity from 42 to 50 per cent, conditions similar to those in our hospital wards.

When the loss of viability of Wood 46 was compared with that of PS 80, that of a Group III antibiotic-resistant strain and that of a penicillin-sensitive strain of Group II, it was found that after 14 days there was no significant loss of viability by PS 80 or the Group III strain, while the count of Wood 46 was reduced by 99 per cent and that of the Group II strain by 90 per cent.

The 37 strains could be divided into two groups: those that showed no loss of viability after 14 days storage and those that showed a significant loss.

Strains of the following phage types showed no loss—Group I: 52A/79, 80/81 and lysogenically converted strains derived from type 80/81 strains (9 strains); Group III: 6/54, 42E, 47 and 77; Group IV: 42D.

Strains that showed significant loss of viability included 6 strains of different patterns in Group I (including the 35-year-old Bundaberg strain), all of 5 strains of Group II that were tested, 3 strains of Group III and 4 non-typable strains. The death rates per day varied from $k = 0.011$ to $k = 0.176$ over periods of time up to 90 days.

It would appear pertinent to the question of differential survival that strains of types frequently implicated in epidemics survived best under these conditions.

While there is not at present sufficient evidence to allow a definite decision as to whether these dried organisms are capable of infecting new hosts, it is probable that this is so. Colbeck (1960) reported that type 81 staphylococci dried on woollen threads and stored at room temperature could induce abscesses when the threads were tied into rabbits. Infected threads dried for 7 days were able to cause abscesses.

Preliminary results (Rountree and Glen) indicate that PS 80 and a type 47 antibiotic-resistant strain dried on silk sutures for 28 days have undiminished viability and undiminished ability to infect mice when the sutures are introduced subcutaneously. In this situation, as was also shown by James and MacLeod (1961), as few as 20 to 50 cocci can initiate lesions.

Many observations on the infection of surgical wounds and on the colonization of the noses of patients entering contaminated wards also suggest that dried organisms present in bedding and in the ward air can be transmitted to new hosts. This evidence from wards is however circumstantial and often difficult to evaluate.

To summarize, some experimental evidence suggests that strains of staphylococci that have been implicated in epidemics are able to survive for considerable periods of time when dried on textiles, that their infectivity is not impaired under these conditions and that this ability to survive may be a character of importance in their spread.

3. *Ability to Set Up the Carrier State*

Another character of possible significance in the survival and transmission of a strain might be the ability to colonize readily (rather than to infect) new hosts. Since one of the chief ecological niches of the staphylococcus is the anterior nares of man, a character that facilitated colonization might allow the perpetuation of a strain until such time as conditions appeared that were suitable for the production of lesions and so of larger numbers of cocci.

In hospital epidemics, many people may be carrying the "epidemic" strain. While such persons can undoubtedly act as a reservoir of infection, their presence in large numbers could be a fortuitous reflexion of widespread contamination of their environment.

Possibly of more significance is a report by White (1961) that quantitative techniques of sampling showed that 77 per cent of 82 carriers of type 80/81 yielded more than 10^4 colonies per swab compared with 64 per cent of 420 carriers of other types.

However, our studies of patients in a surgical ward did not reveal any significant differences in the yield of staphylococci per nasal swab from carriers of epidemic and non-epidemic strains. Profuse carriers were regarded as those whose plates showed semi-confluent growth of *Staph. aureus* on the first quarter of the plate. Only the results of the first positive swab from each patient were used. Out of 739 carriers, 251 carried an antibiotic-resistant type 47 strain. Of these 28.7 per cent were profuse carriers. Of 81 carriers of type 80/81, 23.5 per cent were profuse carriers while the proportion of profuse carriers of 80 non-epidemic strains was 25 per cent. These figures did not support the idea that carriers of type 80/81 and of type 47 had a larger population of staphylococci in their noses than did carriers of other types.

Information was also obtained on the frequency of nasal carriage of these two strains and of other types by the nursing staff of this ward during a period of 12 months. The 104 nurses concerned stayed in the ward for from 2 to 48 weeks and were swabbed each week. At one time or another, 18 carried type 80/81 or 52/52A/80/81 and 29 carried type 47. There were 27 carriers of 18 other phage types. The type 47 strains, which were widely dispersed in the ward, were frequently picked up by the nurses but usually lost just as frequently, only 31 per cent of the swabs from carriers of this strain being positive. On the other hand, 62 per cent of swabs from the type 80/81 carriers were positive and after this strain had been acquired it tended to persist. The significance of the difference between these two strains was, however, rendered doubtful by the observation that 53 per cent of the swabs from the carriers of the other phage types were positive.

To sum up, there is a possibility that some epidemic strains, in particular phage type 80/81 strains, may populate the anterior nares in larger numbers than other strains and that carriage of these strains may be more prolonged than that of other types. Evidence on these points is not, however, conclusive and further observations are required.

SUSCEPTIBILITY OF THE HOST

One final point that should be considered is the question as to how far alterations in the susceptibility of their hosts have influenced the spread of virulent staphylococci.

The increased practice of intravenous infusion has undoubtedly provided a new avenue for infection. Surgical operations are often more extensive and of longer duration. Patients with ischaemic vascular disease whose defence mechanisms are impaired are frequently operated upon. Improvements in the techniques of thoracic surgery have permitted operations that were impossible fifteen years ago. Broad spectrum antibiotics have altered the intestinal flora of patients and cortico-steroids have suppressed normal defence mechanisms.

Nevertheless, while such patients constitute hosts of increased susceptibility, they represent only a small proportion of those infected. Most infections, particularly those of the newborn and their mothers and those outside hospitals, would appear to occur in essentially normal people.

CONCLUSION

One of the features of the staphylococcal population of any place is that it is in a state of flux. During the years that phage typing has been used, the appearance, increase in incidence, and either persistence or disappearance of individual strains have been observed. New strains are being introduced into hospitals continually by both patients and staff. In only rare instances do these new strains establish themselves in this new milieu. To do so they must compete with those strains already in occupation.

The factors that may contribute to their success are the subject of speculation. Some have been considered in this paper. They include penicillinase production and the ability to mutate to antibiotic-resistance, the ability to produce lesions yielding large numbers of organisms, the ability to invade the defences of the host, the ability to set up the carrier state and the ability to retain their virulence after they have shed from the body and dried.

The relative importance of these various properties is unknown. However, certain strains have scored marked epidemiological successes and have added to the reputation of this micro-organism as a genetically adaptable and biologically successful parasite.

REFERENCES

Allison, V. D. 1949. Discussion on food poisoning. Proc. Royal Soc. Med. 42: 214.

Barber, M., and J. E. M. Whitehead. 1949. Bacteriophage types in penicillin resistant staphylococcal infections. Brit. Med. J. 2: 565.

Barbour, R. G. H., and A. Edwards. 1953. Mutation of different bacteriophage types of staphylococci to streptomycin resistance. Aust. J. Exptl. Biol. Med. Sci. 31: 561.

Blair, J. E., and M. Carr. 1960. Distribution of phage groups of *Staphylococcus aureus* in the years 1927 through 1947. Science 132: 1247.

Bynoe, E. T., R. H. Elder, and R. D. Comtois. 1956. Phage-typing and antibiotic-resistance of staphylococci isolated in a general hospital. Can. J. Microbiol. 2: 346.

Chickering, H. T., and J. H. Park. 1919. *Staphylococcus aureus* pneumonia. J. Am. Med. Assoc. 72: 617.

Colbeck, J. C. 1960. Environmental aspects of staphylococcal infections acquired in hospitals. I. The hospital environment—its place in the staphylococcus infections problem. Am. J. Pub. Health 50: 468.

Colebrook, L. 1950. A new approach to the treatment of burns and scalds. Fine Technical Publications, London.

Duthie, E. S. 1957. Generalised staphylococcal epidemics in a hospital group. Symposium on Hospital Coccal Infections 23.

Eichenwald, H. F., O. Kotsevalov, and L. A. Fasso. 1961. Some effects of viral infection on aerial dissemination of staphylococci and on susceptibility to bacterial colonization. Bacteriol. Rev. 25: 274.

Hare, R., and E. M. Cooke. 1961. Self-contamination of patients with staphy-lococcal infections. Brit. Med. J. 2: 233.

Hinton, N. A., J. R. Maltman, and J. H. Orr. 1960. The effect of desiccation on the ability of *Staphylococcus pyogenes* to produce disease in mice. Am. J. Hyg. 72: 343.

Hunt, T. 1852. On carbuncles and boils: with especial reference to their preva-lance as an epidemic. Lancet 2: 149, 190.

Hurst, V., and M. Grossman. 1960. The hospital nursery as a source of staphy-lococcal disease among families of newborn infants. New England J. Med. 262: 951.

James, R. C., and C. J. Macleod. 1961. Induction of staphylococcal infections in mice with small inocula introduced on sutures. Brit. J. Exptl. Path. 42: 266.

Johnson, A., P. M. Rountree, K. Smith, N. F. Stanley, and K. Anderson. 1960. A survey of staphylococcal infections of the skin and subcutaneous tissues in general practice in Australia, May–December, 1958. N.H. M.R.C. Special Report Series No. 10, Canberra.

Lidwell, O. M., and E. J. Lowbury. 1950. The survival of bacteria in dust. II. The effect of atmospheric humidity on the survival of bacteria in dust. J. Hyg. 48: 21.

Maltman, J. R., J. H. Orr, and N. A. Hinton. 1960. The effect of desiccation on *Staphylococcus pyogenes* with special reference to implications concerning virulence. Am. J. Hyg. 72: 335.

Parker, M. T., and J. Kennedy. 1949. The source of infection in pemphigus neonatorum. J. Hyg. 47: 213.

Rountree, P. M., and B. M. Freeman. 1955. Infections caused by a particular phage type of *Staphylococcus aureus*. Med. J. Aust. 2: 157.

Rountree, P. M., and E. Asheshov. 1961. Further observations on changes in the phage-typing pattern of phage type 80/81 staphylococci. J. Gen. Micro-biol. 26: 111.

Rountree, P. M., and M. A. Beard. 1962. Observations on the distribution of *Staphylococcus aureus* in the atmosphere of a surgical ward. J. Hyg. 60: 387.

Sakurai, N., E. Updyke, A. J. Nahmias, and M. R. Gerhardt. 1961. Laboratory observations on the lysogenic properties of hospital staphylococci and their possible epidemiological significance. Am. J. Pub. Health 51: 566.

Shaffer, T. E., R. F. Sylvester, J. N. Baldwin, and M. S. Rheins. 1957. Staphy-lococcal infections in newborn infants. II. Report of 19 epidemics caused by an identical strain of Staphylococcus pyogenes. Am. J. Pub. Health 47: 990.

White, A. 1961. Quantitative studies of nasal carriers of staphylococci among hospitalized patients. J. Clin. Invest. 40: 23.

CORRELATION OF VIRULENCE OF STAPHYLOCOCCI FROM PATIENTS WITH BACTERAEMIA WITH VARIOUS LABORATORY INDICES

KIRSTEN ROSENDAL

Statens Seruminstitut
Copenhagen, Denmark

THE AIM of the present report is to find out if any of the bacterial properties of certain staphylococcal strains examined have a bearing on virulence. The method used has previously been described by Professor Williams as "Prospective Epidemiological Studies in Man."

About 550 human cases of staphylococcal bacteraemia from 1957 to 1961 have been investigated, and certain bacterial properties of the infecting strains have been examined. The material has been divided into comparable groups, and the bacterial properties have been correlated with mortality rates within these groups.

In order to be able to divide the material, certain facts about the patients have been recorded: age, sex, severe complications (diabetes, cancer, etc.), origin of the infection (hospital or community), and portal of entry for the infection. The following properties of the strains isolated were determined: phage type (Williams *et al.*, 1952, 1953), drug resistance (Jensen & Kiær, 1947; Dragsted & Erichsen, 1953), production of lipase (Gillespie & Alder, 1952; Sierra, 1957), alpha-toxin (Jackson, Dowling & Lepper, 1955), hyaluronidase (Faber & Rosendal, 1960), and resistance to mercuric-chloride (Moore, 1960).

Any relation between biochemical properties of micro-organisms and their pathogenicity for man must be confirmed by observations of human infections and not depend solely on animal experiments. This is especially true of staphylococci, the pathogenicity of which is clearly species-dependent.

An attempt has been made to avoid clinical evaluation of the severity of the infections by considering the death or survival of the patient as the measure of pathogenicity. The feature common to all is that staphylococci have gained entrance to the bloodstream. As a result, the material comprises cases of severe septicaemia and less serious bacteraemia, which makes it possible to find out whether the outcome is determined largely by host factors or by measurable bacterial properties.

RESULTS

It was found that mortality rate was higher when the infection originated in the hospital than when it originated outside the hospital (Table 1) even if one considers cases with and without serious complicating diseases. In some cases it was impossible to determine with certainty the origin of infection. Therefore "total material" comprises more infections than those listed as "hospital" + "community."

TABLE 1

ORIGIN OF INFECTIONS CORRELATED WITH MORTALITY RATE

Origin	Number	Mortality rate
Hospital	252	51%
Community	280	26%
Total (incl. unknown origin)	588	37%

	Mortality rate Primary severe conditions	
	+	−
Hospital	59%	46%
Community	47%	20%

The mortality rate could not be correlated with age, sex, or portal of entry for the infection, when groups of the same origin were compared.

Another factor found to influence mortality was the drug resistance of the infecting strain (Table 2). More resistant strains were found among the

TABLE 2

MORTALITY RATE RELATED TO ANTIBIOTIC RESISTANCE OF THE INFECTING STRAINS
(The total number of cases is given in parentheses)

	Penicillin		Tetracyclines	
	Resistant	Sensitive	Resistant	Sensitive
Hospital	58% (207)	14% (29)	66% (56)	49% (180)
Community	28% (170)	19% (99)	25% (16)	25% (253)
Total (incl. unknown)	44% (412)	20% (141)	54% (76)	36% (477)

hospital strains than among the community ones. Infections caused by antibiotic-resistant strains give a higher mortality rate than cases caused by sensitive ones. Within the two groups of origin the difference is still demonstrated but is most pronounced in the case of resistant strains.

At the present moment it can neither be ruled out nor proved that antibiotic-resistant strains which have a better chance of survival in the hospital may, by passages through human beings, add an extra still-unknown virulence factor to their properties. Also, it is a matter of doubt whether resistance to antibiotics is a virulence factor in itself or simply increases the mortality rate because inadequate antibiotic treatment is given. The answer to this can only be obtained by investigating the outcome of a series of untreated cases caused by strains of different antibiotic sensitivity.

TABLE 3

MORTALITY AND EGG-YOLK REACTION IN COMPARABLE GROUPS OF PATIENTS
(Mortality rate in percentages. The total number of patients in each group
is given in parenthesis. S = streptomycin.)

	Hospital		Community	
	S-resistant	S-sensitive	S-resistant	S-sensitive
EY+	60% (89)	26% (57)	32% (59)	19% (135)
EY−	72% (69)	43% (14)	50% (16)	35% (34)
u-value	1.52	0.89	1.02	1.77 Σ = 5.20

A *u* test has been used in order to compare the mortality rate of the infections caused by
EY-positive and EY-negative strains in the four groups. The *u* values do not exceed 2,
when Yate's correction (Hald, 1952) is used, i.e. there is no significance for the single group.
However, if the tendency of all four groups is taken into consideration a new *u* value of
2.60 (5.20/2, because the mean error of the sum of the four *u* values = 2) is found which
expresses the difference of the mortality rates. This value gives a reliable significance
(*p* below 1 per cent).

As a consequence of the higher mortality rate in the hospital group and
among the antibiotic-resistant strains, the material was scrutinized, and it
was found that the various characteristics of the strains were not distributed
evenly. Therefore the following correlations were carried out after the
material was divided into groups of the same origin and the same antibiotic
resistance.

The third factor found to influence mortality is the egg-yolk factor (Table
3). In all instances, mortality rate is highest for infections due to EY-
negative strains. These are chiefly found among the resistant hospital strains.

It may seem peculiar to connect virulence with a negative property.
However, it is possible that some EY-negative strains produce an unknown
substance which destroys the lipase, and that this substance is identical with
the virulence factor. It is a fact that EY-negative strains often give a positive
serum opacity reaction and that some of them inhibit the reaction given by
EY-positive strains on solid medium.

Mortality could not be shown to be influenced by the phage type of the
strains (Table 4). Mortality is only a few per cent higher for infections
caused by type 80 when all the cases are considered, and this small prepon-
derance disappears completely when infections of the same origin and the
same resistance to penicillin are compared.

Type 80 is the type found most frequently in Danish hospitals. Thus it is

TABLE 4

PHAGE TYPE CORRELATED WITH MORTALITY RATE
(Mortality rate in percentages. The number of cases in each group
is given in parenthesis. P = penicillin.)

		Hospital		Community	
	Total	P-resistant	P-sensitive	P-resistant	P-sensitive
Type 80	43% (240)	58% (117)	0% (7)	30% (83)	20% (10)
Other types	35% (314)	59% (90)	4% (20)	26% (84)	20% (85)
TOTAL	38% (554)				

permissible to conclude that it is a strain which has undergone many, if not the most, passages through human beings. The finding that the mortality rate for this type is average does not support the previously mentioned suggestion that the antibiotic-resistant hospital strains might have acquired their increased virulence by passages through man.

However, the distribution of the phage types of the bacteraemia strains might differ from that of strains from other sources. It did not differ from that of 7,000 strains from miscellaneous sources isolated from staff members and patients admitted to hospitals (Jessen et al., 1963), but it did differ from that of about 100 strains isolated from the noses of healthy carriers, where most of the strains were non-typable or unidentified (Jessen et al., 1959a).

Production of alpha-toxin and hyaluronidase could not be correlated with mortality rate.

At first it looked as if resistance to mercuric-chloride could be correlated with mortality (Table 5), but the subdivision of the material into comparable groups made it clear that the correlation was secondary to origin of infection and antibiotic resistance. Resistance to mercuric-chloride was found chiefly among antibiotic-resistant strains: 6 per cent of sensitive strains, 20 per cent of penicillin-resistant strains and 80 per cent of strains resistant to penicillin and streptomycin were resistant to mercury. The difference in mortality is less pronounced if one deals only with strains resistant to penicillin; and among hospital strains it disappears completely, if only strains with the same resistance to streptomycin are considered.

TABLE 5

MORTALITY AND MERCURY RESISTANCE OF THE INFECTING STRAINS
(The total number of cases in each group is given in parenthesis)

	Hg-resistant	Hg-sensitive
Total	48% (247)	30% (264)
Penicillin-resistant		
Total	49% (239)	38% (144)
Hospital	62% (132)	52% (63)
Community	31% (88)	25% (71)
Hospital		
Streptomycin-sensitive	27% (33)	27% (182)
Streptomycin-resistant	55% (186)	54% (39)

An interesting feature of the mercuric-chloride resistance is that the proportion of mercury-resistant strains is greatest among those belonging to types 80 and 83A, even when strains of the same resistance to antibiotics are investigated. At the present moment these types are the ones that give rise most frequently to epidemics in Denmark. This communicability may well be connected with resistance to mercuric-chloride, as suggested by Moore (1960).

Type 83A may reveal interesting facts about the virulence factors of the staphylococci. It combines the properties of EY-negativity and resistance to penicillin, streptomycin and tetracyclines, with resistance to mercuric-chloride.

SUMMARY

On investigating about 550 bacteraemia cases it was found that hospital-acquired infections had a more serious prognosis than infections of any other origin.

Antibiotic resistance of the strain aggravated the prognosis considerably.

Cases of bacteraemia caused by EY-negative strains gave a distinctly higher mortality rate than cases due to EY-positive ones.

The phage type of the infecting strain could not be correlated with mortality.

REFERENCES

Some of the present results have been published previously in the papers marked with an asterisk.

Dragsted, P. J., and I. Erichsen. 1953. Technique for direct resistance determination of bacterial flora in sputa. Acta Pathol. Microbiol. Scand. *32*: 383–392.

Faber, V., and K. Rosendal. 1960. Correlation between phage-type and hyaluronidase-production of *Staphylococcus aureus*. Acta Pathol. Microbiol. Scand. *48*: 367–373.

Gillespie, W. A., and V. G. Alder. 1952. Production of opacity in egg-yolk media by coagulase-positive staphylococci. J. Pathol. Bacteriol. *64*: 187–200.

Hald, A. 1952. Statistical theory, with engineering applications. Wiley, New York.

Jackson, G. G., H. F. Dowling, and M. H. Lepper. 1955. Pathogenicity of staphylococci: Comparison of alpha-hemolysin production with coagulase test and clinical observations of virulence. New England J. Med. *252*: 1020–1025.

Jensen, K. A., and I. Kiær. 1947. Problems concerning the estimation of the chemosensitivity of microbes and measuring of penicillin and streptomycin concentrations in the blood and spinal fluid. Acta Pathol. Microbiol. Scand. *25*: 146–151.

Jessen, O., V. Faber, K. Rosendal, and K. R. Eriksen.* 1959a, b. Some properties of *Staphylococcus aureus* possibly related to pathogenicity. I. A study of 446 strains from different types of human infection. II. In vitro properties and origin of the infecting strains correlated to mortality in 190 patients with *Staphylococcus aureus* bacteremia. Acta Pathol. Microbiol. Scand. *47*: 316–326, 327–335.

Jessen, O., K. Rosendal, V. Faber, K. Hove, and K. R. Eriksen.* 1963. Some properties of *Staphylococcus aureus*, possibly related to pathogenicity. III. Bacteriological investigations of *Staphylococcus aureus* strains from 462 cases of bacteraemia. Acta Pathol. Microbiol. Scand. *58*: 85–98.

Moore, B. 1960. A new screen test and selective medium for the rapid detection of epidemic strains of *Staphylococcus aureus*. Lancet *ii*: 453–458.

Sierra, G. 1957. A simple method for the detection of lipolytic activity of micro-organisms and some observations on the influence of the contact between cells and fatty substrates. Antonie van Leeuwenhoek *23*: 15–22.

Williams, R. E. O., and J. E. Rippon. 1952. Bacteriophage typing of *Staphylococcus aureus*. J. Hyg. *50*: 320–353.

Williams, R. E. O., J. E. Rippon, and L. M. Dowsett. 1953. Bacteriophage typing of strains of *Staphylococcus aureus* from various sources. Lancet *i*: 510–514.

THE PHAGOCYTOSIS OF STAPHYLOCOCCI*

DAVID E. ROGERS

Vanderbilt University School of Medicine
Nashville, U.S.A.

ALTHOUGH STAPHYLOCOCCAL DISEASE has been studied since the early days of microbiology, the factor or factors which serve as primary determinants of pathogenicity among staphylococci are still poorly understood. My colleagues in this symposium have reviewed a number of approaches which have been brought to bear on this problem. While good general correlation exists between the possession of certain biological characteristics such as coagulase or hemolysin production and virulence, the evidence that such extracellular products play a primary role in the establishment of staphylococcal infection is unconvincing. Thus, in the main, virulence for man has been determined retrospectively on the basis of epidemiologic correlations.

The pathogenic strains of many bacterial species which produce acute suppurative infections are characterized by capsules which render them resistant to phagocytosis (1). In the case of pneumococci (2), streptococci (3), and *Klebsiella pneumoniae* (4), it is clear that resistance to phagocytosis plays a primary role in pathogenicity. Despite the many studies on the phagocytosis of staphylococci, until recently, little attention has been directed to the surface structure of pathogenic strains, or their opsonic requirements in phagocytic systems. The majority of experiments employing human cells have not shown significant differences between rates of ingestion of strains isolated from known infection and non-pathogenic strains isolated from other sources. While scattered reports have suggested that encapsulation can occasionally be of importance in pathogenicity (5–7), the majority of staphylococci isolated from human disease have not demonstrated such characteristics.

During the past ten years, we have explored the behavior of staphylococci in phagocytic systems. Our initial studies employed human leukocytes in human serum or plasma. In these experiments, we were unable to obtain significant differences in the rates of phagocytosis of coagulase positive strains isolated from infection, and coagulase negative strains isolated from air or normal skin (8). It was thus our belief that resistance to phagocytosis *per se* was not a characteristic of pathogenicity. However, in 1959, Cohn and Morse showed that certain strains of coagulase positive staphylococci

*Certain studies reported were supported by Grant E-3082 from the Institute of Allergy and Infectious Diseases, National Institutes of Health, Bethesda, Maryland, and the George Hunter Laboratory, Vanderbilt University School of Medicine, Nashville, Tennessee.

were resistant to phagocytosis in systems containing rabbit cells and serum (9). We have thus re-examined staphylococcal phagocytosis utilizing different animal cells and sera. These studies indicate that resistance to phagocytosis can be the primary determinant of virulence of certain strains. Tentative indirect evidence suggests that surface antigens retarding phagocytosis may also play a role in determining virulence among strains producing infection in man.

The Dynamics of the Phagocytic Process

(A time lapse strip taken under phase contrast microscopy was used to demonstrate the dynamics of the phagocytic process.)

When appropriate numbers of viable staphylococci are placed in a drop of human blood mounted in a thin cover slip preparation, the details of the phagocytic process can be readily observed under phase contrast microscopy. In such systems, human polymorphonuclear leukocytes soon become actively motile. Advancing cells extend broad hyloplasm-containing pseudopods which are initially free of granules. As the cell advances, there is a streaming of cytoplasmic granules into the advancing pseudopod. Definite positive chemotaxis toward staphylococci can be observed. When cocci are encountered, the pseudopod flows about the micro-organisms. The engulfing arms of the pseudopod fuse, pinching off a small portion of the leukocyte surface membrane, and bacteria come to lie within a cytoplasmic vacuole. As phagocytosis proceeds, progressive degranulation of the polymorphonuclear leukocyte is evident (10–12). The degree of degranulation has been shown to relate directly to the number of particles ingested and may provide a mechanism for release of digestive enzymes and phagocytin into the vacuole (11). Occasionally, leukocytes egest bacteria after varying periods of residence within the cell (13). The ability of cocci to survive intracellular residence can be determined by disrupting leukocytes by the passage of electric current through such preparations. Viable bacteria subsequently form microcolonies within the cellular debris.

The Outcome of the Phagocytic Process

Utilizing roller tubes containing large populations of staphylococci and leukocytes, or direct observation under phase microscopy, we have shown that strains isolated from infection possess superior survival capacity within phagocytes (8, 14). From 40 to 80 per cent of staphylococci isolated from human disease survive 60 minutes or more within leukocytes. In contrast, non-pathogenic strains of staphylococci are destroyed rapidly and none are culturable after 15 to 20 minutes within cells. Thus it appears that strains capable of producing human disease possess the biologic advantage of resistance to destruction within the cytoplasm of polymorphonuclear leukocytes.

The Immunology of the Phagocytic Process

The serum requirements for phagocytosis of staphylococci were examined using a single strain of staphylococci, the Smith diffuse variant. These studies

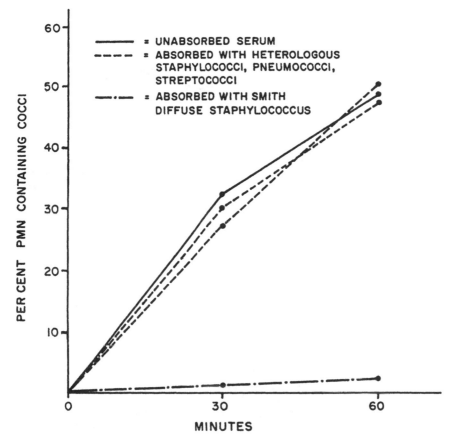

FIG. 1. The specificity of the opsonin present in sera of vaccinated rabbits. Opsonic activity is not removed by absorption with heterologous staphylococci or other microbial species. It is completely removed by absorption with the homologous Smith diffuse variant.

have shown that this staphylococcus behaves like an encapsulated micro-organism (15). When rabbit serum is employed, this micro-organism is not ingested by rabbit or human leukocytes in systems in which non-pathogenic strains are ingested readily. Serum obtained from rabbits immunized with a heat-killed whole cell vaccine induces brisk phagocytosis. The majority of adult human sera also promote phagocytosis of the Smith diffuse variant.

The opsonin present in the serum of immunized rabbits or normal adults behaves like specific antibody. It can be absorbed completely by the homologous strain. It is absorbed incompletely by heterologous staphylococci. It is not removed by absorption with other species of micro-organisms. A representative experiment is shown in Fig. 1.

This phagocytosis-promoting factor is heat-stable. While heated serum from immunized rabbits or adult humans does not induce phagocytosis, the opsonizing properties of heated sera are fully restored by the addition of guinea-pig complement, normal rabbit serum, or serum from agammaglobu-linemic adults (Fig. 2). None of these sera are of themselves capable of

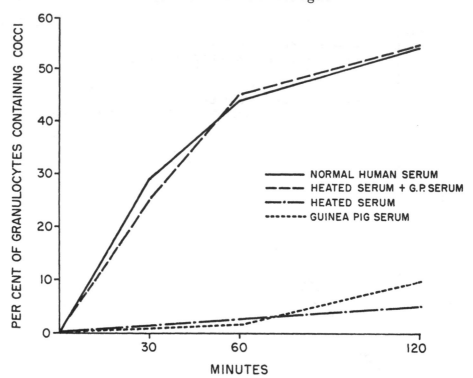

FIG. 2. The heat stability of the opsonin present in the sera of vaccinated rabbits. The opsonic activity of normal adult serum heated to 56 C for 30 minutes is completely restored by the addition of dehydrated guinea pig serum containing complement. (Republished from Yale J. Biol. and Med. 34: 566, 1962, with the permission of the editors.)

promoting phagocytosis. Other encapsulated organisms have similar dual opsonizing requirements (14).

To date, opsonizing antibody has been found in sera obtained from most normal adults. Incomplete studies suggest that the antibody is present in cord blood, disappears from the blood of infants between the ages of 6 weeks and 4 months, and rapidly reappears after 6 months. The amount of antibody added to a phagocytic system appears to be rate determining. As noted in Fig. 3, increasing amounts of antibody increase the speed of the phagocytosis. Similar observations have been made on antibody promoting the phagocytosis of pneumococci (17).

Opsonic Requirements of Other Strains of Staphylococci

The apparent specificity of the opsonizing antibody for the Smith diffuse variant led us to believe that an opsonic system might be utilized for typing staphylococci similar to that utilized in the bacteriocidal test for Group A streptococcal antibody (18). To date, this goal has not been realized. Most strains isolated from human disease have been found to be less resistant to phagocytosis and less specific in their opsonic requirements. As Table 1

EFFECT OF DECREASING AMOUNTS OF RABBIT IMMUNE SERUM IN NORMAL SERUM ON RATE OF PHAGOCYTOSIS

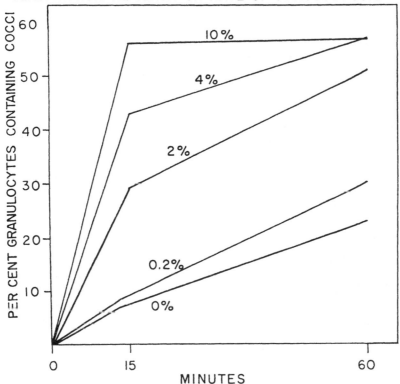

FIG. 3. Increasing concentrations of immune rabbit serum in normal rabbit serum increase the speed of phagocytosis in siliconed roller tubes. (Republished from Yale J. Biol. and Med. *34*: 569, 1962, with the permission of the editors.)

TABLE 1

COMPARATIVE OPSONIC REQUIREMENTS OF THE SMITH DIFFUSE STAPHYLOCOCCUS AND STRAINS RECENTLY ISOLATED FROM INFECTION

	Sera	Smith Strain	Other Strains
Diffuse immune serum	Rabbit	++++*	++++
Heated immune serum	Rabbit	0	++
Normal serum	Rabbit	0	++++
Heated normal serum	Rabbit	0	0
HIRS+NRS†	Rabbit	++++	++++
Adult serum	Human	++++	++++
Heated adult serum	Human	0	+++
Guinea-pig complement	—	0	++++
HHS+GPC†	Human	++++	++++

*Indicates degree of phagocytosis at 30 minutes.
†HIRS = heated immune rabbit serum; NRS = normal rabbit serum; HHS = heated human serum; GPC = guinea-pig complement.

indicates, the majority of isolates from infections are opsonized by *either* Smith antibody *or* heat labile factor resembling complement. While this finding initially suggested that the Smith diffuse variant was an unusual biologic variant of doubtful relationship to human infection, recent experiments have suggested an alternative hypothesis.

In 1961, Tompsett reported studies on four strains of staphylococci of unusual mouse virulence which lacked slide coagulase or clumping factor (19). Study of these additional four strains in our laboratory has shown that they all closely resemble the Smith diffuse variant (20). All are coagulase-positive but lack clumping factor; all produce fatal infections in mice when injected intraperitoneally in numbers which do not produce mortality with most strains; all produce alpha and delta hemolysins; all possess dual opsonic requirements for antibody and heat labile factor. Antibody promoting phagocytosis of all five strains can be evoked with heat-killed vaccine prepared from any one of these strains.

The Relationship of Resistance to Phagocytosis to Virulence

Recent observations show that the mouse virulence of these strains is directly related to their resistance to phagocytosis (20–21). Protection can be evoked by immunization with heat-killed vaccine which promotes rapid phagocytosis, but not by heterologous vaccines which fail to opsonize these micro-organisms. Immunization with alpha toxoid fails to induce phagocytosis, and toxoid vaccinated animals die of progressive intraperitoneal infection despite high levels of protection against alpha hemolysin *per se* (22). Thus, alpha hemolysin does not play an important role in the initiation of these infections.

The Possible Relationship of Resistance to Phagocytosis to Virulence in Man

We thus have five unusual strains of staphylococci which behave like encapsulated bacteria. These strains differ from the majority of pathogenic strains isolated from infection as shown in Table 2. It is clear that these strains are unusual. The characteristics described may be readily explained by possession of a surface antigen similar to or identical with the Smith surface antigen characterized by Morse (23). While these properties are not shared by most strains isolated from human infection, certain indirect

TABLE 2

COMPARATIVE BIOLOGIC CHARACTERISTICS OF 5 MOUSE VIRULENT STAPHYLOCOCCAL STRAINS AND OTHER STRAINS OF STAPHYLOCOCCI ISOLATED FROM INFECTION

Biologic characteristic	Mouse virulent strains	Other staphylococcal strains
1. Clumping factor	Absent	Present
2. Growth in soft serum agar	Diffuse	Compact
3. Intraperitoneal virulence for mice	High	Low
4. Opsonic requirements	Antibody+HLF	Antibody *or* HLF
5. Phage typing	Non-typable	Usually typable

evidence suggests the possibility that other pathogenic staphylococci may acquire similar features during growth in tissues.

First, we have evidence indicating that staphylococci lose virulence during passage *in vitro*. Preliminary work has shown that staphylococci obtained from infected lesions are more virulent for mice after but one intervening growth phase than after serial passage. Similar observations were reported by Van de Velde (24).

Secondly, the fact that virtually all normal adults have serum antibody capable of opsonizing these unusual variants suggests wide human experience with a similar or identical phagocytosis-retarding antigen. It thus seems reasonable to believe that this antigen is more common than suggested by studies on wild type staphylococci. That there are close antigenic relationships between these unusual strains and more common pathogenic strains is suggested by the fact that immunization of rabbits with certain recent staphylococci isolates evokes a heat stable opsonin which promotes phagocytosis of the Smith diffuse variant. Thus apparent differences in antigenic make-up may be quantitative rather than qualitative.

Finally, there are certain precedents to support the thesis that microbial parasites can acquire virulence factors during *in vivo* growth. For example, strains of *Pasteurella pestis* which are indistinguishable from avirulent strains *in vitro* may encapsulate and acquire resistance to phagocytosis during multiplication in the animal body (25).

These scattered bits of evidence have led us to advance the thesis that these unusual strains may represent staphylococci which breed true outside host tissues (20, 26). The acquisition of surface antigens conferring resistance to phagocytosis during *in vivo* growth might explain many of the puzzling features of staphylococcal disease in humans, and appears worthy of further experimental study.

References

1. Wood, W. B., Jr. 1960. Phagocytosis with particular reference to encapsulated bacteria. Bacteriol. Rev. 24: 41.
2. MacLeod, C. M. 1958a. The pneumococci. *In* Dubos, R. J., Bacterial and mycotic infections of man, p. 239. Philadelphia, J. B. Lippincott Company.
3. McCarty, M. 1958. The hemolytic streptococci. *In* Dubos, R. J., Bacterial and mycotic infections of man, p. 248. Philadelphia, J. B. Lippincott Company.
4. MacLeod, C. M. 1958b. Pathogenic properties of bacteria and defense mechanisms of the host. *In* Dubos, R. J., Bacterial and mycotic infections of man, p. 88. Philadelphia, J. B. Lippincott Company.
5. Gilbert, I. 1931. Dissociation in an encapsulated staphylococcus. J. Bacteriol. 21: 157.
6. Price, K. M., and Y. Kneeland, Jr. 1954. A mucoid form of *Micrococcus pyogenes var. aureus* which shows capsular swelling with specific immune serums. J. Bacteriol. 67: 472.
7. Lyons, C. 1937. Antibacterial immunity to *Staphylococcus pyogenes*. Brit. J. Exptl. Pathol. 18: 411.

8. Rogers, D. E., and R. Tompsett. 1952. The survival of staphylococci within human leukocytes. J. Exptl. Med. *95*: 209.

9. Cohn, R. A., and S. I. Morse. 1959. Interactions between rabbit polymorphonuclear leukocytes and staphylococci. J. Exptl. Med. *110*: 419.

10. Robineaux, J., and J. Frederic. 1955. Contribution à l'étude des granulations neutrophiles des polynucléaires par la microcinématographie en contrast de phase. Comp. Rend. Soc. Biol. *149*: 486.

11. Hirsch, J. G., and Z. A. Cohn. 1960. Degranulation of polymorphonuclear leukocytes following phagocytosis of microorganisms. J. Exptl. Med. *112*: 1005.

12. Cohn, Z. A., and J. G. Hirsch. 1960. The influence of phagocytosis on the intracellular distribution of granule-associated components of polymorphonuclear leukocytes. J. Exptl. Med. *112*: 1015.

13. Rogers, D. E., and M. A. Melly. 1961. The dynamics and immunology of the phagocytosis of staphylococci. Trans. Assoc. Am. Phys. *24*: 216.

14. Melly, M. A., J. Thomison, and D. E. Rogers. 1960. Fate of staphylococci within human leukocytes. J. Exptl. Med. *112*: 1121.

15. Rogers, D. E., and M. A. Melly. 1962. Observations on the immunology of pathogenic staphylococci. Yale J. Biol. and Med. *34*: 560.

16. Zinsser, H., J. F. Enders, and L. Fothergill. 1939. The phenomena of phagocytosis in immunity. *In* Principles and applications in medicine and public health, p. 317. New York, Macmillan Company.

17. Ward, H., and J. F. Enders. 1933. An analysis of the opsonic and tropic actions of normal and immune sera based on experiments with the pneumococcus. J. Exptl. Med. *57*: 527.

18. Maxted, W. R. 1956. The indirect bacteriocidal test as a means of identifying antibody to the M antigen of *Streptococcus pyogenes*. Brit. J. Exptl. Pathol. *37*: 415.

19. Tompsett, R. 1961. Relation of clumping factor produced by staphylococci to their phagocytosis and intracellular survival. *In* Finland, M., and G. Savage, Antimicrobial agents and chemotherapy, pp. 67–73. Ann Arbor, Braum-Brumfield, Inc.

20. Koenig, M. G., M. A. Melly, and D. E. Rogers. 1962a. Factors relating to the virulence of staphylococci. II. Observations on four mouse pathogenic strains. J. Exptl. Med. *116*: 589.

21. Koenig, M. G. 1962. Factors relating to the virulence of staphylococci. I. Comparative studies on two colonial variants. Yale J. Biol. and Med. *34*: 537.

22. Koenig, M. G., M. A. Melly, and D. E. Rogers. 1962b. Factors relating to the virulence of staphylococci. III. Antibacterial versus antitoxic immunity. J. Exptl. Med. *116*: 601.

23. Morse, S. I. 1962. Isolation and properties of a surface antigen of *Staphylococcus aureus*. J. Exptl. Med. *115*: 295.

24. Van de Velde, H. 1894. Etude sur le méchanisme de la virulene du *Staphylocoque pyogene*. La Cellule *10*: 401.

25. Burrows, T. W., and G. A. Bacon. 1954. The basis of virulence in *Pasteurella pestis*: Comparative behavior of virulent and avirulent strains *in vivo*. Brit. J. Exptl. Path. *35*: 134.

26. Rogers, D. E. 1962. On staphylococci and man. J. Am. Med. Assoc. *181*: 38.

IMMUNIZATION AGAINST STAPHYLOCOCCAL INFECTIONS

J. B. DERBYSHIRE

Agricultural Research Council, Field Station
Institute for Research on Animal Diseases
Compton, Berkshire, England

IN THIS CONTRIBUTION I wish to discuss staphylococcal virulence from the point of view of immunization against staphylococcal diseases. It will be clear that the subjects of immunity and virulence in any infectious disease are closely related, and it may be that the relative lack of success in staphylococcal immunization is related to the complexity of the virulence mechanisms of staphylococci.

PROBLEMS OF TESTING IMMUNITY TO STAPHYLOCOCCI

Some of the difficulties of assessing the virulence of a strain experimentally, which Professor Williams has mentioned, are applicable to the problem of testing immunity. Since the pathogenesis of infection may vary with species and route of infection it seems important not only that the species used for testing immunity should be the same or closely related to the natural host, but also that the route of challenge infection and the nature of the lesions produced should correspond to those in the natural disease. Clearly these criteria are almost impossible to fulfil experimentally in the human subject, but in the veterinary field more realistic experimental work is possible. In this paper I shall refer frequently to studies that we have been making during the past five years on immunization against mastitis produced experimentally in the dairy goat.

The technique for producing experimental mastitis in the goat has been described in detail elsewhere (Derbyshire, 1955); it is sufficient in the present context to say that in non-immune goats the inoculation of appropriate numbers of staphylococci into the teat canal produces gangrenous or severe suppurative mastitis, but only a mild, transient reaction in immune animals. The value of this experimental system is that it is closely related from the point of view of host and lesions to a natural staphylococcal disease, so that findings based upon it can be applied with some confidence to field experience.

The rather high degree of natural resistance to staphylococcal disease presents a problem in testing immunity, as well as in assessing the virulence of a strain. The proportion of the human and animal population carrying staphylococci in the absence of clinical disease is high, and experimentally, while infection may be produced by small numbers of organisms, relatively large doses of bacteria are required to produce characteristic staphylococcal lesions. We found that in goats with low antibody levels a dose of between 10^8 and 10^9 living organisms had to be used to produce severe mastitis constantly, although small doses sufficed to produce colonization of the mammary gland. Furthermore, approximately equal numbers of bacteria of strains isolated from lesions or from carrier animals were required to produce disease. This type of experience, which is also reported from experiments using other strains of staphylococci in a variety of hosts suggests that apparent virulence of a strain may sometimes be more an expression of depressed natural host resistance.

DIFFUSIBLE ANTIGENS AS IMMUNIZING AGENTS

Knowledge of the diffusible growth products of staphylococci is steadily increasing, and has been accompanied by interest in their possible role in the virulence mechanism of the organisms. Since many of these products are antigenic, crucial evidence for such a function would be provided if they could be demonstrated to have a protective effect against staphylococcal disease when used as vaccines. Such immunological studies have been restricted mainly to the haemolytic toxins, and to leucocidin and coagulase. Other products for which a biological activity has been demonstrated include hyaluronidase, fibrinolysin, proteases and lipases. Although these substances may be antigenic, and their antibodies are sometimes detected in staphylococcal infections, there is as yet no evidence that they exert a protective function in disease. In fact, these products have rarely been specifically included in vaccines. Recent work (Bernheimer & Schwartz, 1961) indicates that this list of diffusible products is by no means complete, and that many more extracellular proteins are produced by staphylococci. The activity of these, and particularly their immunological functions, need to be studied. May we now consider the significance of the immunological studies which have been carried out using the haemolysins, leococidin and coagulase.

Haemolysins. Of all the products of the staphylococcus, greatest attention has been given to the alpha haemolysin and the extensive literature on this subject has been reviewed critically and comprehensively by Elek (1959). It has been recognized for many years that certain small laboratory animals immunized with alpha haemolysin toxoid show an increased survival time in acute experimental infections. The same product has been subjected to clinical trial in man and animals on a rather wide scale, and successful use has been claimed by some workers in certain diseases. Beta and delta haemolysins have received relatively little attention, but it is known that the activity of delta lysin can be non-specifically neutralized by normal serum (Marks, 1951). One of the initial objects of our own work on experimental staphylococcal mastitis in goats (Derbyshire, 1960, 1961a; Derbyshire & Helliwell, 1962) was to characterize the immunological activity of vaccines containing alpha and beta haemolysin with respect to a variety of strains of

TABLE 1
IMMUNIZATION WITH ALPHA AND BETA HAEMOLYSINS

Treatment	Antibody levels when challenged				Level of immunity to challenge	
	Anti-alpha haemo-lysin	Anti-beta haemo-lysin	Anti-leuco-cidin	Anti-coagu-lase	With strain 201	With strain BB
Vaccinated with toxoided alpha plus beta haemolysin	High	High	Low	Nil	High	Low
Vaccinated with toxoided alpha haemolysin	High	Low	Low	Nil	High	Low
Untreated	Low	Low	Low	Nil	Low	Low

staphylococci of bovine origin. Some of the results of these and subsequent studies are summarized in Table 1. This indicates that vaccination with preparations containing alpha haemolysin alone, or alpha plus beta haemolysin, produced a high level of immunity to challenge by certain strains of staphylococci, exemplified by strain 201. Against another group of strains, however, exemplified by strain BB, no such immunity was produced either by alpha haemolysin alone, or by alpha plus beta haemolysins. There appear to be three significant conclusions to be drawn from this work. First, beta haemolysin would appear not to play a significant role in virulence. Secondly, for some staphylococci, alpha haemolysin production seems to be an important virulence determinant and thirdly, other strains are able to produce disease in the presence of anti alpha-haemolysin, and could therefore be regarded as more virulent than the 201 type of strain.

Leucocidin. The specific leucocidin of staphylococci which has recently been characterized biochemically by Woodin (1959) has been somewhat neglected from the immunological aspect, but is currently receiving some attention. Johanovsky (1958) demonstrated a correlation between anti-leucocidin titre and resistance to infection in man, and staphylococcal toxoids have recently been tested for antileucocidin production in clinical trials in man by Mudd and his associates (1962). Our own interest in leucocidin has been in attempts to immunize against the strain BB type of staphylococcus in goats; this work has also involved the use of coagulase.

Coagulase. The work of Duthie and Haughton (1958) on the biochemical characterization of coagulase has supplied techniques for the concentration of the enzyme into a form suitable for vaccination studies. Some time ago Boake (1956) vaccinated rabbits with coagulase, and these animals survived longer than normal controls following intravenous challenge. In our own work we have tried to determine the immunizing effect of coagulase together with leucocidin and alpha haemolysin against strain BB in goats (Derbyshire & Helliwell, 1962). The results of this are summarized in Table 2. Our first attempt to produce antibody to coagulase was unsuccessful, probably because the antigen used was toxoided, but nevertheless this group of goats

TABLE 2

IMMUNIZATION AGAINST STRAIN BB WITH ALPHA HAEMOLYSIN,
LEUCOCIDIN AND COAGULASE

Treatment	Antibody levels at time of challenge			Level of immunity to challenge
	Anti-alpha haemolysin	Anti-leucocidin	Anti-coagulase	
Vaccination with alpha haemolysin	High	Low	Nil	Low
Vaccination with alpha haemolysin + leucocidin + coagulase (inactive)	High	High	Nil	Partial
Vaccination with alpha haemolysin + leucocidin + active coagulase	High	High	High	Partial
Untreated	Low	Low	Low	Low

did show partial immunity to challenge in that a proportion of them showed only a mild, transient reaction, although some individuals were as severely affected as the controls. When anticoagulase as well as antihaemolysin and antileucocidin production was stimulated successfully, a similar level of partial immunity only was produced. Thus it may be concluded that while leucocidin appears to play a significant part in the virulence mechanism of this type of strain, coagulase is less important and does not contribute to immunity.

CELLULAR ANTIGENS AS IMMUNIZING AGENTS

I wish now to mention briefly the subject of the association of cellular factors with virulence and immunity. To summarize the current situation, it appears that vaccines of intact bacterial cells are in general reported to be of little value, and we have confirmed this in our own experiments. Of rather more promise has been the use of various preparations of disintegrated cells, which Stamp (1961) and Greenberg and Cooper (1960) have shown to have immunizing power in rabbits under certain conditions. We have been interested recently to study the immunizing effect of the dornase-lysed vaccine of the type described by Greenberg, against our BB strain in goats, in conjunction with the alpha lysin, leucocidin, coagulase vaccine that I have mentioned earlier. However, we have not been able to demonstrate any greater protection in this test system when goats were immunized in this way than when the three diffusible products were used alone.

IMMUNITY IN STAPHYLOCOCCAL INFECTIONS

The lack of success in producing a high level of immunity to challenge with certain strains of staphylococci leads one to postulate the occurrence of virulence factors in such strains which have so far been unrecognized. It is then necessary to consider whether such unrecognized factors are antigenic, and this can be done by looking for evidence of immunity in actual infections of animals with staphylococci. Under natural conditions, recurrent or persistent staphylococcal disease rather than a single attack in an individual seems to be the rule rather than the exception, although certain antibodies may be detected in quite high titre in such individuals. This situation suggests that natural infection with some strains of staphylococci produces only a low grade of immunity, and is somewhat disheartening from the point of view of artificial immunization. To investigate this experimentally (Derbyshire, 1961b) we have produced subcutaneous abscesses in goats with strain BB and when these were healing the animals were subjected to mammary challenge with the same strain. In this type of experiment, only a partial degree of immunity was produced, as a proportion of the animals developed severe mastitis following challenge. The irregular response resembled that which occurred in goats vaccinated with alpha haemolysin and leucocidin and it may be suggested that for strains of staphylococci of this type it is unlikely that artificial immunization could produce a better level of immunity than this. We have not had the opportunity of measuring the duration of immunity under these circumstances. However, since the "peak" level produced is of a limited order, it may well be that the low level of immunity which does develop is rather transient.

CONCLUSIONS

To conclude, I wish to try to relate these immunological findings to the occurrence and spread of apparently virulent strains of staphylococci in the field.

Disease caused by some strains of staphylococci can apparently be blocked by anti alpha-haemolysin, and significant natural levels of this antibody occur in many individuals. Therefore, such strains would be less likely to produce severe disease in the field, and might thus have less opportunity to spread. They would thus be regarded as relatively avirulent strains.

Other strains of staphylococci have a more complex virulence mechanism, and infection with such strains does not appear to produce a persistent or high level of immunity in the host. Such strains are more likely to produce severe disease in the population, and are thus likely to spread more readily— that is, they would be regarded as highly virulent. Clearly the virulence potential of such strains would be increased if they had the additional property of antibiotic resistance.

REFERENCES

Bernheimer, A. W., and Lois L. Schwartz. 1961. Extracellular proteins of staphylococci. Proc. Soc. Exptl. Biol. Med. *106*: 776–780.

Boake, W. C. 1956. Antistaphylocoagulase in experimental staphylococcal infections. J. Immunol. *76*: 89–96.

Derbyshire, J. B. 1958. The experimental production of staphylococcal mastitis in the goat. J. Comp. Pathol. *68*: 232–241.

Derbyshire, J. B. 1960. Studies in immunity to experimental staphylococcal mastitis in the goat and cow. J. Comp. Pathol. *70*: 222–231.

Derbyshire, J. B. 1961a. Further immunological studies in experimental staphlococcal mastitis. J. Comp. Pathol. *71*: 146–158.

Derbyshire, J. B. 1961b. The immunization of goats against staphylococcal mastitis by means of experimental infections of the skin and udder. Res. Vet. Sci. *2*: 112–116.

Derbyshire, J. B., and B. I. Helliwell. 1962. Immunity to experimental staphylococcal mastitis in goats produced by alpha lysin, coagulase and leucocidin. Res. Vet. Sci. *3*: 56–62.

Duthie, E. S. and G. Haughton. 1958. Purification of free staphylococcal coagulase. Biochem. J. *70*: 125–134.

Elek, S. D. 1959. *Staphylococcus pyogenes* and its relation to disease. E. and S. Livingstone, Ltd., Edinburgh and London.

Greenberg, L. and Margaret Y. Cooper. 1960. Polyvalent somatic antigen for the prevention of staphylococcal infection. Can. Med. Assoc. J. *83*: 143–147.

Johanovsky, J. 1958. Die Bedentung des Antileucozidins und Antitoxins bei der Immunitat gegen Staphylokokkeninfectionen. Z. Immunforsch. *116*: 318–328.

Marks, J. 1951. The standardisation of staphylococcal alpha antitoxin, with special reference to anomalous haemolysins including delta-lysin. J. Hyg. (Lond.) *49*: 52–66.

Mudd, S., G. P. Gladstone, Nancy A. Lenhart, and D. Hochstein. 1962. Titrations of antibodies against alpha-haemolysin and the components of staphylococcal leucocidin in human subjects following immunisation. Brit. J. Exptl. Pathol. *43*: 313–319.

Stamp, Lord. 1961. Antibacterial immunity to *Staphylococcus pyogenes* in rabbits. Brit. J. Exptl. Pathol. *42*: 30–37.

Woodin, A. M. 1959. Fractionation of a leucocidin from *Staphylococcus aureus*. Biochem. J. *73*: 225–237.

SYMPOSIUM XII

MICROBIAL CLASSIFICATION

Chairman: V. ZHDANOV

V. B. D. SKERMAN

Design and Purpose in Classification

S. D. HENRIKSEN

Can We Find a Uniform Base-line for Each Taxonomic Rank?

S. E. LURIA

Molecular and Genetic Criteria in Bacterial Classification

ROMAN PAKULA

Can Transformation be used as a Criterion in Taxonomy of Bacteria?

O. LYSENKO

The Statistical Approach to Bacterial Taxonomy

This symposium was organized by the International Committee on Bacterial Nomenclature and was supported by a grant from the International Union of Biological Sciences.

CHAIRMAN'S REMARKS

V. ZHDANOV

Institute of Virology
Moscow, U.S.S.R.

OPENING THIS SYMPOSIUM which is dedicated to Microbial Classification, I must note that a rapid development of knowledge in biochemistry, genetics, biometry and some other fields of biology has brought many important changes in the principles of taxonomy of micro-organisms.

For this symposium, then, it was considered worth while to discuss the general principles of microbial classification, leaving special topics, such as Leptospirae and Viruses, to be discussed in the various sections and subsections of the International Nomenclature Committee.

Dr. V. B. D. Skerman starts this symposium by pointing out the design and purpose of classification. Another general aspect in classification will be covered by Dr. S. D. Henriksen, who is trying to answer the question: Can we find a uniform base-line for each taxonomic rank?

Molecular biology and genetics in their application to bacterial classification will be discussed in two papers. Dr. S. E. Luria will present broad aspects of the topic just mentioned, and Dr. R. Pakula wants to probe into the more special subject: May interspecific transformations be used as a criterion in taxonomy?

The final paper, which is to be read by Dr. O. Lysenko, deals with the statistical approach to classification.

I hope that the reports to be presented will be fruitful in clarifying some modern approaches to microbial classification.

DESIGN AND PURPOSE IN CLASSIFICATION

V. B. D. SKERMAN

Department of Microbiology
University of Queensland
Brisbane, Australia

SINCE SOME 200,000 words were contributed to Microbial Classification (the 12th Symposium of the Society for General Microbiology) on this problem without providing a solution to it, I may be forgiven for failing to cover this aspect in 2,500. However, in contrast to Ross (1962), who, in dealing with nomenclature, stated that he hoped that his paper "by contributing to an understanding of the difficulties, would help to reduce the irritation, even if it contained little in the way of suggestions for overcoming them," it is my hope that this paper, by contributing towards the solution of the problem, may help to overcome it, even if it does little to remove the irritation.

What is the purpose of classification and how should we design our approach to attain this purpose?

Classification is simply the grouping together of objects which have certain characteristics in common. With micro-organisms it is carried out in a number of stages—the primary grouping of strains into species, the secondary grouping of species into genera and so on. Whether the action has the purely utilitarian aim of subsequently simplifying the process of identifying new strains or the more hallowed one of determining "natural" relationships, the practical problems involved are the same. These are (a) the adequate characterization of the strain, (b) the process of comparison of the strains and (c) the determination of the boundaries of the various taxa.

From personal experience, from consultations with microbiologists in many parts of the world and from statements in the literature, it is apparent that universal agreement is being reached on the fact that the "strain" *is* the practical working unit in microbial classification, that adequate characterization of strains is the first essential of any system of classification and that for such characterization standardization of procedure is essential.

There is, however, considerable diffidence regarding the practicability of achieving uniform application of tests even if agreement was reached on the range of tests to be employed. It is doubted whether it would be practicable for all microbiologists to use the same materials, since standardization of methods necessarily implies the standardization of the ingredients and methods of preparation of media and reagents. It is also doubted whether, even if there were access to the same materials, one can ever expect to obtain uniform interpretation of the results. There is no question that these doubts are formidable and no attempt is being made to hide the fact. However we have very good evidence that where some measure of agreement has been reached on procedures and these procedures have received what amounts to international sanction (as in the characterization of the enterobacteria) the manufacturers of bacteriological media have not been loath to market the products. I have noted that these methods and media have been used widely despite their cost which may be expected to diminish as the demand increases. Can we not then expect that similar action would follow upon an international agreement on a range of tests to be employed in the description of all micro-organisms?

Difficulties which arise from the lack of uniform interpretation of tests may be overcome, particularly when taxonomic as opposed to purely diagnostic questions are being considered, by the concurrent examination of the same collection of strains by a number of different workers. Or can we envisage a central reference laboratory whose function it would be to characterize, but not to burden itself with the storage of, strains for people who are not equipped to handle the material themselves or, like many biochemists, do not wish to do so?

What should the tests be? Should a common series of tests be applied to all bacteria? Should different tests be applied to different groups or should a selected range of tests be used as a common ground for comparison and a supplementary series of tests be applied to the groups so separated? The adoption of the first of these proposals, while perhaps achieving a measure of stability now non-existent, would impede research which, even in taxonomy, is the essence of progress. The second proposal has the highly undesirable effect of eliminating comparative study of micro-organisms which, after all, is the whole crux of classification. With the enterobacteria and the genus *Streptomyces* there have been very constructive moves towards agreement on the range of characters to be determined and the procedures to be adopted. But while considerable progress has been made with the differentiation of the organisms included within these groups, very little information has been obtained on the interrelationships between them and other closely allied groups. The third proposal offers an ideal choice which permits both the basic comparison of all organisms and the specialized study of groups which become separated on the primary analysis. It is ideal also in that it permits the selection of a "central" range of characters from past experience for immediate use for primary differentiation and fits the machinery of modern taxonomy, as will be seen later.

One of the principal objections to the application of some tests which may be selected for the primary analysis is that they have no *importance* within the group under consideration, for example, sugar reactions in the genus *Pseudomonas*. This objection is intimately bound up with the controversial matter of "weighting" of characteristics. In my own experience with the teaching of taxonomic microbiology students have been introduced to the study of a wide range of genera by two methods. In one, selected "taxonomically related" genera have been studied (usually 6 at a time) using for the differentiation of the selected genera only those tests commonly employed for the purpose. In the other, each group of genera was studied over a very wide range of tests which were found necessary (collectively) for the differentiation of all the genera. The former procedure led to difficulties. In the first place a considerable amount of time was spent in explaining the purpose of the different series of tests employed in each practical session. The regular change in materials and methods also led to a great deal of confusion on the part of the students, the more inquiring of whom quite logically asked why the tests were varied from day to day. It was not possible to offer any convincing explanation to the students in the absence of the "unimportant" test material and the other groups of genera. It was also impossible for the students effectively to correlate the day-to-day observations in the absence of strictly comparable evidence. In the second approach, although the students observed the reactions of only a limited number of genera each day, it was possible for them, individually, to evaluate the significance of certain tests as aids to differentiation as the work progressed. It was only *after the work had been completed* that *any* test assumed "importance" in the bacteriological meaning of the term. Quite apart from this, certain characters were revealed in some species which had not previously been attributed to them simply because the tests had never been performed, presumably because of an *a priori* lack of "importance" in the genus concerned. One such example was in the genus *Photobacterium* whose species were found to hydrolyse chitin. This is not an isolated example and it emphasizes the danger of *a priori* reasoning in terms of importance. Nor should we delude ourselves that this is purely a problem encountered by the student. It is a pitfall for the most experienced.

There should be no fear of an "important" character losing its ultimate significance (if it really has any!) through submergence into the common pool. If it is as important as implied, this fact will inevitably be reflected in its correlation with a multiplicity of other characters.

Opponents of the principle of weightlessness of characters should bear in mind the fate of the all-important lactose fermentation test in the classification of the enterobacteria, a character which has been relegated to a position of insignificance in the proposals of Ewing and Edwards (1960).

The selection of characteristics upon which descriptions might be based is a matter for a working party on bacterial systematics. I have provided separately a list* of the numerous morphological, nutritional and biochemical characters which have been used collectively in the description of species recorded in the 7th edition of Bergey's *Manual of Determinative*

---

*Copies are available from the author's laboratory.

Bacteriology. The list may provide a suitable basis for discussion on the types of tests which might profitably be recommended for future use. A decision on this matter would aid materially in the establishment of an international code for punch card records.

PROCESS OF ANALYSIS

It has been the practice in the past for the results of tests on a selected series of strains to be tabulated and a somewhat tedious visual analysis of the table to be made for the extent to which the individual strains could be correlated. On this basis, and by comparison with named cultures and published descriptions of species (themselves only the end-product of a similar activity and not the detailed list of characteristics of the strains which constituted the species), new species have been described. It is now suggested that this tedious process be replaced by machine analysis. In advancing this proposal Sneath (1962) calls for the use of a programme for determining percentage correlation and a subsequent rearrangement of strains in a descending order of correlation. Although these operations can be carried out laboriously by hand they can be performed automatically by the computer. The characters must first be coded onto punch cards (or tape) which are subsequently used as the feed input to the machine. The information is either stored in the "memory" of the machine or passed out for storage on magnetic tape or other device from which it can be retrieved when required.

The computer has to be programmed to analyse the information according to a predetermined programme. It can be programmed to carry out the type of operation advocated by Sneath which is intended for the purpose of classification. It can also be programmed for the much simpler task of direct comparison of a single set of data, such as the coded description of a new strain, with all the data stored in its memory or transferable to it from outside storage, an activity more suited to the problem of identification. It is for this that I advocate that some immediate attention be given to the problem of selection of characters for strain description and the standardization of methods to be employed. If this were done and the code established it would be possible to proceed with the filing of the information pending some agreement on the actual method of analysis which should be used. In view of the rapidity with which new equations are being proposed and the note of caution sounded by Silvestri *et al.* (1962) it is doubtful whether common agreement will be reached on this matter faster than it is being reached on the methods of description. In the meantime, however, simple comparison of strains for precise or partial agreement with recorded data can go on unhindered. The stored data could be analysed at any time, now or a century hence, by any method desired.

Notwithstanding the highly desirable features of the computer-performed analysis there are serious practical limits to its application. According to

Sneath (personal discussions) the existing computers lend themselves to the analysis of about two hundred strains only at a time. This means, in effect, that the ideal of permitting the computer to perform an unbiased analysis of *all* the characteristics of *all* the bacteria cannot be realized. Some break-down of the great array of bacterial strains has to be made before any detailed analysis can be made of any selected group. Research to date has, significantly, been applied to selected groups which one could justifiably argue were selected on weighted characteristics in the first place (the chromobacteria on pigment and the *Streptomyces* on morphology) although in both cases a few foreign organisms were included to offset this rejoinder!

While one may expect some improvement in the design of computers it is doubtful whether the capacity can be increased without an inordinate increase in operating costs and a code once formulated would be very diffi-cult to change because of the expense involved. For this reason there appears to be no real justification for further delay in laying down proposals for the characters to be determined.

The existing type of punch card suited for use with the computer is adequate in its capacity to meet all requirements well beyond the foreseeable future. It would permit (i) successive numbering of strains up to 1,000,000,000 (ii) recording of mutants to each strain up to 1,000 per strain (iii) recording of the location of storage or isolation for up to 10,000 locations, and still leave space for the registration of 564 characters. This is simply an example of the use to which the card could be put. It is not a recommendation. The minimum rate of direct comparison is of the order of 400 descriptions per minute. This can be increased considerably. The pro-cedure permits the rapid comparison of details of descriptions of strains from different collections, a means of determining when wild types from one collection equate with mutants from another and the permanent storage of the sort of detailed strain data which are indispensable for classification studies but which, largely because of editorial policy, lie buried in inac-cessible files in laboratories all over the world.

DETERMINATION OF THE BOUNDARIES OF THE VARIOUS TAXA

It was mentioned earlier that the strain is the practical working unit in taxonomy. It determines its own behaviour and there its responsibility ends. The taxonomic activity is a human one largely designed for human ends. Since there are no rules to govern the grouping of strains and no arbiter other than (bacteriological) public opinion has functioned in the past to pass judgement on the conclusions of taxonomists, it is gratifying to find that numerical analysis, despite some disagreement on the details of pro-cedure, appears to yield essentially the same results on the same material in the hands of different workers. In this the method shows considerable promise and seems certain of ultimate universal application. However the decision as to where to draw the line in the delimitation of species has still to be made and the nomenclature problem of applying names to the newly defined groups and determining their relationship to existing names has to be solved.

It is well to realize that one inevitable outcome of numerical analysis will be a great lumping of strains into groups larger in content and smaller in number than at present existing. Attendant to this will be a diminishing of the number of characters which all the strains in a particular group will share. Although the characters which were selected in the preparation of my key for the Identification of the Genera of Bacteria would hardly be considered as "random" in the statistical sense, they covered about 80 characters of a biochemical, nutritional and serological nature and about 60 optically determinable characters (mostly morphological) and were therefore as "random" as any other selection which has been used since. But despite this there were so few common characters within each group that the keys had to be prepared from an analysis of the individual descriptions. Had the descriptions been of strains (as in the genus *Paracolobactrum*) the keys would have been a strain analysis. Since this situation existed with the "split" state of affairs it will be aggravated by an increase in "lumping." I do not see much hope for the successful development of keys based on the shared characters as defined by numerical analysis and wish to emphasize the contention of van Niel (1940) that identification and classification should be treated apart. It is indeed fortunate that the coded data stored in the computer can, with equal facility, be used for both.

Finally some consideration must be given to the problem facing laboratories without computing facilities. Here the problem is twofold. Where a large survey of a restricted ecological group is being made and the amount of data to be analysed is considerable, the only solution is to enlist the aid of some centre willing to code the data and do the analysis. This is being done quite widely. Where the interest of the individual is in the identification of isolated strains the problem is similar in many respects to the identification of the serotypes of the genus *Salmonella*. For the latter, laboratories have become accustomed to the maintenance of a limited range of diagnostic sera sufficient to identify the serotypes which normally occur locally. If these fail the culture is forwarded to a larger centre. The position with the more general problem of identification is somewhat similar except that the small group of diagnostic sera is replaced by a collection of duplicate punch cards supplied by a centre to cover the limited field required. Fortunately a computer is not essential for the handling of small parcels of cards, comparisons with which can be made, albeit more slowly, with very much less expensive card-sorting machines. Cards which failed to match the limited series would then be referred to the centre.

In the absence of a card sorter the position is indeed difficult since this type of punch card cannot be sorted by hand.

598   XII. CLASSIFICATION: *V. B. D. Skerman*

REFERENCES

Bergey's Manual of Determinative Bacteriology. 7th ed., 1957.   Williams & Wilkins.

Ewing, W. H., and P. R. Edwards.   1960.   Intern. Bull. Bacteriol. Nomencl. Taxonomy, *10*: 1–12.

Ross, R.   1962.   *In* Microbial classification, 12th Symposium Soc. Gen. Microbiol., pp. 394–404. Cambridge University Press.

Sneath, P. H. A.   1962.   *Ibid.*, pp. 289–332.

Silvestri, L., M. Turri, L. R. Hill, and E. Gilardi.   1962.   *Ibid.*, pp. 333–360.

Van Niel, C. B.   1946.   Cold Spring Harbor Symp. Quant. Biol. *11*: 285–301.

CAN WE FIND A UNIFORM BASE-LINE FOR EACH TAXONOMIC RANK?

S. D. HENRIKSEN

Kaptein W. Wilhelmsen og Frues Bakteriologiske Institutt
Oslo University and Rikshospitalet
Oslo, Norway

IN SPITE OF THE TITLE of this symposium I propose to deal only with bacterial classification. There are two main difficulties which face us in bacterial classification. The first is lack of adequate information about many bacteria. This is a difficulty which is in the process of rapid elimination, and the many new techniques for the study of bacteria which have become available in recent years make it virtually certain that we shall soon have accumulated all the information that is needed.

The second difficulty is that until very recently a biological yardstick for the measurement of relationships between bacteria has been missing, with the consequence that it has been impossible to define any uniform base-line. After the discovery of genetic recombination in bacteria such a yardstick seems to have come within reach, but it may yet take a long time before it can be applied to classification in a rational manner. Before this can be done, it is necessary to find out just what this new yardstick measures.

I. GENETIC COMPATIBILITY AS A BASE-LINE IN CLASSIFICATION

Dr. Luria is going to speak about genetic criteria in bacterial classification, and I apologize to him for trespassing, but I feel that a discussion of base-lines in bacterial classification which leaves out any reference to genetic evidence is impossible at the present time. By utilizing genetic evidence combined with other kinds of evidence it may eventually be possible to sort out groups of bacteria which have real or potential access to common genetic pools. Without going into the philosophy of classification, which has been adequately covered in recent symposia (Ainsworth & Sneath, 1962; Lwoff, 1958; Vendrely, 1958a; Schaeffer, 1958; Renoux, 1958; Le Minor, 1958; Thibault, 1958), it may be postulated that the species is a useful concept in classification, and that it can only be a stable and uniform concept if defined on some criterion of fundamental biological significance. Genetic compatibility or genetic homology is such a criterion, which could be utilized in defining the base-line of the bacterial species.

Sneath (Ainsworth & Sneath, 1962) has shown that natural classifications can be based on Adansonian principles, and this may become increasingly useful in bacterial classification as our knowledge about bacteria increases, but it may be doubted that Adansonian classification could give us a definition of the species which would satisfy every one. Any degree of over-all similarity can be expressed numerically, but the choice of the level where the species should be located would remain arbitrary in the absence of some guiding biological principle. Our best hopes for finding a generally acceptable base-line, therefore, rest on the mechanisms for genetic recombination. And the prospects look bright. Transformation has already been reported in ten of the present genera (Ravin, 1961), and two more can be added, since work in our institute has shown that transformation is possible both in the genus *Moraxella* (Bövre & Henriksen, 1962) and in *Pasteurella* (Henriksen, 1962). Transduction and conjugation also have succeeded in a number of genera, and yet the study of these phenomena is only in its early infancy.

I shall only mention that results already obtained in these studies suggest that our classification may be due for revision at several points, and that in some instances the species may have been devaluated to an unreasonably low level (Schaeffer, 1958; Cowan, 1959). But even though the results of recombination studies may eventually be applied to taxonomy, it should be emphasized very strongly that we should be in no kind of hurry in revising the classification. I believe that there has generally been too much hurry in bacterial taxonomy. A lot of work remains to be done before we can even begin to evaluate the genetic relationships of bacteria. The main thing is that we should try to anticipate the development ahead of us, and that we should avoid introducing changes at this stage, which would be at cross-purposes to the natural trends.

Although it is possible that studies of recombination may help us define some kind of base-line for the species, it remains to be seen whether this will be a sharp line at a uniform level or a broad and diffuse band. There is even a possibility that some genera may come to be defined as groups of species showing some degree of incomplete genetic homology. But with respect to higher taxonomic ranks it is difficult to see any possibility that they could be based on anything but Adansonian principles. It is reasonable to believe that the question of how many different taxonomic ranks of higher order should be employed and how they should be circumscribed will remain a matter of convenience. It may be unrealistic to insist upon any kind of common base-line for these higher ranks, but when the time is ripe for a revision of the system of classification, it may be useful to discuss whether there really is any need for all the ranks between the genus and the class.

II. PROPOSITION OF AN INTERIM POLICY IN BACTERIAL CLASSIFICATION

The criteria of genetic homology may not be applicable to all bacteria. Furthermore, it must be expected to take a long time before these criteria can be used in classification, even where they do apply. For these reasons there is a need for an interim policy in bacterial taxonomy, while waiting for a new base-line to materialize. It is the main purpose of this paper to formulate the principles of such a policy in general terms.

The first principle that I should like to advocate is conservatism in taxonomy. The system of classification has been revised often, sometimes for little apparent reason. At this stage we might call a truce and postpone all major changes until the possibility of a new, truly biological base-line has been fully explored. Later very radical revisions may be needed, but until then we should use the system we have with as little change as possible.

The second principle is informality. In the present state of knowledge it may be better to speak about informal groups, as some of the *Enterobacteriaceae* people have been doing, than to be concerned with formal names and exact taxonomic rank.

We should be prepared to accept a certain degree of diversity within the species. The species, if defined genetically, would be assumed to have arisen through mutations and selection (Ravin, 1960), and although genetic homology should exist within the species in the sense that the individuals can exchange genes, this does not mean that they are genetically identical.

Bacteria, therefore, should not be placed in separate species on account of differences due to mutation of a single, or even of several characters. In general there has been a tendency to place bacterial species within too narrow bounds. As pointed out by Ewing and Edwards (1960), separation of bacteria in different species on the basis of differences in a single character, such as lactose fermentation, leads to unreasonable results. It is as important to recognize the mutation range of a species as to describe its typical behaviour.

Serological criteria, although very useful in diagnosis and epidemiology, may not be as suitable for formal classification. Most antigens used in grouping and typing owe their specificity to polysaccharides. But examples of partial cross-reactions between polysaccharides due to entirely accidental structural similarity are now so numerous that partial cross-reactions between bacterial antigens should not be interpreted as signs of relationship without supporting evidence.

Kauffmann (1959) proposed that the serotype should be the species in the *Enterobacteriaceae*, and Kauffmann, Lund and Eddy (1960) proposed to consider the serotype of the pneumococcus as the species. Rauss (1962) has voiced a corresponding opinion with respect to the Proteus-Providence group. Exception has already been taken to these proposals by Taylor (1959) and by Cowan (1959), and it has been pointed out that these proposals would create a major nomenclaturial headache. And even more serious arguments against these proposals can be given. The facts that any pneumococcal type can be transformed into any other type, and that, as with *Haemophilus influenzae*, even artificial double types can be produced in the laboratory (Austrian & Bernheimer, 1959), suggest that the serotype is not a sufficiently stable character to be used as the basis of the species. The transformation experiments with pneumococci, streptococci and staphylococci (Bracco, Krauss, Roe & MacLeod, 1957; Pakula, Hulanicka & Walczak, 1958; Perry & Slade, 1962) suggest that these proposals would be steps in the wrong direction.

In the *Enterobacteriaceae* (Taylor, 1959) identical antigens can be found in many different serotypes and even in different biochemical groups now considered to be genera. Some antigenic determinants, such as Salmonella O-factors 1, 15, 34 and 27 (Le Minor, Le Minor & Nicolle, 1961), are produced only in the presence of bacteriophage, and others, for example the flagellar antigens, can be transduced.

Thus the serotypes are only different combinations of certain sets of antigens, and they can be changed, in some cases even back and forth, by such extraneous influences as bacteriophages. These serological criteria, therefore, can hardly be suitable for the definition of species, even if the impossible consequences in nomenclature are left out of consideration. Serological groups and serotypes are useful as such, and they do not become any more useful if their taxonomic rank is altered.

The highly interesting results obtained by Kauffmann and his collaborators (Kauffmann, Krüger, Lüderitz & Westphal, 1960; Kauffmann, Braun, Lüderitz, Stierlin & Westphal, 1960; Kauffmann, Krüger, Lüderitz & Westphal, 1961) in the study of the O-antigens suggest that when strains mutate from S to R their antigenic specificity may become identical. This suggests that the O-antigens are variations of the same theme, arising by the addition of side chains to a common polysaccharide skeleton. But the fact that all these antigens have a common backbone, so to speak, could be more significant in classification than the fact that they are different in the S-form. In any case, to consider the serotypes as species would be to put the species in a straightjacket.

In brief, my conclusions are that for the time being we should be conservative and at the same time informal in bacterial taxonomy. Further devaluation of the species should be avoided, and future developments will show whether a formal, hierarchical system is suitable in bacterial classification.

REFERENCES

Ainsworth, G. C., and P. H. A. Sneath. 1962. *In* Microbial classification. 12th Symposium Soc. Gen. Microbiol. Cambridge University Press.

Austrian, R., and H. P. Bernheimer. 1959. Simultaneous production of two capsular polysaccharides by pneumococcus. I. Properties of a pneumococcus manifesting binary capsulation. J. Exptl. Med. *110*: 571–584.

Bracco, R. M., M. R. Krauss, A. S. Roe, and C. M. MacLeod. 1957. Transformation reactions between pneumococcus and three strains of streptococci. J. Exptl. Med. *106*: 247–259.

Bövre, K., and S. D. Henriksen. 1962. An approach to transformation studies in *Moraxella*. Acta Path. Microbiol. Scandinav. *56*: 223–228.

Catlin, B. W., and L. S. Cunningham. 1961. Transforming activities and base contents of deoxyribonucleate preparations from various *Neisseriae*. J. Gen. Microbiol. *26*: 303–312.

Cowan, S. T. 1959. Nonconformism in nomenclature. Intern. Bull. Bacteriol. Nomencl. Taxonomy *9*: 131.

Ewing, W. W., and P. R. Edwards. 1960. The principal divisions and groups of *Enterobacteriaceae* and their differentiation. Intern. Bull. Bacteriol. Nomencl. Taxonomy *10*: 1–12.

Henriksen, S. D. 1962. Transformation of streptomycin resistance in *Pasteurella*. Acta Path. Microbiol. Scandinav. *55*: 496.

Kauffmann, F. 1959. On the principles of classification and nomenclature of *Enterobacteriaceae*. Intern. Bull. Bacteriol. Nomencl. Taxonomy 9: 1–6.

Kauffmann, F. 1959. Definition of genera and species of *Enterobacteriaceae*. Intern. Bull. Bacteriol. Nomencl. Taxonomy 9: 7–8.

Kauffmann, F., E. Lund, and B. E. Eddy. 1960. Proposal for a change in the nomenclature of *Diplococcus pneumoniae* and a comparison of the Danish and American type designations. Intern. Bull. Bacteriol. Nomencl. Taxonomy *10*: 31–40.

Kauffmann, F., L. Krüger, O. Lüderitz, and O. Westphal. 1960. Zur Immunchemie der O-antigene von *Enterobacteriaceae*. I. Analyse der Zuckerbausteine von Salmonella-O-antigenen. Zbl. Bakteriol. I. Orig. *178*: 442–458.

Kauffmann, F., O. H. Braun, O. Lüderitz, H. Stierlin, and O. Westphal. 1960. Zur Immunchemie der O-antigene von *Enterobacteriaceae*. IV. Analyse der Zuckerbausteine von Escherichia-O-antigenen. Zbl. Bakteriol. I. Orig. *180*: 180–188.

Kauffmann, F., L. Krüger, O. Lüderitz, and O. Westphal. 1961. Zur Immunchemie der O-antigene von *Enterobacteriaceae*. VI. Vergleich der Zuckerbausteine von Polysacchariden aus Salmonella-S- und R-Formen. Zbl. Bakteriol. I. Orig. *182*: 57.

Leidy, G., E. Hahn, and H. E. Alexander. 1953. In vitro production of new types of *Hemophilus influenzae*. J. Exptl. Med. 97: 467–482.

Le Minor, L. 1958. La notion d'éspèce dans le groupe *Salmonella*. Ann. Inst. Pasteur 94: 207–212.

Le Minor, L., S. Le Minor, and P. Nicolle. 1961. Conversion des cultures de *Salmonella schwarzengrund* et *Salmonella bredeney*, dépourvues de l'antigène 27 en cultures 27 positives par la lysogénisation. Ann. Inst. Pasteur *101*: 571–589.

Lwoff, A. 1958. L'espèce bactérienne. Ann. Inst. Pasteur 94: 137–141.

Pakula, R., E. Hulanicka, and W. Walczak. 1958. Transformation between streptococci, pneumococci and staphylococci. Bull. Acad. Polon. Sci. Classe II, *6*: 325–328.

Perry, D., and H. D. Slade. 1962. Transformation of streptococci to streptomycin resistance. J. Bacteriol. *83*: 443–449.

Ravin, A. R. 1960. The origin of bacterial species: Genetic recombination and factors limiting it between bacterial populations. Bacteriol. Rev. *24*: 201–220.

Ravin, A. R. 1960. The genetics of transformation. In Advances in genetics, ed. E. W. Caspari and J. M. Thoday, *10*: 62–163. Academic Press.

Renoux, G. 1958. La notion d'espèce dans le genre *Brucella*. Ann. Inst. Pasteur 94: 179–206.

Rauss, K. 1962. A proposal for the nomenclature and classification of the Proteus and Providencia groups. Intern. Bull. Bacteriol. Nomencl. Taxonomy *12*: 53–64.

Schaeffer, P. 1956. Transformation interspécifique chez les bactéries du genre *Hemophilus*. Ann. Inst. Pasteur *91*: 192–211.

Schaeffer, P. 1958. La notion d'espèce après les recherches récentes de génétique bactérienne. Ann. Inst. Pasteur 94: 167–178.

Taylor, J. 1959. Why christen a *Salmonella*? Intern. Bull. Bacteriol. Nomencl. Taxonomy 9: 159–164.

Thibault, P. 1958. La notion d'espèce dans le groupe *Shigella*. Ann. Inst. Pasteur 94: 213–218.

Vendrely, R. 1958. La notion d'espèce à travers quelques données biochimiques récentes et le cycle L. Ann. Inst. Pasteur 94: 142–166.

MOLECULAR AND GENETIC CRITERIA IN BACTERIAL CLASSIFICATION

S. E. LURIA

Department of Biology
Massachusetts Institute of Technology
Cambridge, U.S.A.

IN RECENT YEARS, bacterial genetics has become a major branch of genetics because of its close integration with the study of the genetic materials at the molecular level. Yet, in bacteriology as in other branches of systematic biology, genetics cannot advance claims to provide a basis for a natural classification. Its main contribution must be to enlighten the systematist about the organization of the hereditary materials and about the unit processes of hereditary change which underlie evolution, so that the trees of classification that are devised, besides serving the practical purposes of identification, will also reflect as much as possible the phylogenetic relationships of the various organisms, that is, the amount of their common ancestry and their potential common posterity. In specific cases, genetics can warn against adoption of poor criteria of classification, such as differences known to be readily altered by mutation or by naturally occurring processes of genetic recombination.

In addition, recent advances in bacterial genetics and in molecular biology have provided a significant body of comparative information on the chemical and biological basis of bacterial heredity in a number of organisms. In the following sections I shall attempt to evaluate the relevance of these findings for the systematics of bacteria.

DEOXYRIBONUCLEIC ACID COMPOSITION AND BACTERIAL CLASSIFICATION

The classical papers by Lee, Wahl and Barbu (1956) and by Belozersky and Spirin (1958) first pointed out the remarkable spread in the mean composition of deoxyribonucleic acid (=DNA) of different bacterial groups. The so-called GC content of DNA, that is, the ratio $(G + C) / (G + C + A + T)$, where G, C, A, and T stand for the molar concentrations of guanine, cystosine, adenine and thymine, ranges from 0.27 to 0.75 in different bacteria (Sueoka, 1961). This is in marked contrast with the situation in higher plants and in vertebrates and invertebrates, where the mean GC content is relatively uniform (0.35 to 0.48). As shown in Table 1, in bacteria there is a fairly good over-all correlation between GC content and systematic position, with several outstanding exceptions, such as *Micrococcus lysodeikticus*.

TABLE 1

The Guanine-Cytosine Content of the DNA in Representative Bacteria
(mostly from data compiled by Sueoka, 1961)

G + C content, %	Organisms
26–32	*Clostridium perfringens, C. bifermentans; Micrococcus pyogenes*
34–38	*Micrococcus asaccharolyticus; Streptococcus faecalis, S. foetidus, S. pyogenes; Diplococcus pneumoniae; Bacillus cereus, B. megaterium, B. thuringiensis; Proteus vulgaris*
40	*Neisseria catarrhalis; Bacillus laterosporus*
42–44	*Bacillus subtilis, B. polymyxa; Vibrio cholerae*
50–52	*Neisseria gonorrheae, N. meningitidis; Salmonella enteritidis, S. gallinarum, S. typhimurium; Escherichia coli; Shigella dysenteriae, S. paradysenteriae; Bacillus macerans*
56–58	*Aerobacter aerogenes; Serratia marcescens; Brucella abortus*
64–68	*Pseudomonas fluorescens, P. aeruginosa, P. saccharophila*
72	*Sarcina lutea; Micrococcus lysodeikticus*
74	Various *Actinomyces* sp.

Significantly, some groups of organisms that are considered as closely related by the systematist, for example, the Escherichia-Shigella-Salmonella group, have nearly identical GC contents. Yet other members of the *Enterobacteriaceae*, such as *Aerobacter aerogenes, Serratia marcescens*, and *Proteus vulgaris*, are very different. Also, members of the genus *Bacillus* have GC contents ranging from 0.32 to 0.50 (Marmur *et al.*, 1962).

Two physico-chemical methods have made possible a closer analysis of the molecular composition of bacterial DNA: the *temperature denaturation method* (Marmur & Doty, 1959), which correlates GC content with the temperature dependence of strand separation; and the *equilibrium density gradient centrifugation method* (Meselson *et al.*, 1957), which correlates GC content to specific gravity of DNA in a solution of CsCl or of other heavy salts. These two methods make it possible to study the spread in base composition among the DNA molecules extracted from each bacterial strain. Both methods reveal a remarkable situation: the molecules or segments of DNA from a given bacterium, and even their mechanically produced fragments down to average molecular weights of about 10^6, are very homogeneous in GC content (Sueoka *et al.*, 1959; Rolfe & Meselson, 1959). Thus, if two organisms differ by 10 per cent in mean GC content, they will have practically no large DNA fragments of similar composition.

This is indeed an astounding discovery: if DNA carries the genetic information and if different bacteria have a certain amount of genetic information in common, there ought to be certain DNA molecules in common. Among the many interpretations proposed (unsuspected types of genetic code; variety of different codes in different organisms; presence of excess nongenetic DNA [see Sueoka, 1962]), recent evidence favors the hypothesis that the genetic code is indeed universal or quasi-universal, but that organisms with different GC ratios do not have large segments of common genetic information. In fact, in organisms with dissimilar GC contents, proteins with identical functions have different structures and serological specificities. This is true, for example, for the β-D-galactosidases of *E. coli* and *A. aerogenes* and for the alkaline phosphatases in *E. coli* and *S. marcescens* (Signer *et al.*, 1961). Thus, the identity of function of the respective enzymes in these organisms has presumably evolved either by convergence, that is, by the accumulation under natural selection pressure of mutations leading to an optimal function, or by selective persistence of important functions despite a divergent evolution of the genetic material. Sueoka (1962) has outlined a theory of the evolution of bacterial DNA in which the main source of variation is postulated to be the occurrence of "transitional" mutations (G-C $\rightleftarrows$ A-T); the controlling factors would be the ratio of the two mutation rates and the selection pressures; a shift in mutation rate ratio, for example, by certain mutagens, could alter the GC content without necessarily increasing its heterogeneity. Rates of evolution computed on the basis of reasonable mutation and growth rates can account for slow emergence of differences in GC content, explaining the observed stability of GC content in contemporary groups of bacteria. If the code is not strictly universal, owing to mutational changes in the system that translates nucleic acid information into protein structure (Benzer & Champe, 1961; Yanofsky *et al.*, 1961), then changes in code will favor shifts in GC content. The existence of some more adaptive sets of translating systems could explain any tendency of the mean GC content values in bacteria to cluster around certain preferred modes (Lanni, 1960). More information on this subject should be forthcoming rapidly in the next few years.

HYBRIDIZATION OF HEATED DNA AS A TEST OF GENETIC HOMOLOGY

The single strands of DNA present in heat-denatured DNA can be "renatured" by slow cooling, with reformation of single stranded DNA (Marmur & Lane, 1960). Using mixtures of DNA's labelled or unlabelled with N^{15} or deuterium, that is, heavy or light DNA's, the renatured DNA can be detected as bands of hybrid density in a CsCl density gradient. Schildkraut *et al.* (1961) and Marmur *et al.* (1961) have applied this method

TABLE 2

CORRELATION OF GENETIC RECOMBINATION AND HYBRID DNA FORMATION

Organisms	Recombination process	Extent hybrid DNA formation
B. subtilis × *B. natto*	Transformation ++++	++++
B. subtilis × *B. polymyxa*	" +	+
B. subtilis × *B. brevis*	" −	−
E. coli B × *E. coli* K-12	Conjugation, transduction ++++	++++
S. dysenteriae × *E. coli*	Conjugation, transduction ++	++
S. typhimurium × *E. coli*	Conjugation +	−
E. freundii #5610-52 × *E. coli*	?	−
E. freundii #17 × *E. coli*	?	+
E. carotovora × *E. coli*	?	−

to mixtures of heated DNA's from different bacterial strains and species. The hypothesis in this work is that the amount of hybrid density DNA formed reflects the degree of homology in the base sequences of two DNA samples. The renaturation data are compared with the occurrence of genetic transfers by transformation or by conjugation, taken as an indication of genetic homology. The results, some of which are presented in Table 2, show that hybrid DNA formation is excellent among *E. coli* strains; is low but significant between *E. coli* and *S. dysenteriae*; and is non-detectable between *E. coli* and *S. typhimurium*, as well as between *E. coli* and one strain of *E. freundii* (another strain gives some hybrid DNA with *E. coli*). Similar relations obtain among members of the genus Bacillus and in the Pneumo-coccus-Streptococcus group. The results correlate well but not completely with those of genetic hybridization (see below). If indeed hybrid DNA formation and genetic hybridization reflect, respectively, base sequence homology and genetic homology, and if the two homologies have the same molecular basis, then the hybrid DNA formation is the less sensitive of the two tests: genetic hybridization occurs, however rarely, between strains that give no detectable hybrid DNA. One may well conceive that the amount of molecular homology needed to secure at least some genetic synapsis would be less than that needed to produce detectable molecular hybridization *in vitro*.

GENETIC TRANSFERS AND BACTERIAL SYSTEMATICS

A variety of mechanisms for genetic exchanges among bacteria have been discovered and analysed in the last fifteen years (Hartman & Goodgal, 1959; Jacob & Wollman, 1961). Presumably, additional mechanisms will be revealed by further study. Two questions concern us here: what do genetic exchanges tell us about relationships among bacterial groups? and what role do such exchanges play in bacterial evolution?

Three categories of genetic transfers have been recognized in bacteria, depending on the vehicle of transfer: transformation by free DNA; cell-to-cell conjugation; and bacteriophage infection. The genetic material transferred is DNA in all known cases, except for a group of recently discovered RNA phages (Loeb & Zinder, 1961).

(a) *Transformation* has been reported to occur in a variety of organisms (Ravin, 1961). Its occurrence appears to be determined mainly by the competence of the bacterial cells to accept free DNA through their surface layers, as well as by the ability of the transferred DNA to express its functions and to integrate itself in the recipient cells.

(b) *Conjugation* depends on the possession of certain specialized genetic elements, which we shall call "conjugons" and which determine the ability to pair and to establish a cell-to-cell transfer channel: the fertility (=F) factors found in *E. coli* and in *P. aeruginosa* (Holloway & Jennings, 1958), the colicinogenic factors (Ozeki & Howarth, 1961; Meynell, 1962), and the resistance transfer factor (RTF; see Watanabe & Fukasawa, 1961) of *Entero-bacteriaceae.* Some of these conjugons are episomes (Jacob *et al.*, 1960), that is, accessory genetic elements that can either multiply autonomously in the bacterial cells or assume a lineom-associated state.[1] The genetic material transferred in conjugation may be the conjugon only, or a set of lineomal genes, or both. When lineom is transferred, the transfer is generally partial, presumably because of breakage in the lineom in transfer (merozygosis; Jacob & Wollman, 1961). The genetic length of the transferred segment is directly correlated with the amount of DNA transferred. Those conjugons that are episomes may be physically associated and cotransferred with smaller or larger portions of the lineomal genes (as in F-duction; Jacob & Adelberg, 1959).

(c) *Phage infection* depends on the specificity of phage-receptors on the bacterial surface. The genetic material introduced by a phage may be either the specific phage genome or a fragment of lineom. In many cases, the phage genome itself carries genes that express themselves by alteration of bacterial properties; this results in "conversion" phenomena (Uetake *et al.*, 1958). When a phage carries lineomal genes (or other genetic factors, such as the F conjugon) the transfer is called "phage-mediated transduction" or "transduction" *tout court* (Zinder, 1953). A transduced lineomal fragment may be associated with the phage genome (Arber *et al.*, 1957; Luria *et al.*, 1960).

An important distinction concerns the fate of the transferred genetic materials. Three possibilities exist:

1. The transferred genes may persist in functional form, but without multiplication or integration into the recipient cell's lineom; this is observed mainly in abortive transduction (Lederberg, 1955) and in phage infection of a lysogenic, immune bacterium (see Bertani, 1958).

2. The transferred genes may multiply without becoming integrated into the lineom (extralineomal replication). The multiplication can lead to lysis, as with virulent phage, or to indefinite replication in non-integrated form—the most frequent outcome of the transfer of conjugons into compatible recipients.

3. Some or most of the transferred genes may become integrated into the lineom, as observed following transformation, conjugation and transduction. With temperate phages, integration is the reduction of the phage genome to prophage at some specific location on the bacterial lineom (lysogenization; Lwoff, 1953). Genes that have been transferred abortively or that are replicating in extralineomal form can occasionally become integrated into the lineom of the cells that carry them.

In relation to genetic transfers between different bacteria, the following generalizations appear to be valid:

1. Genetic transfers can occur between bacteria of different GC content,

---

[1]In this paper the genetic structure of the bacterial cells is referred to as the *lineom* (Kühn, 1961) rather than the chromosome, because the former term is less committal than the latter.

as between *Escherichia* (or *Salmonella*) and *Serratia* (Falkow *et al.*, 1961).

2. Extralineomal replication may occur even in cases when the transferred DNA has a different GC content from the DNA of the recipient. Thus, phages with a whole range of GC contents can grow in the same bacterium. More significantly, an episome like the F factor associated with a group of *E. coli* genes (GC content 0.5) can multiply indefinitely in *S. marcescens* (GC content 0.58) (Signer *et al.*, 1961).

3. Integration into the lineom appears to occur only when the transferred DNA has the same composition as the recipient bacterium. This holds true in all reported instances of transfer of lineomal fragments and of episomes; even lysogenization has been found only when phage and host-bacterium have DNA's of similar GC contents (Luria, 1959; Lanni, 1960). The frequency of integration and its dependence on taxonomic relationship between donor and recipient bacterium will be discussed in the following section.

In line with current ideas of molecular biology, the interpretation of the findings stated above is probably as follows. Genetic transfer requires compatibility of surfaces; functionally similar surface structures may have arisen in genetically distant organisms by convergence, or may have persisted during evolution despite extensive divergence at the genetic and molecular level. DNA uptake, phage adsorption, and conjugation reflect only the compatibility of the surface mechanisms and need not bespeak any close relationship. Thus, for example, coliphage P1 adsorbs onto, penetrates, and kills many strains of *P. aeruginosa*, but apparently does not multiply within them (Amati, 1962). Once DNA has successfully penetrated, its replication has somewhat stricter requirements, but may ultimately be conditioned only by the ability of the exogenous DNA to be effectively copied by the DNA polymerase(s) of the recipient bacterium and to be sheltered from its nucleases. Whether such stranger DNA will function will depend also on its ability to be read by the resident RNA polymerase to give functional messengers. The most elegant evidence on this point comes from the study of a strain of *S. marcescens* that has received an F factor derived from *E. coli* and carrying the structural gene for the enzyme alkaline phosphatase (Levinthal *et al.*, 1962). In this organism, the *E. coli* genes never become integrated; they multiply with the F factor and can be removed by treatment with acridine dyes (Hirota, 1960). This organism produces normal *S. marcescens* phosphatase and normal *E. coli* phosphatase; in addition, it makes also some hybrid phosphatase. The *coli* and *marcescens* phosphatases are both dimers of polypeptide monomers; the hybrid phosphatase is a dimer of *coli* and *marcescens* monomers. In such organisms, the exogenous DNA fragment can actually be detected by CsCl density gradient centrifugation as a small DNA fraction with the typical lower density of *E. coli* DNA among the bulk of the heavier *S. marcescens* DNA (Marmur *et al.*, 1961).

These remarkable findings show that *Escherichia* genes can be read correctly by the protein-making machinery of *Serratia* and indicate that the genetic code must be very closely similar, and possibly identical, in these two groups despite the different GC contents of their DNA's. Since the different monomers of the *coli* and *marcescens* phosphatases can still dimerize to give a functional enzyme, it seems likely that evolution from a common ancestor, including many changes in genetic code and amino acid sequence, has preserved those features of the polypeptide needed for proper dimerization and enzyme activity (Levinthal *et al.*, 1962).

A clear-cut situation is that of the Neisseria genus (Catlin and Cunningham, 1961). Members of six species of this genus have equal GC contents, 0.5, and give interspecific transformation, although generally at lower frequency than the intraspecific one. Cultures of a seventh species, *N. catarrhalis*, have a GC content of 0.4 and give no transformation with strains of other species.

FREQUENCY OF GENETIC INTEGRATION AND RELATIONSHIP BETWEEN BACTERIA

As mentioned in the preceding section, integration of exogenous genetic determinants into the bacterial lineom occurs only when the corresponding DNA's have similar GC contents. Presumably, base sequence homology is a prerequisite for the homologous pairing leading to integration. In most cases of transformation and recombination after conjugation, integration is the replacement of resident genetic determinants with the newly entered ones, by mechanisms that are still unclarified. In the case of episomes such as the F factors and temperate phages, there probably is actual addition of a certain amount of genetic material; whether or not some lineomal element is actually replaced by the episome remains a matter for speculation (Campbell, 1962). The same requirement for equal GC content appears to exist for integration of lineomal genes into an episome, such as transducing phage, as for integration into a recipient cell's lineom.

Frequency of integration provides a subtle measure of genetic homology. In general, the closer the genetic relationship between donor and recipient strain, the higher the integration frequency. This is true in transformation, conjugation, and transduction. The following regularities are observed: integration frequency is highest for transfer between derivatives of the same strain; may be lower between different strains of the same species; is generally much lower between strains classified as different species; and is not uniform for different genetic determinants.

Some informative examples are presented in Table 3. The frequencies of integration after transformation, transduction, or conjugation are lower in interspecific than in intraspecific transfers. Moreover, in transfers between strains classified in different species or genera, some genetic markers altogether fail to become integrated. In some instances, as in conjugation between an *E. coli* donor and *Salmonella typhimurium*, the apparent difficulty of integration leads to persistent partial diploidy, with occasional

TABLE 3
Frequencies of Integration after Intraspecific and Interspecific Hybridization

Process	Markers	Donor	Recipient	Integration frequency
Conjugation	lac⁺, ara⁺	E. coli	E. coli	1
		"	S. dysenteriae	10^{-2}
	mal⁺, ind⁺	"	E. coli	1
		"	S. dysenteriae	$<10^{-7}$
Transformation	str-r	H. influenzae	H. influenzae	1
		"	H. parainfluenzae	10^{-4}
	hem	H. parainfluenzae	H. influenzae	$<10^{-7}$
	str-r	N. meningitidis	N. meningitidis	1
		"	N. perflava	10^{-1}
		"	N. subflava	2×10^{-2}
		"	N. catarrhalis	$<10^{-5}$
		N. catarrhalis	"	1
		"	N. meningitidis	$<10^{-6}$
	try⁺	B. subtilis	B. subtilis	1
		"	B. natto	3
		"	B. niger	10^{-4}

Symbols: *lac, ara, mal* = lactose, arabinose, maltose utilization; *hem, try* = hematin and tryptophan biosynthesis; *str-r* = streptomycin resistance.

integration of some lineomal segments to form a truly hybrid lineom (Baron *et al.*, 1959; Miyake and Demerec, 1959).

Integration of exogenous genetic determinants may involve regions of various length. Once a segment of the lineom has become integrated it retains the characteristics of the strain from which it has derived and thereby influences the specificity of successive transfers in which the original recipient bacteria act as donors. The following is an instructive example (Zinder, 1960). A large lineomal segment including the *ara⁺* or *ara⁻* marker, transferred from *E. coli* into *S. typhimurium* by conjugation, can become integrated into it. Then, the transduction of these *coli* markers by a *S. typhimurium* phage is compared with that of analogous *typhimurium* markers. The results are clear-cut: the phage can donate a *coli ara⁺* marker to an *ara⁻* segment derived from *E. coli*; it can donate a *typhimurium ara⁺* marker to a *typhimurium ara⁻* segment; but it does not introduce a *coli ara⁺* marker into a *typhimurium ara⁻* region, or vice versa. Clearly, the fragment of *E. coli* DNA has remained homologous to *coli* DNA even when incorporated into the *typhimurium* lineom.

An interesting observation is that the determinant for hematin independence from *Hemophilus parainfluenzae*, whose absence in *H. influenzae* is a stable enough character to serve as a major taxonomic criterion, fails to appear following transformation of *H. influenzae* with DNA from *H. parainfluenzae*, whereas many other traits are transformed (Schaeffer, 1961). A similar failure to be integrated is observed for the ability to produce gas from fermentable substrates after conjugation of *E. coli* donors with *Shigella* strains as recipients (Luria and Burrous, 1957). This suggests that differences such as "loss" of hematin synthesis in *H. influenzae* or of aerogenesis in *S. dysenteriae* are due either to major changes in the organization of the genetic material such as deletions, or to changes in several not closely linked genes.

That low integration frequencies reflect low degrees of homology in the structure of the genetic material is in agreement with the already cited results of DNA hybrid formation, which is less complete with strains that give lower frequencies of genetic integration (Marmur *et al.*, 1961).

When genetic transfer mechanisms are recognized in two related organisms, one can compare the large-scale genetic organization of their lineoms. This can be done, for example, for *E. coli* and *S. typhimurium* using both transduction and conjugation. The genetic maps of these two organisms look very much alike (Miyake & Demerec, 1959; Zinder, 1960). It is at a finer level that we may expect to find evidence for the process of micro-evolution which is leading to integrative incompatibility and presumably also to adaptive divergence.

In this respect, recent studies on the comparative structure of the genetic segment controlling lactose-utilization (*lac* region) in the *E. coli–S. dysenteriae* groups are informative. In *E. coli*, this region consists of four adjacent loci: *i*, controlling adaptability; *o*, the operator gene; *z*, determining β-D-galactosidase enzyme; and *y*, determining β-galactoside permease. In conjugation between *E. coli* donors and *S. dysenteriae* recipients, the *E. coli* genes can be transferred in a group, although infrequently, to the recipient lineom (Luria & Burrous, 1957). Transduction by phage P1 reveals that the *lac*⁺ genes of *E. coli*, when introduced into strains of *S. dysenteriae*, can function immediately but are only rarely integrated; often they persist and multiply as part of a defective P1*dl* prophage (Luria *et al.*, 1960). Transduction of various *E. coli lac*⁻ mutants as recipients using phage P1 grown on strains of *S. dysenteriae* reveals that these typically lactose-negative organisms possess defective genetic *lac* regions; they have apparently a deletion of the permease gene, that is, are y^{del}, but are $i^+o^+z^+$ and can generally make some β-D-galactosidase (Li *et al.*, 1961; Franklin & Luria, 1961). In a typical instance, that of *S. dysenteriae* #60, the galactosidase is serologically related to that of *E. coli* strains but differs from it in a number of properties, such as heat stability, turnover number, etc. (Sarkar & Luria, 1963). By transduction one can obtain hybrid strains in which recombination has occurred within the *z* gene; these hybrids have galactosidase enzymes intermediate in properties between those of *E. coli* and *S. dysenteriae* #60; the differences involve at least 5 or 6 genetic sites, probably more. Thus, in the *S. dysenteriae* group, we observe what may be a series of stages in the mutational elimination of one genetic function, that of the z^+ locus, when this is not needed any more (probably owing to the loss of the *y* locus). *E. coli* mutants that have lost parts of the *lac* region by genetic deletions behave somewhat like *S. dysenteriae*; the frequency of genetic integration of the *lac*⁺ genes following transduction is decreased.

These examples show that transduction analysis can be used to compare the genetic microstructure of related bacterial strains.

GENETIC ANALYSIS AND BACTERIAL CLASSIFICATION

The main finding in studies of genetic and molecular homologies among bacteria validate by and large the classical groupings; this indicates that in bacteria, as well as in other groups of organisms, the choice of major criteria of classification, however empirical, has been altogether wise. Some of the relations suggested specifically by molecular genetics, for example, the closer similarity of *M. lysodeikticus* to *Sarcina* than to other members of the genus *Micrococcus*, and the close relationship among certain members of the genus *Bacillus*, had already been surmised by astute systematists.

Claims of abrupt major evolutionary changes, as in the transmutation of enteric bacteria into cocci and alkali-producing nonfermentors (Spirin & Belozersky, 1956), have been rendered even more suspicious by the reported data on DNA composition. Some current groupings will ultimately require important revisions if the criteria of molecular genetics are introduced into systematics. Thus, if the mean GC content of DNA is indeed a slowly evolving character, and if its distribution includes significantly clustered groups of values, these clusterings may be useful guides for major subdivisions. If such criteria of classification should conflict with the classical major criteria of morphology and structural organization, it should be kept in mind that similar morphological characters may have arisen secondarily and independently in different groups of bacteria: for example, transition from rods to cocci, and gains or losses of sporulation, may belong in this class. On the other hand, GC content of DNA may have evolved relatively rapidly within a group of related bacteria, while other characteristics changed more slowly. For example, there are indications that the soluble RNA, that is, the translation mechanism for the genetic code, is more nearly the same in different *Enterobacteriaceae*, irrespective of their GC content, than in other bacterial groups (A. Rich, personal communication). Such basic features as the translation mechanism and the configuration of important enzymes may have been preserved more stubbornly than other features during the diverging evolution of the bacterial groups.

An important question concerns the impact of the recently discovered mechanisms of genetic transfer for bacterial classification. At variance with some other geneticists, this writer does not favor considering as members of the same species all organisms between which genetic transfers can occur, not even those in which such transfers can lead to formation of an integrated recombinant lineom. The critical question is whether enough gene flow occurs in nature to balance and counteract the diversifying influences of the internal and external milieu. Even though transformation and conjugation probably do occur in nature (see Ravin, 1961), their frequency and effectiveness in producing gene flow between different strains may easily be overestimated. Phage-mediated transduction may be a slightly more effective natural means of genetic exchange.

Instead, genetic analysis suggests a number of potential and actual pitfalls that can mar the value of any classification aiming at practical applications. Thus, for example, the antigenic characters used in distinguishing among members of the genus *Salmonella* are known to be interconverted not only by transduction (Lederberg, 1955), but also by lysogenization with converting phages (Iseki & Sakai, 1953). Another example is that of enteric pathogens, which are generally screened as non-lactose fermenters; but lactose fermentation can be introduced into dysentery bacilli from *E. coli* by conjugation or transduction (Luria & Burrous, 1957; Luria *et al.*, 1960). Also, *S. flexneri* strains of various serotypes can give rise to new serotypes by hybridization with *E. coli* (Luria & Burrous, 1957). These findings, and others bound to emerge as bacterial genetics develops, ought to receive careful consideration in the continuous process of revision and improvement of bacterial classification.

REFERENCES

Amati, P.   1962.   Abortive infection of *Pseudomonas aeruginosa* and *Serratia marcescens* with coliphage P1. J. Bacteriol. *83*: 433–434.

Arber, W., G. Kellenberger, and J. Weigle.   1957.   La defectuosité du phage lambda transducteur. Schweiz. Z. allg. Path. Bakt. *20*: 659–665.

Baron, L. S., W. F. Carey, and W. M. Spilman.   1959.   Genetic recombination between *Escherichia coli* and *Salmonella typhimurium*. Proc. Nat. Acad. Sci. (U.S.) *45*: 976–984.

Belozersky, A. N., and A. S. Spirin.   1958.   A correlation between the compositions of deoxyribonucleic and ribonucleic acids. Nature *182*: 111–112.

Benzer, S., and S. P. Champe.   1961.   Ambivalent mutants of phage T4. Proc. Nat. Acad. Sci. (U.S.) *47*: 1025–1038.

Bertani, G.   1958.   Lysogeny. Adv. in Virus Research *5*: 151–193.

Campbell, A.   1962.   Episomes. Adv. in Genetics *11*: 101–145.

Catlin, B. W., and L. S. Cunningham.   1961.   Transforming activities and base contents of deoxyribonucleate preparations from various *Neisseriae*. J. Gen. Microbiol. *26*: 303–312.

Falkow, S., J. Marmur, W. F. Carey, W. M. Spilman, and L. S. Baron.   1961.   Episomic transfer between *Salmonella typhosa* and *Serratia marcescens*. Genetics *46*: 703–706.

Franklin, N. C., and S. E. Luria.   1961.   Transduction by bacteriophage P1 and the properties of the *lac* genetic region in *E. coli* and *S. dysenteriae*. Virology *15*: 299–311.

Fredericq, P.   1957.   Colicins. Ann. Rev. Microbiol. *11*: 7–22.

Hartman, P. E., and S. H. Goodgal.   1959.   Bacterial genetics (with particular reference to genetic transfer). Ann. Rev. Microbiol. *13*: 465–504.

Hirota, Y.   1960.   The effect of acridine dyes on mating type factors in *Escherichia coli*. Proc. Nat. Acad. Sci. (U.S.) *46*: 57–64.

Holloway, B. W., and P. A. Jennings.   1958.   An infectious fertility factor for *Pseudomonas aeruginosa*. Nature *181*: 855–856.

Iseki, S., and T. Sakai. 1953. Artificial transformation of O antigens in *Salmonella-E.* group. II. Antigen-transforming factor in bacilli of subgroup E_2. Proc. Japan Acad. *29*: 127–131.

Jacob, F. 1961. Discussion of paper by Signer *et al.* (1961).

Jacob, F., and E. A. Adelberg. 1959. Transfert de caractères génétiques par incorporation au facteur sexuel d'*Escherichia coli.* Compt. rend. *249*: 189–191.

Jacob, F., P. Schaeffer, and E. L. Wollman. 1960. Episomic elements in bacteria. Symp. Soc. Gen. Microbiol. *10*: 67–91.

Jacob, F., and E. L. Wollman. 1961. Sexuality and the genetics of bacteria. Academic Press, New York.

Kühn, A. 1961. Grundriss der Vererbungslehre. 2nd., p. 112. Fisher.

Lanni, F. 1960. Genetic significance of microbial DNA composition. Perspectives in Biol. and Med. *3*: 418–432.

Lederberg, J. 1955. Recombination mechanisms in bacteria. J. Cell. Comp. Physiol. *45*, suppl. 2: 75–107.

Lederberg, J., and P. R. Edwards. 1953. Serotypic recombination in *Salmonella.* J. Immunol. *71*: 232–240.

Lee, K. Y., R. Wahl, and E. Barbu. 1956. Contenu en bases puriques et pyrimidiques des acides désoxyribonucléiques des bactéries. Ann. Inst. Pasteur *91*: 212–224.

Levinthal, C., E. R. Signer, and K. Fetherolf. 1962. Reactivation and hybridization of reduced alkaline phosphatase. Proc. Nat. Acad. Sci. (U.S.) *48*: 1230–1237.

Li, K., L. Barksdale, and L. Garmise. 1961. Phenotypic alterations associated with the bacteriophage carrier state of *Shigella dysenteriae.* J. Gen. Microbiol. *24*: 355–367.

Loeb, T., and N. D. Zinder. 1961. A bacteriophage containing RNA. Proc. Nat. Acad. Sci. (U.S.) *47*: 282–288.

Luria, S. E. 1959. Genetic transfers by viruses. *In* Brookhaven Symp. in Biol., No. 12, Structure and function of genetic elements, pp. 95–102.

Luria, S. E., J. N. Adams, and R. C. Ting. 1960. Transduction of lactose-utilizing ability among strains of *E. coli* and *S. dysenteriae* and the properties of the transducing phage particles. Virology *12*: 348–390.

Luria, S. E., and J. W. Burrous. 1957. Hybridization between *Escherichia coli* and *Shigella.* J. Bacteriol. *74*: 461–476.

Lwoff, A. 1953. Lysogeny. Bacteriol. Rev. *17*: 269.

Marmur, J., and P. Doty. 1959. Heterogeneity in desoxyribonucleic acids. I. Dependence on composition of the configurational stability of desoxyribonucleic acids. Nature *183*: 1427–1429.

Marmur, J., and D. Lane. 1960. Strand separation and specific recombination in deoxyribonucleic acids: Biological studies. Proc. Nat. Acad. Sci. (U.S.) *46*: 453–461.

Marmur, J., R. Rownd, S. Falkow, L. S. Baron, C. Schildkraut, and P. Doty. 1961. The nature of intergeneric episomal infection. Proc. Nat. Acad. Sci. (U.S.) *47*: 972–979.

Marmur, J., C. L. Schildkraut, and P. Doty. 1961. The reversible denaturation of DNA and its use in studies of nucleic acid homologies and the biological relationships of microorganisms. J. Chim. Phys., 1961: 945–955.

Marmur, J., E. Seaman, and J. Levine. 1963. Interspecific transformation in *Bacillus.* J. Bacteriol. *85*: 461–467.

Meselson, M., F. Stahl, and J. Vinograd. 1957. Equilibrium sedimentation of macromolecules in density gradients. Proc. Nat. Acad. Sci. (U.S.) *43*: 581–588.

Meynell, G. G. 1962. *Salmonella enteritidis* as a genetic donor in intraspecific and interspecific crosses initiated by colicine factors. J. Gen. Microbiol. *28*: 169–176.

Miyake, T., and M. Demerec. 1959. *Salmonella-Escherichia* hybrids. Nature *183*: 1586.

Ozeki, H., and S. Howarth. 1961. Colicine factors as fertility factors in bacteria. Nature *190*: 986–987.

Ravin, A. W. 1961. The genetics of transformation. *In* Advances in Genetics, ed. E. W. Caspari and J. M. Thoday, *10*: 61–163. Academic Press.

Rolfe, R., and M. Meselson. 1959. The relative homogeneity of microbial DNA. Proc. Nat. Acad. Sci. (U.S.) *45*: 1039–1043.

Sarkar, S., and S. E. Luria. 1963. Regulation of biosynthesis of a heat sensitive β-d-galactosidase in *Shigella dysenteriae*. Biochim. Biophys. Acta *68*: 506–508.

Schaeffer, P. 1958. La notion d'espèce après les recherches récentes de génétique bactérienne. Ann. Inst. Pasteur *94*: 167–178.

Schaeffer, P. 1961. Les réactions hétérospécifiques de la transformation bactérienne. Thesis, Univ. of Paris, Faculty of Sciences.

Schildkraut, C. L., J. Marmur, and P. Doty. 1961. The formation of hybrid DNA molecules and their use in studies of DNA homologies. J. Mol. Biol. *3*: 595–617.

Signer, E. R., A. Torriani, and C. Levinthal. 1961. Gene expression in intergeneric merozygotes. Cold Spring Harbor Symp. Quant. Biol. *26*: 31–34.

Spirin, A. S., and A. N. Belozersky. 1956. Composition of nucleic acids in experimental mutability of bacteria of the coli group [trans. title]. Biochimia *21*: 768–775.

Sueoka, N. 1961. Variation and heterogeneity of base composition of deoxyribonucleic acids: A compilation of old and new data. J. Mol. Biol. *3*: 31–40.

Sueoka, N. 1962. On the genetic basis of variation and heterogeneity of DNA base composition. Proc. Nat. Acad. Sci. (U.S.) *48*: 582–592.

Sueoka, N., J. Marmur, and P. Doty. 1959. Heterogeneity in deoxyribonucleic acids. II Nature *183*: 1429–1431.

Uetake, H., S. E. Luria, and J. W. Burrous. 1958. Conversion of somatic antigens in *Salmonella* by phage infection leading to lysis or lysogeny. Virology *5*: 68–91.

Watanabe, T., and T. Fukasawa. 1961. Episome mediated transfer of drug resistance in *Enterobacteriaceae*. J. Bacteriol. *81*: 669–683.

Yanofsky, C., D. R. Helinski, and B. D. Maling. 1961. The effects of mutation on the composition and properties of the A protein of *Escherichia coli* tryptophan synthetase. Cold Spring Harbor Symp. Quant. Biol. *26*: 11–24.

Zinder, N. D. 1953. Infective heredity in bacteria. Cold Spring Harbor Symp. Quant. Biol. *18*: 261–269.

Zinder, N. D. 1960. Hybrids of *Escherichia* and *Salmonella*. Science *131*: 813–815.

CAN TRANSFORMATION BE USED AS A CRITERION IN TAXONOMY OF BACTERIA?

ROMAN PAKULA

Department of Bacteriology
State Institute of Hygiene
Warsaw, Poland

BACTERIA are asexually reproducing organisms and genetic criteria have so far played no direct role in their classification. However, development of bacterial genetics in the post-war period brought to light evidence in favor of exchange of genetic material between bacteria and of recombination of this material with the genome of the recipient cell. This makes it possible to verify, at least in some instances, how well genetic criteria of relationship accord with the current classification of bacteria.

Three routes of transfer of genetic material are known; these are conjugation, transduction and transformation.

By means of conjugation, genetic elements can be transmitted beyond the boundaries of groups recognized as species. A number of *Shigella* strains and also some strains of various *Salmonella* are fertile as recipients in mixed cultures with *E. coli* F+ strains (Luria & Burrous, 1957; Baron, Spilman & Carey, 1959). As a result of these conjugations, hybrids occur which combine characters typical of the donor with characters typical of the recipient.

Transfer of multiple drug resistance of *E. coli* to all genera of *Enterobacteriaceae* was reported by Japanese workers (Harada *et al.*, 1960; Mitsuhashi *et al.*, 1960). The resistance to three or four drugs of *Shigella, Salmonella* and *Citrobacter*, which was infected from *E. coli*, is transmitted reversibly to drug-sensitive *E. coli*.

The specificity of bacteriophages in infecting bacterial hosts limits the possibility of exchange of genetic information between different species by means of transformation. Some bacteriophages of broad host range are, however, known and these are capable of effecting transduction between species and even genera (Lederberg & Edwards, 1953; Lennox, 1955).

Interspecific transformation reactions between various species or types have been investigated within four genera of bacteria: *Hemophilus, Neisseria, Bacillus* and *Streptococcus*. In most of these investigations streptomycin-resistance was the only genetic marker used.

Detailed studies on interspecific transformations within the genus of *Hemophilus* were carried out by Schaeffer (1956, 1958) and by Leidy, Hahn and Alexander (1956, 1959). Schaeffer (1958) found that the frequency of intraspecific transformation, with *H. influenzae* as recipient, is of the order of 3×10^{-3} cells. The frequencies of interspecific transformations with DNA's from *H. parainfluenzae* and *H. suis* are, however, only 1×10^{-5} and 3×10^{-7} respectively.

Similar quantitative results of heterologous transformations between *H. influenzae* and *H. parainfluenzae* were reported by Leidy *et al.* (1959). As in the experiments of Schaeffer, the numbers of cells transformed by heterologous DNA were only a small fraction of those transformed by homologous DNA. However, in a recipient population of *H. influenzae* or of *H. aegyptius*, the number of cells transformed by either *H. influenzae* or *H. aegyptius* DNA is of the same order of magnitude.

A suggestion was made by the foregoing workers that in a given population of *Hemophilus* the ratio of the number of transformants induced by heterologous DNA to the number transformed by homologous DNA might be a numerical index of relationship.

Catlin and Cunningham (1961) investigated reciprocal transformations between various strains of *Neisseria*, characterized in Bergey's *Manual* (1957) as separate species. Transformations to streptomycin-resistance were carried out with representatives of the following seven species: *N. meningitidis*, *N. flava*, *N. perflava*, *N. subflava*, *N. flavescens*, *N. sicca* and *N. catarrhalis*. Representatives of all seven species were transformed by homologous DNA preparations extracted from strains of corresponding species. With the exception of *N. catarrhalis*, interspecific transformations were produced for all possible combinations of recipient cells and transforming DNA's, derived from strains of the six remaining species. Ratios of heterologous to homologous transformations were 0,01 or higher. *N. catarrhalis* cells, which exhibited high frequency of intraspecific transformation, could not be transformed by any DNA of the six other heterologous species. DNA of *N. catarrhalis* exhibited no transforming activity for recipient cells of the other *Neisseria* species.

The bases adenine, thymine, guanine and cytosine were present in about equal proportions in DNA preparations of the six *Neisseria* species. In DNA of *N. catarrhalis*, adenine and thymine predominated. The ratio of adenine + thymine to cytosine + guanine was 1.4 for DNA of *N. catarrhalis* but only about 1.0 for the other DNA's.

Marmur, Seaman and Levine (1961) reported recently interspecific transformations within the genus *Bacillus*. The following genetic markers were used: indol$^-$→indol$^+$, argine$^-$→arginine$^+$ and erythromycin-resistance. Of twenty-two DNA preparations, extracted from twenty-two different strains, designed as separate species or variants of *B. subtilis*, only four were active in heterologous transformation with *B. subtilis* as recipient. These are DNA preparations of *B. subtilis* var. *aterrimus*, *B. substilis* var. *niger*, *B. natto* and *B. polymyxa*.

The auxotrophic mutant of *B. subtilis* was transformed to the wild type by DNA's of *B. natto* and of *B. subtilis* var. *aterrimus* at a higher frequency than by homologous DNA. The frequency of the heterologous transformations, induced by DNA's of the remaining donors, were 10^3–10^4 times lower than the homologous transformation of B. subtilis.

The content of guanine+cytosine in DNA preparations of Bacillus species, effective in heterologous transformations with B. subtilis cells as recipients, varied between 42.5 — 44.0 per cent, as compared to 43 per cent in DNA of B. subtilis. However, DNA preparations of two other species, with a guanine + cytosine content of 42.5 and 43.5 per cent, were not active in interspecific transformations.

In 1957, Bracco, Krauss, Roe and MacLeod reported reciprocal transformations to streptomycin-resistance between a pneumococcus and two strains of viridans streptococci.

The frequency of the homologous transformation of one of the streptococcal strains, indicated as a percentage of the total recipient population, was 1.0 but only 0.04 for the intraspecific transformation of the pneumococcus. In the pneumococcal recipient population, the efficiency of homologous transformation was at least 10^3 higher than that of the heterologous one, induced by streptococcal DNA. One per cent of transformants were, however, produced in the streptococcal recipient population with either homologous or pneumococcal DNA. Bracco et al. conclude, therefore, that efficiency of transformation does not necessarily reflect the degree of relationship.

The technique used by the above workers seems to be inadequate for measuring efficiencies of transformation since the recipient populations were exposed to DNA for a period of eight hours. Under these conditions one is calculating the number not only of transformants but also of their progeny.

Heterospecific transformations between different species of streptococci, between pneumococci and streptococci and between streptococci and staphylococci were reported by Pakula et al. (1958). Results to be presented are an extention of our previous work. In this study, DNA preparations carrying three markers, namely streptomycin-, cathomycin- and erythromycin-resistance, were used in genetic transformation.

In these experiments, efficiency of heterospecific, as compared to homospecific, transformation is the only possible indication of a relationship between the recipient and donor. Adequate experimental design must, therefore, be applied to eliminate errors and should include: exposure of a recipient population of known competency to different DNA preparations used in the same, preferably saturating concentration, short time duration of exposure, use of a proper time period for phenotypic expression, and, finally, assay of the number of transformants in a medium containing a suitable concentration of the selective agent when drug resistance is used as genetic marker. In addition, the use of different DNA preparations, extracted from the same donor, may also result in fluctuations which should be considered. Our experiments were carried out with all these in mind.

We used as recipients: the R36A pneumococcus strain, a group H hemo-

TABLE 1

TRANSFORMATIONS OF (A) STREPTOCOCCUS STRAIN CHALLIS; (B) *Streptococcus sanguis*; (C) *D. pneumoniae*, STRAIN R36A, TO STREPTOMYCIN-, CATHOMYCIN- AND ERYTHROMYCIN-RESISTANCE

(The homospecific transformation is assigned a value of 100 per cent.)

Donors	Markers					
	Sm-resistance		Cath-resistance		Ery-resistance	
A.						
Group H hem. streptococcus, Challis*	100%		100%		100%	
S. sanguis, type I/II	100	(70–120)	95	(70–130)	110	(80–125)
S. mitis, Br	4.8	(3.0–7.5)	1.3	(1.15–1.45)	0.01	(0.003–0.03)
S. mitis, 158	2.5	(0.5–7.1)	2.3	(1.8–2.9)	0.01	(0.002–0.02)
D. pneumoniae, R36 A	2.9	(0.7–6.4)	0		0.01	(0.002–0.02)
S. pyogenes, G III	0.5	(0.15–0.85)	0		not tested	
S. salivarius, 167	0.28	(0.25–0.4)	0.1	(0.02–0.2)	1.2	(0.7–1.4)
Group C hem. streptococcus, C_4	0.15	(0.1–0.2)	0.18	(0.12–0.26)	5.5	(4.3–6.3)
S. faecalis, D_3	0.06	(0.03–0.08)	not tested		not tested	
Staph. aureus, St. 70	0.006	(0.002–0.009)	not tested		not tested	
B.						
S. sanguis, type I/II	100%		100%		100%	
Group H hem. streptococcus, Challis*	120	(90–150)	120	(80–130)	1.5	(1.0–2.0)
D. pneumoniae, R36 A	6.4	(0.9–9.6)	0.2	(0.1–0.24)	0.02	(0.01–0.05)
S. mitis, Br	5.8	(1.1–7.9)	2.5	(1.1–5.2)	0.17	(0.14–0.21)
S. mitis, 158	3.8	(1.0–5.9)	4.9	(1.3–11.5)	0.03	(0.01–0.4)
S. pyogenes, G III	0.9	(0.6–1.3)	not tested		not tested	
S. salivarius, 167	0.9	(0.8–1.2)	0.09	(0.01–0.25)	0.9	(0.2–2.2)
Group C hem. streptococcus, C_4	0.4	(0.25–0.5)	0.2	(0.06–0.4)	3.1	(2.7–7.4)
S. faecalis, D_3	0.08	(0.07–0.09)	not tested		not tested	
Staph. aureus, St. 70	0.004	(0.003–0.005)	not tested		not tested	
C.						
D. pneumoniae, R36 A	100%		100%		100%	
S. mitis, Br	6	(1.6–13.2)	0		0.15	(0.12–0.2)
S. mitis, 158	12	(2.8–24.8)	2.9	(1.5–5.0)	0.5	(0.2–1.6)
Group H hem. streptococcus, Challis	6	(1.4–8.6)	0		0	
S. sanguis, type I/II	6	(1.8–10.8)	0		31	(7.5–49)
S. salivarius, 167	0.9	(0.5–1.1)	0		7.3	(2.7–13)
S. pyogenes, G III	0.8	(0.4–1.3)	0		not tested	
Group C hem. streptococcus, C_4	0.44	(0.35–0.5)	0		13.6	(3.6–23)

*This strain is a mutant in regard to Sm- and Cath-resistance but the Ery-resistance marker was introduced by DNA from an Ery-resistant mutant of *S. sanguis*.

lytic streptococcus, designated as Challis, and a type I/II strain of *Streptococcus sanguis*. We used as donors: the three strains mentioned and two strains of *Streptococcus mitis*, one strain of *Streptococcus salivarius*, one group A hemolytic streptococcus, one group C hemolytic streptococcus, one enterococcus strain and one strain of *Staphylococcus aureus*. Transformations were carried out with recipient populations preserved in the deep freeze and prepared for use according to the procedure of Fox and Hotchkiss, recommended for pneumococci (1957).

Results of homo- and of hetero-specific transformations of the two streptococcal strains and of the pneumococcus, used as recipients, are presented in Table 1. Each figure in the tables is the mean of at least three experiments with a given DNA preparation and experiments were carried out with at least two DNA preparations derived from the same donor.

The streptomycin-resistance markers of all donors, including that of the staphylococcus, infect recipient cells of the strain Challis. We failed to introduce into this recipient the cathomycin-resistance character of the pneumococcus and of the group A streptococcus. The strain Challis is transformed to erythromycin-resistance by homologous DNA, derived from a spontaneous mutant, at a very low efficiency of 1–2 per cent of the number of transformants to either streptomycin- or cathomycin-resistance. However, DNA preparations extracted from transformants, infected with the erythromycin-resistance marker of *S. sanguis*, produce numbers of transformants of the same order as those obtained in homospecific transformation to streptomycin- and cathomycin-resistance.

In principle, similar quantitative results were obtained in homo- and heterospecific transformations of the *S. sanguis* strain (Table 1). This strain, in contrast to strain Challis, can be infected with the cathomycin-resistance marker of the pneumococcus.

Table 1 illustrates results of transformations of the pneumococcus recipient with homologous and heterologous DNA. We succeeded in infecting this strain with the streptomycin-resistance character of all donors, with the exception of the enterococcus and staphylococcus.

Cathomycin-resistant transformants were obtained only with homologous DNA and with DNA of the viridans streptococcus 158. Erythromycin-resistance could also be infected from other donors, namely from the *S. sanguis* strain and from the group C streptococcus.

The failure to introduce some characters of heterologous bacteria into the pneumococcus is certainly an indication of lack of microhomology of corresponding sites in DNA of the donor and recipient. However, it should be pointed out that the competence of the pneumococcus used in these transformation experiments was low as compared to the competence of the streptococcal recipients. While the two streptococcal strains were transformed to drug resistance at an efficiency of 3–10 per cent, efficiencies of only 0.2–1.3 per cent of the entire recipient population were obtained in homologous transformations of the pneumococcus. It is likely that low competence of the recipient is a factor limiting the probability of heterospecific transformation.

What conclusions may be drawn from the data represented in the tables? If introduction of one to three markers provides an adequate basis for comparison of genetic relationship, all the recipients and donors are to some extent related. The group H hemolytic streptococcus and the *S. sanguis* type I/II strain behave in reciprocal transformation reactions as one would expect from two strains belonging to the same species. Genetic evidence of relationship is in this case in close agreement with physiological and immunological data reported by Dodd (1949) and by Porterfield (1950). Despite minor differences existing between these two representatives, there seems to be good reason for combining group H streptococci and *S. sanguis* into one group.

The streptomycin- and cathomycin-resistance markers of pneumococci infect one or the other of the streptococcal recipients with higher efficiency than the analogous markers of *S. salivarius* or of group A and C streptococci. The pneumococcus recipient, on the contrary, is transformed to streptomycin- and cathomycin-resistance by DNA of viridans streptococci, *S. salivarius*, *S. sanguis* and of group A and C streptococci. Moreover, in earlier experiments with one viridans streptococcus strain as recipient, it was found that this strain is transformed to streptomycin-resistance by pneumococcal DNA at a higher frequency than by any DNA preparation of four heterologous species or types of streptococci (Pakula, 1961). These data are in agreement with the classification of Topley and Wilson (1955) who did not find justification for separation of pneumococci from streptococci by forming a genus *Diplococcus*.

Enterococci differ from other streptococci with regard to many physiological traits and poor efficiencies of heterospecific transformations of streptococci with DNA of enterococci provide direct genetic evidence that these bacteria are distantly related to other streptococci.

The frequency of transformation of streptococci with staphylococcal DNA was found to be even lower than with DNA of enterococci. This result is in accordance with current taxonomic criteria by which staphylococci and streptococci are classified as belonging to different families.

In general, results of transformation between streptococci, pneumococci and staphylococci supported expectations based on current taxonomic criteria.

Data presented by Marmur *et al.* (1961) and by Catlin and Cunningham (1961) indicate that similarity of over-all base content of DNA seems to be a minimum requirement of genetic compatibility of donors and recipients. Poor efficiencies of heterospecific transformations are due, as suggested by Schaeffer (1958), to incomplete homology of DNA molecules (or their parts) of the donor and recipient, carrying the locus under test. The degree of homology may differ for various loci. This is evident from different frequencies of transformation for individual markers with a given DNA carrying three markers (Table 1; see also Marmur *et al.*, 1961).

Summarizing, one may conclude from all data available that genetic exchange between bacteria is a useful tool in the study of their relationship.

It is a general feeling that criteria of bacterial classification are arbitrary and, in some cases, divergencies between current classification and genetic data may be expected. We therefore find justification in the opinion of Marmur *et al.* (1961) that "the use of interspecific transformation offers an important criterion for taxonomic relatedness and approaches the use of genetic compatibility in the definition of species for higher plants and animals."

The extent of the phenomenon of transformation is rather limited and so obviously are the possibilities for the use of transformation in bacterial classification. The question may, therefore, be asked what are the perspectives of extension of transformation to hitherto non-transformed bacteria?

Studies carried out in this laboratory on the nature of competence of transformable streptococci revealed that sterile supernatants of competent cultures contain a factor provoking competence. This factor and also its crude concentrates, obtained by precipitation with ammonium sulphate, provoke transformation of cells grown in the absence of either albumin or serum necessary to produce transformation of these bacteria (Pakula *et al*, 1962). A similar factor was found in cultures of pneumococci and it is probably also present in cultures of H. *influenzae* as one may conclude from the studies of Goodgal and Herriott (1961).

The factor in question is heat-sensitive. A loss of about 50 per cent initial activity was found after 10 minutes heating at 65 C. The reversion of non-competent cells into competent ones by addition of this factor is concomitant with an enzymatic reaction. The process is time- and temperature-dependent, with a maximum at 37 C, and is also specific. Supernatants of cultures of strain Challis, acting on homologous bacteria, are unable to provoke or to enhance transformation of closely related cells of S. *sanguis*, but supernatants of S. *sanguis* cultures do not act on cells of the strain Challis. However, crude concentrates of this factor, derived from culture supernatants of strain Challis, are capable of provoking transformation of 2-4 per cent of the cells of the non-transformable strain Wicky, a group H streptococcus. These concentrates result also in a very significant increase of transformability of another group H streptococcus (strain 3437), characterized by low competence.

Even if the hypothetical enzyme, produced by competent bacteria, could be used to provoke transformation of non-transformable bacteria, as one may conclude from the data presented, the phenomenon will probably be limited because of its specificity. In spite of this limitation, some extension of bacterial transformation and also its use in classification may be expected.

REFERENCES

Baron, L. S., W. M. Spilman, and W. F. Carey. 1959. Hybridization of *Salmonella* species by mating with *Escherichia coli*. Science *130*: 566–567.

Bergey's Manual of Determinative Bacteriology. 7th ed. 1957. Williams & Wilkins.

Bracco, R. M., M. R. Krauss, A. S. Roe, and C. M. MacLeod. 1957. Transformation reactions between pneumococcus and two strains of streptococci. J. Exptl. Med. *106*: 247–259.

Catlin, B. W., and L. S. Cunningham. 1961. Transforming activities and base contents of deoxyribonucleate preparations from various *Neisseriae*. J. Gen. Microbiol. *26*: 303–312.

Dodd, R. L. 1949. Serological relationship between *Streptococcus* group H and *Streptococcus sanguis*. Proc. Soc. Exptl. Biol. Med. 70: 598–599.

Fox, M. S., and R. D. Hotchkiss. 1957. Initiation of bacterial transformation, I. Nature *187*: 1002–1003.

Goodgal, S. H., and R. M. Herriott. 1961. Studies on transformation of *Hemophilus influenzae*. I. Competence. J. Gen. Physiol. *44*: 1201–1227.

Harada, K., M. Suzuki, M. Kameda, and R. Egawa. 1960. Japan. J. Exptl. Med. *30*: 301–306.

Lederberg, J., and P. R. Edwards. 1953. Serotypic recombination in *Salmonella*. J. Immunol. *71*: 232–240.

Leidy, G., E. Hahn, and H. E. Alexander. 1956. On the specificity of the desoxyribonucleic acid which induces streptomycin resistance in *Hemophilus*. J. Exptl. Med. *104*: 305–320.

Leidy, G., E. Hahn, and H. E. Alexander. 1959. Interspecific transformation in *Hemophilus*: A possible index of relationship between *H. influenzae* and *H. aegyptius*. Proc. Soc. Exptl. Med. Biol. *102*: 86–88.

Lennox, E. S. 1955. Transduction of linked genetic characters of the bacteriophage P1. Virology *1*: 190–206.

Luria, S. E., and J. W. Burrous. 1957. Hybridization between *Escherichia coli* and *Shigella*. J. Bacteriol. *74*: 461–476.

Marmur, J., E. Seaman, and J. Levine. 1963. Interspecific transformation in *Bacillus*. J. Bacteriol. *85*: 461–467.

Pakula, R., Z. Fluder, E. Hulanicka, and W. Walczak. 1958. Studies on transformation of streptococci. Bull. Acad. Polon. Sci. Classe II, *6*: 319–323.

Pakula, R. E. Hulanicka, and W. Walczak. 1958. Transformation reactions between streptococci, pneumococci and staphylococci. Bull. Acad. Polon. Sci. Classe II, *6*: 325–328.

Pakula, R. 1961. Interspecific transformation as a mean of determining genetic relationship of streptococci. Acta Microb. Polon. *10*: 249–254.

Pakula, R., M. Piechowska, E. Bankowska, and W. Walczak. 1962. A characteristic of DNA mediated transformation system of two streptococcal strains. Acta Microb. Polon. *11*: 205–222.

Porterfield, J. S. 1950. Classification of streptococci of subacute bacterial endocarditis. J. Gen. Microb. *4*: 92–101.

Schaeffer, P. 1956. Transformation interspécifique chez des bactéries du genre *Hemophilus*. Ann. Inst. Pasteur *91*: 323–337.

Schaeffer, P. 1958. Interspecific reactions in bacterial transformations. Symposia Soc. Exptl. Biol. *12*: 60–74.

Topley's and Wilson's Principles of Bacteriology and Immunity. 1955.

THE STATISTICAL APPROACH TO
BACTERIAL TAXONOMY

O. LYSENKO

Department of Insect Pathology
Institute of Entomology CSAV, Prague
Czechoslovakia

THE LAST PAPER of this symposium is dedicated to the statistical approach to bacterial taxonomy. No less interesting, and I think more instructive, would be to speak about the statistical approach to bacterial taxonomists, because taxonomy lives by its practice, a practice which is expressed by microbiologists. Even microbiologists are human and their opinions may be influenced by national, educational and disciplinary traditions, or by their own experience and personal bias. In their opinions people are even more variable than bacteria and the faults we attribute to bacteria perhaps should be redirected to people. Cowan (1956), quoting a colleague, wrote that "bacteria are difficult to classify, because they have not yet heard of the Bergey Manual"; it would, perhaps, be better to note that they have not yet heard of the individuality and different opinions of bacteriologists. There are no statistical records about the techniques used and the opinions expressed by taxonomists; if there were most of our problems might be clearer. Nevertheless, I shall pursue my subject and will try to give an outline of some problems connected with the statistical approach to bacterial taxonomy.

I shall draw attention only to the more general and not yet answered questions and problems, because time is limited and more comprehensive reviews (Sneath, 1961, 1962; Sokal & Sneath, 1963), as well as a part of the Society for General Microbiology Symposium (1962), have been devoted to this topic. I shall not deal with the mathematical side of the subject as that is outside the understanding of most biologists.

Every taxonomist who tries to create a taxonomic scheme uses statistical methods. Determination of the frequency of a character in several strains is a statistic in itself, even though a very simple one. The statistical analysis is made to determine the diagnostic value of the character, or we look for a correlation of characters, i.e., we try to define a taxon. In both cases we sort and sometimes weight the evidence. Whether we realize it or not we are making a statistical assessment.

From the early attempts (e.g., Winslow & Rogers, 1906; Levine, 1918) a working method has developed in zoology (Michener & Sokal, 1957; Cain & Harrison, 1960) or in botany (Rogers & Tanimoto, 1960) and in microbiology (Sneath, 1957). If we may judge by the number of papers published, it has found the greatest use in microbiology; these have dealt with the application of the methods to the taxonomy of larger bacterial groups (Sneath & Cowan, 1958; Brisbane & Rovira, 1961) and to smaller ones, such as actinomycetes (Silvestri *et al.*, 1962), mycobacteria (Cerbòn & Bojalil, 1961; Bojalil *et al.*, 1962), bacilli (Sneath, 1962), micrococci (Hill, 1959; Pohja, 1960), streptococci (Blondeau, 1961), lactobacilli (Cheeseman & Bedridge, 1959), pasteurellae (Talbot & Sneath, 1960), enterobacteria (Lysenko & Sneath, 1959), chromobacteria (Sneath, 1957) and pseudomonads (Shewan *et al.*, 1960; Colwell & Liston, 1961; Rhodes, 1961; Lysenko, 1961). Besides bacteria this method has also been used for the taxonomy of viruses (Andrewes & Sneath, 1958). These papers have been discussed by Sneath (1962). It is noteworthy that even though the different authors have used different material and different modifications of the method, their results are in general agreement, an achievement which shows the practical usefulness of these methods.

Up to now I have dealt with application of statistical methods in the taxonomies of particular bacterial groups. What role can these methods play in solving some of the general taxonomic problems of microbiology, and what are these problems? I shall try to point out some of them.

The view that bacteria form a huge spectrum of slightly different and continuously changing forms (Edwards & Ewing, 1955) is now accepted. But a basic problem remains: how do we determine the centres that form the taxa, for without their definition we cannot make a classification. Further, it is necessary to define the borders and connecting links of these taxa, for without defining the neighbours the definition of the taxon itself is incomplete and subject to change. Even though my comparison is a rough one, I would compare taxonomy with the work of a cartographer who tries to map an area. I believe that our present taxonomy is analogous to a map of Africa in Roman times or perhaps the Middle Ages; in many cases all that is missing is the well-known "Hic sunt leones."

There are groups of bacteria about which we know sufficient to dispense with the statistical approach in our diagnostic practice, but on the other hand we may not know how these groups are linked one to another. We lack general methods for treating, arranging and sorting the information we have. The amount of these details will rapidly increase and we are in danger of being overwhelmed by data. This situation is brought about not only by convention or by lack of standard laboratory methods; it is a question of basic general method. The statistical expression of these relationships, the introduction of standard diagnostic methods, and a general plan of further research could help us. We require the mutual correlation of characters and have reached the conclusion that the taxon should be defined by the sum of its characters as one unit, but frequently we do not know how these characters or their mutual relationships can be expressed simply. This, it seems to me, is only possible by the use of statistics.

The application of these methods creates new problems. One is the definition of the unit character. From the standpoint of numerical taxonomy Sneath (1962) had defined it as ". . . a taxonomic character of two or more states which within the study at hand cannot be further subdivided logically. . . ." But two characters which appear to be distinct may be a cause and a consequence of one and the same phenomenon, or the external expression of the same mechanism or metabolic pathway (e.g., the production of acid from glucose and the Methyl Red test). Here we need to know better and in detail the mechanisms of our diagnostic characteristics. This is important when Adansonian principles are employed; without this knowledge, it would be possible to prefer one character to the other. This requirement to prevent and exclude possible duplication has both practical and theoretical limitations. The micro-organism is not only the sum of particular characters but also a result of their mutual integration. The same is valid for a taxon.

The next problem is how to code and incorporate in our statistical expressions the ecological factor of the natural occurrence of the microbe. The variability of micro-organisms, which is an indivisible part of their way of life, is closely connected with their ecology. On the contrary, the frequency of one or a set of features is a guide to the allocation and definition of our centres (taxa) around which other forms are clustered. An example will make it clearer. If physiological properties are being used, the loss of ability to form acid from dextrose does not mean that the micro-organism should automatically be transferred to another group, just as, even though the comparison may seem absurd, the diabetic does not cease to be a man because his sugar metabolism is changed. The frequency of certain features or their correlation may characterize a taxon; other combinations with a lower frequency may be regarded as anomalous or in another way defined as exceptions. For this purpose, we want to know the ecological distribution of different types of similar bacteria. This ecological aspect should be incorporated in our taxonomy and the statistical methods could take it into account. In the same way the genetic, serological and other similar properties should be taken into consideration in characterizing a bacterium.

The next problem is in the continuity and discontinuity of our taxonomic groups. Here I am going back to the theory of bacteria as a huge spectrum of intergrading forms. To be able to use our system, we want to define certain centres (taxa) in this spectrum; without them, our spectrum will be useless. Statistical methods, especially cluster analysis, can help us to find and define these centres. It still remains a question whether definition is a matter of convention, or whether there are natural rules governing their distribution and relationships. In other words, is this chaos the objective mode of their existence or only the result of our inadequate knowledge?

Most numerical taxonomic analyses in microbiology employ statistical methods that originate from Adamsonian principles. Analogously other principles may be used, for example, the census of the weighted coincidences and noncoincidences of qualitative specific characters (Smirnov, 1960), or the *a priori* discriminative appreciation of characters.

Other similar theoretical assumptions could be given but we should bear in mind that statistics are and will only be methods which produce numerical, graphic or tridimensional expressions, which, in turn, are only expedients to help us to understand the existing relationships better. Statistics are the methodical way by which information can be sorted and evaluated, but this information could be obtained and fully examined subjectively. Statistical methods do not guarantee that the same result is always obtained because the data used may be false.

Although it is not possible to make a direct comparison between the biological and the physical sciences, I have tried to show that statistical methods can be applied to solving some of the problems encountered by the practical bacteriologist. It is true that their use is not new, but on the other hand we should keep in mind that used with computers these methods may be invaluable in treating and sorting an enormous mass of data without which aid the material could not be worked up. Let us not make premature judgments for time will show us to what extent these electronic and other devices will be of help to us.

It is possible to summarize. Statistical methods can be a useful aid for both concrete and theoretical taxonomic work. Their application is not yet fully appreciated, and ecology, genetics and other characters may have to be taken into consideration. The objectivity of the results is dependent on the characters chosen. Standard diagnostic methods and the standard coding of data for use in computer systems will enable statistical methods to come into general use for mapping of the whole system of bacteria. They could give us a wider view of the bacterial kingdom as a unit.

REFERENCES

Andrewes, C. H., and P. H. A. Sneath. 1958. The species concept among viruses. Nature *182*: 12.

Blondeau, H. 1961. Utilisation des ordinateurs électroniques pour l'étude de l'homogénéité de l'espèce *Streptococcus faecalis*: Application à la détermination de l'origine de la contamination des semi-conserves de viande. Maurice Fabre, Lyon.

Bojalil, L. F., J. Cerbón, and A. Trujillo. 1962. Adansonian classification of mycobacteria. J. Gen. Microbial. *28*: 333.

Brisbane, P. G., and A. D. Rovira. 1961. A comparision of methods for classifying rhizosphere bacteria. J. Gen. Microbiol. *26*: 379.

Cain, A. J., and G. A. Harrison. 1960. Phyletic weighting. Proc. Zool. Soc. Lond. *135*: part 1, p. 1.

Cerbón, J., and L. F. Bojalil. 1961. Physiological relationships of rapidly growing mycobacteria: Adansonian classification. J. Gen. Microbiol. *25*: 7.

Cheesemann, G. C., and N. J. Beridge. 1959. The differentiation of bacterial species by paper chromatography. VII. The use of electronic computation for the objective assessment of chromatographic results. J. Appl. Bacteriol. *22*: 307.

Colwell, R. R., and J. Liston. 1961. Taxonomic relationships among the pseudomonads. J. Bacteriol. 82: 1.

Cowan, S. T. 1956. "Ordnung in das Chaos" Migula. Can. J. Microbiol. 2: 212.

Edwards, P. R., and W. H. Ewing. 1955. Identification of *Enterobacteriaceae*. Burgess Publ. Co., Minneapolis, Minn.

Hill, L. R. 1959. The Adansonian classification of staphylococci. J. Gen. Microbiol. 20: 277.

Levine, M. 1918. A statistical classification of the colon-cloacae group. J. Bacteriol. 3: 253.

Lysenko, O. 1961. *Pseudomonas*—an attempt at a general classification. J. Gen. Microbiol. 25: 379.

Lysenko, O., and P. H. A. Sneath. 1959. The use of models in bacterial classification. J. Gen. Microbiol. 20: 284.

Michener, C. D., and R. R. Sokal. 1957. A quantitative approach to a problem in classification. Evolution 11: 130.

Pohja, M. S. 1960. Micrococci in fermented meat products: Classification and description of 171 different strains. Suom. Maataloust. Seur. Julk. no. 96: 1.

Rhodes, M. E. 1961. The characterisation of *Pseudomonas fluorescens* with the aid of an electronic computer. J. Gen. Microbiol. 25: 331.

Rogers, D. J., and T. T. Tanimoto. 1960. A computer program for classifying plants. Science 132: 1115.

Shewan, J. M., G. Hobbs, and W. Hodgkiss. 1960. A determinative scheme for the identification of certain genera of gram-negative bacteria, with special reference to the *Pseudomonadaceae*. J. Appl. Bacteriol. 23: 379.

Silvestri, L., M. Turri, L. R. Hill, and E. Gilardi. 1962. A quantitative approach to the systematics of Actinomycetes based on overall similarity. *In* Microbial classification, 12th Symposium Soc. Gen. Microbiol., pp. 333–360. Cambridge University Press.

Smirnov, E. S. 1960. Taxonomic analysis of a genus (in Russian). Zhur. Obshchei Biol. 21: 89.

Sneath, P. H. A. 1957. The application of computers to taxonomy. J. Gen. Microbiol. 17: 201.

Sneath, P. H. A. 1961. Recent developments in theoretical and quantitative taxonomy. Systematic Zool. 10: 118.

Sneath, P. H. A. 1962. The construction of taxonomic groups. *In* Microbial classification, 12th Symposium Soc. Gen. Microbiol. pp. 289–332. Cambridge University Press.

Sneath, P. H. A., and S. T. Cowan. 1958. An electro-taxonomic survey of bacteria. J. Gen. Microbiol. 19: 551.

Society for General Microbiology. 1962. Microbial classification, 12th Symposium of the Society, ed. G. C. Ainsworth and P. H. A. Sneath, Cambridge University Press. 483 pp.

Sokal, R. R., and P. H. A. Sneath. 1963. The principle of numerical taxonomy (in preparation).

Talbot, J. M., and P. H. A. Sneath. 1960. A taxonomic study of *Pasteurella septica*, especially of strains isolated from human sources. J. Gen. Microbiol. 22: 303.

Winslow, C. E. A., and A. F. Rogers. 1906. A statistical study of generic characters in the Cocceae. J. Infect. Dis. 3: 485.

SYMPOSIUM XIII

INFLUENCE OF THE ENVIRONMENT
ON THE EPIDEMIOLOGY
OF MYCOSES

Chairman: C. W. EMMONS

N. van UDEN

Factors of Host-Yeast Relationship

P. K. C. AUSTWICK

The Ecology of *Aspergillus fumigatus* and the Pathogenic Phycomycetes

ROGER O. EGEBERG

Factors Influencing the Distribution of *Coccidioides immitis* in soil

E. S. McDONOUGH

Studies on the Growth and Survival of *Blastomyces dermatitidis* in Soil

JUAN E. MACKINNON

Ambient Temperature and Some Deep Mycoses

F. MARIAT

Notes Epidémiologiques à Propos des Mycétomes

This symposium was organized by the International Society for Human and Animal Mycology.

CHAIRMAN'S REMARKS

C. W. EMMONS

National Institute of Allergy and Infectious Diseases
National Institutes of Health
Bethesda, Maryland, U.S.A.

THE SYSTEMIC MYCOSES, with very rare exceptions, are not contagious and their infectious agents grow as saprophytes in soil, or organic debris in man's environment. This has long been common knowledge for such fungi as *Aspergillus fumigatus* and some of the Phycomycetes which occasionally cause disease. Recognition of similar environmental relationships for fungi known primarily as pathogens of man came more recently. An environmental source of infection in Valley fever was revealed in 1932 when Stewart and Meyer isolated *Coccidioides immitis* from soil near a building which housed patients with coccidioidomycosis. Ten years later Coccidioides was found again in desert soil and in rodents. The classic studies of Dickson, Gifford and Smith related the epidemiology of coccidioidomycosis to this environmental source of infection.

Interest in this peculiar epidemiologic aspect of systemic mycoses was renewed and stimulated when *Histoplasma capsulatum* was isolated from soil in 1949 on the eastern seaboard of the United States. This was followed by the isolation of *Cryptococcus neoformans* from soil in 1951 and from pigeon manure in 1955. Isolations of *Sporotrichum schenckii*, from water and timbers of gold mines in Africa, and of *Nocardia asteroides, Allescheria boydii*, and the etiologic agents of mycetoma and chromoblastomycosis from soil or wood have now supported epidemiologic evidence that the systemic and subcutaneous mycoses are caused by fungi which are normal components of the extremely complex microflora of soil and the organic debris with which it is contaminated. A few dermatophytes also have been isolated from soil by an old mycological technique known as "baiting" (i.e., supplying a selective medium such as keratin in the case of chytrids and dermatophytes), but the role of contaminated soil in the epidemiology of dermatophytosis is not yet clear.

Ecological studies indicate that some of the pathogenic fungi are sharply delimited in distribution with respect to substratum and space. These observations have stimulated and sustained an interest in the environmental factors which influence the geographic and local distribution of these pathogens. Lack of contagious transmission in systemic mycoses and their dependence upon environmental exposure by inhalation or by traumatic subcutaneous implantation of spores of pathogenic fungi require continued attention to the nature and peculiarities of environmental sources of infection. Interest in this subject and some recent significant advances in our knowledge of the ecology of pathogenic fungi led to our selection of the subject, "Influence of the Environment on the Epidemiology of Mycoses" for this symposium.

FACTORS OF HOST-YEAST RELATIONSHIP[*]

N. VAN UDEN

Department of Microbiology
Botanical Institute
University of Lisbon, Portugal

THE YEASTS which occur in the digestive tract of man and other warm-blooded animals constitute three different ecological groups (di Menna, 1954; van Uden & Carmo-Sousa, 1957; Parle, 1957). Group one is composed of the transients; these are not truly intestinal yeasts; they don't multiply noticeably in the digestive tract and usually occur there only in low numbers; their habitat is outside the animal body. Group two is composed of the facultative saprophytes. These yeast species have their habitat both outside and inside the animal body; they are capable of growing in the digestive tract and building up populations with relatively high densities. Some of these facultative saprophytes, such as *Candida tropicalis* and *C. parapsilosis*, are potential pathogens. Group three is composed of the obligatory saprophytes. Though some of them may survive for some time outside the animal body, their habitat is the digestive tract where they grow and attain under favourable conditions population densities of many millions of cells per gram intestinal contents. Most of them appear to be harmless; *Saccharomycopsis guttulata*, *Torulopsis pintolopesii* and *C. slooffii* are examples. Others, such as *C. albicans* and *T. glabrata*, are potential pathogens (Table 1).

TABLE 1
INTESTINAL YEASTS OF MAN AND WARM-BLOODED ANIMALS

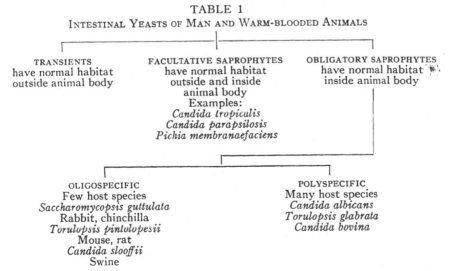

TRANSIENTS	FACULTATIVE SAPROPHYTES	OBLIGATORY SAPROPHYTES
have normal habitat outside animal body	have normal habitat outside and inside animal body Examples: *Candida tropicalis* *Candida parapsilosis* *Pichia membranaefaciens*	have normal habitat inside animal body

OLIGOSPECIFIC	POLYSPECIFIC
Few host species *Saccharomycopsis guttulata* Rabbit, chinchilla *Torulopsis pintolopesii* Mouse, rat *Candida slooffii* Swine	Many host species *Candida albicans* *Torulopsis glabrata* *Candida bovina*

[*]This work was subsidized by the Calouste Gulbenkian Foundation, Lisbon, Portugal.

The obligatory saprophytes may be subdivided on the basis of their host specificity into oligospecific and polyspecific species. The polyspecific yeast species are those that occur as obligatory saprophytes in a wide range of hosts. *T. glabrata* and *C. albicans* belong to this subgroup. *T. glabrata*, for example, may be found in such divergent host species as baboons and crows, men and sea gulls, swine and cattle. The oligospecific yeasts on the other hand are adapted only to closely related host species. Examples are *S. guttulata* adapted to rabbits and chinchillas, *T. pintolopesii* adapted to mice and a few other small rodents and *C. slooffii* adapted to wild and domestic pigs.

Can the saprophytes of the digestive tract be distinguished from other yeast species by their known physiological properties? The answer is yes for the oligospecific obligatory saprophytes. This group of yeasts is highly specialized for life in warm-blooded hosts, has lost the capacity for growth at room temperature and displays a pronounced dependency on external growth factors. All other saprophytes, however, including the polyspecific obligatory saprophytes, such as *C. albicans* and the facultative saprophytes such as *C. tropicalis*, grow well at room temperature and are no more dependent on external growth factors than many yeast species that have their habitat outside the animal body.

However, we have found a correlation of physiological properties that seems to be characteristic for all saprophytic yeasts of the warm-blooded host's digestive tract. Castelo Branco and I (unpublished results) determined the maximum temperature that allowed growth for all the described species of the genus *Candida* and the genus *Torulopsis*. Belo Correia and I (unpublished results) then determined in the same species the minimum pH at which growth still occurs. A number of isolates were tested in each species. We found that in the great majority of *Candida* and *Torulopsis* species the maximum temperature and the minimum pH are fixed within a narrow range. Usually the variation in the maximum temperature from isolate to isolate of the same species does not exceed 3 C, and the variation in the minimum pH rarely goes beyond 0.2.

From species to species, however, considerable differences were found. *T. nodaensis* and *T. halophilus*, for example, only grow at pH values higher than 3.6. *C. slooffii* and *T. pintolopesii*, on the other hand, grow at a pH as low as 1.1. All *Candida* and *Torulopsis* species which are obligatory or facultative saprophytes of the digestive tract grow at pH values lower than 2.3. But many other species also have a low minimum pH; *T. bacillaris* with a minimum pH of 1.5 and *C. parapsilosis* var. *intermedia* with a minimum pH of 1.8 are examples.

Also, the maximum temperature differs from species to species. *C. marina* and *T. norvegica*, for example, do not grow above 31 C. All *Candida* and *Torulopsis* species that are saprophytes of the digestive tract, on the other hand, grow above 40 C. But many other species, such as *C. silvicola* and *C. rugosa*, have their maximum temperature above 40 C.

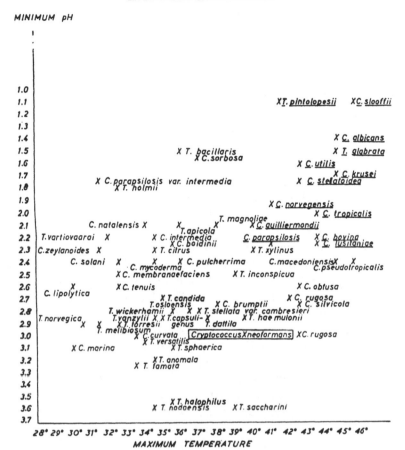

FIG. 1. Correlation between high maximum temperature for growth and low minimum pH for growth found in yeast species (underlined) that occur as saprophytes in the digestive tract of warm-blooded animals.

When the maximum temperature for growth of the *Candida* and *Torulopsis* species is plotted against the minimum pH for growth, it is seen (Fig. 1) that many species, including the saprophytes of the digestive tract, can grow above 40 C and at pH values below 2.3. The simultaneous occurrence of both properties, however, was found exclusively in those *Candida* and *Torulopsis* species which are saprophytes of the digestive tract of warm-blooded animals, including the oligospecific obligatory saprophytes *T. pintolopesii* and *C. slooffii*, the polyspecific obligatory saprophytes *C. albicans*, *C. bovina* and *T. glabrata*, and the facultative saprophytes *C. tropicalis*, *C. krusei*, *C. parapsilosis*, *C. lusitaniae*, *C. utilis*, *C. norvegensis* and *C. guilliermondii*. *C. stellatoidea*, which apparently is an obligatory saprophyte of the human vagina, is also found in this same group.

It appears from these results that, at least in the genera *Candida* and *Torulopsis*, there is a strict correlation between habitat in the digestive tract, high maximum temperature and low minimum pH. That yeasts which live in association with warm-blooded animals have a maximum temperature a few degrees above the body temperature of the host is not surprising. The meaning of the low minimum pH, however, is less evident. There is some evidence, provided by other workers, that capacity for growth in the stomach is important in the maintenance of the cycle of certain species. Shifrine and Phaff (1958) studied the obligatory saprophyte of the rabbit, *Saccharomycopsis guttulata*, and found that both the budding of the vegetative cells and the germination of the ascopores of this yeast occur mainly in the contents of the stomach. A still more intimate relationship with the stomach was found by Mackinnon (1959) for *T. pintolopesii*. Mackinnon observed this yeast regularly in the stomach of mice, not simply in the contents of the stomach but on the surface of the epithelium of the glandular part and in the lumen of the tubular glands. Also, Rolle and Mehnert (1957) observed the occurrence of yeasts in the stomachs of a number of host species.

The very low minimum pH of 1.1 we found for *T. pintolopesii* agrees well with Mackinnon's observations. *C. slooffii* has the same extremely low minimum pH and it would therefore not be surprising if this saprophyte of the swine's digestive tract were also found in intimate connection with the glands of its host's stomach.

Since we found that all yeast saprophytes of warm-blooded hosts are capable of growth at low pH values, varying from 1.1 to 2.3, the general question should be raised whether this reflects capacity for growth in the more or less acid parts of the stomach and its contents and whether such capacity might be an essential attribute of yeasts which habitually live in the digestive tract. *Cryptococcus neoformans*, which is pathogenic but does not occur in the digestive tract of warm-blooded animals as a saprophyte, has a minimum pH as high as 2.8–3. This suggests that a low minimum pH for growth is not a necessary attribute of yeasts capable of tissue invasion but rather of yeasts which have a saprophytic habitat in the digestive tract.

Besides the physiological properties of the yeasts, other factors are of importance in host-yeast relationships. Among them are factors inherent to the host species. With regard to yeasts, mammals and birds may be divided into two main groups (Table 2). Group one is composed of the species which are not suitable as hosts; their digestive tracts harbour either no yeast at all or only transients. Examples are the hippopotamus, the Californian sea lion, and species of bats and of insectivorous birds. Group two is composed of the warm-blooded species which are suitable as hosts for yeasts. These species harbour obligatory saprophytes and transients as well. Within this group several subgroups may be distinguished. In many species only a relatively small proportion of the individuals harbour their saprophytes. Man, fowl and the sparrow, for example, characteristically harbour *Candida albicans*, but with an incidence that usually does not surpass 35 per cent of the individuals and may be as low as 5 per cent. Other host species show a somewhat higher incidence. About 50 per cent of domestic pigs, for

TABLE 2
WARM-BLOODED ANIMALS AS HOSTS FOR INTESTINAL YEASTS

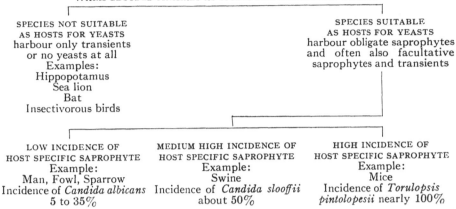

SPECIES NOT SUITABLE AS HOSTS FOR YEASTS harbour only transients or no yeasts at all Examples: Hippopotamus Sea lion Bat Insectivorous birds		SPECIES SUITABLE AS HOSTS FOR YEASTS harbour obligate saprophytes and often also facultative saprophytes and transients
LOW INCIDENCE OF HOST SPECIFIC SAPROPHYTE Example: Man, Fowl, Sparrow Incidence of *Candida albicans* 5 to 35%	MEDIUM HIGH INCIDENCE OF HOST SPECIFIC SAPROPHYTE Example: Swine Incidence of *Candida slooffii* about 50%	HIGH INCIDENCE OF HOST SPECIFIC SAPROPHYTE Example: Mice Incidence of *Torulopsis pintolopesii* nearly 100%

example, harbour *C. slooffii*. Still other species have an extremely high incidence of their characteristic saprophyte; nearly 100 per cent of the world's rabbits harbour *Saccharomycopsis guttulata*, and the incidence of *Torulopsis pintolopesii* in mice and rats is equally high (Mackinnon, 1959). Parenthetically it should be noted that in mice and rats *Candida bovina*, which is closely related to *T. pintolopesii*, is sometimes found.

Two general questions may be raised: (1) Why are certain warm-blooded species suitable as hosts for yeasts whereas others are not? and (2) Why do certain individuals of a suitable host species harbour a characteristic saprophyte, whereas other individuals of the same species do not? In work already reported we had obtained evidence that animals that feed mainly on cellulosic material, such as hippopotami, sheep and goats, are less suitable as hosts for yeasts than species which have a high intake of food rich in starch and simple carbohydrates, such as man, baboons and swine (van Uden, 1960). It had also been found that in a suitable host species like the domestic pig, animals that had been held on a diet rich in starch harboured *C. slooffii* more frequently, and in higher numbers, than animals that had been fed a diet rich in proteins or in cellulose (van Uden & Carmo-Sousa, 1962).

We have continued the study of the possible influence of diet composition on host suitability along two lines: (1) quantitative and qualitative yeast surveys of free living mammals and birds with various types of natural diets; (2) feeding experiments with mice.

Cormorants and Californian sea lions are fish eaters. No yeasts were found in the intestinal content of eight specimens of each species caught off the coast of Baja California, Mexico (van Uden & Castelo Branco, unpublished results).

Around Lisbon, Portugal, we caught a number of insect-eating mammals and birds including 18 bats, 14 barn swallows, 7 swifts, 8 pied flycatchers, 1 reed warbler and 8 melodious warblers. *Hanseniaspora valbyensis* was isolated from two melodious warblers and one reed warbler in numbers ranging from 15,000 to 150,000 viable cells per gram of wet intestinal contents. *H. valbyensis* is not known as a saprophyte of the digestive tract, though it appears occasionally, like so many other yeast species, as a transient. For the time being the significance of its occurrence in rather high numbers in the three insectivorous birds is not known. All the other insectivorous birds as well as the bats were negative for yeasts (van Uden & Vidal Leiria, unpublished results). So, from a total of 72 free-living mammals and birds, belonging to 8 fish- or insect-eating species, no yeasts known as saprophytes of the digestive tract were isolated. I think that these results constitute further evidence that diets rich in proteins and poor in carbohydrates are unfavourable to the establishment of an intestinal yeast flora. Parle's (1957) findings on the absence of yeasts in the digestive tract of the cat points in the same direction.

Results with omnivorous and grain-eating birds were illuminating in this respect.

The intestinal yeast flora of 28 specimens of the African pied crow, an omnivorous scavenger, shot in North Mozambique, was studied (Carmo-Sousa & van Uden, unpublished results). A total of 42 isolates was obtained, belonging to 8 species as follows: *Candida albicans* 5; *Torulopsis glabrata* 1; *C. krusei* 16; *C. tropicalis* 8; *C. lusitaniae* 4; *C. guilliermondii* 2; *Trichosporon cutaneum* 5; and *Saccharomyces cerevisiae* 1. All 8 species are known as saprophytes of the digestive tract: the first two are obligate, the others facultative. The pied crow being a scavenger, its diet differs from that of fish- and meat-eating birds by the additional intake of food rich in starch and simple carbohydrates and I suppose that its intestinal yeast flora is, at least in part, a consequence of a stimulating influence of carbohydrate rich food on intestinal yeast growth. It might be argued, however, that the yeasts isolated from the pied crows were in this case only transients which had been ingested with the highly polluted food which these birds don't refuse. It is reasonable to suppose that transients are usually present only in low numbers whereas saprophytes multiply in the digestive tract and attain high population densities. Similar reservations apply to the interesting findings of Saëz (1959). This author, by the use of a quantitative technique, isolated *C. albicans* and other yeasts from the faeces of captive specimens of warm-blooded species, which feed on a diet low in starch and simple carbohydrates, including the insectivorous species *Myrmecophaga jubata* (Great anteater) and the fish-eating species *Lutra lutra* (common otter), *Lutra cinerea* (clawless otter) and *Aptenodybes patagonica* (King penguin). However, *C. albicans* and other saprophytes of the digestive tract of certain warm-blooded species may occur as transients in other warm-blooded species. One way to distinguish between the two modalities is a comparison of the respective yeast population densities by the use of a quantitative technique.

Such a quantitative study was undertaken with another scavenger species, the Western sea gull (*Larus occidentalis*), of which fourteen specimens were shot off the coast of Baja California, Mexico (van Uden & Castelo-Branco, unpublished results). Five gulls were negative for yeasts, another had low numbers of a species of *Prototheca*, an achloric yeastlike alga; *C. tropicalis* was isolated from 3 birds and *C. krusei* from two. In 6 gulls, that is about 45 per cent of the total, the obligate saprophyte *Torulopsis glabrata* was isolated in numbers ranging from 25,000 to 344,000 per gram of intestinal contents, average 100,000. So the Western gull, and possibly other gull species, is a host for the obligatory saprophyte *Torulopsis glabrata* which has only twice been isolated from sources outside the animal body. Phaff, Mrak and Williams (1952) obtained this yeast from the surface of shrimp in the Gulf of Mexico, and Bhat and Kachwalla (1955) isolated it from the Indian Ocean. Possibly in both cases the samples had recently been polluted by gulls. So, while the cormorant, which eats only fish, had been found yeast-free, the Western gull, which will take, besides fish, anything edible including fruit, bread and other carbohydrate rich food, was found to harbour typically intestinal yeasts in rather high numbers.

That food rich in starch may have something to do with a warm-blooded host's suitability for harbouring yeasts was further confirmed in a study of grain-eating birds. Buckley and van Uden (unpublished results) found that the common sparrow (*Passer domesticus*), probably the most cosmopolitan of all wild birds, is a natural host for *Candida albicans*. Of 37 sparrows caught around Lisbon, 11 harboured *C. albicans*, an incidence of about 30 per cent, and quite similar to the incidence of this yeast in many groups of man and fowl. The number per gram of wet faeces varied; 3 sparrows contained 170–530, 1 contained 26,000 but 7 contained 1 to 14 million per gram.

With Abranches and Vidal Leiria (unpublished results) I have obtained some experimental evidence of the influence of diet on intestinal yeast populations. Mice are well suited for such work because their faeces contain large numbers of yeasts and the incidence is practically 100 per cent. The predominant species is *T. pintolopesii*. We used two diets, one rich in starch, the other rich in protein. Both contained a complete vitamin mixture, 4 per cent of salt mixture U.S.P. no. 2, 2 per cent brewers yeast U.S.P. and 8 per cent olive oil. The starch-rich diet contained 68 per cent starch and 18 per cent casein, the protein-rich diet 64 per cent casein and 22 per cent starch. The results I can present now are only preliminary and incomplete. In one experiment 17 mice were fed for two weeks on the high starch diet, after which time their faeces contained an average of 10,000,000 viable yeast cells per gram. The mice were then fed the high protein diet for two weeks. The yeast count fell to an average of only 330,000 yeast cells per gram faeces. They were again put on the high starch diet and after two weeks the average count had climbed to 8,000,000 cells per gram faeces. What probably happens is the following. The stomach of the mouse constitutes a permanent reservoir of *T. pintolopesii*. Small numbers of the yeast regularly enter the small intestine and are transported rapidly to the caecum where a much slower transport towards the anus is initiated. The only carbon source that allows vigorous growth of *T. pintolopesii* is glucose. When the diet of the mouse is rich in starch, correspondingly large amounts of glucose are formed in the small intestine and sufficient amounts are carried over to the large intestine to allow vigorous growth of the yeast. When, on the other hand, the diet is poor in starch, the level of glucose in the large intestine remains low and yeast growth is limited.

These experimental results seem to confirm our field observations. Species of mammals and birds that naturally live on a diet poor in starch and simple carbohydrates, including fish-eating, insectivorous and grass-eating species, are unsuitable as hosts for intestinal yeasts. Warm-blooded species that feed on a diet rich in starch and/or simple carbohydrates, including omnivorous and grain-eating species, are suitable hosts for such yeasts. In the omnivorous species such as mice and swine the population density and/or the incidence of intestinal yeasts responds to the proportion of starch in the diet. It should be kept in mind, however, that composition of the diet of the host is only one of several factors which govern host-yeast relationship.

SUMMARY

All *Candida* and *Torulopsis* species, which occur in the digestive tract of warm-blooded animals as obligatory or facultative saprophytes, can grow above 40 C and at pH values below 2.3. Though many other *Candida* and *Torulopsis* species are capable of growth at similar values of temperature or pH, none has both properties simultaneously. The dual capacity for growth (1) at the body temperature of the host and (2) in its stomach, is certainly characteristic for some and possibly for all saprophytic yeasts of the digestive tract.

Fish-eating and insectivorous species of mammals and birds are apparently not suitable as hosts for intestinal yeasts. This was observed in 72 free-living specimens of the following species: *Phalocrocorax penicillatus* (cormorant), *Zalophus califormanus* (Californian sea lion), *Rhinolophus hipposideros* (bat), *Hirundo rustico* (barn swallow), *Apus apus* (swift), *Muscicapa hypoleuca* (pied flycatcher), *Acrocephalus scirpaeus* (reed warbler) and *Hypolais polyglotta* (melodious warbler).

Grain-eating species and omnivorous species are apparently suitable as hosts for intestinal yeasts. This was oberved in 79 free-living specimens of the following species: *Passer domesticus* (house sparrow), *Corvus albus* (pied crow) and *Larus occidentalis* (Western gull). The house sparrow and the pied crow are hosts for *Candida albicans*, the Western gull for *Torulopsis glabrata*.

Feeding experiments with white mice showed that a high starch–low protein diet increases the population density of intestinal yeasts, whereas a low starch–high protein diet has a depressing effect.

REFERENCES

Bhat, J. V. and N. Kachwalla. 1955. Marine yeasts off the Indian coast. Proc. Indian Acad. Sci. B*41*: 9–15.

Mackinnon, J. E. 1959. A yeast in the stomach of the mouse. Mycopathologia *10*: 207–208.

Menna, M. E. Di. 1954. Non-pathogenic yeasts of the human skin and alimentary tract: A comparative study. J. Pathol. Bacteriol *68*: 89–99.

Parle, J. N. 1957. Yeasts isolated from the mammalian alimentary tract. J. Gen. Microbiol. *17*: 363–367.

Phaff, H. J., E. M. Mrak, and O. B. Williams. 1952. Yeast isolated from shrimp. Mycologia *44*: 431–451.

Rolle, M., and B. Mehnert. 1957. Hefen als Symbionten bei Säugetieren. Z. Bakteriol. I Orig. *160*: 268.

Saëz, H. 1959. Contribution à l'étude de la mycoflore intestinal des animaux sauvages en captivité. Rev. Mycol. *24*: 426–433.

Shifrine, M., and H. J. Phaff. 1958. On the isolation, ecology and taxonomy of *Saccharomycopsis guttulata*. Leeuwenhoek ned. Tijdschr. *24*: 193–209.

Uden, N. Van. 1960. The occurrence of *Candida* and other yeasts in the intestinal tracts of animals. Ann. N.Y. Acad. Sci. *89*: 59–68.

Uden, N. Van, and L. do Carmo-Sousa. 1957. Yeasts from the bovine caecum. J. Gen. Microbiol. *19*: 435–445.

Uden, N. Van, and L. do Carmo-Sousa. 1962. Quantitative aspects of the intestinal yeast flora of swine. J. Gen. Microbiol. *27*: 35–40.

ECOLOGY OF *ASPERGILLUS FUMIGATUS* AND THE PATHOGENIC PHYCOMYCETES

P. K. C. AUSTWICK

Central Veterinary Laboratory
Weybridge, England

ECOLOGY, EPIDEMIOLOGY AND ENVIRONMENT

ECOLOGY expresses the mutual relations of organisms in physical, chemical and temporal terms. Thus it includes both the epidemiology of an infectious disease and the relationship of the parasite to its environment. This environment is of primary importance to pathogenic fungi because most of them, including even dermatophytes, exist independently of their animal hosts, in which infection is incidental and plays no part in their survival. In studying the epidemiology of mycoses we are therefore concerned first with fungal activity on such substrates as soil and plants and secondly with host activity in acquiring infection. This contribution describes some of the environmental factors influencing epidemiology in aspergillosis and phycomycosis and relates them to the ecology of the causal fungi.

The environment of a fungus consists of physical, chemical and biotic factors, with green plants as the ultimate source of nutrients. These factors influence the fungus in (*a*) the external environment in which it grows, reproduces and is dispersed through the medium of air, water, animals or man and (*b*) the internal environment, reached as soon as the inoculum is retained in or on the body following inhalation, ingestion or contact.

THE EXTERNAL ENVIRONMENT

1. Habitat

Compilation of the records of *Aspergillus fumigatus* and the pathogenic phycomycetes from non-living substrates gives little information as to the most favourable habitats but two common substrates are considered here, namely soil and fodder.

Soil. Although *A. fumigatus* has been reported about fifty times from soil, its optimum growth conditions on this substrate have not yet been discovered (though Nicot, 1960, reported it as dominant in one zone of desert sand). Possibly its spores are washed into the soil from the surface (Burges, 1958), making it a "soil invader" (Garrett, 1955). Alternatively it may be a "soil inhabitant" of specialized substrates. Among the pathogenic phycomycetes, *Absidia ramosa*, *A. corymbifera*, *Mucor pusillus*, *M. racemosus* and several *Rhizopus* spp. have also been isolated from the soil, but the first

TABLE 1

SPORE CONTENT OF HAY OF DIFFERENT QUALITIES, 22 DAYS AFTER BALING
(Expressed as millions of spores/gram dry weight)

	"Good"	"Poor"	"Very Poor"
Moisture content at baling	16%	28%	42%
Maximum temperature reached	35° C	44° C	64° C
Aspergillus spp.	0.07	21.99*	0.62
Mucoraceae	0.00	1.51	3.69
Total moulds	0.19	23.51	4.43
Actinomycetes	0.24	0.27	199.46

*Mainly *A. glaucus.*

three species, together with *R. cohnii*, were isolated originally from mouldy bread (Lichtheim, 1884; Lindt, 1886), and shown to be pathogenic some years before their presence in natural systemic disease was established.

Hay and straw. Sixty years ago both Renon (1897) and Lucet (1897) knew that *A. fumigatus* grew well in hay and straw but the reason for this luxuriant growth remained unexplained. Experimental work carried out at Rothamsted Experimental Station (Gregory & Bunce, 1960) (Table 1) has now shown that the succession of micro-organisms in hay is determined mainly by the moisture content at the time of baling, because airborne spores of all the potential mould fungi have probably already been deposited on the grass by the time of cutting and are ready to germinate.

A. fumigatus and the pathogenic Mucoraceae were the main fungi in the "very poor" hay which matured at a maximum temperature of 64 C after baling at 42 per cent moisture content. Aerobic actinomycetes were also extremely abundant, often growing directly on the mould mycelium. "Poor" hay developed from hay baled at 28 per cent moisture content in which the

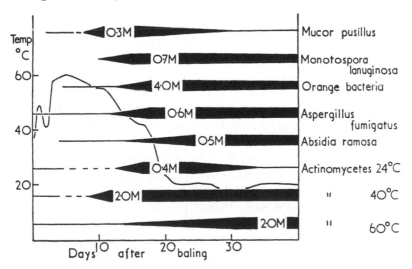

FIG. 1. Relationship of the development of fungi to time and temperature in hay baled at 46 per cent water content. Numbers of colonies in millions per gram of hay.

temperature reached about 44 C, and contained mainly A. *glaucus* type spores. "Good" hay baled at 16 per cent moisture content produced few organisms. Fig. 1 shows a rapid development of fungi and sometimes a decline with replacement of one group of organisms by another.

These results were obtained both by cultural examinations and by a standard procedure of shaking small quantities of hay in a wind tunnel at a wind speed of 4.2 m/sec for 3 min, and sampling the air to estimate the number of airborne spores set free. Mouldy hays often release as many as 1×10^8 mould spores/g dry wt of hay (as well as 12×10^8 spores of actinomycetes).

2. *Medium of dispersal*

Fungus spore dispersal depends (*a*) on the characters of the spore itself (including its attachment or "presentation") and (*b*) on the efficiency of mechanisms for getting it into the air. In this discussion the air is considered the only important medium of dispersal.

The spore and its take-off. A. *fumigatus* conidia average 3 μ in diameter and have dry, verrucose walls, probably composed of polysaccharide spines with lipid material between (Burges, 1962). They are difficult to wet and their water-repelling properties seem to increase with age. The sporangio-spores of the pathogenic phycomycetes are easily wettable, but probably disperse in the dry state as smooth, slightly collapsed bodies, 2–8 μ in size. Special adaptations favouring take-off are unknown in these fungi and the spores of both A. *fumigatus* and the pathogenic phycomycetes are liberated chiefly by the bending and breaking of spore-covered stems and leaves during the handling or eating of hay or straw.

The airborne spore. The many published studies on this subject give little specific information on these fungi, but their spores must follow the laws of aerodynamics according to their size, density, shape and surface charac-ters (Gregory, 1961). Sampling by exposing Petri dishes is notoriously non-quantitative, but has given valuable information on the kinds of viable spores present in the atmosphere. Quantitative methods, such as the Hirst trap, are of little use for spores of the Aspergilli and Mucorales, because these cannot be identified visually with certainty in dust deposits on trap slides, on which they are usually few compared with other components of outdoor air spora such as *Cladosporium.*

Outdoor air. At Rothamsted, in the summer months of 1952, the mean total outdoor air spore concentration was estimated by Gregory and Hirst (1957) at 12.5×10^3 spores/m³. *Aspergillus* and *Mucor* types were ignored but cannot have averaged more than 5 per cent of the total, i.e. an upper limit of 600 per cubic metre. Hamilton (1959) found in 1954 an average 92 *Aspergillus-Penicillium* spores /m³ in the air at Rothamsted Experimental Station and 165/m³ in South Kensington where in 1955 she obtained 419 of these spores /m³. During the winter of 1959–60, a Hirst spore trap was run at the London Zoo with pectin jelly as an adhesive. At least one colony of *A. fumigatus* was found on each day tested, and the concentration ranged from 0.25 to 7 spores /m³; *Mucor pusillus* ranged from 0 to 2 spores, and *Absidia ramosa* from 0 to 4 spores /m³ (Fiennes & Austwick, 1960).

Indoor air. The air-spora of a cowshed at Weybridge (Baruah, 1961) increased whenever the hay and straw were handled and fed to the cows, with the concentrations of *Aspergillus* and *Mucor* type spores rising from $0.1 \times 10^6/m^3$ to $16 \times 10^6/m^3$ within a few minutes. In other observations by Gregory and Bunce (1961), the concentrations of mould spores increased from $0.2 \times 10^6/m^3$ to $68 \times 10^6/m^3$ (and actinomycete spores to $780 \times 10^6/m^3$) when a sample of mouldy hay was shaken in a barn, but in both the air-spora returned soon to the original concentration (Table 2). Cultures obtained with the Andersen sampler while shaking the hay showed *A. fumigatus* and *Absidia ramosa* to be the commonest moulds, with *Aspergillus terreus* and *Mucor pusillus* also present. While eating such hay, animals will probably be exposed temporarily to even higher concentrations of spores. A recent estimation of *A. fumigatus* in the air of a London hospital ward by Clayton and Noble (1962) shows a range of concentrations from 0.3 to 2,300 spores/m³ but one can only speculate as to their source.

TABLE 2

SPORE CONTENT OF INDOOR AIR OF COWSHEDS (millions/m³)

	Normal hay in cowshed (Baruah's data)		Mouldy hay in barn at Banwell, Somerset, 1961		
	Off-peak period	Peak period	Before shaking	During shaking	20 min later
Aspergillus type	0.03	12.39	0.06	21.57	3.44
Mucor type	0.03	1.22	0.04	28.88	1.15
Total moulds	0.10	16.50	0.19	67.97	7.60
Actinomycetes	(not counted)		0.74	758.84	112.79

THE INTERNAL ENVIRONMENT

A fungus spore leaves the external environment in which it has been produced as soon as it enters the animal body. Conditions in its new environment may vary according to its entry point but our chief concern here is with the respiratory tract.

The sequence of events following the inhalation of different concentrations of airborne micro-organisms depends on the following factors: (1) susceptibility of the host, as determined by species, age, health and individual resistance; (2) total intake of inoculum; (3) rate of intake; and (4) amount of inoculum retained. These factors determine whether the animal remains unaffected, becomes infected, or becomes sensitized.

Susceptibility of the host. Mammals and birds are most prone to aspergillosis in the first week of life, but adult water birds, and animals weakened by other infections (particularly viral) or by cortisone treatment are also very susceptible (Sidransky & Friedman, 1959). Phycomycosis in man is associated frequently with uncontrolled diabetes or with leukaemia (Baker, 1957) and its ulcerative gastric form in calves and piglets appears to follow digestive disturbance. In bovine mycotic abortion apparently only the placental tissue is invaded (Austwick & Venn, 1962).

Inhalation. Although A. *fumigatus* and the pathogenic phycomycetes may invade the gastric mucosa (Gitter & Austwick, 1959), the respiratory route of infection is assumed to be commoner in the former organism. The total volume and the rate of respiration thus govern the number of spores entering the body from any given concentration in the air.

An active man with minute volume of 30 l. would inhale 43.2 m³ air/day. Exposed to a mean summer outdoor concentration of 12,500 spores/m³ (Gregory & Hirst, 1957), he would inhale 5.7×10^7 spores of all types daily at a rate of 2.2×10^4/hr, but *Aspergillus* and *Mucor* type spores would comprise less than 8 per cent of the total. In the cowshed studied by Baruah the same minute volume would provide 1.7×10^5 spores/hr during off-peak periods, and 2.8×10^7/hr during peak periods. A man working 3 hr during the peak periods would thus inhale 8.4×10^7 spores of which 82 per cent might be *Aspergillus* and *Mucor* types. The daily respiratory intake of a cow in this building was estimated at 2.9×10^8 spores. These figures give some measure of the resistance of healthy adult animals to normal inhaled levels of potentially pathogenic fungi.

Retention of spores in the respiratory tract. It is accepted that the respiratory tract acts as a filtering system in which particles over 10μ diameter are mainly caught in the nasal mucosa, those between 5μ and 10μ are deposited in the trachea, bronchi and bronchioles, and those below 5μ penetrate to the alveolar ducts (Mitchell, 1960). The alveolar system appears extremely efficient in retaining 90 per cent of particles between 1μ and 5μ in diameter, with a maximum efficiency at about 2μ but all these values will vary with the rate of respiration. A. *fumigatus* and the mucoraceous spores fall roughly into the $2–8\mu$ diameter size group, and a high proportion of single spores would be expected to be retained deep enough in the lung to escape removal by bronchial ciliary action.

Relation of spore intake to disease. The levels of spore intake which lead to disease have not yet been determined experimentally for any animal, but the infection pattern in pulmonary aspergillosis can be defined in general terms.

Very high spore concentrations from mouldy straw have apparently caused the death of adult poultry within 24 hours. Acute haemorrhagic congestion of the lungs was produced by experimental exposure of birds to a bale of straw from such an outbreak, which liberated 36×10^6 spores/g, mainly A. *fumigatus* and *Mucor pusillus*. Samples of straw and hay associated with an outbreak of acute aspergillosis in piglets, had slightly fewer spores (32×10^6 spores/g) (Gregory & Bunce, 1961). In other experiments 12-week-old chickens, which inhaled 16–70 million A. *fumigatus* spores during 5 minutes died from acute aspergillosis within 4 days, whereas exposures for

1 minute in the same atmosphere (with estimated intakes of 5–10 million spores) did not kill similar birds (Austwick & Appleby, 1961). If mycotic abortion is eventually shown to result from the inhalation of airborne spores, intake levels will probably also lie in this region, but the cumulative effect of repeated and long exposures may be important. Intravenous injection of 30 million spores of A. *fumigatus* led to uterine infection in pregnant heifers but an estimated lung intake of 3,000 million spores did not (Venn & Austwick, 1959).

Respiration in a medium concentration of airborne spores may lead to subclinical aspergillosis and this condition has recently been detected in 66 per cent of dairy cow lungs (Austwick, 1962). The minute lesions contained characteristic "asteroid" bodies which enclosed viable hyphae of A. *fumigatus*.

The low concentrations of *Aspergillus* (and *Penicillium*) type spores in outdoor air (10 to 10,000 /m³) do not seem to cause infection in man but allergic responses probably occur in sensitized persons even at these levels. The estimated range of A. *fumigatus* spore concentrations in the penguin enclosure at the London Zoo (0.25–7 spores/m³) might also seem too low to be associated with the occurrence of chronic aspergillosis in these birds, but no other source of spores appears to be easily available (Fiennes & Austwick, 1960). There is no evidence that the pathogenic phycomycetes commonly cause acute pulmonary disease, as is seen in aspergillosis, but the respiratory route of infection through the nasal sinuses has been suggested in orbital and cerebral disease. The occurrence of gastro-intestinal lesions in this disease may also indicate more frequent entry via the alimentary tract in phycomycosis (Baker, 1957).

CONCLUSIONS

This survey is an attempt to relate the ecology of *Aspergillus fumigatus* and the pathogenic phycomycetes to the diseases they cause. The relationship between the quantity of a pathogenic fungus in an environment and the incidence and severity of the infection has been emphasized particularly because it indicates that the quantitative methods now commonly used in plant and animal ecology must be adopted in mycology. Histoplasmosis and coccidioidomycosis as well as aspergillosis and mucormycosis are in need of such an approach because in these diseases individual animals become infected from a common external source. This source may be localized in mouldy bales of hay and straw in aspergillosis and yet produce such a profusion of spores that other natural sources can be virtually discounted in an agricultural region.

In aspergillosis the environment clearly plays the major epidemiological role by determining the number of spores produced and their concentration in the air, i.e. the size of the potential inoculum. Variation in susceptibility of individual hosts then determines the course of events. Fig. 2 is an attempt

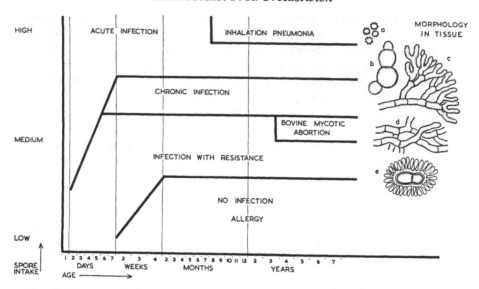

FIG. 2. Diagram of the suggested relationship between the numbers of *Aspergillus fumigatus* spores inhaled and the development of infection: (*a*) ungerminated spores; (*b*) swollen hyphae from acute lesion; (*c*) "actinomycetoid" branch from early chronic lesion; (*d*) "vegetative" type hyphae from bovine placenta; (*e*) "asteroid" containing swollen hyphae from bovine lung.

to express this concept graphically: towards the top left, rising spore concentrations cause acute infection and death; towards the bottom right, lowering spore concentrations either have no effect or set up an allergic response. Between is an area where infection occurs but is resisted successfully. This may occasionally happen following the acute and chronic disease or else the infection may become localized, for example in the uterus.

Much more experimental work will be necessary in aspergillosis and mucormycosis before there is information comparable to that of Henderson (1952) and of Rosebury (1947) on airborne anthrax and brucellosis, but the pattern of natural infections in mycoses seems to hint that the key to their control may lie in a study of the ecology of their causal fungi.

ACKNOWLEDGEMENTS

I am greatly indebted to Dr. P. H. Gregory and Mrs. M. E. Lacey (*née* Bunce) without whose data and constant help this contribution could not have been prepared, and also to Mr. R. J. Parker for preparing Fig. 2.

REFERENCES

Austwick, P. K. C. 1962. The presence of *Aspergillus fumigatus* in the lungs of dairy cows. Lab. Invest. *11*: 1062–1072.
Austwick, P. K. C., and E. C. Appleby. 1961. Unpublished data.
Austwick, P. K. C., and J. A. J. Venn. 1962. Mycotic abortion in England and Wales, 1954–1960. Proc. 4th Int. Congr. Anim. Reprod. *3*: 562–568.

Baker, R. D.   1957.   Mucormycosis—a new disease? J. Am. Med. Assoc. *163*: 805–808.

Baruah, H. K.   1961.   The air spora of a cowshed. J. Gen. Microbiol. *25*: 483–491.

Burges, A.   1958.   Micro-organisms in the soil, Hutchinson, London. 188 pp.

Burges, A.   1962.   Personal communication.

Clayton, Y., and W. C. Noble.   1961.   Personal communication.

Fiennes, R. N. T. W., and P. K. C. Austwick.   1960.   Unpublished data.

Garrett, S. D.   1955.   Microbial ecology of the soil. Trans. Brit. Mycol. Soc. *38*: 1–9.

Gitter, M., and P. K. C. Austwick.   1959.   Unpublished data.

Gregory, P. H.   1961.   The microbiology of the atmosphere. Leonard Hill, London. 251 pp.

Gregory, P. H., and J. M. Hirst.   1957.   The summer air-spora at Rothamsted in 1952. J. Gen. Microbiol. *17*: 135–152.

Gregory, P. H., and M. E. Bunce.   1960.   Microfloral succession in hay. Rept. Rothamsted Exp. Sta. 1959: 109–110.

Gregory, P. H., and M. E. Bunce.   1961.   Personal communication.

Hamilton, E. G.   1959.   Studies on the air spora. Acta allerg., Kbh. *13*: 143–175.

Henderson, D. W.   1952.   An apparatus for the study of airborne infection. J. Hyg. *50*: 53–68.

Lichtheim, L.   1884.   Ueber pathogene Schimmelpilze. II. Ueber pathogene Mucorineen und die durch sie erzeugten Mykosen des Kaninchens. Ztschr. klin. Med. 7: 140–177.

Lindt, W.   1886.   Mitteilungen über einige neuer pathogene Schimmelpilze. Arch. exp. Path. Pharmak. *21*: 269–298.

Lucet, A.   1897.   De l'*Aspergillus fumigatus* chez animaux domestiques et dans les œufs en incubation: Étude clinique et expérimentale. Paris, Ch. Mendel. 108 pp.

Mitchell, R. I.   1960.   Retention of aerosol particles in the respiratory tract: A review. Am. Rev. Resp. Dis. *82*: 627–639.

Nicot, J.   1960.   Some characteristics of the microflora in desert sands. *In* The ecology of soil fungi, ed. D. Parkinson & J. S. Waid, pp. 95–97.

Rénon, L.   1897.   Etude sur l'aspergillose chez les animaux et chez l'homme. Paris, Masson et cie, 301 pp.

Rosebury, T.   1947.   Experimental airborne infection. Williams and Wilkins, Baltimore. 222 pp.

Sidransky, H., and L. Friedman.   1959.   The effect of cortisone and antibiotic agents on experimental pulmonary aspergillosis. Am. J. Pathol. *35*: 169–184.

Venn, J. A. J., and P. K. C. Austwick.   1959.   Unpublished data.

FACTORS INFLUENCING THE DISTRIBUTION OF *COCCIDIOIDES IMMITIS* IN SOIL

ROGER O. EGEBERG*

Los Angeles County Hospital
and
University of Southern California School of Medicine
Los Angeles, California, U.S.A.

IN 1956, Egeberg and Ely reported the recovery of *Coccidioides immitis* in a high percentage of surface soil samples collected in a small six-acre area of virgin land in the southwestern part of the San Joaquin Valley. We had studied soils for the presence of *C. immitis* at four times of the year, in samples collected from animal burrows and randomly from the surface and from four-, eight- and twelve-inch depths. We had recovered the organism from 3 to 7 per cent of animal burrow samples, rarely in the sub-surface samples and not at all in the surface samples taken in midsummer, autumn or midwinter (the rainy season). However we had cultured *C. immitis* from 25, 39 and 28 per cent of surface soil samples collected in the spring of three successive years—1955, 1956 and 1957—shortly after the rainy seasons were over and the warm weather had arrived.

We raised the following questions in 1957: "Could it be that the scorching summer heat is necessary to the life of *C. immitis*? Does it prepare a thin layer of relatively sterile surface soil which needs only moisture to favor invasion by the fungi living below it? Could heat be an ally of *C. immitis* which produces, for a brief period of time, a growth medium undisturbed by antagonists and competitors?"

To study the pattern more closely we collected and cultured the soils from this same area near Buttonwillow on a monthly basis. In 1958 we recovered *C. immitis* from only three soil samples and recovered none in 1959, 1960 and 1961, years when the mean and average temperatures showed no appreciable deviation and there was no apparent change in the vegetation, despite the collection and study of 36 to 72 separate samples each month. More recently it has appeared again and in the May 1962 soils we recovered *C. immitis* from seven of thirty-six surface samples: 19.5 per cent. Smith, Plunkett (personal communications), Lubarsky and Plunkett (1955), and others, including our group, have shown that *C. immitis* survives well in sterile soil, but all who have searched for it in the soil *in situ* have found its

*This paper describes work in which Ann F. Elconin, M.D., and Margaret C. Egeberg were equal collaborators. The work was supported by grants from the National Institutes of Health, Bethesda, Maryland, and the Attending Staff Association of the Los Angeles County Hospital.

occurrence in an endemic area to be extremely spotty, so a layer of sterile soil would not seem to be the entire answer. Hundreds of square miles of San Joaquin Valley surface soil receive the same sterilizing temperature for three or four months each summer and yet of more than 5,000 soil samples studied from the southern San Joaquin Valley and other endemic areas we had been able to recover *C. immitis* from only two spots and 99 per cent of our positive samples had come from this one location, near Buttonwillow.

This extremely spotty distribution of *C. immitis* in the soil, its dramatic seasonal variation and apparent cyclical swing suggested that more needs to be learned about the environmental needs of an organism which, in the laboratory, could survive under amazing ranges of pH, organic nutritional substances, inorganic constituents, moisture and temperature, as shown by Hampson (1954), Friedman *et al.* (1956), and others.

As one listed the possible influencing factors from trace elements to the broad spectrum of inorganic and organic constituents of soil, and considered antagonists and competitors among other fungi, yeasts or bacteria; as one thought of phages and plants, of animals and reptiles as secondary hosts, and of rain and sun in different sequences and intensities: as one considered all these factors the possible permutations and combinations of requirements for an overtly undiscriminating but subtly fastidious fungus seemed to verge on the astronomical.

It was necessary to evolve several hypotheses and to test them if one wanted an answer to the question.

First we thought it well to clarify three questions: (*a*) Was the sterilization of the soil by the summer sun important? (*b*) What effect did moisture have on the presence of *C. immitis*? (*c*) Could *C. immitis* live in soils from non-endemic regions?

(*a*) Twenty-four recently collected soils from which *C. immitis* had been isolated were stored in the laboratory at room temperature with the jar covers loose. After 6 months we were unable to recover *C. immitis* again from the soil, even with repeated efforts at culturing and through animal inoculation over a period of a year. Eighteen soils from the same Buttonwillow area were sterilized by intermittent treatment in the autoclave at 20 lb pressure, and then lightly seeded with *C. immitis* and stored in the laboratory with loose covers. *C. immitis* can still be recovered from all these soils after 2 years.

(*b*) To evaluate the effect of moisture, 27 samples of soil from the Buttonwillow area were sterilized and lightly seeded with *C. immitis*. Nine were kept uncovered in a desiccator, 9 were kept moderately moist by adding 3–5 ml of water every 3 months, and 9 were kept in a wet muddy state. At the end of 15 months, *C. immitis* could be recovered from each of the 27 samples.

(*c*) Lubarsky and Plunkett (1955), Ajello (personal communication), and others had placed *C. immitis* cultures in soils from many regions and countries where the disease did not occur, and recovered it easily at a later time. We repeated this in a variety of sterilized soils and could recover the organism a year later.

It now appeared that *C. immitis* could tolerate a great variation in the moisture content of its environment, that it could live in a variety of soils and that it persisted easily in sterilized soil, but disappeared in six months from soils taken freshly from the Buttonwillow area.

We therefore concluded that the presence of *C. immitis* in the soil of an endemic area was not dependent upon strict qualities of nutritional elements or limits of moisture in the soil, but that its presence was influenced by biologic elements or the products of living biologic elements that could in turn be destroyed by sterilizing heat.

Since the anticoccidioidal effect was probably microbiological, soil samples were cultured on Sabouraud's agar and, after ten days incubation, the mixed flora was extracted with chloroform or with water. Clear zones, up to one inch in diameter, were obtained around filter paper discs soaked in the extracts; the chloroform extracts were more active than aqueous extracts. The mixed flora from soil taken just after *C. immitis* disappeared was more active than that from soil containing the pathogen.

Pure cultures were also tested and, of 36 isolates, 6 fungi, 1 yeast and 2 bacteria had an antibiotic effect against *C. immitis*.

It was then evident that microbial antagonists did influence the survival of *C. immitis* in soil. However, as we rarely observed this antagonism on our plates, we thought that non-biological factors may play a part and decided to analyse the soil chemically.

Groups of samples from the Buttonwillow area from which we had not recovered *C. immitis* and groups of samples from which this organism had occurred in 20 per cent or more of the samples were examined. Pooled samples of the positive and pooled samples of the negative soils were prepared and analysed.

No correlation was found between the presence of *C. immitis* and pH, organic matter, nitrogen, phosphorus, potassium, calcium, magnesium or zinc. However, in the soils from which *C. immitis* had been recovered in three different years, there was 4 to 12 times as much soluble salts as in the coccidioides-free soils; values for the saturation extract conductivity were 5 to 13 times the optimum concentration for the growing of crops.

The soluble minerals in the extract were therefore examined (Table 1). The concentration of calcium, potassium and sulphates was 2 to 5 times greater in the positive than in the negative soils. The amount of sodium, however, was 8 to 75 times greater in the *C. immitis* positive soils; chlorides 10 to 240 times and boron 3 to 25 times greater.

This finding suggests that the very great increase of the soluble salts, particularly sodium and the chlorides, in the soils in which *C. immitis* was found is at least temporarily inimical to the antagonists and competitors of *C. immitis* while being well tolerated by *C. immitis* itself.

TABLE 1
SOLUBLE MINERALS IN SATURATION EXTRACT

Samples no.			(1)	(2)*	(3)	(4)	(5)*	(6)*
Calcium	(Ca)	ppm	1440	2880	520	645	1550	970
Magnesium	(Mg)	,,	45	18	38	29	98	188
Sodium	(Na)	,,	100	7650	187	290	2400	5380
Potassium	(K)	,,	39	201	54	54	100	200
Chloride	(Cl)	,,	52	12650	353	249	3950	4840
Sulphate	(SO₄)	,,	3620	5000	1370	1710	2600	6100
Boron	(B)	,,	0.50	12.1	2.65	2.43	7.27	7.44

*C. immitis positive soils.

This may help in clarifying the spotty distribution of C. immitis with respect to location and its evanescence in areas where it is known to exist.

SUMMARY

In view of the ability of C. immitis to live under grossly variable conditions of moisture and nutrition, and of the antibiotic effect of a number of soil organisms against C. immitis and of the very great elevation of soluble salts, particularly sodium and chlorides, during periods when C. immitis is recovered readily from the soil, it would appear that C. immitis exists in a biologically hostile environment. To increase in number it needs two allies: (1) the summer sun with its sterilizing effect on the uppermost soil and, (2) a chemical ally that inhibits the growth of the organisms hostile to and competitive with C. immitis. This chemical ally would appear to be one or more of the water-soluble salts found in the soil.

REFERENCES

Egeberg, R. O., and Ann F. Ely. 1956. *Coccidioides immitis* in the soil of the southern San Joaquin Valley. Am. J. Med. Sci. 23: 151–154.

Friedman, L., C. E. Smith, D. Pappagianis, and R. J. Berman. 1956. Survival of *Coccidioides immitis* under controlled conditions of temperature and humidity. Am. J. Publ. Health. 46: 1317–1324.

Hampson, C. R. 1954. Sporulation capacity of *Coccidioides immitis* affected by cultural conditions. J. Bacteriol. 67: 739–740.

Lubarsky, R., and O. A. Plunkett. 1955. Some ecological studies of *Coccidioides immitis* in soil. *In* Therapy of fungus diseases, ed. T. G. Sternberg and V. D. Newcomer, pp. 308–310. International Symposium. Boston, Little.

STUDIES ON THE GROWTH AND SURVIVAL OF *BLASTOMYCES DERMATITIDIS* IN SOIL

E. S. McDONOUGH

Biology Department, Marquette University
Milwaukee, Wisconsin, U.S.A.

SCHWARTZ AND BAUM (1951) and many other investigators (reviewed by: Abernathy, 1959; Baum & Schwartz, 1959; Harrell & Curtis, 1959; Chick, Denton & Boring, 1960) have shown that a majority of the human cases of North American blastomycosis have a primary pulmonary focus. Since the disease is not contagious, the occurrence of primary lung infection suggests that the infectious elements of *Blastomyces dermatitidis* are produced in nature, are disseminated readily into the environment and taken into the lungs. Soil or some other non-living substratum may be the habitat if *B. dermatitidis* exists in nature as a saprophyte.

The demonstration by Stewart and Meyer (1932) that *Coccidioides immitis* occurs in soil and the subsequent isolation by Emmons of *Histoplasma capsulatum* (Emmons, 1949) and *Cryptococcus neoformans* (Emmons, 1951) from soil have led to numerous investigations resulting in the generally accepted idea that the soil is the natural habitat of all the airborne etiologic agents of fungus diseases in man (Ajello, 1962).

In spite of the apparently clear epidemiological picture of the soil as the natural habitat of *B. dermatitidis* and in spite of numerous attempts to isolate this fungus from such a source, only one positive soil sample has been reported (Denton, McDonough, Ajello & Ausherman, 1961). This sample was collected in a tobacco shed which had harbored, two years previously, a dog with blastomycosis.

Attempts to duplicate this isolation have not been successful. Thirty soil samples were collected within a radius of three feet from the site where the original positive sample had been obtained. Twelve samples were taken as nearly as possible from the exact place. Altogether 101 samples taken from the tobacco stripping shed were tested for the presence of the fungus by both intraperitoneal and intravenous injection into mice and also by plating out at 37 C and at 25 C. Collections were made on four different occasions, two of these being at the same time of year as the original collection.

What seems to have been established by the successful isolation of *B. dermatitidis* is that the fungus can exist in soil in nature for an extended length of time (two years at least). Whether or not the positive sample was indicative of the natural habitat of the fungus has yet to be determined.

In order to learn more about the relation of *B. dermatitidis* to soil and possibly to find the type of soil most favoring the growth of the mold, a number of experiments with natural soil have been undertaken. Some of the results will be given here.

METHODS

The two strains of *B. dermatitidis* used were known to be pathogenic for mice. One (B533) had been isolated from a human case of blastomycosis, the other (Den) was the Kentucky soil isolate.

The soil tested in the experiment reported here had been collected in the same location in the tobacco shed from which the sample yielding the natural soil isolate had been obtained. This experimental soil had been assayed for the presence of *B. dermatitidis* without positive results.

Since it has been reported that *B. dermatitidis* grows only at a high relative humidity (Menges, Furcolow, Larch & Hinton, 1952) all soil cultures were made in 20 × 150 mm sterile glass Petri dishes sealed with water-repelling tape.

Approximately 20-gram portions of soil were incorporated into cultures in four different ways. "Natural soil" samples were prepared by spreading in a Petri dish a portion of the soil and moistening it throughout with sterile distilled water, a drop at a time, so as not to flood the soil. At the end of each month the culture was moistened with sterile distilled water. One milliliter of a suspension of approximately 600,000 mycelial elements was placed on the soil in the center of the dish in an area having a diameter of about 1 inch.

"Autoclaved soil" cultures were prepared by autoclaving the soil on 3 successive days and allowing the soil to stand for 2 weeks previous to inoculation with *B. dermatitidis*.

"Natural soil on SABD agar" and "Autoclaved soil on SABD agar" samples were prepared by placing a portion of the soil on a 2-week-old culture of the fungus on Sabouraud dextrose agar in a Petri dish. Twenty-five milliliters of agar were used for each plate and inoculated by placing a small amount of mycelium on the agar in the center of each dish.

Two weeks, 6 weeks and 14 weeks after the fungus had been brought into contact with the soil a segment comprising one-fourth of the soil culture was suspended in physiological salt solution containing penicillin and streptomycin. The ability of *B. dermatitidis* to grow or survive on the soil culture was assayed by using samples of the suspension to culture directly on 6 plates and to inoculate into 6 mice with subsequent culturing of lung, brain, spleen and liver (McDonough *et al.*, 1961; Denton, McDonough, Ajello, & Ausherman, 1961).

Altogether, directly and indirectly, 72 cultures were made from each soil sample segment.

658   XIII. MYCOSES: *E. S. McDonough*

RESULTS

The results are summarized in Table 1. It will be noticed that, while both strains of *B. dermatitidis* were recovered from the natural soil after exposure to it for 2 weeks, no isolations were obtained at later periods. This apparent failure of the fungus to grow in natural soil could not be attributed to a lack of food in view of the results obtained when the natural soil was layered on Sabouraud dextrose agar before inoculation. On this substratum the "Den" strain was recovered after 6 weeks and after 14 weeks. The small number of positive cultures, however, suggested prolonged survival rather than increased growth. Noteworthy also in this connection was the excellent growth of both strains on autoclaved soil with and without the agar supplement.

Visual evidence was also obtained that the natural soil had an inhibitory effect on the growth and survival of *B. dermatitidis*. When 20 grams of

TABLE 1
EFFECTS OF NATURAL SOIL ON *Blastomyces dermatitidis*

Soil treatment	Inoculum	% Cultures containing B. dermatitidis*		
		2 weeks	6 weeks	14 weeks
Natural Soil				
Sample 1	None	0	0	0
" 2	None	0	0	0
" 3	Strain B533	0	0	0
" 4	Strain B533	6	0	0
" 5	Den strain	5 −	0	0
" 6	Den strain	3 −	0	0
Natural Soil on SABD agar				
Sample 1	None	0	0	0
" 2	None	0	0	0
" 3	Strain B533	0	0	0
" 4	Strain B533	0	0	0
" 5	Den strain	6	11	3 −
" 6	Den strain	6 −	3 −	4 +
Autoclaved soil				
Sample 1	None	0	0	0
" 2	None	0	0	0
" 3	Strain B533	4 +	4 +	1 +
" 4	Strain B533	3 −	80	20
" 5	Den strain	82	64	54
" 6	Den strain	90	86	56
Autoclaved soil on SABD agar				
Sample 1	None	0	0	0
" 2	None	0	0	0
" 3	Strain B533	40	73	87
" 4	Strain B533	18	67	80
" 5	Den Strain	82	80	86
" 6	Den strain	90	82	72

*Cultures were made from the soil sample after 2 weeks, after 6 weeks, and after 14 weeks.

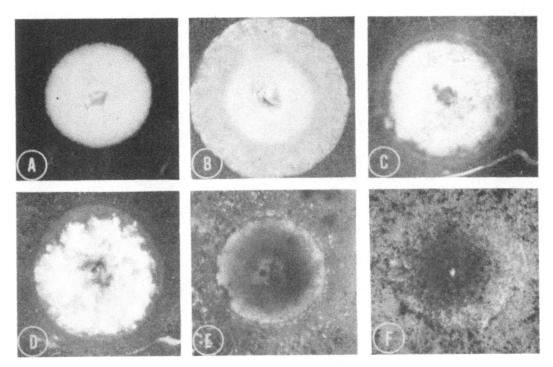

PLATE I. Lytic action of natural soils on *Blastomyces dermatitidis*. *A*, a two-week-old colony covered with black soil as seen through the bottom of a Petri dish. *B*, a control. The gray outer growth was produced after a colony had been covered with black auto-claved soil two weeks previously. *C–F*, lytic action by four different soils. In *F* the original growth had been almost completely destroyed. Photographs by Stanislaus Ratajczak.

autoclaved soil were placed on a colony of the fungus growing on Sabouraud dextrose agar, an increase in growth occurred (Plate I, *A* and *B*). On the other hand, when natural soil was placed on a similar colony, lysis of at least a part of the colony occurred within two weeks. This destructive action was found to be general with soils from different places (Plate I, *C–F*).

DISCUSSION

The inhibitory and lytic action of natural soil on *B. dermatitidis* as demonstrated in this study is not unique among fungi.

A "widespread fungistasis" in soil was described by Dobbs and Hinson in 1953, and lysis of young mycelium in unsterilized soil was described by Novogrudsky in 1948 and Chinn in 1953. Since these early investigations, numerous confirming reports have shown the phenomena to be of common occurrence (reviewed by Brian, 1960; Dobbs, Hinson & Bywater, 1960). A few papers have been published that show similar phenomena with human or animal pathogenic fungi. Grin (1959) reported that the mycelium of *Trichophyton violaceum* in hairs was destroyed on 15 natural soils. Vanbreuseghem, Dekeyser and Lauwers (1960) observed that *Tricophyton mentagrophytes* and *Microsporum canis* produced mycelium on the hairs of animals in natural soil. *T. mentagrophytes*, however, failed to develop on unsterilized earth to which fowl or human faeces had been added.

To date, 26 soil samples taken from different locations have been shown to inhibit the growth of *B. dermatitidis*. This does not prove that this fungus will not grow or persist in some unsterilized soils. What it does seem to show is that the widespread mycolysis found in most soils is operative in regard to *B. dermatitidis*, as is true of a large number of fungi.

Of interest in this connection was the demonstration by Lockwood (1960) that the mycelium of most of a group of 20 plant pathogenic fungi was almost completely destroyed when covered for 1 to 2 weeks with field soil. Some of the 20 fungi, including *Rhizoctonia solani*, were well-recognized root rot pathogens and known inhabitants of soil. In spite of this, approximately 50 per cent of the mycelium of *R. solani* was destroyed in 14 days. It has been shown, however (Boosalis & Scharen, 1959), that the mycelium of this root rot fungus can carry on an active saprophytic life in plant debris in soil.

It may well be that *B. dermatitidis* is able to grow and survive in certain soils or in favorable particles scattered in soil.

Further support for the idea that *B. dermatitidis* may yet be shown to grow with some regularity in debris in soil, or in favorably conditioned soil, may be inferred from studies which are to be published in detail elsewhere. In these studies the mycelium of *Allescheria boydii* (and especially that of *Histoplasma capsulatum*) has been shown to be inhibited in growth or to be lysed by natural soils. Yet there is no doubt that these fungi normally inhabit soils.

SUMMARY

Conidia and mycelial fragments of *Blastomyces dermatitidis* were inoculated directly onto natural soils in Petri dishes. The fungus was recovered from such samples after 2 weeks but not after 6 weeks or 14 weeks.

When natural soil was placed directly on growing mycelium the latter underwent lysis. This lytic activity was substantiated by culture studies and mouse inoculation and comparison with controls using autoclaved soils. The lytic phenomenon was thought to be similar to the widespread mycolysis described by others for saprophytic and plant pathogenic fungi.

ACKNOWLEDGMENT

This investigation was supported in part by awards E-2211 (C2 and C3) from the National Institute of Allergy and Infectious Diseases.

The technical assistance of Mr. John Bartizal, Mr. Gregory Chan, Miss Mary Grochowski, and Miss Virginia Peterson is gratefully acknowledged.

REFERENCES

Abernathy, R. S. 1959. Clinical manifestations of pulmonary blastomycosis. Ann. Internal Med. *51*: 707–727.

Ajello, L. 1962. Epidemiology of human fungous infections. *In* Fungi and fungous diseases, ed. B. Dalldorf, pp. 69–83. Charles C. Thomas, Springfield, Ill.

Baum, G. L., and J. Schwartz. 1959. North American blastomycosis. Am. J. Med. Sci. *238*: 661–683.

Boosalis, M. G., and A. L. Scharen. 1959. Methods for microscopic detection of *Aphanomyces euteiches* and *Rhizoctonia solani* associated with plant debris. Phytopathology *49*: 192–198.

Brian, P. W. 1960. Antagonistic and competitive mechanisms limiting survival and activity of fungi in soil. *In* The ecology of soil fungi, ed. D. Parkinson and J. S. Waid, pp. 115–129. Liverpool University Press, Liverpool, England.

Chick, E. W., H. J. Peters, J. F. Denton, und W. D. Boring. 1960. Die nordamerikanische blastomykose. Ergeb. allgem. Pathol. u pathol. Anat. *40*: 34–98.

Chinn, S. H. F. 1953. A slide technique for the study of fungi and actinomycetes in soil, with special reference to *Helminthosporium sativum*. Can. J. Bot. *31*: 718–724.

Denton, J. F., E. S. McDonough, L. Ajello, and R. J. Ausherman. 1961. Isolation of *Blastomyces dermatitidis* from soil. Science *133*: 1126–1127.

Dobbs, C. G., and W. H. Hinson. 1953. A widespread fungistasis in soils. Nature *172*: 197–199.

Dobbs, C. G., W. H. Hinson, and J. Bywater. 1960. Inhibition of fungal growth in soils. *In* The ecology of soil fungi, ed. D. Parkinson and J. S. Waid, pp. 130–147. Liverpool University Press, Liverpool, England.

Emmons, C. W. 1949. Isolation of *Histoplasma capsulatum* from soil. Public Health Repts. (U.S.) *64*: 892–896.

Emmons, C. W. 1951. Isolation of *Cryptococcus neoformans* from soil. J. Bacteriol. *62*: 685–690.

Grin, E. I. 1959. Upliv zemlje injezine micropopulacije na patogene dermatofite u inficiranoij dlaci. Rad. Nauč. Društ. Bosne-Hercegovine 12: 5–22. (English summary)

Harrell, E. R., and A. C. Curtis. 1959. North American blastomycosis. Am. J. Med. 27: 750–766.

Lockwood, J. L. 1960. Lysis of mycelium of plant pathogenic fungi by natural soil. Phytopathology 50: 787–789.

McDonough, E. S., L. Ajello, R. J. Ausherman, A. Balows, J. T. McClellan, and S. Brinkman. 1961. Human pathogenic fungi recovered from soil in an area endemic for North American blastomycosis. Am. J. Hyg. 73: 75–83.

Menges, R. W., M. L. Furcolow, H. W. Larsh, and A. Hinton. 1952. Laboratory studies on histoplasmosis. J. Infectious Diseases. 90: 67–70.

Novogrudsky, D. M. 1948. The colonization of soil bacteria on fungal hyphae. Mikrobiologiya 17: 28–35.

Schwartz, I., and G. L. Baum. 1951. Blastomycosis. Am. J. Clin. Pathol. 21: 999–1029.

Stewart, R. A., and K. F. Meyer. 1932. Isolation of Coccidioides immitis (Stiles) from the soil. Proc. Soc. Exptl. Biol. Med. 29: 937–938.

Vanbreuseghem, R., P. Dekeyser, et R. Lauwers. 1960. Culture sur terre non stérile de divers dermatophytes. Ann. Soc. Belge Méd. Trop. 40: 415–422.

AMBIENT TEMPERATURE AND SOME
DEEP MYCOSES*

JUAN E. MACKINNON

Instituto de Higiene
Montevideo, Uruguay

THE STUDY of the experimental disease of the guinea-pig produced by *Paracoccidioides brasiliensis* (1, 3, 9, 17) induced us to consider the influence of ambient temperature on some aspects of South American blastomycosis (12) and some other mycoses (2, 10, 11). The maximal temperature for growth of some fungi causing deep mycoses is close to the deep body temperature of man and laboratory animals. The temperature of the body is not homogeneous. Some segments, organs and regions are more easily cooled than others and the life of some pathogens might be possible in cooled regions and impossible in warmer organs or segments. Moreover, environmental temperature causes variations of the deep body temperature which, although slight, may be important because they occur in a thermal zone critical for the pathogen. The experiments reported in this paper have been carried out since 1959.

METHODS AND RESULTS

Maximal Temperature for Growth

Maximal temperature for growth was studied in Sabouraud glucose agar, in nutrient agar with 1 per cent glucose and 20 per cent horse serum and in blood agar in an atmosphere of 100 per cent relative humidity. It was found to be: for 3 strains of *Paracoccidioides brasiliensis*, 3 strains of *Sporotrichum schenckii* and 6 strains of *Madurella grisea*, between 38 and 39 C; for 3 strains of *Histoplasma capsulatum*, between 39 and 40 C; for 2 strains of *Blastomyces dermatitidis*, between 41 and 42 C; and for 2 strains of *Allescheria boydii* between 41 and 42.5 C. Moreover, all 6 strains of *Madurella mycetomi* grew well at 42.5 C.

Experiments with Paracoccidioides brasiliensis in guinea-pigs

During the winter of 1959 we inoculated 12 guinea-pigs by the intracardiac route (3) with a suspension of a yeast-phase culture. Fifteen to 30 days later the animals showed lesions in the eyes and testes, in some areas of the skin such as the eyelids, ears, muzzle and perigenitalia as well

*This work was aided by a grant of the Universidad de la República, Montevideo, Uruguay.

as in the rectum. Some guinea-pigs died and a notable finding was the absence or rare occurrence of lesions in the lungs, spleen, liver, brain, etc.; when found they were very small in size. Only the terminal segment of the intestinal tract was involved distinctly. Moreover, all 12 guinea-pigs showed nodular lesions in the muscles of the buttocks, forearms and legs while no lesions were visible in other groups of striated muscles. The selective involvement of some regional groups of muscles, of the testes and eyes was a very striking feature. Because the maximal temperature for growth of the fungus was lower than the deep body temperature of the guinea-pig, the influence of a cooling regional effect of environmental temperature was suspected. The experiment was carried out at an undetermined ambient temperature but according to meteorological data it was estimated as varying between 6 and 13 C.

In order to substantiate the foregoing hypothesis new experiments were conducted. Twenty-one guinea-pigs were inoculated by the cardiac route and divided at random into three equal groups. One group was placed in a room at 14–20 C; 7 weeks later, lesions of the skin were seen in the muzzle, eyelids and perineal region of all 7 animals. The second group was placed at 28–30 C; all the animals developed skin lesions but at the end of the experiment 4 had recovered. The third group was kept at 14–20 C for 12 days when lesions were visible in all; the animals were then transferred to a room at 37 C and a rapid healing of skin lesions was observed.

In another experiment 22 guinea-pigs were inoculated in the heart and distributed into two groups. Of 12 animals kept at 15–16 C, 9 developed lesions of the skin and uveitis while none of the 10 animals kept at 37 C showed such lesions.

As none of the guinea-pigs kept at an ambient temperature between 14 and 20 C developed the myositis observed in our first experiment, 7 inoculated animals were kept at 5–9 C and the myositis was observed in 5.

Comments. Our results are believed to demonstrate that a low ambient temperature is decisive for the production of lesions by *P. brasiliensis* in the guinea-pig and that high environmental temperatures suppress all visible effects of the infection. A comparison between the maximal temperature for growth of the pathogen and the temperature of different segments of the body (12) clearly suggests that the observed features were due to an inhibitory effect of the temperature of the tissues.

Experiments with Sporotrichum schenckii in rats

Young male rats were inoculated intraperitoneally and distributed into two groups. One group was placed at 31 C and the other at 10–20 C. The 11 animals in each group all showed lesions in the testes and epididymis but the lesions in the group at 31 C were milder than in the group at low temperature. Lesions in the bones of the paws and tail were seen in 10 out of the 11 animals kept at the lower temperature, while none of the 11 animals at 31 C showed such lesions. The absence of lesions in the paws and tail of animals kept at 31 C might be due to lack of metastasis from the milder lesions of the testes or because the fungus was not able to develop in the bones.

Thirty-six young male rats, weighing 50 to 70 g, were inoculated intra-cardially and distributed at random into two groups of 18. One group was kept at 31 C and the other at 5–15 C. Some animals died within 60 hours of inoculation, the groups being thus reduced to 13 and 15 animals respectively. Lesions of the paws and tail appeared between the 9th and 15th day in 13 out of the 15 animals kept at low ambient temperature while no lesions were seen on the paws or tails of the animals kept at 31 C.

Comments. Since the maximal temperature for growth of *S. schenckii* ranged from 38 to 39 C and inasmuch as the deep body temperature of the rat is 37.7 C, the distal segments of the limbs being very susceptible to cool-ing, it was assumed that the inhibitory effect of high environmental tempera-ture on the disease was due to changes from the optimal conditions for the growth of the pathogen (11).

Experiment with Histoplasma capsulatum in mice

We studied the regression of the infection in two groups of 60 mice inoculated in the peritoneum and kept at 10 C and at 35–37 C (10). After 90 days the surviving mice—58 at 10 C and 54 at 35–37 C—were killed. From the liver of each mouse 0.3 to 0.5 g was cultivated on 6 Sabouraud glucose agar slants. *H. capsulatum* was recovered from 55 per cent of the animals kept at 10 C and from 15 per cent of those kept at 35–37 C.

Comments. The deep body temperature of the mouse is 37.2 C but it rises above 39 C in mice kept at 35–37 C. As the inoculated fungus grew poorly at 39 C and did not grow at all at 40 C it was thought that the difference between rates of recovery of *H. capsulatum* from the two groups of mice was related to changes in the inner temperature of the body.

Experiment with Blastomyces dermatitidis in guinea-pigs

A yeast-phase culture was inoculated into the heart of 50 guinea-pigs, 20 males and 30 females but seven animals died within 72 hours. The two groups were thus reduced to 25 animals—10 males and 15 females—at 10–20 C and 18 animals—8 males and 10 females—at 35–37 C.

Twelve out of the 25 animals at 10–20 C, 6 males and 6 females, died 7 to 34 days after inoculation with nodular lesions in the upper surface of the brain and in the concavity of the cranial vault. The testicles were involved consistently, but not other viscera. Survivors were killed between the 46 and 50th days but no lesions were visible to the naked eye and brain cultures were negative.

None of the animals kept at 35–37 C showed symptoms of disease, nor were lesions visible to the naked eye at the end of the experiment but *B. dermatitidis* was isolated from the brain of 8 animals, 3 males and 5 females.

Comments. Low environmental temperature had a decisive influence on the course of the disease. High ambient temperature reduced the infection to latency, at least for the duration of the experiment: 45 days (2).

The yeast-phase of the inoculated strain grew well *in vitro* between 37 and 39 C, poor growth was seen at 41 C and no growth at 42 C. These data and the localization of the lesions in the testicles and in the upper surface of the brain do not contradict the assumption that *B. dermatitidis* grew in tissues cooled by the environmental temperature.

DISCUSSION

Pasteur's classic pioneer experiments on hens inoculated with *Bacillus anthracis* will at this point undoubtedly be evoked by all of us and might contribute to a better understanding of some aspects of deep mycoses. Kuhn (7) related the resistance of the rabbit to *Cryptococcus neoformans* to high deep-body temperature. This pathogen does not grow at 40 C. Kuhn reported that mice inoculated intravenously with *C. neoformans* and kept at 35–36 C survived longer than those kept at 24–27 C. Kligman, Crane and Norris (6) reported 90.8 per cent mortality in chick embryos inoculated intravenously with *C. neoformans* and incubated at 37 C while increased rates of survival were recorded at 39, 40 and 41 C. The use of fever therapy has not been encouraging in cryptococcosis (8).

Our results demonstrate that high ambient temperature suppresses the effect of the infection of guinea-pigs with *P. brasiliensis* and some of the effects of the inoculation of *S. schenckii* into rats, that it reduces to latency the infection of guinea-pigs with *B. dermatitidis* and favours the regression of the infection of the mouse with *H. capsulatum.* These features may facilitate the understanding of some epidemiological and clinical aspects of the deep mycoses in man. Actually histoplasmosis differs in different climates and countries. Sixty-five cases of histoplasmosis have been recorded at the latitude of Uruguay (10) and Argentina (13) with moderate skin test rates. In Honduras, Central America, Hoeckenga and Tucker (5) found 40 per cent of positive reactors to histoplasmin but only one case of histoplasmosis was known. Tucker (16) reported a similar result in Panama and recently Shirokov (15) has pointed out that only one clinical case was observed in a Panamanian, in contrast with the fact that ⅔ or ⅘ of the population reacts to histoplasmin. Further north the problem of histoplasmosis reappears especially in zones of the United States with hot-humid and cold seasons. A rather similar influence may be expected from altitude in mountainous countries, such as Mexico.

Environmental conditions, such as high temperature and high relative humidity, have a double effect. They favour the growth of some pathogenic fungi, such as *S. schenckii* and *H. capsulatum,* under natural conditions but on the other hand they may prevent the clinical manifestations of the infection. These effects render conceivable the assumption that the correlations between skin test rates and the clinical manifestations vary according to different climatological conditions.

The influence of cooling should be investigated in South American blastomycosis. The clinical manifestations might be more severe in temperate zone of southern Brazil and Uruguay than in very hot zones. The classic zone of South American blastomycosis, São Paulo, belongs to the humid tropics according to vegetational criteria but it is a temperate zone according to climatological standards (4). Working in cold ambient temperatures, or migration to temperate or cold countries, may affect potential patients.

In order to evaluate the antifungal effects of chemotherapeutic compounds and antibiotics, in animals and in man, we must consider temperature as a parameter.

Silva (14) remarks that the maximal temperature for growth of *Phialophora* (*Fonsecaea*) *pedrosoi* lies between 35 and 40 C and suggests the artificial raising of temperature as a possible method of therapy in chromoblastomycosis. Some deep mycoses, such as chromoblastomycosis, sporotrichosis and exogenous mycetomas, are usually localized in segments of the limbs. Local heating is easy and it seems to have been useful in a case of sporotrichosis (11). We suspect that a number of so-called spontaneous cures may have been due to ambient temperature. Local heating in mycetomas by species showing a low maximal temperature for growth, such as *Madurella grisea*, deserves thorough trial.

SUMMARY

High ambient temperature counteracts the effects of intracardiac inoculation of guinea-pigs with *Paracoccidioides brasiliensis*, prevents osteoarthritis in rats inoculated intraperitoneally or in the heart with *Sporotrichum schenckii*, favours the regression of the infection in mice inoculated intraperitoneally with *Histoplasma capsulatum* and reduces to latency the infection of guinea-pigs with *Blastomyces dermatitidis*. Environmental conditions such as high temperature and humidity which favour the growth of some pathogenic fungi under natural conditions have an unfavourable effect on their parasitic life, in laboratory animals. These two compensatory effects of high temperature make it conceivable that the correlations between skin test rates and the clinical manifestations in some mycotic infections may differ in countries with different climates.

Hence we should consider the possible effects of ambient temperature when evaluating the antifungal effects of chemotherapeutic compounds and antibiotics in laboratory animals and man.

REFERENCES

1. Conti-Díaz, I. A. 1960. Lesiones oculares en la blastomicosis sudamericana. Hospital (Rio de J.) 58: 903–914.

2. Conti-Díaz, I.A., and J. E. Mackinnon. 1961. Infección evolutiva e infección latente del cobayo con *Blastomyces dermatitidis* condicionadas a la temperatura ambiente. An. Fac. Med. Montevideo *46*: 280–282.

3. Conti-Díaz, I. A., L. A. Yarzabal, and J. E. Mackinnon. 1959. Lesiones cutáneas, orofaríngeas, rectales y musculares por inoculación intracardíaca de *Paracoccidioides brasiliensis* al cobayo y al conejo. An. Fac. Med. Montevideo *44*: 601–607.

4. Fosberg, F. R., B. J. Garnier, and A. W. Küchler. 1961. Delimitation of the humid tropics. Geogr. Rev. *51*: 333–347.

5. Hoeckenga, M. T., and H. A. Tucker. 1960. Sensibilidad a la histoplasmina y a la coccidioidina en Honduras. Bol. Of. Sanit. Panamer. *29*: 1135–1138.

6. Kligman, A. M., A. P. Crane, and R. F. Norris. 1951. Effect of temperature on survival of chick embryos infected intravenously with *Cryptococcus neoformans*. Am. J. Med. Sci. *221*: 273–278.

7. Kuhn, L. R. 1949. Effect of elevated body temperature on cryptococcosis in mice. Proc. Soc. Exptl. Biol. (N.Y.) *71*: 341–343.

8. Litman, M. L., and L. E. Zimmerman. 1956. Cryptococcosis. Grüne & Stratton, New York and London.

9. Mackinnon, J. E. 1961. Miositis en la blastomicosis sudamericana y en la histoplasmosis. Mycopathol. et Mycol Appl. (Den Haag) *15*: 171–176.

10. Mackinnon, J. E., and I. A. Conti-Díaz. 1962. The effect of ambient temperature on the experimental histoplasmosis of the mouse. Sabouraudia *2*: 31–34.

11. Mackinnon, J. E., and I. A. Conti-Díaz. 1962. The effect of temperature on sporotrichosis. Sabouraudia *2*: 56–59.

12. Mackinnon, J. E., I. A. Conti-Díaz, L. A. Yarzabal, and N. Tavella. 1960. Temperatura ambiental y blastomicosis sudamericana. An. Fac. Med. Montevideo *45*: 310–318.

13. Negroni, P. 1960. *Micosis profundas*. Vol. II, *Histoplasmosis*. Artes Gráficas B. V. Chiesino, Buenos Aires.

14. Silva, Margarita. 1958. The saprophytic phase of the fungi of chromoblastomycosis: Effect of nutrients and temperature upon growth and morphology. Trans. N.Y. Acad. Sci., Ser. II, *21*: 46–57.

15. Shirokov, E. P. 1961. Histoplasmosis in Panama. J. Am. Med. Assoc. *177*: 297–299.

16. Tucker, H. A. 1950. Histoplasmin, tuberculin and coccidioidin sensitivity on the isthmus of Panama. Preliminary report of 500 patients. Am. J. Trop. Med. *30*: 865–870.

17. Yarzabal, L. A. 1961. Rectitis y lesiones perianales en la blastomicosis sudamericana experimental. G. E. N. (Caracas) *16*: 1–10.

NOTES EPIDEMIOLOGIQUES A PROPOS DES MYCETOMES

F. MARIAT

Institut Pasteur, Paris, France

LES DIVERS AUTEURS qui se sont intéressés au problème des mycétomes se sont bien souvent interrogés sur l'influence que pouvait avoir le milieu, sur l'apparition et le développement de cette maladie. La première grande enquête épidémiologique dans ce domaine, a été conduite par J. E. Bocarro (1893) ; elle comportait l'analyse de cent mycétomes observés au cours de dix années, dans la région de Hyderabad. D'autres travaux similaires ont été effectués depuis, portant sur un nombre plus ou moins élevé de cas. Rappelons plus spécialement la thèse de P. H. Abbott (1954), les travaux de F. Latapí (1956), de F. Latapí et Yolanda Ortiz (1961) et de M. Rey (1961). Ce dernier, dans une thèse récente, préparée à l'Institut Pasteur de Dakar sous la direction de R. Camain, a étudié plus de deux cents mycétomes du Sénégal et de Mauritanie ; la partie épidémiologique de ce travail est très complète et nous nous y sommes largement documentés.

Lorsque des travaux semblables auront analysé un nombre suffisant de cas, il sera alors plus aisé de vérifier les hypothèses de travail formulées actuellement. Il nous a paru utile, dans cet esprit, de réunir des observations effectuées par des travailleurs isolés et d'en tirer d'éventuels enseignements. Ce rapport rend donc essentiellement compte, des résultats d'une enquête conduite dans les milieux connus pour s'intéresser aux mycétomes.

I. ENQUÊTE SUR LES MYCÉTOMES

Au début du mois de mars de 1962, nous avons adressé à 131 correspondants répartis dans le monde entier, un questionnaire se rapportant aux mycétomes éventuellement rencontrés (nombre et nature des mycétomes ; âge, sexe et race des malades ; avis du correspondant sur certains facteurs épidémiologiques, etc...) A la date du premier juillet 1962, 77 correspondants nous avaient retourné le questionnaire dûment rempli. La liste de ces correspondants se trouve à la fin de ce rapport ; les numéros entre parenthèses reportent à leur documentation. A notre grand regret nous n'avons pas reçu de réponse de certaines régions réputées riches en mycétomes.

Le tableau 1 donne quelques précisions sur les réponses reçues, mentionnant 854 mycétomes étudiés au cours des vingt dernières années. Comme il ne peut être question dans une telle enquête, de discuter la détermination

TABLEAU 1

Données générales se rapportant à l'enquête effectuée

	Amérique du Nord et Centrale	Amérique du Sud	Afrique et Madagascar	Asie	Océanie	Europe	TOTAUX
Nombre de questionnaires envoyés	21	19	43	24	12	12	131
Nombre de réponses reçues	14	10	28	9	11	5	77
Réponses donnant au moins 1 mycétome	10	9	21	8	5	2	55
Réponses ne donnant aucun mycétome	4	—	2	1	5	3	15
Réponses sans information	—	1	5	—	1	—	7
Mycétomes fongiques	19	58	245	5	—	11	338
Mycétomes actinomycosiques	214	49	196	23	2	3	487
Mycétomes sans étiologie	5	1	19	—	4	—	29
TOTAUX mycétomes	238	108	460	28	6	14	854

proposée par nos correspondants, c'est celle-ci qui figure dans le tableau 2. Dans de très rares cas, il est possible qu'il y ait chevauchement de certains résultats. Cela ne semble pas devoir modifier grandement les résultats d'ensemble ; ce risque d'erreurs est évalué à 1 ou 2 pour cent du total au grand maximum.

Les chiffres des tableaux sont uniquement ceux fournis par nos correspondants ; nous avons volontairement omis toute référence à la bibliographie. Par ailleurs, nous n'avons pris en considération que les seules réponses chiffrées, ignorant les mentions imprécises telles par exemple « prépondérance de mycétomes à... » « nombreux mycétomes à... », etc...

1. *Localisation géographique*

Le tableau 2 rapporte à la fois la distribution géographique des mycétomes et des espèces. La maladie est fréquente au Mexique. En Amérique du Sud, c'est au Venezuela et en Argentine que les cas rapportés par nos correspondants sont en plus grand nombre. En Afrique les mycétomes sont nombreux dans la bande de territoires qui s'étend du Sénégal aux Somalis. Les chiffres mentionnés confirment l'existence d'une zone de grande endémie avec plusieurs foyers importants. Au nord comme au sud de cette aire, se rencontrent également des mycétomes mais ils y sont souvent sporadiques, dispersés et en nombre peu élevé. On note cependant un foyer relativement important au Tanganyika. A Madagascar, les mycétomes observés proviennent en grande partie du sud de l'Ile.

Le tableau 2 pourrait faire apparaître l'Asie comme un continent où les mycétomes n'existent qu'en nombre restreint. Cela s'explique par le peu de réponses qui nous sont parvenues de cette immense région ; on sait bien cependant que, dans certaines parties de l'Inde par exemple, la maladie est endémique.

En Océanie les mycétomes semblent peu nombreux et dispersés ; quant à l'Europe on y rencontre la maladie à l'état sporadique dans les régions méridionales et notre enquête ne la signale qu'en Roumanie et en Bulgarie. Nous savons qu'ils existent également au Portugal et en Italie. Dans ce continent, les cas mentionnés par la littérature sont souvent d'origine extra-européenne.

Les mycétomes sont donc une maladie essentiellement endémique des régions avoisinant le Tropique du Cancer mais ils peuvent également déborder cette aire préférentielle.

2. *Les agents des mycétomes et leur distribution géographique*

La distribution des diverses espèces est représentée dans le tableau 2 et dans la figure 1.

Madurella mycetomi est responsable de 18 pour cent des cas. C'est un champignon rencontré à peu près partout où il y a des mycétomes. En Afrique Occidentale, cette espèce prédomine dans la région du Fleuve Sénégal (31, Rey 1961).

TABLEAU 2

DISTRIBUTION DES MICROORGANISMES AGENTS DE MYCÉTOMES D'APRÈS LES RÉSULTATS DE L'ENQUÊTE EFFECTUÉE

(Les chiffres entre parenthèses suivant la localité reportent à la liste des correspondants à la fin du rapport.)

| | MYCÉTOMES FONGIQUES | | | | | | | | | | MYCÉTOMES ACTINOMYCOSIQUES | | | | | | | | | | |
| | Mycétomes à grains noirs | | | | | Mycétomes à grains blancs | | | | | Mycétomes à grains blancs | | | | | | | | | | |
Localité	Maduerella mycetomi	M. grisea	Leptosphaeria senegalensis	Mycétomes à gr. noirs divers	Totaux mycétomes à gr. noirs	A. boydii ou M. apiospermum	Cephalosporium	Mycétomes à gr. blancs divers	Totaux mycétomes à gr. blancs	Totaux mycétomes fongiques	S. madurae	S. somaliensis	N. asteroides	N. brasiliensis	Totaux mycétomes dits « à petits » grains (N.a et N.b)	Autres mycétomes à gr. blancs	S. pelletierii	Mycétomes actinomycosiques non précisés	Totaux mycétomes actinomycosiques	Mycétomes sans autres données	Totaux généraux
U.S.A. (10)		2			2					2			1		1				1		3
,, (20)						1			1	1	1	1		1	1				3		4
,, (9)						1			1	1			1		1				1		2
,, (1)						1			1	1										5	6
,, (5)						1			1	1	1			1	1				2		3
,, (12)						1	1		2	2											2
,, (14)						1			1	1											1
,, (23)													1		1				1		1
Puerto Rico, Virgin I., St-Thomas (21)				2[a]	2					2							2		2		4
Mexique F.L. (15)						2	2		4	4	12	2		188	188				202		206
TOTAUX Amérique du Nord et Centrale		2		2	4	8	3		11	15	14	3	3	190	193		2		212	5	232
AMÉRIQUE DU SUD																					
Venezuela (4, 7, 18)	4	19[b]		1	24	4	1		5	29	12	1	9	15	24		1		38	1	68
Colombie (6)	2				2					2											2
Pérou (11)		1			1					1				2	2				2		3
Brésil (Nord 8)						3			3	3				3	3	1	1		5		8
Brésil (Sud 16)													2		2				2[c]		2
Uruguay (17)													1	1	2				2		2
Argentine (24)	14	4			18	5			5	23											23
TOTAUX Amérique du Sud	20	24	0	1	45	12	1	0	13	58	12	1	12	21	33	1	2		49	1	108
TOTAUX AMÉRIQUE	20	26	0	3	49	20	4	0	24	73	26	4	15	211	226	1	4		261	6	340

TABLEAU 2 (*suite*)

| AFRIQUE | MYCÉTOMES FONGIQUES | | | | | | | | | | MYCÉTOMES ACTINOMYCOSIQUES | | | | | | | | | | |
| | Mycétomes à grains noirs | | | | | Mycétomes à grains blancs | | | | | Mycétomes à grains blancs | | | | | | | | | | |
	Madurella mycetomi	*M. grisea*	*Leptosphaeria senegalensis*	Mycétomes à gr. noirs divers	Totaux mycétomes à gr. noirs	*A. boydii* ou *M. apiospermum*	*Cephalosporium*	Mycétomes à gr. blancs divers	Totaux mycétomes à gr. blancs	Totaux mycétomes fongiques	*S. madurae*	*S. somaliensis*	*N. asteroides*	*N. brasiliensis*	Totaux mycétomes dits à «petits» grains (N.a et N.b)	Autres mycétomes à gr. blancs	*S. pelletierii*	Mycétomes actinomycosiques non précisés	Totaux mycétomes actinomycosiques	Mycétomes sans autres données	Totaux généraux
Colomb Béchar (35)				12[d]	12					12											12
Sénégal (31)	57		44	7[d]	108		3	14	17	125	16	19			8		46		89		214
Niger (34)	6			1	7					7	1	1			1		4		7		14
Tchad (36, 27, 38, 40)	14		1	15[e]	30		1		1	31	9	5					8		22		53
Haute-Volta (28)	1				1					1	2						2		4		5
Ethiopie (1)	4				4					4											4
Cote Fse des Somalis (37, 44)	12			1[f]	13					13	3	16				1			20		33
Somalia (48)	22			1[f]	23	1		5[g]	6	29		13			1		3		17		46
Cameroun (25)								2[h]	2	2				2	5				5		7
Ouganda (52)								1	1	1			7		7			2	9		10
Congo Leop. (51)		1			1	5		1	6	7	2			2	4				6		13
Tanganyika (50)																				19[m]	19
TOTAUX	116	1	45	37	199	6	4	23	33	232	33	54	7	4	26	1	63	2	179	19	430
Madagascar (29)	12	1			13			4	4	17	1	1					13	2	17		34
TOTAUX AFRIQUE ET MADAGASCAR	128	2	45	37	212	6	4	27	37	249	34	55	7	4	26	1	76	4	196	19	464

	Total
ASIE	
Arabie (1)	2
Liban (59)	1
Israël (Yemen) (60)	6
Sud Viet Nam (55)	1
Indonésie (58)	4
Japon (Kanazawa) (56)	5
Japon (Fukuska) (57)	2
Japon (Kuruma) (61)	9
TOTAUX	30
OCÉANIE	
Nlle Guinée Holland. (65)	2
Australie et Nlle Guinée (64)	2
Nouvelles Hébrides (69)	1
Iles Fiji (70)	1
Tahiti (62)	1 [n]
TOTAUX	6
EUROPE	
Bulgarie (73)	5
Roumanie (77)	9
TOTAUX	14
TOTAUX GENERAUX	854

a Madurella americana.
b Pyrenochaeta romeroi.
c Ne tient pas compte des mycétomes actinomycosiques marqués « environ 40 ».
d dont peut-être Curvularia lunata et Pyrenochaeta romeroi.
e dont 1 à P. romeroi.
f P. romeroi.
g 3 à Neotestudina rosatii, 1 à Scedosporium sclerotiale.
h dont Neotestudina rosatii et peut-être un Fusarium.
i Trichophyton ferrugineum.
j Mortierella mycetomi.
k Geotrichum candidum.
l chiffre comprenant des mycétomes fongiques non précisés.
m dont certains maintenant identifiés sur coupes: 5 à Madurella mycetomi, 1 à P. romeroi, 1 à Monosporium (?), 1 à S. somaliensis, 1 à S. pelletierii et 1 à petits grains.
n maintenant identifié sur coupe à M. apiospermum.

Madurella grisea est une espèce relativement rare rencontrée presque exclusivement en Amérique du Sud où Mackinnon, Ferrada—Urzúa et Montemayor (1949) l'ont décrite. Elle n'a été observée dans aucune des grandes enquêtes africaines récentes. Nous ne la trouvons mentionnée qu'une fois au Congo-Léopoldville (51) et une fois à Madagascar (29).

Leptosphaeria senegalensis n'a surtout été observé qu'en Afrique Occidentale (31) où il est responsable de 44 des 125 mycétomes à grains noirs. Il est également reconnu comme étant l'agent d'un mycétome au Tchad (36).

L'espèce *Pyrenochaeta romeroi*, décrite au Venezuela, se trouve au Sénégal (3 mycétomes), au Tchad (1 mycétome) et en Somalia (1 mycétome). Avec P. Destombes, nous venons de l'identifier sur la coupe d'un des mycétomes du Tanganyika que nous a adressée le Dr. W. R. G. Thomas (50).

Curvularia lunata a été isolé de deux mycétomes à grains noirs à Dakar.

Les mycétomes à *Monosporium apiospermum* (ou à *Allescheria boydii*) sont relativement rares en Afrique ; ils se rencontrent surtout en Amérique. Un mycétome des Nouvelles Hébrides (69) semble dû à cette espèce. Les mycétomes à *Cephalosporium* qu'il est difficile de différencier sur coupe de ceux dûs à *Monosporium apiospermum* sont rares. Il en existe quelques cas en Amérique, au Sénégal et au Tchad.

Parmi les autres agents mentionnés dans le tableau 2 comme responsables de mycétomes à grains blancs, citons *Neotestudina rosatii*. Ce champignon a été isolé de deux mycétomes de Somalia (48).

Streptomyces madurae est l'actinomycète responsable de mycétome, le plus cosmopolite. Les réponses reçues le signalent surtout en Afrique mais également au Mexique (15).

Streptomyces somaliensis a une distribution beaucoup plus limitée. On l'observe surtout dans la partie orientale de la zone nord-tropicale africaine (37, 44, 48). Cet actinomycète est également isolé en Mauritanie (31), signalé à Dar-es-Salam (50) et plus curieusement au Mexique (15) et même aux Etats Unis.

S. pelletierii est une espèce essentiellement africaine où elle prédomine dans l'Ouest. Elle est en cause dans 21,5 pour cent des mycétomes étudiés par Camain *et al.* (31). On sait par ailleurs que la même espèce est fréquente dans le nord de la Nigeria (33). La fréquence des mycétomes à grains rouges en Afrique diminue d'Ouest en Est ; ils sont rares dans le secteur oriental où nous n'en connaissons que 3 en Somalia (48) et 1 au Tanganyika (50). Ils semblent fréquents à Madagascar (29).

Les mycétomes à « petits grains », provoqués par *Nocardia brasiliensis* et *N. asteroides* représentent plus de 31 pour cent du total général (tableau 2). C'est l'existence de l'important foyer mexicain qui est la raison de ce pourcentage élevé. *N. brasiliensis* est en effet la cause de 90 pour cent des mycétomes mexicains. Cette espèce se rencontre également en Afrique où Vanbreuseghem, Courtois, Thys et Doupagne (1956) l'ont isolée pour la première fois. Cockshot (33) signale que dans le sud de la Nigeria cette espèce provoque la plupart des mycétomes.

N. asteroides ne doit plus être maintenant discuté comme agent de mycétome puisqu'il est à l'origine de 33 des cas du tableau 2. On le trouve disséminé dans le monde, au Japon, en Amérique, mais également en Afrique où il est notamment à l'origine de 7 des 9 mycétomes à petits grains observés par Wilson en Ouganda (52).

On a remarqué, à l'énoncé des différentes espèces mentionnées ci-dessus que de nouveaux champignons pathogènes certains sont apparus: *Leptosphaeria senegalensis* (Segretain, Baylet, Darasse, Camain, 1959), *Pyrenochaeta romeroi* (Borelli, 1959), *Neotestudina rosatii* (Segretain et Destombes, 1961). Il semble que le nombre restreint d'espèces admises par les auteurs modernes doit maintenant s'augmenter de ces nouveaux agents. Au moins en ce qui concerne les mycétomes fongiques, il devient évident que des espèces variées, saprophytes du sol ou des végétaux, peuvent être à l'origine de ce syndrome.

II. CONSIDÉRATIONS ÉPIDÉMIOLOGIQUES

Nos observations dans ce domaine s'appuient, d'une part sur nos informations, réunies lors de l'étude de mycétomes africains et mexicains et, d'autre part, sur les renseignements fournis par nos correspondants. Abbott (1954), Latapí (1956), Vanbreuseghem (1958), Destombes, André, Segretain, Mariat, Camain et Nazimoff (1958) et Rey (1961) ont rendu compte d'observations que nous ne pouvons, le plus souvent, que reprendre à notre compte.

1. De l'influence des climats et des sites géographiques

Les mycétomes ne semblent, dans la grande majorité des cas, se développer que sous des climats caractérisés par l'alternance d'une saison sèche et d'une saison humide et par des précipitations pluviales annuelles allant de 50 à 1000 mm (figure 1). Certaines espèces provoquent des mycétomes dans des régions à chutes de pluies plus abondantes (jusqu'à 2000 mm). C'est dans la zone limitée par les isohyètes 50 et 500 mm que la fréquence des mycétomes est la plus grande. On distingue nettement cette zone préférentielle dans la région nord tropicale de l'Afrique. Elle s'étend de Dakar à Djibouti, parallèlement au Tropique du Cancer, puis s'infléchit le long de la côte orientale jusqu'à l'Equateur. Les précipitations pluviales semblent d'ailleurs gouverner la répartition de certains agents de mycétomes.

Streptomyces somaliensis est isolé essentiellement dans les régions arides ne recevant que 50 à 250 mm de pluie. Cette espèce se rencontre rarement au-dessus de 500 mm, mais c'est notamment le cas pour les deux mycétomes mexicains (15).

Madurella mycetomi prédomine entre les isohyètes 250 et 500 mm mais on peut également les trouver dans des zones tempérées chaudes. Ils sont plus rares dans les régions équatoriales. Au Sénégal, Rey (1961) note qu'ils sont surtout nombreux dans la région du Fleuve Sénégal mais qu'on peut les trouver en plein Sahara (Atar) comme dans les régions humides de Haute Volta ou du Togo. *Leptosphaeria senegalensis* et *Pyrenochaeta romeroi* ont une distribution voisine de celle de *M. mycetomi*.

Les mycétomes à grains rouges dûs à l'espèce *Streptomyces pelletierii* s'observent principalement au-dessus de l'isohyète 250 et jusqu'à 800 à 1000 mm. Ils deviennent rares sous des précipitations plus abondantes mais peuvent éventuellement se rencontrer dans des zones très humides.

Dans les régions qui reçoivent de 500 à 2000 mm d'eau, on rencontre des mycétomes provoqués généralement par des germes différents des précédents et en particulier par *Monosporium apiospermum* (ou A. *boydii*), *Nocardia brasiliensis* et *N. asteroides*. Rey (1961) pense que peut-être *M. apiospermum* serait un agent rencontré dans des zones relativement humides (plus de 1000 mm) et que *Cephalosporium* serait plus xérophile.

Les deux *Nocardia* peuvent exister en zone semi aride mais se présentent avec une relative fréquence, dans des territoires chauds et humides d'Afrique, d'Amérique et d'Asie. Le climat subtropical d'altitude du centre du Mexique (isohyétes 500 à 1500) convient parfaitement aux mycétomes à *N. brasiliensis*.

Les sites géographiques peuvent, dans une certaine mesure, intervenir dans la distribution des mycétomes s'ils constituent par exemple, des microclimats ou bien encore, dans le cas des vallées, s'ils sont soumis aux inondations saisonnières. Au Tchad comme au Sénégal, les mycétomes sont plus nombreux dans les régions que les eaux recouvrent au cours de crues annuelles. La proximité de la mer peut également agir sur la répartition des mycétomes. Rey (1961) note qu'ils disparaissent presque complètement dans les 100 à 150 derniers kilomètres de la vallée du Sénégal, au voisinage de la mer.

2. *Des facteurs liés à l'hôte*

Les hommes sont, sans conteste plus fréquemment atteints que les femmes (504 hommes pour 109 femmes dans le tableau 3, soit 82,2 pour cent d'hommes). Les chiffres rapportés par d'autres auteurs non cités dans notre enquête sont assez voisins: Bocarro (1893): 92 pour cent d'hommes à Hyderabad ; Boyd et Crutchfield (1921) : 90 pour cent dans le sud des Etats Unis et le nord du Mexique; Abbott (1954): 83,1 pour cent au Soudan. Dans les chiffres rapportés par ailleurs mais inclus dans notre enquête citons ceux de Rey (1961): 86 pour cent au Sénégal et ceux de Latapí (1956): 81 pour cent au Mexique.

Nous ne pensons pas que cette haute proportion d'hommes soit seulement due au mode de vie comme on l'a souvent avancé. Si l'homme travaille souvent au champ, dans de nombreuses régions la femme y travaille souvent autant et quelquefois plus. Abbott (1954) et Latapí (1956) suggèrent que peut-être les hommes ont plus de facilités pour consulter, mais Rey (1961) note à ce propos qu'en pays Toucouleur, à Podor, au Sénégal, le cahier de

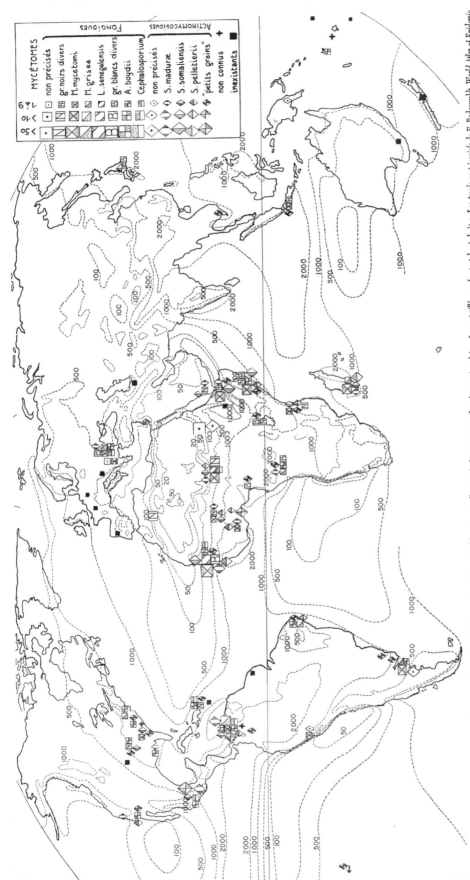

FIG. 1. Carte montrant la répartition géographique des espèces. Cette carte est établie avec les chiffres du tableau 2 mais elle tient également compte des réponses imprécises. Les pointillés représentent les isohyètes. Les tracés sont inspirés de E. Rodenwaldt, *World Atlas of Epidemic Disease* Part III, Falk, Hambourg, 1961.

MYCÉTOMES

	1 à 9	< 10	< 50
non précisés			
gr. noirs divers			
M. mycetomi			
M. grisea			
L. senegalensis			
gr. blancs divers			
A. boydii			
Cephalosporium			

Fongiques

non précisés			
S. madurae			
S. somaliensis			
S. pelletieri			
"petits grains"			

Actinomycosiques

non connus +
inexistants ■

TABLEAU 3

RÉPARTITION DES MYCÉTOMES SUIVANT LE SEXE ET L'ÂGE

	Amérique du Nord et Centrale	Amérique du Sud	Afrique et Madagascar	Asie	Océanie	Europe	TOTAUX
Nombre d'hommes atteints	159	4	321	17	1	2	504
Nombre de femmes atteintes	42	—	62	4	—	1	109
Ages 0–10 ans	—	1	—	—	—	—	1
11–20 ans	8	1	13	—	—	—	27
21–30 ans	36	—	43	5	—	—	89
31–40 ans	27	—	34	3	—	—	64
41–50 ans	15	—	15	8	—	—	38
51–60 ans	10	—	22	—	—	—	32
61–70 ans	6	—	5	—	—	—	11
TOTAUX	102	2	142	16	0	0	262

consultations porte plus de femmes que d'hommes ce qui pourtant ne renverse pas la proportion habituelle. Il est probable que des facteurs hormonaux interviennent pour rendre l'homme plus sensible aux mycétomes (comme d'ailleurs aux mycoses en général).

L'âge des patients est très variable (tableau 3). Les mycétomes peuvent s'observer à tous les âges de la vie mais sont surtout fréquents chez les adultes, à l'époque la plus active. La maladie peut apparaître chez de jeunes enfants comme chez des vieillards mais il semble qu'on en observe très rarement avant la puberté. Là aussi, il se pourrait qu'un facteur hormonal intervint. A l'appui de cette hypothèse, citons deux exemples mexicains. Le premier est celui d'une jeune fille de 18 ans qui aurait présenté un mycétome (dont elle porte encore les traces) lors de son tout jeune âge. Les lésions qui avaient totalement disparu ont réapparu après (ou lors de) la puberté. Le second exemple est donné par une malade du Dr Lavalle atteinte d'un mycétome de la région fessière. Une nouvelle grossesse a provoqué une nouvelle poussée de ce mycétome pourtant cliniquement guéri par des médicaments actifs.

De mauvaises conditions physiques, une dénutrition éventuelle découlant souvent d'un état de misère, interviennent sans doute également. A l'encontre de cette observation il nous faut reconnaître que les malades que nous avons observés à Mexico paraissaient souvent en excellentes conditions.

3. *Des traumatismes*

On admet généralement que les mycétomes se développent à la suite d'un traumatisme. Nos correspondants mentionnent le plus souvent des piqûres par échardes ou épines de plantes variées mais également des piqûres par écailles ou nageoires de poissons, des morsures de serpents, des piqûres d'insectes, des coups de pieds de cheval ou de bovidés, des blessures par des instruments aratoires ou des outils, des coupures de machettes, des piqûres par des clous ou des fils de fer, des coups de pierre, des blessures provoquées par des fragments de verre ou de métal. Ils citent également des traumatismes plus curieux, des fractures par exemple ou encore de simples érosions cutanées dues à des techniques de colportage ou des nécessités professionnelles. La contamination de la blessure par de la terre ou des poussières paraît constamment probable. Un seul de nos correspondants pense que les traumatismes ne sont pour rien dans l'origine des mycétomes.

Les blessures par épines sont si souvent citées que certains auteurs (J. A. Gammel, 1927) ont pensé que les agents de mycétomes vivent en parasite sur les plantes et qu'après inoculation à l'homme ils deviennent pathogènes pour ce dernier. Cette hypothèse serait valable si les mycétomes apparaissaient uniquement à la suite d'un traumatisme par un organe végétal, or nous avons vu qu'il n'en est rien. Il est évident que la présence de nombreux épineux augmente le risque des inoculations traumatiques, mais elle n'est pas, seule, responsable des mycétomes. On sait d'ailleurs qu'il existe des zones à épineux où les mycétomes sont absents et réciproquement.

Il s'avère en fait certain que le traumatisme ne fait que permettre l'entrée d'un germe potentiellement pathogène, d'origine tellurique. C'est en réalité le sol qui constitue la source d'infections.

4. *De la présence des agents de mycétomes dans la nature*

Divers champignons pathogènes ont été isolés du sol. Parmi ceux-ci figurent certains agents de mycétomes. *Allescheria boydii* isolé en particulier par L. Ajello (1952) et par Emmons (1950), est trouvé avec une relative fréquence. Borelli (4) a isolé par deux fois *Madurella grisea*. Les autres champignons n'ont pas encore été isolés du sol, hormis des souches de *Cephalosporium* qui est un saprophyte très fréquent.

R. E. Gordon et W. A. Hagan (1936) ont isolé du sol *Nocardia asteroides*. N. M. McClung (1960), à partir de 102 échantillons de sols du sud des Etats Unis a isolé 64 *Nocardia* dont 48 *N. asteroides*. A. González Ochoa et Maria de Los Angeles Sandoval (1960) ont isolé de 21 échantillons de sols mexicains 10 souches rapportées aux espèces *N. brasiliensis* et *N. asteroides*.

Nous avons, à plusieurs reprises, avec G. Segretain, tenté d'isoler des agents de mycétomes à partir de sols africains (Sénégal et Tchad). Aucun des champignons isolés ne pouvait être rapproché des espèces pathogènes. Parmi les nombreux actinomycètes obtenus, un seul (terre des environs de Fort Lamy), présentait des caractères qui aurait pu évoquer l'espèce S. *pelletierii*. A plusieurs reprises nous avons isolé fortuitement des souches saprophytes ayant tous les caractères de *N. asteroides*.

Les agents de mycétomes ne sont en fait pas encore tous isolés de sol (L. Ajello, 1962). Il faut voir dans les nombreux insuccès la faillite des techniques utilisées. Des méthodes plus sélectives permettront d'apporter la preuve que tous ces microorganismes sont des hôtes du sol, ce dont nous avons des preuves indirectes. Il faut aussi insister sur la difficulté de démontrer le pouvoir pathogène des germes isolés et surtout celui de former des grains chez l'animal d'expérience. Plusieurs auteurs ont obtenu la formation de grains expérimentaux avec certains champignons ou actinomycètes, il serait maintenant utile de pouvoir provoquer aisément la formation du syndrome mycétome.

Il n'est pas impossible que les microorganismes qui nous intéressent existent également sur les végétaux. Quelques essais d'isolement ne nous ont pas permis de le démontrer. R. Baylet, R. Camain et M. Ray (1961) ont ensemencé 37 lots d'épines ou de fragments végétaux du Sénégal; six sont demeurés stériles. Des 31 lots restant ils ont isolé 85 souches de champignons divers dont seulement deux (*Curvularia* sp. et *Cephalosporium* sp.) pourraient à l'extrême rigueur provoquer des mycétomes.

III. CONCLUSION

Les conditions climatiques qui, dans certaines régions où les mycétomes sont nombreux, permettent le développement d'une flore caractéristique, permettent également le développement d'une microflore responsable de l'endémicité de la maladie. L'alternance des saisons, les précipitations pluviales, la température de l'air et du sol sont les principaux responsables. Le cycle d'inondation de grandes surfaces de terrain, puis de dessiccation presque totale des sols intervient grandement, dans la sélection d'une microflore particulière. C'est là, à notre avis, qu'il faut voir l'origine des grands foyers d'endémies mycétomiques. Ces conditions n'agissent sans doute pas sur le seul pouvoir pathogène de microorganismes qui, en d'autres lieux, seraient inoffensifs. Il sera sans doute possible, à l'avenir, de dresser des cartes où des zones à microflore nettement différenciées se superposeront aux zones de grande endémie des mycétomes.

Il nous faut évoquer pour terminer un problème que Vanbreuseghem (1958) a fort bien posé : Comment se fait-il que dans des régions où les agents des mycétomes sont probablement présents en quantité dans le sol, et les chances d'inoculation traumatique nombreuses, la maladie ne soit pas plus fréquente ? La réponse ne nous est pas encore connue et peu d'explications valables ont été proposées jusqu'alors. C'est là qu'interviennent peut-être des facteurs physiologiques liés à l'hôte, d'ordre hormonal, immunologique ou autres. Dans ce domaine également le champ de recherche est vaste et l'étude de l'importante question des mycétomes est loin d'être terminée.

RÉSUMÉ

Une enquête a permis de réunir des informations sur 854 mycétomes dont 39,6 pour cent sont fongiques et 57 pour cent actinomycosiques. Le rapport rend compte de la distribution géographique de la maladie et de la répartition des microorganismes agents de mycétomes, telles qu'elles ressortent des résultats de l'enquête. Des considérations épidémiologiques font envisager l'influence des conditions climatiques (alternance des saisons, précipitations pluviales, etc...), des sites géographiques, des facteurs liés à l'hôte. On montre que les traumatismes généralement mentionnés à l'origine des mycétomes permettent la pénétration de germes pathogènes d'origine tellurique. Ces champignons et actinomycètes sont recherchés dans le sol d'où il n'a été possible d'en isoler que quelques rares espèces : *Monosporium apiospermum* (ou *Allescheria boydii*), *Madurella grisea*, *Nocardia brasiliensis* et *N. asteroides*.

Les conditions climatiques en contribuant à la sélection d'une microflore particulière aux régions incriminées sont reconnues comme étant la cause principale des foyers de grande endémie. Les conditions physiologiques de l'hôte doivent également jouer un rôle très important qu'il reste à préciser.

REMERCIEMENTS

Nous adressons nos très vifs remerciements à tous les correspondants qui ont bien voulu répondre à nos questionnaires. Les information qu'ils nous ont transmises constituent la matière première sans laquelle ce rapport n'aurait pas été possible.

LISTE DES CORRESPONDANTS

Amérique

(1) L. Ajello, Atlanta, U.S.A.
(2) L. Antuñez, Tegucigalpa, Honduras
(3) Audebaud, Guadeloupe
(4) D. Borelli, Caracas, Venezuela
(5) S. Browne, Berkeley, U.S.A.
(6) Calle V. et Angela Restrepo, Medellin, Colombia
(7) H. Campins, Barquisimeto, Venezuela
(8) Chaves Batista, Recife, Brésil
(9) N. F. Connant, Durham, U.S.A.
(10) C. W. Emmons, Bethesda, U.S.A.
(11) H. Florez, Lima, Pérou
(12) K. Friedman, New Orleans, U.S.A.
(13) M. L. Furcolow, Kansas City, U.S.A.
(14) C. Halde, San Francisco, U.S.A.
(15) F. Latapí, Mexico, Mexique
(16) A. T. Londero, Santa Maria, Brésil
(17) J. E. Mackinnon, Montevideo, Uruguay
(18) L. de Montemayor, Caracas, Venezuela
(19) E. Montestruc, Fort de France, Martinique
(20) M. Moore, St-Louis, U.S.A.
(21) Margarita Silva, New York, U.S.A.
(22) C. R. Silvérie, Cayenne, Guyane française
(23) T. H. Sternberg, Los Angeles, U.S.A.
(24) R. C. Zapater, Buenos Aires, Argentine

Afrique

(25) Blaché, Douala, Cameroun
(25) Gamet, Yaoundé, Cameroun
(26) A. Boujnah, Tunis, Tunisie
(27) Breaud, Largeau, Tchad
(28) V. Brumpt, Bobo-Dioulasso, Haute Volta
(29) E. R. Brygoo, Tananarive, Madagascar
(30) Public Health Laboratory, Bulawayo, Rhodésie Nyasaland
(31) R. Camain, Dakar, Sénégal
(32) A. Chippaux, Bangui, Oubangui-Chari
(33) W. P. Cockshott, Ibadan, Nigeria
(34) J. Darrigol, Niamey, Niger
(35) Delahaye, Colomb-Béchar
(36) Destombes, André, Segretain, Mariat, Fort-Lamy, Tchad
(37) Destombes, Dutour, Djibouti, Côte française des Somalis
(38) J. Fourré, Fort-Lamy, Tchad
(39) P. Ledoux, Atar, Mauritanie
(40) Le Henaff, Fort Archambault, Tchad
(41) J. B. Lynch, Khartoum, Soudan
(42) Martin de Mirandol, St-Denis, La Réunion
(43) Hôpital de Nairobi, Kenya
(44) J. Orio, Djibouti, Côte française des Somalis

(45) R. Park, Salisbury, Rhodésie Nyasaland
(46) Revel, Ouagadougou, Haute Volta
(47) Rollier, Casablanca, Maroc
(48) L. Rosati, Mogadiscio, Somalia
(49) C. Sérié, Addis Abeba, Ethiopie
(50) W. R. G. Thomas, Dar es Salaam, Tanganyika
(51) R. Vanbreuseghem, Congo-, Léopoldville
(52) A. M. M. Wilson, Kampala, Ouganda

Asie

(53) Baltazard, Teheran, Iran
(54) E. T. Cetin, Istanbul, Turquie
(55) Duong-Hông-Mô, Saïgon, Sud Viet-Nam
(56) R. Fukushiro, Kanazawa, Japon
(57) K. Higuchi, Fukuoka, Japon
(58) Lie Kian J., Djakarta, Indonésie
(59) Madet, Beyrouth, Liban
(60) Raubitschek, Jerusalem, Israël
(61) H. Urabe, Kurume, Japon

Océanie

(62) Borries, Tahiti
(63) E. B. Durie, Crows Nest, N.S.W., Australie
(64) B. R. V. Forbes, Sydney, Australie
(65) H. Harms, Hollandia, Nouvelle Guinée hollandaise
(66) G. Loison, Nouméa, Nouvelle Calédonie
(67) H. A. Macdonald, Guam, Iles Marianne
(68) M. J. Marples, Dunedin, Nouvelle Zélande
(69) W. H. Rees, Vila, Nouvelles Hébrides
(70) Director of Medical Services, Suva, Fiji
(71) S. Tapa, Tonga, Archipel de Polynésie
(72) J. C. Thieme, Apia, Western Samoa

Europe

(73) V. A. Balabanoff, Sofia, Bulgarie
(74) S. Cajkovac, Zagreb, Yougoslavie
(75) H. Götz, Essen, Allemagne
(76) P. Pereiro Miguens, Santiago de Compostella, Espagne
(77) St. Gh. Nicolau et A. Avram, Bucarest, Roumanie

BIBLIOGRAPHIE

Abbott, P. H.   1954.   Mycetoma: Clinical and epidemiological study. MD Thesis. Cambridge University Press.
Ajello, L.   1952.   The isolation of *Allescheria boydii* an etiologic agent of mycetomas from soil. Am. J. Trop. Med. Hyg. *1*: 227–238.
Ajello, L.   1962.   Epidemiology of human fungous infections. *In* Fungi and fungous diseases, ed. B. Dalldorf, pp. 69–83. Charles C. Thomas, Springfield, Ill.
Baylet, R., R. Camain et M. Rey.   1961.   Champignons de mycétomes isolés des épineux au Sénégal. Bull. Soc. Méd. Afr. noire de langue française *6*: 317–319.
Bocarro, J. E.   1893.   An analysis of 100 cases of mycetoma. Lancet: 797–798.
Borelli, D.   1959.   *Pyrenochaeta romeroi* n.sp.   Rev. Dermat. Venezolana *1*, no 4.

Boyd, M. F., and E. D. Crutchfield. 1921. A contribution to the study of mycetoma in North America. Am. J. Trop. Med. *1*: 215–289.

Brygoo, E. R. 1962. Revue critique des recherches mycologiques à Madagascar et bibliographie pour les années 1946–60. Mycopathol. et Mycol. Appl. *16*: 362–372.

Cockshott, W. P., and A. M. Rankin. 1960. Medical treatment of mycetoma. Lancet, Nov. 19: 1112–1114.

Delahaye, R. P., et J. Moutonnet. 1962. Les mycétomes au Sahara septentrional à propos de 11 observations. Sté Med. Milit. Française, Bull. mensuel *56*: 55–64.

Destombes, P., M. André, G. Segretain, F. Mariat, R. Camain et O. Nazimoff. 1958. Contribution à l'étude des mycétomes en Afrique française. Bull. Soc. Pathol. Exot. *51*: 815–875.

Destombes, P., F. Mariat, O. Nazimoff et J. Satre. 1961. A propos des mycétomes à *Nocardia*. Sabouraudia *1*: 161–172.

Emmons, C. W. 1949. Isolation of *Histoplasma capsulatum* from soil. Public Health Repts. (U.S.) *64*: 892–896.

Emmons, C. W. 1950. The natural occurrence in animals and soil of fungi which cause disease in man. Proc. 7th Intern. Bot. Congress, Stockholm: 416–421.

Emmons, C. W. 1962. Soil reservoirs of pathogenic fungi. J. Washington Acad. Sci. *52*: 3–9.

Gammel, J. A. 1927. The etiology of maduromycosis. Arch. Derm. Syph. (N.Y.) *15*: 241–284.

González Ochoa, A., et M. de L. A. Sandoval. 1960. Aislamiento de *Nocardia brasiliensis* y *asteroides* a partir de suelos. Rev. Inst. Salubr. Enferm. Trop. *20*: 147–151.

Gordon, R. E., and W. A. Hagan. 1936. A study of some acid fast actinomycetes from soil with special reference to pathogenicity for animals. J. Infectious Diseases *59*: 200–206.

Latapí, F. 1956. Micetoma. Analisis de 100 cases estudiados en la Ciudad de México. Mem. III Congr. Iber. Latino amer. Dermatol.: 203.

Latapí, F., F. Mariat, P. Lavalle et Y. Ortiz. 1961. Micetoma por *S. somaliensis* localizado a un dedo de la mano: Comprobación en México del primer caso extra africano. Dermatologia, Rev. Mex. *5*: 257–270.

Latapí, F. et Y. Ortiz. 1961. Los Micetomas en México. Datos nuevos clinicos y epidemiológicos relativos a 197 casos. 1er Congreso Mexicano Dermatol. Réimpression 1963. Mexico D.F.: 126–144.

McClung, N. M. 1960. Isolation of *Nocardia asteroides* from soils. Mycologia *52*: 154–156.

Mackinnon, J. E. 1954. A contribution to the study of the causal organisms of maduromycosis. Trans. Roy. Soc. Trop. Med. Hyg. *48*: 470–480.

Mackinnon, J. E. 1951. Los agentes de maduromicosis de los generos *Monosporium, Allescheria, Cephalosporium* y otros de dudosa identitad. Ann. Fac. Med. Montevideo *36*: 153–180.

Mackinnon, J. E., L. V. Ferrada-Urzúa et L. Montemayor. 1949. *Madurella grisea* n.sp. Mycopathol. *4*: 384–393.

Mackinnon, J. E., L. V. Ferrada-Urzúa et L. Montemayor. 1949. Investigaciones sobre las maduromicosis y sus agentes. Ann. Fac. Med. Montevideo *34*: 231–300.

Murray, I. G., E. T. C. Spooner, and J. Walker. 1960. Experimental infection of mice with *Madurella mycetomi*. Trans. Roy. Soc. Trop. Med. Hyg. *54*: 335–341.

Rey, M. 1961. Les mycétomes dans l'ouest Africain. Thèse Med. Paris. Foulon, Paris 1962.

Segretain, G., J. Baylet, H. Darasse et R. Camain. 1959. *Leptosphaeria senegalensis* n.sp. agent de mycétomes à grains noirs. Compte Rend. Acad. Sci. *248*: 3730–3732.

Segretain, G., et P. Destombes. 1961. Description d'un nouvel agent de maduromycose *Neotestudina rosatii* n.gen. n.sp. isolé en Afrique. Comp. Rend. Acad. Sci. *253*: 2577–2579.

Segretain, G., et F. Mariat. 1958. Contribution à l'étude de la mycologie et de la bactériologie des mycétomes du Tchad et de la Côte des Somalis. Bull. Soc. Pathol. Exot. *51*: 833–862.

Vanbreuseghem, R. 1958. Epidémiologie et thérapeutique des pieds de Madura au Congo Belge. Bull. Soc. Pathol. Exot. *51*: 793–814.

Vanbreuseghem, R., et J. P. Bernaerts. 1955. Production expérimentale de grains maduromycosiques par *Monosporium apiospermum* et *Allescheria boydii*. Ann. Soc. Belge Méd. Trop. *35*: 451–456.

Vanbreuseghem, R., C. Courtois, A. Thys et S. Doupagne. 1956. Deux cas de mycétomes congolais par *Nocardia brasiliensis*. Ann. Soc. Belge Méd. Trop. *36*: 479–486.

Vanbreuseghem, R., et M. Van Brussel. 1952. Emploi et signification de cultures de dermatophytes sur terre et milieu à base de terre. Ann. Parasitol. *32*: 541–556.

ACKNOWLEDGEMENTS

Many institutions, organizations and individuals have supported the Congress in various ways. We are grateful for the contributions made by the various departments of the Government of Canada, the National Research Council, Provincial Governments, McGill University, Université de Montréal, the City of Montreal, the Montreal Tourist and Convention Bureau, and others, too numerous to mention here. The many services provided by the National Research Council have been greatly appreciated by the Secretariat.

We are particularly grateful to the Members of the Canadian Society of Microbiologists, each of whom made a voluntary annual contribution from 1958 to 1962 and thus provided funds for operating expenses in the early stages of planning.

Financial and other assistance from the following organizations is gratefully acknowledged:

International Council of Scientific Unions
International Union of Biological Sciences
The Council for International Organizations of Medical Sciences

Government of Canada

Province of Alberta
Province of Manitoba
Province of Nova Scotia
Province of Ontario
Province of Quebec
Province of Saskatchewan

Anonymous
The Alberta Wheat Pool
American Agar & Chemical Company
Anglo-Canadian Pulp & Paper Mills Ltd.
Ayerst, McKenna & Harrison Limited
B-D Laboratories, Inc.
Bathurst Power & Paper Company Ltd.
Bellco Glass Company
Borden Company Ltd.
Borden Foods Company
Brinkmann Instruments, Inc.
Bristol Laboratories of Canada Ltd.
Buckman Laboratories, Inc.
Burroughs Wellcome & Co. (Canada) Ltd.

City of Montreal
Montreal Tourist and Convention Bureau

American Institute of Biological Sciences
National Science Foundation

National Research Council of Canada

McGill University
Université de Montréal
Institut de Microbiologie et d'Hygiène

Canadian Society of Microbiologists
Canadian Committee on Culture Collections of Micro-organisms

The Bank of Montreal

Canada Malting Company Ltd.
Canada Packers Foundation
Canada Vinegars Ltd.
Canadian Aniline & Extract Co. Ltd.
Canadian International Paper Co.
Canadian Laboratory Supplies, Ltd.
Canadian Milk Powder Manufacturers Association
Canadian Wine Institute
Catelli Food Products Ltd.
Ciba Company Limited
Continental Can Company of Canada Ltd.
Cordon Bleu Limitée
Corning Glass Works

DeLaval Company Ltd.
Difco Laboratories
Distillers Corporation Limited
Dominion Brewers Association
Dominion Rubber Company Ltd.
Dominion Tar & Chemical Co. Ltd.
Dow Brewery Ltd.
Dow Chemical of Canada Ltd.
DuPont of Canada Ltd.
T. Eaton Co. Ltd.
Elmhurst Dairy Limited
Falstaff Brewing Corporation
Federated Co-op Ltd.
Fine Chemicals of Canada Ltd.
Fisher Scientific Co. Ltd.
Fisons (Canada) Limited
Charles E. Frosst & Co.
Geigy (Canada) Limited
The Great West Life Assurance Co.
Green Giant of Canada Ltd.
The Griffith Laboratories Ltd.
Guaranteed Pure Milk Co.
H. J. Heinz Company of Canada Ltd.
Hygrade Food Products Inc.
Imperial Oil Limited
Imperial Tobacco Company of Canada Ltd.
Intercontinental Packers Ltd.
Jersey Production Research Co.
Kraft Foods Limited
Labatt's Brewery Ltd.
Labline Inc.
Lederle Laboratories
Lever Brothers Limited
Eli Lilly & Co.
McCain Foods Limited
Merck, Sharp and Dohme
Microbiological Associates Inc.

Molson's Brewery Quebec Ltd.
The Ogilvie Flour Mills Co. Ltd.
Parke, Davis & Co. Ltd.
S. B. Penick and Co.
Pfizer Corporation
Philips Roxane, Inc.
Pillsbury Canada Limited
Potash Co. of America
Price Brothers' Company Ltd.
Procter & Gamble Co. of Canada Ltd.
Procter & Gamble Co. (U.S.A.)
James Richardson & Sons Limited
Saskatchewan Wheat Pool
The F. M. Schaefer Brewing Co.
R. P. Scherer Limited
The Schering Corporation
Schneider Ltd.
Joseph E. Seagram & Sons Ltd.
Seven-Up Montreal Ltd.
Shell Oil Company of Canada Ltd.
Silverwood Dairies Ltd.
Slack Brothers Ltd.
Smith Kline & French Inter-American Corporation
Sun Life Assurance Company of Canada
Ivan Sorval Inc.
Squibb Institute for Medical Research
Standard Brands Limited
Sun Oil Company
Union Milk Company Limited
United Dairies Limited
Upjohn Company
Vinegars Ltd.
Hiram Walker & Sons Ltd.
Wallerstein Company
Warner-Lambert Canada Ltd.
Winnipeg Clinic

ADDENDUM

Ce supplément comprend les Statuts, les Sociétés Nationales constituantes et les Comités du Travail de l'Association, ainsi que le procès-verbal de l'Assemblée Générale du 24 août 1962.

I. STATUTS

Les Statuts suivants ont été adoptés à l'Assemblée Générale du 8e Congrès international de microbiologie, qui a eu lieu à Montréal en 1962, et remplacent ceux formulés à Rome au cours du 6e Congrès.

Article 1

Le nom de l'Association est « Association internationale des Sociétés de Microbiologie (AISM) ».

Article 2

Les buts de l'Association sont les suivants:

(a) assurer la continuité des Congrès internationaux de Microbiologie et organiser toute autre réunion ou colloque ;

(b) promouvoir la recherche microbiologique ;

(c) favoriser la création de bourses pour permettre au microbiologistes des nations participantes de poursuivre des études ou des recherches à l'étranger ;

(d) entretenir des rapports avec les Sociétés de Microbiologie du monde entier ;

(e) assurer la permanence d'un comité international de nomenclature et constituer éventuellement des comités ou des sections s'occupant de tout sujet de la compétence de l'AISM ;

(f) maintenir des rapports avec les organisations compétentes des Nations Unies.

Article 3

Il existe deux catégories de membres. Les membres nationaux et les membres bienfaiteurs. Les demandes d'adhésion sont soumises au Comité Exécutif qui décide de l'acceptation ou du rejet des candidatures.

(A) Un membre national est, soit une Société nationale de Microbiologie, soit, —s'il n'existe pas dans un pays de Société nationale de Microbiologie—une institution scientifique s'intéressant à la Microbiologie, ceci jusqu'à ce que soit formée une société de Microbiologie représentative qui pourra demander une revision de la situation. Chaque pays ne pourra être représenté que par une seule société, organisation ou institution scientifique.

La cotisation unitaire annuelle pour chaque société ou institution nationale sera de 50 dollars U.S.A. Chacune des sociétés membres décide elle-même, en fonction de l'importance de son activité scientifique, du nombre d'unités qui constituera sa contribution. L'Assemblée Générale a le pouvoir de modifier l'unité de cotisation annuelle des sociétés membres.

ADDENDUM

Included in this Addendum are the Statutes, the Constituent National Societies and the Working Committees of the International Association of Microbiological Societies as well as the Minutes of the General Assembly, August 24, 1962.

I. STATUTES

At the General Assembly of the 8th International Congress for Microbiology held in Montreal, 1962, the following Statutes were adopted and replace those formulated at the 6th Congress which met in Rome.

Article 1

The name of the Association is International Association of Microbiological Societies (IAMS).

Article 2

The objectives of the Association are:

(*a*) To ensure the continuity of International Congresses for Microbiology and organize other meetings and symposia;

(*b*) to encourage research in microbiology;

(*c*) to encourage the establishment of fellowships to enable microbiologists of component nations to pursue study and investigation abroad;

(*d*) to maintain contact with microbiological societies throughout the world;

(*e*) to maintain an international committee on nomenclature and other committees and sections on such subjects as may be appropriate;

(*f*) to maintain contact with relevant United Nations Organizations.

Article 3

There are two classes of members: National Members and Supporting Members. Application for membership should be submitted to the Executive Committee, which is entitled to accept new members.

(A) A National Member is either a National Microbiological Society, an organization of microbiological societies, or, from countries where there is no microbiological society, a scientific institution interested in microbiology until such time as a representative microbiological society is formed and requests a review of the membership. Membership shall be recognized to only one society, organization or scientific institution from any given country.

The unit annual contribution from each adhering National Society or Institute for the period between Congresses shall be fifty (50) U.S. dollars. Each Member Society can choose the number of units it is prepared to pay in accordance with the scope of its scientific activities. Should change in the annual unit contribution from adhering societies seem advisable, such change can be made by action of a General Meeting.

Tout membre national qui n'aura pas versé sa cotisation pendant trois années consécutives sera, après avertissement donné par le Trésorier, considéré comme démissionnaire. Le montant des cotisations dues sera considéré comme créance à recouvrer.

(B) Les membres bienfaiteurs sont des personnes morales ou physiques désireuses d'aider financièrement l'Association. Les membres bienfaiteurs n'ont pas droit de vote mais chacun d'eux peut envoyer un délégué aux assemblées générales. Ils ont le droit de recevoir gratuitement les publications de l'Association. Une assemblée générale décidera du montant de l'unité de base des membres bienfaiteurs. L'unité de base pourra être modifiée par une assemblée générale. Chacun des membres bienfaiteurs décide lui-même du nombre d'unités qui constituera sa contribution annuelle.

Article 4

Si les sociétés d'une région donnée le jugent utile, elles peuvent se grouper en organisations régionales de l'AISM.

Article 5

Le bureau de l'Association sera constitué par les délégués nationaux réunis en Assemblée Générale, par le Comité exécutif et par le Comité consultatif.

(A) L'Assemblée Générale est constituée par l'ensemble des délégués des sociétés nationales membres. Chacune des sociétés peut déléguer un à trois membres (maximum) mais ne dispose que d'un seul bulletin de vote. Le délégué ayant droit de vote est tenu de présenter à chaque séance sa lettre de créance au Secrétaire Général.

L'Assemblée Générale dispose de tous les pouvoirs et peut prendre des décisions concernant toute activité de l'Association; elle doit élire le Comité Exécutif et approuver les comptes. Le Secrétaire Général devra communiquer aux membres, au moins six mois avant la date de l'Assemblée, un ordre du jour provisoire pour la première assemblée générale ainsi qu'un compte rendu de la situation budgétaire.

Les résolutions sont adoptées à la majorité simple des membres présents. Deux assemblées générales se tiendront pendant la durée de chaque congrès de microbiologie.

(B) Le Comité Exécutif est composé du Président, du Président sortant, du Vice Président, du Secrétaire Général, du Secrétaire Général sortant et du Trésorier. Ce comité demeure en fonction jusqu'à l'élection d'un nouveau comité par l'Assemblée Générale du Congrès suivant. Le Vice Président est de droit Président du Comité Consultatif. Un membre du Comité Exécutif ne peut remplir plus de deux fois la même fonction.

Le Secrétaire Général du futur Congrès recevra copie de la correspondence du Comité Exécutif relative aux membres de l'Association, aux comités, aux souscomités et aux affaires intéressant le congrès.

Le Comité Exécutif assure l'exécution des décisions de l'Assemblée Générale, approuve le budget et dirige les affaires de l'Association entre les Congrès conformément à l'article 2, il transmet toute proposition d'un comité ou d'une section de l'AISM impliquant l'intervention d'organismes internationaux ; il soumet le bilan et rend compte de son activité à l'Assemblée Générale de chacun des

A National Member which has not paid its contribution for three successive years shall be regarded, on notice having been given by the Treasurer, as having resigned, the three annual payments being debts outstanding.

(B) Supporting Members are organizations or individuals interested in furthering the aims of the Association by means of financial assistance. Supporting Members have no voting power but may each send one representative to the General Meetings. Supporting Members are entitled to receive free of charge the publications sponsored or edited by the Association. A General Meeting shall determine the unit contribution of the Supporting Members for the periods between consecutive Congresses. Each Supporting Member shall determine the number of units he or it is prepared to pay.

Article 4

National Members may group themselves into regional organizations within the IAMS, should such an arrangement seem desirable to the Societies of a given region.

Article 5

The administrative bodies of the Association shall be constituted by the national representatives assembled in General Meeting, by the Executive Committee and by the Advisory Council.

(A) The General Meeting shall be formed by one, or at a maximum three, delegate(s) representative of each National Member, but each National Member shall be entitled to only a single vote. At each General Meeting the voting delegate shall establish his credentials with the Secretary General.

The General Meeting is endowed with full power and may pass resolutions on all activities concerning the Association; it shall elect the Executive Committee and approve the budget of the Association. The Secretary General shall provide the members with a tentative agenda for the First General Meeting and with a statement of budget no later than six months before this meeting.

The resolutions will be taken by a simple majority of the members present. Two General Meetings shall be held at every Congress for Microbiology.

(B) The Executive Committee shall be composed of a President, Past President, Vice-President, Secretary General, Past Secretary General, and Treasurer; it shall remain in power until the next Congress. The Vice-President shall also be Chairman of the Advisory Council. No Officer shall serve more than two terms in the same office. The Secretary General of the next Congress shall receive copies of correspondence addressed to the Executive Committee so that he may be informed of actions of the Committee, particularly as it applied to Member Countries, Committees and Subcommittees, and matters dealing with Congress policy.

The Executive Committee shall oversee implementation of motions of the General Meeting, approve budget, and direct the affairs of the Association between congresses in compliance with Article 2; it shall pass on any proposal involving interaction with international bodies by a Permanent Committee or Section of IAMS; it shall submit the balance-sheet to the next following General Meeting and shall be responsible for its activities to the General Meetings. The members of the Executive Committee are allowed to pass resolutions by correspondence.

congrès. Les membres du Comité Exécutif sont autorisés à prendre des décisions par correspondance.

(C) Le Comité Consultatif est composé d'un Président, d'un Secrétaire et de Membres. Son Président est le Vice Président de l'Association, son Secrétaire le Secrétaire Général de l'Association, ses Membres seront le Président (ou son représentant) de chacun des comités et sections de l'Association, ainsi que six membres élus au cours d'une Assemblée Générale par les délégués nationaux qui tiendront compte de la répartion géographique des sociétés nationales.

Le Comité Exécutif pourra demander l'avis du Comité Consultatif sur toute question relative à l'AISM. Les questions intéressant une section ou un comité permanent ou une région géographique donnés peuvent être soumises, pour avis, par le Comité Exécutif à l'examen du Président ou du Membre compétent. Tout comité permanent ou section et toute société nationale a le droit de faire des suggestions au Comité Exécutif.

Le Comité Exécutif et les Membres du Comité Consultatif (à l'exception des Présidents des sections et des comités permanents qui sont élus par les différents comités et sections) seront élus lors de la deuxième Assemblée Générale de chaque congrès.

(D) Pour les élections, on procèdera comme suit : à la première Assemblée Générale un comité de nomination sera constitué qui comprend tous les membres du Comité Exécutif présents au Congrès et un nombre égal de délégués nationaux élus par l'Assemblée. A la deuxième Assemblée Générale, ce comité proposera des candidats pour les postes de Président, Vice Président, Secrétaire Général et Trésorier de l'Association. D'autres candidats pour ces postes, ainsi que pour les six membres du Comité Consulatif, pourront être proposés par les représentants nationaux présents. Le bureau serra alors élu à la majorité par les représentants nationaux à l'Assemblée Générale.

(E) Si, entre deux congrès, il se présente une vacance, pour raison de santé ou par démission, au Comité Exécutif les membres restants du Comité Exécutif pourront proposer un remplaçant. La nomination sera faite par les membres du Comité Consultatif qui voteront par correspondance. S'il se produit une vacance au Comité Consultatif, il sera pourvu an remplacement par, suivant les cas, le Comité permanent, la section ou la région géographique intéressée.

Article 6

Le siège social de l'Association est l'institution où le Secrétaire Général exerce son activité. Normalement l'Association est représentée par le Président ou par le Secrétaire Général. Avec l'approbation du Comité Exécutif d'autres microbiologistes peuvent être désignés pour représenter l'Association.

Article 7

Les règlements de l'Association sont arrêtés au cours d'une Assemblée Générale. Tout membre national peut proposer des modifications au règlement à condition d'en avoir informé le Secrétaire Général au moins six mois avant la date du congrès.

(C) The Advisory Council shall consist of a Chairman, Secretary, and Members. The Chairman shall be the Vice-President of the Association. The Secretary shall be the Secretary General of the Association. Members shall be the President or Chairman of each established and provisional Committee and Section of the Association or his representative together with six Members-at-Large elected by the National Representatives at a General Meeting, with due consideration to geographical distribution.

Questions relevant to IAMS as a whole may be submitted for advice, at the discretion of the Executive Committee, to the Advisory Council. Questions relevant to the interests of any Permanent Committee or Section or to any geographical region may be submitted, at the discretion of the Executive Committee, to the appropriate President, Chairman or Member-at-Large for advice. Advice to the Executive Committee may also be given on the initiative of any Permanent Committee or Section or any geographical region, or on the initiative of any National Society.

The Executive Committee and Members of the Advisory Council (exclusive of Presidents or Chairmen of the Permanent Committees and Sections, who are elected by the several Committees and Sections), shall be elected at the second General Meeting at each Congress.

(D) Election procedure shall be as follows: At the first General Meeting a Nominating Committee shall be constituted of all members of the Executive Committee present at the Congress and an equal number of National Representatives elected from the floor. This Committee shall submit to the second General Meeting nominations for President, Vice-President, Secretary General and Treasurer of the Association. Other nominations for Officers may be made from the floor if desired. Nominations for Members-at-Large shall be made from the floor. The Officers and Members-at-Large shall then be elected by vote of a majority of the National Representatives at the General Meeting.

(E) Should a vacancy on the Executive Committee occur between Congresses by reason of health or resignation, nomination for replacement may be made by the remaining members of the Executive Committee. Election shall be by mail ballot of the Advisory Council.

Should a vacancy occur on the Advisory Council, replacement shall be by the Permanent Committee, Section or geographic region in question. The Executive Committee shall be duly apprised of this replacement.

Article 6

The Association shall have its legal seat where the Secretary General has his headquarters.

It shall be normally represented by the President or by the Secretary General. With the approval of the Executive Committee any other microbiologists may be appointed to represent the Association.

Article 7

The rules of the Association shall be laid down at a General Meeting. Any National Member shall be entitled to propose an alteration in the rules by giving at least six months' notice to the Secretary General.

II. SOCIÉTÉS NATIONALES CONSTITUANTES

Les noms sous-mentionnés sont ceux des membres du bureau des diverses sociétés au mois de janvier 1963, ou des personnes qui peuvent donner des renseignements sur leur Société. La lettre (S) indique le secrétaire, d'après nos plus récentes informations.

ARGENTINA ARGENTINE	Asociación Argentina de Microbiología	Prof. Dra. Teresa Satriano de Daurat (S) Avda Santa Fé 1145, Buenos Aires
		Dr. L. C. Verna Universidad de Buenos Aires Paraguay 2155, Buenos Aires
AUSTRALIA AUSTRALIE	Australian Society for Microbiology	Mr. J. R. Harris (S) Soil Microbiology Section C.S.I.R.O., Div. of Soils Private Mail Bag No. 1, G.P.O. Adelaide
		Dr. V. B. D. Skerman Univ. of Queensland Herston, Brisbane
AUSTRIA AUTRICHE	Oesterreichische Gesell-schaft für Mikrobio-logie und Hygiene	Dr. Kurt Berger (S) Possingergasse 38, Wien 16
		Prof. Dr. J. Michalka Bacteriology Department Veterinary School of Vienna, Wien
BELGIUM BELGIQUE	Société Belge de Microbiologie	Dr. E. Nihoul (S) Laboratorium voor Bacteriologie en Virologie, Apoteekstraat 5, Gent
BRAZIL BRÉSIL	Sociedade Brasileira de Microbiologia	Dr. Rudolf L. Hausmann (S) Instituto de Microbiologia da Universidade do Brasil Av. Pasteur 250, Rio de Janeiro
		Dr. Genesio Pacheco Instituto Oswaldo Cruz Caixa Postal 926, Rio de Janeiro
CANADA	Canadian Society of Microbiologists Société canadienne des Microbiologistes	Dr. V. Portelance (S) Institut de Microbiologie et d'Hygiène, Université de Montréal C.P. 6128, Montréal
		Dr. M. Panisset Institute of Microbiology & Hygiene 2900 Mt. Royal Blvd., Montreal, Quebec

II. CONSTITUENT NATIONAL SOCIETIES

The names given are of Officers of the Society as of January 1963, or of persons who should be in a position to give information about the Society. (S) indicates the Secretary according to our latest information.

CHILE CHILI	Instituto de Microbiolo- gia e Immunologia de la Facultad de Medicina de la Uni- versidad de Chile	Dr. H. Vaccaro Casilla 370, Santiago
COSTA RICA	Asociacion Costarricense de Microbiologia	Dr. F. Montero-Gei (S) Apartado 1404, San Jose
CZECHOSLOVAKIA TCHÉCOSLOVAQUIE	Czechoslovak Society for Microbiology	Dr. J. Stárka (S) Dept. of Microbiology Faculty of Science, Charles Univ. Viničná 5, Prague 2 Dr. I. Málek Czechoslovak Academy of Sciences Institute of Microbiology Na cvičišti 2, Prague 6
DENMARK DANEMARK	Danmarks Mikrobiologiske Selskab	Dr. E. J. Petersen Den Kongelige Veterinaer- og Landbohøjskole, Rolighedsvej 23, København V
FINLAND FINLANDE	Societas Biochemica, Biophysica et Microbiologica Fenniae	Dr. J. K. Miettinen (S) Biochemical Institute Kalevankatu 56, Helsinki Dr. A. J. Virtanen Biochemical Institute Kalevankatu 56, Helsinki
FRANCE	Association des Microbiologistes de Langue Française	Prof. ag. L. Le Minor (S) Institut Pasteur 28, rue du Dr. Roux Paris XVe, France Dr. E. Wollman Institut Pasteur 25, rue du Docteur Roux Paris XVe, France
GERMANY ALLEMAGNE	Deutsche Gesellschaft für Hygiene und Mikrobiologie	Prof. Dr. Werner Herrmann (S) Hygienisch-bakteriologisches Inst. Robert-Koch-Haus, Städt. Krankenanstalt. Hufelandstr. 55, Essen Prof. Dr. Walter Kikuth Institut für Hygiene und Mikrobiologie der Med. Akademie, Witzelstr. 109, Düsseldorf

GREAT BRITAIN
GRANDE-
  BRETAGNE
	Society for General
	Microbiology
		Dr. S. T. Cowan (Gen. Secretary)
		National Collection of Type
		  Cultures
		Central Public Health Laboratory
		Colindale Ave., London N.W.9

		Prof. E. F. Gale (International Representative) Biochemistry School Cambridge, England
GREECE GRÈCE	Greek Society of Microbiology	Professor C. Moutoussis Dept. of Microbiology National University of Athens 4 Dimokritou St., Athens
INDIA INDE	Association of Micro- biologists of India	Dr. S. Mukerjee (S) Indian Institute of Biochemistry and Experimental Medicine Calcutta 13
		Dr. B. N. Singh Central Drug Research Inst. Lucknow
ISRAEL ISRAËL	The Microbiological Society of Israel	Dr. A. L. Olitzki The Hebrew University–Hadassah Medical School P.O.B. 1172, Jerusalem
ITALY ITALIE	Società Italiana di Microbiologia	Prof. V. Puntoni Istituto di Igiene Citta Universitaria, Rome
		Prof. A. Cimmino (S) Istituto di Microbiologie Citta Universitaria, Rome
JAPAN JAPON	National Committee of Microbiology of Japan	Dr. T. Akiba Dept. of Bacteriology Medical School, Univ. of Tokyo Bunkyo-ku, Tokyo
MOROCCO MAROC	La Société des Sciences Naturelles et Physiques du Maroc	Dr. A. Sasson Dept. de Biologie Végétale Faculté des Sciences Avenue Moulay Chérif, Rabat
MEXICO MEXIQUE	La Asociacion Mexicana de Microbiologia	Dr. Luis Felipe Bojalil Unidad de Patologia Hospital General, Mexico 7
NETHERLANDS PAYS-BAS	Nederlandse Vereniging voor Microbiologie	Dr. H. Veldkamp (S) Laboratorium voor Microbiologie Hesselink van Suchtelenweg 4 Wageningen

NEW ZEALAND
NOUVELLE
  ZÉLANDE
	New Zealand Micro-
	biological Society
		Dr. D. E. Gardner (S)
		Wallaceville Animal Research
		  Station
		Private Bag, Wellington

		Prof. J. A. R. Miles Microbiology Department Medical School, Dunedin

NORWAY NORVÈGE	Norwegian Society for Microbiology	Mag. Scient Emmy Möllerud (S) Kolstien 41b, Bergen
		Docent Jostein Goksöyr University of Bergen, Bergen
POLAND POLOGNE	Polskie Towarzystvo Mikrobiologow	Dr. H. Meisel State Inst. of Hygiene Chocinska Str. 24, Warszawa
ROUMANIA ROUMANIE	Society of Infectious Pathology of the Union of Medical Sciences Societies	Dr. V. Prodescu (S) 8, rue Progresul, Bucharest Prof. S. Milcu 8, rue Progresul, Bucharest
SPAIN ESPAGNE	Sociedad de Microbió- logos Españoles	Prof. Dr. Vilas Lopez (S) Catédra de Microbiología Facultad de Farmacia Ciudad Universitaria, Madrid
		Prof. Dr. G. Clavero del Campo Facultad de Medicina Ciudad Universitaria, Madrid
		Dr. R. de Vicente Jordana Instituto "Jaime Ferrán" de Microbiologia, Joquín Costa 32 Madrid 6
SWEDEN SUÈDE	Svenska Föreningen för Mikrobiologi	Dr. L. Philipson (S) Institute of Virology, Uppsala
		Prof. Gunnar Löfström Department of Bacteriology University of Uppsala, Uppsala
		Prof. S. Gard Institute of Virology Karolinska Institutet, Stockholm
		Dr. C.-G. Hedén Institute of Bacteriology Karolinska Institutet, Stockholm
SWITZERLAND SUISSE	Schweizerische Mikrobiologische Gesellschaft Société Suisse de Microbiologie	Dr. H. U. Gubler c/o Dr. A. Wander AG Mikrobiolog. Abt. Bern Dr. F. Kradolfer c/o Ciba Ag., Basil
THAILAND THAÏLAND	The Microbiological Society of Thailand	Dr. Prakorb Tuchinda (Gen. Sec.) Government Pharmaceutical Laboratories, Bangkok
		Khun Ketudat Vidhyaphyadhi 359 Near Pran Nok Market Dhonburi
		Dr. C. Puranananda Queen Soavabha Memorial Institute Bangkok

TURKEY TURQUIE	Turk Mikrobiyoloji Cemiyeti	Dr. Z. M. Tuncman Divonyolu No. 103, Istanbul

UNITED ARAB
  REPUBLIC
RÉPUBLIQUE
  ARABE UNIE
	Society for General
	Microbiology of
	Egypt
		Dr. Hussein Mazloum (S)
		Faculty of Medicine
		Alexandria

U.S.A. ETATS UNIS D'AMÉRIQUE	American Society for Microbiology	Dr. P. Gerhardt (S) University of Michigan Ann Arbor, Mich.
U.S.S.R. U.R.S.S.	Scientific Medical Metchnikov's Society of Epidemiologists, Microbiologists & Infectionists of the U.S.S.R.	Prof. V. I. Vashkov (S) Central Scientific Research Institute of Disinfection Miusskaya place 3/8, Moscow A-47 Prof. V. D. Timakov Academy of Medical Sciences 14 Solyanka, Moscow Dr. V. M. Zhdanov Institute of Virology 1st Shchukinsky proyezd 24, Moscow D98

III. COMITÉS DU TRAVAIL

A. COMITÉ EXÉCUTIF DE L'AISM (CEAISM)

Président :   Dr. A. Lwoff
Président sortant : Dr. S. Mudd
Vice Président :   Dr. C.-G. Hedén
Membre* :   Prof. V. D. Timakov
Trésorier :   Dr. M. Welsch
Secrétaire   Dr. N. E. Gibbons
   Générale   Division de Biologie Appliquée
                 Conseil National de Recherches
                 Ottawa 2, Canada

B. COMITÉ CONSULTATIF DE L'AISM (CCAISM)

Président :   Dr. C.-G. Hedén
Secrétaire: Dr. N. E. Gibbons
Membres :   Dr. P. R. Brygoo, Comité Permanent de Documentation Micro-
              biologique et Immunologique
          Dr. S. T. Cowan, Comité de Nomenclature : Comité Judiciare
          Dr. J. Craigie, Comité international de Lysotypie Entérique
          Dr. M. Ingram, Section Permanente de Microbiologie et d'Hy-
              giène des Matières Alimentaires
          Dr. A. Lafontaine, Section Permanente de Standardisation
              Microbiologique
          Dr. M. J. Johnson, Section de Microbiologie Economique et
              Appliquée
          Prof. T. Asai, Japon
          Prof. E. F. Gale, Grande-Bretagne
          Prof. G. Löfström, Suède
          Prof. A. Pomales-Lebron, Puerto Rico
          Dr. L. A. Verna, Argentine
          Dr. V. B. D. Skerman, Australie

   *Un membre a été choisi parce que le Secrétaire Générale sortant a été élu
le Vice Président.

URUGUAY	Instituto de Higiene, Montevideo	Prof. Juan E. Mackinnon Instituto de Higiena Av. Alfredo Navarro 3051 Montevideo
VENEZUELA	Sociedad venezolana de Microbiologia	Dr. A. L. Briceno Rossi Instituto Nacional de Higiene Ciudad Universitaria, Caracas
YUGOSLAVIA YOUGOSLAVIE	Yugoslav Society for Microbiology	Dr. Dragoljub Popović Institut de Santé Publique de la R.P. de Serbie, Dr Subotića 3, Belgrade
		Prof. Dr. Marko Radojćević Faculté de Médecine Vétérinaire Bul. J.N.A. 18, Belgrade

III. WORKING COMMITTEES

A. IAMS' EXECUTIVE COMMITTEE (ECIAMS)

President: Dr. A. Lwoff
Past President: Dr. S. Mudd
Vice-President: Dr. C.-G. Hedén
Member-at-Large:°   Prof. V. D. Timakov
Treasurer: Dr. M. Welsch
Secretary General: Dr. N. E. Gibbons
     Division of Applied Biology
     National Research Council
     Ottawa 2, Canada

B. IAMS' ADVISORY COUNCIL (ACIAMS)

Chairman: Dr. C.-G. Hedén
Secretary: Dr. N. E. Gibbons
Members: Dr. P. R. Brygoo, Permanent Committee for Microbiological & Immunological Documentation
     Dr. S. T. Cowan, Nomenclature Committee & its Judicial Commission
     Dr. J. Craigie, International Committee for Enteric Phage Typing
     Dr. M. Ingram, Permanent Section on Food Microbiology & Hygiene
     Dr. A. Lafontaine, Permanent Section of Microbiological Standardization
     Dr. M. J. Johnson, Section on Economic & Applied Microbiology

Members-at-Large:
     Prof. T. Asai, Japan
     Prof. E. F. Gale, Great Britain
     Prof. G. Löfström, Sweden
     Prof. A. Pomales-Lebron, Puerto Rico
     Dr. L. A. Verna, Argentina
     Dr. V. B. D. Skerman, Australia

°A Member-at-Large was chosen because the Past Secretary General was elected Vice-President.

c. comité de nomenclature. *Président*: Dr. S. T. Cowan
comité judiciare. *Président*: Prof. R. E. Buchanan

Secrétaires Associés Permanents
  Bactériologie Médicale et Vétérinaire
    Dr. H. P. R. Seeliger
    Hygiene Institut der Universität
    53 Bonn, Venusberg, Allemagne.

  Bactériologie Non-médicale
    Dr. Wm. A. Clark
    American Type Culture Collection
    2112 M. Street N.W.
    Washington 7, D.C., U.S.A.

Secrétaire de la Rédaction :
    Dr. E. F. Lessel
    American Type Culture Collection
    2112 M. Street N.W.
    Washington 7, D.C., U.S.A.

Sous-comité :	*Président* :	*Secrétaire* :
1. Actinomy-cetes	Prof. D. Gottlieb	Prof. E. Küster University College, Ardmore House, Stillorgan Rd. Dublin 4, Ireland.
2. Brucella	Dr. A. W. Stableforth	Dr. Lois M. Jones Dept. of Bacteriology University of Wisconsin Madison 6, Wisc., U.S.A.
3. Enterobac-teriaceae	Dr. Joan Taylor	Dr. K. Patricia Carpenter Central Public Health Lab. Colindale Ave., London, N.W. 9, England.
4. Lactobacilli & organismes apparentés	Dr. M. Elisabeth Sharpe	Dr. P. Arne Hanson University of Maryland College Park, Md., U.S.A.
5. Leptospira	Prof. J. W. Wolff	Dr. L. H. Turner The Wellcome Laboratory of Tropical Medicine, The Wellcome Building, Euston Rd. London, N.W.1, England.
6. Mycobac-terium	Dr. P. Hauduroy	Dr. G. Penso Istituto Superiore di Sanita Viale Regina Elena 299 Roma, Italy.
7. Neisseriaceae	Dr. M. J. Pelczar	Dr. med. Ulrich Berger Bakteriologisches Laboratorium der Universitätsklinik Martinstrasse 52 Hamburg 20, Germany.

C. NOMENCLATURE COMMITTEE. *Chairman*: Dr. S. T. Cowan
JUDICIAL COMMISSION. *Chairman*: Prof. R. E. Buchanan

Permanent Joint Secretaries:
for Medical & Veterinary Bacteriology
  Dr. H. P. R. Seeliger
  Hygiene Institut der Universität
  53 Bonn, Venusberg, Germany.

for Non-medical Bacteriology
  Dr. Wm. A. Clark
  American Type Culture Collection
  2112 M. Street N.W.
  Washington 7, D.C., U.S.A.

Editorial Secretary
  Dr. E. F. Lessel
  American Type Culture Collection
  2112 M. St. N.W.
  Washington 7, D.C., U.S.A.

Subcommitte on	*Chairman*	*Secretary*
1. Actinomycetes	Prof. D. Gottlieb	Prof. E. Küster University College, Ardmore House Stillorgan Rd., Dublin 4, Ireland.
2. Brucella	Dr. A. W. Stableforth	Dr. Lois M. Jones Dept. of Bacteriology University of Wisconsin Madison 6, Wis., U.S.A.
3. Enterobacteriaceae	Dr. Joan Taylor	Dr. K. Patricia Carpenter Central Public Health Laboratory Colindale Ave., London, N.W.9, England.
4. Lactobacilli & Closely Related Organisms	Dr. M. Elisabeth Sharpe	Dr. P. Arne Hansen University of Maryland College Park, Md., U.S.A.

5. Leptospira	Prof. J. W. Wolff	Dr. L. H. Turner
		The Wellcome Laboratory of
		  Tropical Medicine,
		The Wellcome Building, Euston
		  Road
		London, N.W.1, England.

6. Mycobacterium	Dr. P. Hauduroy	Dr. G. Penso Istituto Superiore di Sanità Viale Regina Elena 299, Roma, Italy.
7. Neisseriaceae	Dr. M. J. Pelczar	Dr. med. Ulrich Berger Bakteriologisches Laboratorium der Universitatsklinik, Martinstrasse 52, Hamburg 20, Germany.

8. Taxonomie Numérique	Dr. V. B. D. Skerman	Dr. P. H. A. Sneath National Institute for Medical Research, Mill Hill, London N.W.7, England. Prof. L. G. Silvestri, Istituto "P. Stazzi" via Celoria 10, Milano 4, Italy.
9. Pseudomonas & organismes apparentés	Dr. J. M. Shewan	Dr. W. C. Haynes USDA, Northern Utilization Research & Development Division Peoria, Ill., U.S.A.
10. Lysotypie de Staphylo-coques	Dr. J. E. Blair	Dr. M. T. Parker Central Public Health Laboratory, Colindale Ave. London, N.W.9, England.
11. Streptococcus & Pneumo-coccus	Dr. R. E. O. Williams	Dr. A. T. Wilson Alfred I. duPont Inst. of the Nemours Foundation Wilmington 99, Delaware, U.S.A.
12. Bactéries sulfato-réductrices	Dr. J. Senez	Dr. J. R. Postgate Microbiological Research Est., Porton, Wilts., England.
13. Toxoplasma	Dr. J. Ch. Siim	
14. Nomen-clature des Vibrios	Dr. R. Hugh	Dr. J. C. Feeley National Institutes of Health, Bethesda, Md., U.S.A.
15. Virus	Sir Christopher Andrewes	

Il y aura bientôt des sous-comités sur les Staphylococcus & Micrococcus, et sur l'Haemophilus.

D. COMITÉ INTERNATIONAL DE LYSOTYPIE ENTÉRIQUE

Coprésidents :   Dr. J. Craigie
                 Dr. E. S. Anderson
Secrétaire :   Dr. P. Nicolle
                 Institut Pasteur
                 25 rue du Docteur Roux
                 Paris XVe, France

E. SOCIÉTÉ INTERNATIONAL DE MYCOLOGIE HUMAINE ET ANIMALE

Secrétaire :   Dr. R. Vanbreuseghem
                 Institut de Médecine Tropicale
                 155 rue National
                 Antwerp, Belgique

F. SECTION PERMANENTE DE MICROBIOLOGIE ET D'HYGIÈNE DES MATIÈRES ALIMENTAIRES

Président :   Dr. M. Ingram
Secrétaire :   Dr. D. A. A. Mossel
                 61 Catharijnesingel
                 Utrecht, Pays Bas

8. Numerical Taxonomy	Dr. V. B. D. Skerman	Dr. P. H. A. Sneath, National Institute for Medical Research, Mill Hill, London, N.W.7, England.
		Prof. L. G. Silvestri, Istituto "P. Stazzi" via Celoria 10, Milano 4, Italy.
9. Pseudomonas & Related Organisms	Dr. J. M. Shewan	Dr. W. C. Haynes USDA, Northern Utilization Research & Development Division, Peoria, Ill., U.S.A.
10. Phage Typing of Staphylococcus	Dr. J. E. Blair	Dr. M. T. Parker Central Public Health Laboratory Colindale Ave., London, N.W.9, England.
11. Streptococcus & Pneumococcus	Dr. R. E. O. Williams	Dr. A. T. Wilson Alfred I. duPont Inst. of the Nemours Foundation, Wilmington 99, Delaware, U.S.A.
12. Sulphate Reducing Bacteria	Dr. J. Senez	Dr. J. R. Postgate Microbial Research Est., Porton, Wilts., England.
13. Toxoplasma	Dr. J. Ch. Siim	
14. Nomenclature of Vibrios	Dr. R. Hugh	Dr. J. C. Feeley National Institutes of Health Bethesda, Md., U.S.A.
15. Viruses	Sir Christopher Andrewes	

Subcommittees on Staphylococcus & Micrococcus and on Haemophilus are being formed.

D. INTERNATIONAL COMMITTEE FOR ENTERIC PHAGE TYPING

Joint Chairmen: Dr. J. Craigie
Dr. E. S. Anderson
Secretary: Dr. P. Nicolle
Institut Pasteur
25 rue du Docteur Roux
Paris XV, France.

E. INTERNATIONAL SOCIETY FOR HUMAN AND ANIMAL MYCOLOGY

Secretary: Dr. R. Vanbreuseghem, Institut de Médecine Tropicale, 155 rue National, Antwerp, Belgium

F. PERMANENT SECTION ON FOOD MICROBIOLOGY & HYGIENE

President: Dr. M. Ingram
Secretary: Dr. D. A. A. Mossel, 61 Catharijnesingel, Utrecht, Netherlands

Comité des Spécifications microbiologique d'aliments
Président : Dr. F. S. Thatcher
Secrétaire : Dr. D. S. Clark
Division de Biologie Appliquée
Conseil National de Recherches
Ottawa 2, Canada

G. COMITÉ PERMANENT DE DOCUMENTATION MICROBIOLOGIQUE ET IMMUNOLOGIQUE

Président : Dr. P. R. Brygoo
Secrétaire : Dr. G. Tunevall
Boîte Postale 177   ou   Boîte No. 4
Stockholm, Suède   NGO Room, UNESCO, Paris

H. SECTION PERMANENTE DE STANDARDISATION MICROBIOLOGIQUE

Président : Dr. A. Lafontaine
Secrétaire Général : Mr. E. C. Hulse
Central Veterinary Laboratory, Weybridge, Surrey, England

I. SECTION DE MICROBIOLOGIE ECONOMIQUE ET APPLIQUÉE

Président : Dr. M. J. Johnson
Secrétaire : Dr. A. E. Humphrey, Towne Building 311-A
University of Pennsylvania, Philadelphia 4, Pa., U.S.A.
Cette Section a été approuvé par l'Assemblée Générale à Montréal.

J. SECTION DES COLLECTIONS DE CULTURES

Président : Dr. V. B. D. Skerman
Secrétaire : Dr. K. H. Steel
Central Public Health Laboratory
Colindale Ave., London, N.W.9, England
Cette Section a été approuvé par CEAISM en décembre 1962, par correspondance.

IV. ASSEMBLÉE GÉNÉRALE ET SÉANCE PLENIÈRE DE L'AISM
Le 24 août 1962

I. ASSEMBLÉE GÉNÉRALE (Délégués officiels)

Le Dr S. Mudd occupait le fauteuil présidentiel.

1. Le Comité des nominations a proposé, pour le Comité exécutif, les candidatures suivantes:

A. Lwoff	Président
S. Mudd	Président sortant
C.-G. Hedén	Vice-Président et Président du Comité consultatif
V. D. Timakov	Membre
M. Welsch	Trésorier
N. E. Gibbons	Secrétaire général et Secrétaire du Comité consultatif

Les délégués nationaux présents n'ayant pas proposé d'autres candidatures, les personnalités ci-dessus ont été élues à l'unanimité.

Committee on Microbiological Specifications for Food
Chairman: Dr. F. S. Thatcher
Secretary: Dr. D. S. Clark, Division of Applied Biology, National Research
          Council, Sussex Drive, Ottawa, Canada.

G. PERMANENT COMMITTEE FOR MICROBIOLOGICAL AND IMMUNOLOGICAL
   DOCUMENTATION

Chairman: Dr. P. R. Brygoo
Secretary: Dr. G. Tunevall, Box 177, Stockholm, Sweden, or Box No. 4,
              NGO Room, UNESCO, Paris.

H. PERMANENT SECTION FOR MICROBIOLOGICAL STANDARDIZATION

President: Dr. A. Lafontaine
Secretary General: Mr. E. C. Hulse, Central Veterinary Laboratory, Weybridge,
              Surrey, England

I. SECTION ON ECONOMIC & APPLIED MICROBIOLOGY

President: Dr. M. J. Johnson
Secretary: Dr. A. E. Humphrey, Towne Building 311-A
              University of Pennsylvania, Philadelphia 4, Pa., U.S.A.

This Section was approved by the General Assembly at Montreal.

J. SECTION ON CULTURE COLLECTIONS

President: Dr. V. B. D. Skerman
Secretary: Dr. K. J. Steel, Central Public Health Laboratory
              Colindale Ave., London, N.W.9, England.

This Section was approved by ECIAMS, by mail vote, December 1962.

IV. IAMS GENERAL MEETING AND PLENARY SESSION

August 24, 1962

I. GENERAL MEETING (Official Delegates)

The President, Dr. S. Mudd, in the Chair.

1. The Nominating Committee proposed the following list of candidates:
   A. Lwoff   *President*
   S. Mudd   *Past President*
   C.-G. Hedén   *Vice President and Chairman of Advisory Council*
   V. D. Timakov   *Member-at-Large*
   M. Welsch   *Treasurer*
   N. E. Gibbons   *Secretary General and Secretary of Advisory Council*

There were no further nominations from the floor and the above committee was
elected unanimously.

2. Le Comité des nominations a proposé, pour le Comité consultatif, les six membres ci-dessous:

T. Asai	Japon
E. F. Gale	Grande-Bretagne
G. Löfström	Suède
A. Pomales-Lebron	Puerto Rico
L. A. Verna	Argentine
V. B. D. Skerman	Australie

Aucune autre proposition n'ayant été faite les membres susnommés ont été élus à l'unanimité.

La composition du Comité consultatif est donc la suivante:

C.-G. Hedén	Président
N. E. Gibbons	Secrétaire
P. R. Brygoo	Comité permanent de documentation microbiologique et immunologique
S. T. Cowan	Comité de nomenclature et son comité judiciaire
J. Craigie	Comité international de lysotypie entérique
M. Ingram	Section permanente de microbiologie et d'hygiène des matières alimentaires
M. J. Johnson	Section de microbiologie économique et appliquée
A. Lafontaine	Section permanente de standardisation microbiologique

et les six membres nouvellement élus.

3. Après une brève discussion, il a été proposé que la contribution unitaire des membres bienfaiteurs soit la même que celle des sociétés membres, c'est-à-dire cinquante (50) dollars américains.
La proposition a été acceptée à l'unanimité.

4. Du fait que le nouveau Président était absent et que le nouveau Vice-Président avait des responsabilités de secrétaire il a été décidé que le Dr Mudd assumerait la présidence de la Séance plénière qui faisait suite à l'Assemblée générale.

II. SÉANCE PLÉNIÈRE

1. Aucun commentaire n'a été fait au sujet des décisions prises par l'Assemblée générale.

2. Le Dr Hedén a fait savoir que la première Assemblée générale ayant eu lieu le 22 août avait (i) approuvé son rapport dont un résumé figure ci-dessous ; (ii) passé en revue la situation financière de l'AISM et approuvé le rapport du Trésorier ; et (iii) adopté les statuts proposés compte tenu de certains amendements suggérés par la CEAISM (voir la version finale à la page 688).
Le rapport du Secrétaire Générale sur les activités de l'AISM et de la CEAISM, de 1958 à 1962, est résumé ci-dessous :

(a) Le VIIe Congrès international de microbiologie a eu lieu à Stockholm du 4 au 9 août 1958. Les comptes rendus ont été publiés sous le titre « Recent Progress in Microbiology ».

(b) Sections
(i) La Section permanente de standardisation microbiologique a été réorganisée. Elle a mis sur pied plusieurs réunions internationales dont les procès-verbaux ont été publiés. (Bruxelles 1958, Jérusalem et Opatija 1959, Wiesbaden 1960, Londres 1961). De nouveaux statuts discutés à Jérusalem sont maintenant approuvés. Il y est indiqué que le but de la Section est d'étudier les problèmes de

2. The Nominating Committee proposed the following six Members-at-Large for the Advisory Council:

T. Asai	Japan
E. F. Gale	Great Britain
G. Löfström	Sweden
A. Pomales Lebron	Puerto Rico
L. A. Verna	Argentina
V. B. D. Skerman	Australia

There being no further nominations the above were elected unanimously.

The Advisory Council therefore consists of:

C.-G. Hedén	*Chairman*
N. E. Gibbons	*Secretary*
P. R. Brygoo	*Permanent Committee for Microbiological & Immunological Documentation*
S. T. Cowan	*Nomenclature Committee and its Judicial Commission*
J. Craigie	*International Committee for Enteric Phage Typing*
M. Ingram	*Permanent Section on Food Microbiology & Hygiene*
M. J. Johnson	*Section on Economic and Applied Microbiology*
A. Lafontaine	*Permanent Section of Microbiological Standardization*

plus the six above-named Members-at-Large.

3. Following a brief discussion, it was proposed that the unit contribution for supporting members be the same as for member societies, i.e. fifty (50) U.S. dollars.

Carried unanimously.

4. In the absence of the new chairman and as the new Vice President had Secretarial duties, it was agreed that Dr. Mudd remain in the chair for the Plenary Session which followed immediately.

II. PLENARY SESSION

1. There were no comments on the actions taken by the General Meeting.

2. Dr. Hedén reported that the first General Assembly, which met on August 22, had (i) approved his report, which is summarized below; (ii) discussed the financial position of IAMS and approved the Treasurer's report; and (iii) had adopted the proposed Statutes, with some amendments suggested by ECIAMS (the final version is given on page 689).

The Secretary General's report on the activities of IAMS and of ECIAMS from 1958 to 1962 is summarized as follows:

(a) The VII International Congress for Microbiology was held in Stockholm, August 4–9, 1958. The Symposia were published under the name "Recent Progress in Microbiology."

(b) Sections

(i) The Permanent Section for Microbiological Standardization had been reorganized. It had organized several international meetings and the proceedings had been published. (Brussels 1958, Jerusalem and Opatija 1959, Wiesbaden 1960, London 1961.) New Statutes were discussed in Jerusalem and have now been approved. These indicate that the general object of the Section is to study

standardisation des sérums, vaccins et autres substances préparées à partir de matières biologiques, et de collaborer avec les organisations internationales ayant des activités dans le même domaine.

(ii) Le Comité permanent de documentation microbiologique et immunologique créé à Stockholm, a été très actif. Sa mission est d'étudier tous les problèmes relatifs à la diffusion et à l'exploitation des données scientifiques et d'organiser un réseau international d'information concernant la microbiologie et l'immunologie. Par ailleurs il coopère avec les organismes internationaux ayant des intérêts connexes.

(iii) Pour avoir des précisions au sujet des activités du Comité international de nomenclature bactériologique et de son comité judiciaire on devra consulter le Bulletin international de Taxonomie et de Nomenclature bactériologique, une revue trimestrielle publiée pour l'AISM avec l'aide de l'UNESCO et de l'UISB (Union internationale des sciences biologiques).

Le Dr Cowan a assumé la présidence d'un Sous-comité sur l'Allocation des Fonds des Collections de Cultures. L'Association lui est très reconnaissante de la façon dont il a réparti les fonds très modestes dont on disposait. Le sous-comité qui est maintenant dirigé par le Dr W. A. Clark conseille la CEAISM quant à la répartition des subventions octroyées par l'UISB pour les collections de cultures.

Depuis 1959 l'AISM patronne le Centre international d'information et de distribution des cultures types (19, Avenue César Roux, Lausanne, Suisse) lequel reçoit également une importante subvention de l'OMS (Organisation mondiale de la santé). Le Centre de Lausanne assure un service gratuit pour les souches microbiennes.

(iv) Par l'intermédiaire de sa Section de microbiologie et d'hygiène des matières alimentaires, l'AISM a été représentée à plusieurs conférences comme la réunion européenne concernant l'emploi des radiations ionisantes pour la conservation des aliments (Harwell, 1958), et elle a collaborée avec l'OAA dans l'organisation de la Réunion Européenne sur la microbiologie des aliments irradiés, qui a eu lieu à Paris en 1960.

(c) L'AISM a maintenu des contacts presque constants avec l'OMS et elle a été représentée aux assemblées générales de cette organisation. L'AISM est également membre du CIOMS (Conseil des organisations internationales des sciences médicales) depuis 1960 et elle a été representée par son trésorier à l'Assemblée générale du CIOMS à Paris en 1961. Une subvention a été demandée à cette organisation pour une réunion sur le toxoplasma qui doit avoir lieu à Copenhague cette année. L'AISM a fourni certaines données pour « l'Enquête concernant les principales tendances des recherches dans le domaine des sciences naturelles », enquête établie par l'UNESCO de concert avec le CIOMS.

Par le truchement de l'un de ses vice-présidents et de son Secrétaire général, l'Association a pris une part active à l'Assemblée générale de l'UISB à Amsterdam en 1961.

Par l'intermédiaire de son Secrétaire général l'Association est représentée au Comité exécutif de l'UISB et au groupe consultatif concernant les effets nuisibles possible des expériences spatiales de COSPAR (Comité pour les recherches spatiales).

(d) Le Comité exécutif s'est occupé de toutes les questions par correspondance à l'exception d'une réunion à Londres en septembre 1961 et d'une réunion qui a eu lieu immédiatement avant le Congrès. Lors de la réunion de Londres le Président du Comité permanent de documentation microbiologique et immunologique le Dr Brygoo a fait des propositions intéressantes visant à la mécanisation de la documentation et la CEAISM a approuvé en principe le programme. Le Comité exécutif s'est montré conscient de l'importance des méthodes mécaniques et

problems of standardization of sera, vaccines, and other products prepared from biological materials, and to offer assistance to international organizations active in the field.

(ii) The Permanent Committee for Microbiological and Immunological Documentation created in Stockholm, has been very active. Its mission is to study all problems relative to the diffusion and exploitation of scientific information and to organize an international network of scientific information in microbiology and immunology. It is co-operating with international bodies with similar interests.

(iii) For activities of the International Committee on Bacteriological Nomenclature and its Judicial Commission, reference should be made to the International Bulletin of Bacteriological Nomenclature and Taxonomy, a quarterly published for IAMS with assistance from UNESCO and IUBS.

Dr. Cowan has functioned as chairman of a Subcommittee on the Allocation of Funds to Culture Collections and the Association owes him much gratitude for his valuable assistance in handling the meagre funds available for distribution. This subcommittee, now under the chairmanship of Dr. W. A. Clark, advises ECIAMS with regard to IUBS grants for this purpose.

Since 1959 IAMS sponsors the International Center for Information on and Distribution of Type Cultures (19 Avenue César Roux, Lausanne, Switzerland) which also receives a substantial grant from WHO. This operates as a free service center for microbial strains.

(iv) Through its Permanent Section on Food Microbiology & Hygiene, IAMS has been represented on various occasions, e.g. at the "European Meeting on the use of ionizing radiations for food preservation" (Harwell, 1958) and collaborated with FAO in organizing the "European meeting on microbiology of irradiated foods" in Paris in 1960.

(c) IAMS has been in almost constant contact with WHO and has been represented at the General Assemblies of the Organization. IAMS has also been a member of CIOMS since 1960 and was represented by its Treasurer at CIOMS' General Assembly in Paris, 1961. This organization has also been approached for a grant to a Toxoplasma meeting in Copenhagen this year. IAMS has furnished certain data for the "Survey on the main trends of inquiry in the field of natural sciences" drawn up by UNESCO in collaboration with CIOMS.

Through one of its Vice Presidents and its Secretary General, the Association took an active part in IUBS' General Assembly in Amsterdam 1961.

Through its Secretary General the Association is represented in the Executive Committee of IUBS and in COSPAR's Consultative Group on Potential Harmful Effects of Space Experiments.

(d) The Executive Committee has handled all matters by correspondence with the exception of one meeting in London, September 1961, and one just before this Congress. At the London meeting, the President of the Permanent Committee for Microbiological and Immunological Documentation, Dr. Brygoo, proposed an interesting approach to mechanized documentation and ECIAMS approved the program in principle. The Executive Committee was conscious of the importance of mechanical and automatic methods in the treatment of scientific information and was convinced of the necessity of forming teams of specialists in prospect of this development. In consequence the Executive Committee recommended that a working group be established in Paris and it authorized this group to undertake officially, in the name of IAMS, the research work leading toward realization of an international pilot center for automatic, mechanized documentation.

automatiques dans le traitement des informations scientifiques et convaincu de la nécessité de former des équipes de spécialistes en vue de cette mécanisation. C'est pourquoi le Comité exécutif a recommandé qu'un groupe de travail soit établi à Paris et il a autorisé ce groupe à entreprendre officiellement pour le compte de l'AISM des études visant à la réalisation d'un centre pilote international pour la documentation automatique et mécanisée.

De plus, la CEAISM a patronné le travail de ce groupe afin de l'aider à obtenir l'aide financière nécessaire à la réalisation de son programme en s'adressant à des organismes susceptibles d'être intéressés à fournir une telle aide.

Les activités du Comité exécutif ont fait l'objet d'un compte rendu dans deux Bulletins de nouvelles envoyées aux membres, l'une au printemps de 1960 et l'autre en 1962. Cette dernière contenait une proposition visant à modifier les statuts afin de parvenir à une représentation et à une participation plus étendues dans les affaires de l'AISM et d'assurer une meilleure stabilité financière à l'Association. Jusqu'à présent les finances de l'Association ont été renforcées par son généreux président et par le fait que ses dirigeants ont payé eux-mêmes la plupart de leurs dépenses de voyage, une situation qui ne pourrait pas continuer indéfiniment.

(e) Au cours de la période considérée dans le présent rapport l'AISM a eu le plaisir d'accepter sept nouvelles sociétés membres :

La Société argentine de microbiologie
The Australian Society for Microbiology
La Société brésilienne de microbiologie
The New Zealand Microbiological Society
L'Institut d'hygiène de Montévidéo, Uruguay
La Société des Sciences Naturelles et Physiques du Maroc
La Société norvégienne de microbiologie.

Cette dernière remplace l'association norvégienne de pathologie qui a démissionnée.

(f) J'aimerais pour conclure faire une déclaration générale à l'effet que durant la période allant de 1958 à 1962 l'Association a connu une période d'affermissement de sa situation. Cet affermissement s'est manifesté autant dans les organismes intérieures que dans les relations avec les plus grandes organisations internationales.

Les délégués doivent maintenant décider de quelle façon l'instrument que représente l'Association doit être manié afin d'obtenir le meilleur résultat possible pour la microbiologie et pour l'humanité. Ceci est, je crois, lié à une seule question : Comment trouvera-t-on les fonds nécessaires pour financer les activités ?

3. Rapport du Comité de nomenclature et de son comité judiciare (par le Dr S. T. Cowan)

A la première réunion du Comité le Professeur E. G. D. Murray, a démissionné et le Dr S. T. Cowan a été élu pour prendre sa place comme Président du Comité. Les rapports des sous-comités de spécialistes ont été reçus et seront publiés dans le Bulletin international de nomenclature bactériologique et de taxonomie. Plusieurs nouveaux sous-comités de spécialistes ont été autorisés. Par suite de l'augmentation des travaux de secrétariat impliqués le Dr E. F. Lessel, Jr a été nommé comme Secrétaire supplémentaire auquel des responsabilités d'édition ont été confiées : comme les secrétaires médicaux et non-médicaux le Dr Lessel n'est pas compté dans le quota national d'aucun pays.

Lors d'une réunion du Comité judiciare on a décidé que le Président du Comité de nomenclature serait automatiquement vice-président du Comité judiciaire. Le Professeur E. G. D. Murray a été élu comme membre en reconnaissance des services qu'il a rendus au Comité de nomenclature.

Furthermore ECIAMS sponsored the work of the group in order to help it to obtain the financial aid required to accomplish its program, from bodies susceptible of giving it material support for this purpose.

The activities of the Executive Committee have been reported in two "Newsletters" to the members, one sent out in the spring of 1960 and one in 1962, the last one containing a proposal to change the statutes to give broader representation and participation in the affairs of IAMS and to make more adequate provision for financial stability of IAMS. So far the economy of the Association has been bolstered by its generous President and by the fact that the officers of the Association have covered most of the essential travel expenses, a situation which can hardly be expected to continue indefinitely.

(e) During the period covered by this report IAMS has had the pleasure of accepting seven new members:

> The Argentine Association of Microbiology
> The Australian Society for Microbiology
> The Brazilian Society of Microbiology
> The New Zealand Microbiological Society
> The Institute of Hygiene, Montevideo, Uruguay
> The Society of Natural & Physical Sciences of Morocco and
> The Norwegian Society for Microbiology

the last replacing the Norwegian Association for Pathology which has resigned.

(f) I should like to make the concluding general statement that in the life of the Association the period 1958 to 1962 has represented a phase of consolidation. This has covered both the inner organization and the relations with the major international organizations.

It now remains for the delegates to decide how the instrument, which the Association represents, shall be handled to the maximum benefit of microbiology and of mankind. This I think is a matter which essentially boils down to one question: How shall the means be found to finance the activities?

3. Report of the Nomenclature Committee and its Judicial Commission (by Dr. S. T. Cowan)

At the first meeting of the Committee, the Chairman, Professor E. G. D. Murray, resigned and Dr. S. T. Cowan was elected to take his place as chairman of the Committee. Reports of the Specialist Subcommittees were received and will be published in the International Bulletin of Bacteriological Nomenclature and Taxonomy. Several new Specialist Subcommittees were authorized. In view of the increased secretarial work involved, Dr. E. F. Lessel, Jr., was appointed as an additional secretary, with editorial responsibilities: like the medical and non-medical secretaries, Dr. Lessel does not count against the national quota of any country.

At a meeting of the Judicial Commission it was decided that the Chairman of the Nomenclature Committee should automatically be Vice-Chairman of the Judicial Commission. Professor E. G. D. Murray was elected a Member-at-Large in recognition of his services to the Nomenclature Committee.

4. Report of the Permanent Section on Food Microbiology and Hygiene (by Dr. M. Ingram)

(a) A symposium on "The Microbiology of Non-Alcoholic Beverages," was held at Evian (France) in September 1960. The full proceedings were published as Vol. XI of the Annales de l'Institut Pasteur de Lille.

4. Rapport de la Section permanente de microbiologie et d'hygiène des matières alimentaires (par le Dr M. Ingram)

(*a*) Un colloque concernant « La microbiologie des boissons non-alcooliques » a eu lieu à Evian, France, en septembre 1960. Les comptes rendus de ce colloque ont été publiés au complet dans le Vol. XI des Annales de l'Institut Pasteur de Lille.

(*b*) Un groupe international composé d'une douzaine d'experts a été convoqué immédiatement avant le VIII^{ieme} Congrès afin d'étudier la microbiologie des aliments congelés. Ce groupe a fait des recommandations unanimes au sujet de la qualité microbiologique des oeufs congelés, des crevettes et de la chair de crabe congelées et des plats cuits congelés : ces recommandations doivent être publiés dans le *Journal of Applied Bacteriology*. Une proposition a été préparée et a été soumise au Congrès afin que cette étude soit poursuivie par un Comité permanent.

(*c*) En rapport avec la Campagne mondiale contre la Faim de l'OAA (Organisation des Nations-Unies pour l'alimentation et l'agriculture) une résolution a été rédigée en vue de son adoption par la Séance plénière du VIII^{ieme} Congrès. Cette résolution concerne la contribution de la microbiologie aux approvisionnements alimentaires du monde.

(*d*) La Section a été responsable de l'organisation du colloque sur Les Microorganismes psychrophiliques à ce Congrès.

(*e*) Au début du Congrès une réunion administrative de la Section a eu lieu au cours de laquelle les questions (*b*) et (*c*) ci-dessus ont été approuvées et on a décidé de préparer un colloque international en 1964, probablement en Suède, concernant l'emploi et l'action des agents de conservation antimicrobiens pour les aliments.

Le Comité des spécifications microbiologiques d'aliments mentionnés en (*b*) ci-dessus a été approuvé en principe par le CEAIMS à l'unanimité.

5. Le Dr. Ingram a lu la résolution concernant la Campagne mondiale contre la Faim de l'OAA. Cette résolution concernant la contribution de la microbiologie aux approvisionnements alimentaires du monde a été adoptée à l'unanimité. Elle figure à la page 719.

6. Rapport de la Section permanente de standardisation microbiologique (par le Dr. E. C. Hulse)

L'adoption par le CEAIMS des nouveaux statuts de cette Section a été annoncée. Les nouveaux statuts stipulent que les buts de cette Section sont les suivants :

(*a*) de provoquer et de coordonner entre ses membres les recherches intéressant la standardisation des sérums, vaccins et autres produits d'origine microbienne, sanguine ou tissulaire, ainsi que de toutes méthodes de contrôle microbiologique ;

(*b*) de recueillir et de porter à la connaissance de ses membres les faits et documents d'intérêt général concernant la legislation, le contrôle et éventuellement la production de ces produits biologiques ;

(*c*) de contribuer à la diffusion des étalons internationaux établis par l'OMS ; de faire préparer et de faire mettre à la disposition de ses membres des sous-étalons ajustés sur les étalons internationaux ; de developper les techniques de laboratoire pour l'évaluation des produits biologiques ;

(*d*) de recueillir, à propos des nécessités que les étalons spécifiques internationaux font surgir, les opinions de groupes représentatifs d'experts ; de charger

(b) An international group of a dozen experts was convened just before the VIIIth Congress, to consider the microbiology of frozen foods. It made agreed recommendations about the microbiological quality of frozen egg, frozen shrimps and crab meat, and frozen pre-cooked meals: these recommendations are to be published in the Journal of Applied Bacteriology. A proposal was prepared for submission to the Congress, to continue this activity by means of a Standing Committee.

(c) In connection with the FAO Freedom from Hunger Campaign, a resolution was drafted for adoption by the plenary session of the VIIIth Congress, on "The contribution of microbiology to world food supplies."

(d) The Section was responsible for organizing the Symposium on "Psychrophilic Microorganisms" at this Congress.

(e) Early in the Congress, a Business Meeting of the Section was held at which items (b) and (c) above were approved and it was agreed to plan for an international symposium in 1964, probably in Sweden, on the use and action of antimicrobial preservatives for foods.

The Committee on Microbial Specifications for Foods, mentioned in (b) above had been approved in principle by ECIAMS and there was no dissent.

5. Dr. Ingram read the resolution in connection with the FAO Freedom from Hunger Campaign.

This resolution, the Contribution of Microbiology to World Food Supplies, was adopted unanimously. It is reproduced on page 719.

6. Report of the Permanent Section of Microbiological Standardization (by Dr. E. C. Hulse)

The adoption by ECIAMS of the New Statutes of this Section was reported. These indicated that this Section will be concerned with the following activities:

to foster and coordinate, within its membership, research in connection with the standardization and distribution of sera and other products prepared from microbial material, blood or tissue, as well as any methods of microbiological control;

to collect and distribute to members facts and documents of general interest about legislation, control and possibly also production of these biological products;

to promote the use of international standards established by WHO;

to have prepared and made available to its members working standards calibrated against international standards, to develop laboratory techniques for the evaluation of biological products;

to express the considered opinion of representative groups of experts on the need for specific international standards;

to request the IAMS to transmit these opinions either to the WHO or to the IOE when substances of medical and veterinary importance are concerned, or to other international bodies when substances of importance in other fields are concerned;

to arrange for the exchange of materials and the conduct of comparative assays, in order to collect experimental results, gather data and routine experience, which may contribute to the basis for international standardization and for the formulation of international requirements;

l'AISM de transmettre ces opinions, soit a l'OMS ou à l'OIE lorsqu'il s'agit de substances biologiques d'importance médicale ou vétérinaire, soit à d'autres organismes internationaux compétents, lorsqu'il s'agit d'autres produits ; d'organiser des essais comparatifs et de diriger les échanges de matériaux pour recueillir tous les renseignements que les faits, la routine, et l'expérimentation sont susceptibles de fournir en vue d'étayer la standardisation et la formulation d'exigences internationales ;

(*e*) de travailler à l'unification des méthodes de contrôle dans les divers pays ;

(*f*) d'organiser entre ses membres des rencontres sous forme de congrès, réunions scientifiques, groupes ou centres d'étude, cours de perfectionnement etc., et de publier des rapports sur ces rencontres ;

(*g*) de financer les programmes de ces activités.

7. Rapport du Comité permanent de documentation microbiologique et immuno-logique (par le Dr P. R. Brygoo).

(*a*) On prépare à l'heure actuelle une « Liste mondiale des Périodiques con-cernant la Microbiologie ». Lorsqu'elle sera complète cette liste sera envoyée aux sociétés nationales pour qu'elles l'approuvent officiellement.

(*b*) Selon un programme déjà approuvé par le Comité exécutif un Centre pilote pour l'étude des méthodes de mécanisation dans la documentation sera formé en partie en Europe en collaboration avec le Bulletin de l'Institut Pasteur et en partie aux Etats-Unis en collaboration avec les *Biological Abstracts*.

On cherchera à obtenir de l'aide financière auprès d'organismes internationaux et nationaux de façon à conserver l'entière autonomie et l'indépendance financière du Centre.

(*c*) Le Comité a accepté les recommandations de CIUS-FID-ISO-UNESCO telles qu'elles figurent dans « Basis for a Code of Good Practice for Scientific Publications » et il a souligné l'importance de la reconnaissance générale des règles et des normes actuelles qui ont été proposées par des organismes interna-tionaux compétents et qui devraient être suivies dans la rédaction des articles concernant la microbiologie.

(*d*) L'établissement d'un Catalogue de films scientifiques et la détermination d'une largeur de film standard pour ce genre de films sont actuellement envisagés.

8. Rapport du Comité international de lysotypie entérique (par le Dr J. Craigie)

On a lu un bref rapport recommandant que le Enteric Reference Laboratory of the *Public Health Service of England and Wales* (Londres) continue de servir de laboratoire international de référence pour la lysotypie entérique.

9. Section de microbiologie économique et appliquée

Le Dr Hedén a fait savoir qu'une réunion avait été convoquée au Congrès pour discuter de la création d'une Section de microbiologie économique et appliquée et que les résolutions suivantes avaient été proposées :

(i) Une Section permanente de microbiologie économique et appliquée est souhaitable ;

(ii) La Section proposée doit organiser un colloque sur les répercussions de la microbiologie appliquée (Stockholm, du 29 juillet au 3 août 1963) ;

(iii) Du fait qu'il est souhaitable que des contacts améliorés soient établis entre les laboratoires des divers pays la Commission exécutive provisoire et le Conseil devraient prêter beaucoup d'attention à la possibilité de former un

to promote uniform control methods throughout the world;

to organize meetings between members in the form of congresses, scientific gatherings, study groups, study centres, advanced study courses etc., and to publish reports of such meetings;

to finance this programme of activities.

7. Report of the Permanent Committee for Microbiological and Immunological Documentation (by Dr. P. R. Brygoo)

(*a*) A "World List of Periodicals Relevent to Microbiology" is being prepared. The List will be submitted to the National Member Societies when completed, for their official approval.

(*b*) According to a program already approved by the Executive Committee a Pilot Centre for the Study of Mechanized Methods in Documentation will be formed, partly in Europe, in collaboration with Bulletin de l'Institut Pasteur, and partly in U.S.A. together with Biological Abstracts.

Financial support will be sought from International and National bodies in such a way as to safeguard the full autonomy and financial independence of the Center.

(*c*) The Committee has concurred in the recommendations of ICSU-FID-ISO-UNESCO, as stated in "Basis for a Code of Good Practice for Scientific Publications," and stresses the importance of a general recognition of existing rules and standards proposed by competent international bodies to be followed in the writing of microbiological articles.

(*d*) The production of a Catalogue of Scientific Films and the issuing of a recommendation of a standard film width for such films is being considered.

8. Report of the International Committee for Enteric Phage Typing (by Dr. J. Craigie)

A brief report was read recommending that the Enteric Reference Laboratory of the Public Health Service of England and Wales (London) continue to act as the International Reference Laboratory for Enteric Phage Typing.

9. Section on Economic and Applied Microbiology

Dr. Hedén reported that a meeting had been convened at the Congress to discuss the creation of a Section on Economic and Applied Microbiology and had proposed the following resolutions:

(i) a permanent Section on Economic and Applied Microbiology is desirable;

(ii) the proposed section convene a symposium on "Global Impact of Applied Microbiology," (Stockholm, July 29–August 3, 1963)

(iii) because of the desirability of improved contacts between laboratories in various countries the provisional Executive Board and Council should give close attention to the possibility of forming an international body for biotechnology and take whatever action they may see fit in this connection. Support from such international bodies as UNESCO should be sought to create a mechanism or organization to stimulate biotechnology.

(iv) the meeting declared itself the First General Assembly of the proposed Section if accepted by an IAMS General Meeting.

organisme international de biotechnologie et de prendre toutes mesures qu'ils jugeront appropriées à cet égard. On devrait rechercher l'aide d'organismes internationaux comme l'UNESCO afin de créer un secrétariat ou une organisation pour stimuler la biotechnologie.

(iv) La réunion s'est déclarée être la première Assemblée générale de la Section proposée sous réserve d'approbation par l'Assemblée générale de l'AIMS. La réunion a adopté ces résolutions et elle a pris les décisions suivantes :

L'Association internationale des Sociétés de microbiologie établit une Section de microbiologie économique et appliquée. Les affaires de cette Section seront réglées par une Commission exécutive provisoire et un Conseil provisoire ainsi constitués :

La Commission : M. J. Johnson, *Président*
C. G. Hedén, *Vice-Président*
I. Malek, *Vice-Président*
A. E. Humphrey, *Secrétaire général*
G. Gualandi, *Trésorier*

Le Conseil : K. Arima (Japon), K. Bernhauer (Allemagne), C. Casas-Campillo (Mexique), E. B. Chain (Grande-Bretagne/Italie), Fang-Sin-Fang (Chine), F. Philippe (France), T. K. Ghose (Inde), M. Herold (Tchécoslovaquie), J. J. H. Hastings (Grande-Bretagne), N. D. Ierusalimski (URSS), H. Katznelson (Canada), K. Kitahara (Japon), J. O. Lampen (Etats-Unis), E. N. Mishustin (URSS), M. Shilo (Israël), J. C. Sylvester (Etats-Unis), T. O. Wikén (Hollande).

Les structures provisoires fonctionneront jusqu'à ce que des statuts soient adoptés par une Assemblée générale de la Section qui doit en principe se réunir en avril 1964. Après avoir approuvé les statuts du nouvel organisme et passé en revue ses activités le Conseil exécutif de l'AIMS pourra lui accorder le statut de Section permanente en août 1964.

Aucune discussion n'a eu lieu à cet égard et la proposition a été adoptée à l'unanimité.

10. Le Dr H. Cox a proposé la résolution suivante :

« Au nom de tous les délégués officiels des nombreux pays représentés au VIIIe Congrès international de microbiologie je désire exprimer nos remerciements et notre profonde gratitude à tous les comités canadiens qui ont fait un excellent travail dans tous les domaines pour organiser et pour administrer ce Congrès. Nos remerciements s'adressent tout particulièrement aux membres du Comité féminin si habilement présidé par Madame A. Frappier et Mrs. D. H. Starkey. »

La résolution a été ovationnée.

11. Le Dr A. Pomales-Lebron a présenté un rapport sur l'Association Américano-Latine de microbiologie, une association de sociétés microbiologiques qui groupe un certain nombre de pays d'Amérique latine et qui avait déjà tenu deux congrès l'un au Mexique et l'autre au Costa Rica se propose d'en avoir un troisième en Colombie en 1964. L'Association espère que ces congrès pourront servir d'un moyen d'éliminer les frontières du nationalisme académique.

12. Le nouveau Secrétaire général, le Dr. N. E. Gibbons, a fait ensuite une brève déclaration. Il a fait remarquer qu'on avait proposé la création de plusieurs sections et comités. Cependant le Comité exécutif considère que ces nouveaux organismes ne devraient pas être mis sur pied à moins qu'ils ne présentent un intérêt incontestable et qu'ils soient dirigés par des personnes soucieuses de leur donner l'orientation qui convient au sein de l'AISM.

The meeting adopted these resolutions and made the following decision:

The International Association of Microbiological Societies initiates a Section on Economic and Applied Microbiology. The affairs of the Section shall be handled by a provisional Executive Board and a Provisional Council, the administrative bodies formed to have the following composition:

Board: M. J. Johnson, *President*
C.-G. Hedén, *Vice-President*
I. Malék, *Vice-President*
A. E. Humphrey, *Secretary General*
G. Gualandi, *Treasurer*

Council: K. Arima (Japan), K. Bernhauer (Germany), C. Casas-Campillo (Mexico), E. B. Chain (Great Britain/Italy), Fang-Sin-Fang (China), F. Philippe (France), T. K. Ghose (India), M. Herold (Czechoslovakia), J. J. H. Hastings (Great Britain), N. D. Ierusalimski (USSR), H. Katznelson (Canada), K. Kitahara (Japan), J. O. Lampen (USA), E. N. Mishustin (USSR), M. Shilo (Israel), J. C. Sylvester (USA), T. O. Wikén (Netherlands).

The provisional governing bodies shall function until statutes are adopted by a General Assembly of the Section which is expected to meet in April 1964. After adoption of the statutes and a general review of its activities, IAMS' Executive Committee can grant the new body status as a permanent section in August 1964.

There was no discussion on the above and the proposal carried unanimously.

10. Dr. H. Cox moved the following resolution:
"In the name of all the official delegates from the many countries attending this VIII International Congress of Microbiology, I would like to express our thanks and deep appreciation to each and all of the Canadian Committees who have done such an excellent job in all ways in organizing and conducting this Congress— and particular thanks to the members of the Ladies Committee so ably headed by co-chairmen Madame A. Frappier and Mrs. D. H. Starkey."

There was a standing vote of thanks.

11. Dr. A. Pomales-Lebron reported on the Association Latino Americana de Microbiologie, an association of microbiological societies in a number of Latin American countries which had already held two congresses, one in Mexico and one in Costa Rica, and proposed a third in Columbia in 1964. The association hopes these congresses may be a means of erasing the boundaries of academic nationalism.

12. The new Secretary General, Dr. N. E. Gibbons, then made a brief statement. He pointed out that several new sections or committees had been proposed. However it was the feeling of the Executive Committee that these should not be set up unless there was adequate interest and a cadre of persons who are willing to provide the necessary impetus and to assure that the proposed section could perform a worthwhile function in the organization.
One of the criticisms of IAMS had been the lack of information about its activities and it was hoped that a Newsletter could be initiated to provide information on Executive decisions and items of interest to the member societies. The Secretary General pointed out that he had to have information before he could pass it on and requested the officials of the National Societies to inform him of their officers and of changes as they were made, and to supply the organizers

L'une des critiques formulées à l'égard de l'AIMS a été l'absence d'information au sujet de ses activités aussi a-t-on exprimé l'espoir qu'un Bulletin de Nouvelles soit éditée pour fournir aux sociétés-membres des renseignements sur les décisions du Comité exécutif et sur d'autres questions d'intérêt général. Le Secrétaire général a fait remarquer qu'il lui faudrait recevoir des informations avant d'en faire part aux intéressés et il a demandé aux responsables des sociétés nationales de lui faire connaître les noms de leurs dirigeants et de le tenir au courant de tous changements à mesure qu'ils sont faits, et que les organisateurs du prochain Congrès devraient recevoir les noms des représentants nationaux au moins 6 mois à l'avance. Il demandait aussi aux secrétaires des comités et sous-comités de l'AISM de l'avertir de toutes modifications en ce qui concerne les membres.

13. Le Président a fait remarquer qu'il était souhaitable de connaître longtemps à l'avance les dates et les emplacements des prochains congrès et il a suggéré qu'on les définisse le plus tôt possible pour les trois prochains congrès.

Aucune information officielle n'a été soumise pour le prochain Congrès mais on a parlé de Moscou. (Une invitation officielle est maintenant parvenue pour que le prochain Congrès ait lieu à Moscou en 1966 et cette invitation a été acceptée.)

L'ordre du jour étant épuisé le Président a confié la réunion au Dr. E. G. D. Murray, Président du Congrès, qui a exprimé les remerciements de la Société canadienne des microbiologistes et du Comité d'organisation du Congrès à tous les délégués pour leur bons souhaits et il a officiallement clôturé le Congrès.

of the next Congress with the names of the National representatives at least six months before the Congress. He also requested secretaries of IAMS committees and subcommittees to inform him of changes in membership.

13. The chairman pointed out the desirability of having well in advance the time and place of the next congress and suggested that as soon as possible information on the next three congresses should be worked out.

No official information had been submitted for the next congress but there was a possibility that it might be held in Moscow. (An invitation to hold the next Congress in Moscow in 1966 has now been received and accepted.)

There being no further business the chairman turned the meeting over to Dr. E. G. D. Murray, President of the Congress, who expressed the appreciation of the Canadian Society of Microbiologists and the Organizing Committee of the Congress to the delegates for their kind wishes and declared the Congress officially closed.

THE CONTRIBUTION OF MICROBIOLOGY TO WORLD FOOD SUPPLIES

A resolution prepared by the
Permanent Section on Food Microbiology & Hygiene and
adopted unanimously by the Plenary Session of IAMS, August 24, 1962

1. The International Association of Microbiological Societies, in sympathy with the FAO. Freedom from Hunger Campaign, notes with concern the widening gap between the global rates of increase of population and of food supply, at a time when there already exists famine or near-famine in many parts of the world. The Association has accordingly considered how microbiology might help towards a future need, clearly indicated, to increase world food production by all conceivable means.

2. One attack on this problem is to improve the fertility of soils, in which connection the following would be helpful:

(a) A study of thermophilic and mesophilic microorganisms capable of more rapidly transforming such non-food wastes as sawdust, straw, weeds, leaves, sludge, etc. into suitable organic matter of manurial value.

(b) Research on the effect of herbicides, fungicides and other chemicals on microorganisms, in order to attempt to control soil populations.

(c) Further studies on the effectiveness and wider distribution of Azotobacters, Rhizobia and other microorganisms capable of fixing atmospheric nitrogen.

3. There is also the possiblity of producing, from appropriate microorganisms, agriculturally useful substances like plant growth factors and inhibitors.

4. Another obvious line of attack is to prevent spoilage of food by microorganisms. There are well-proven ways of doing this like drying, salting, refrigeration or canning; and there are new methods of promise, like the use of antibiotics or irradiation; all these are worth investigating. On a world view, however, it is much more urgent to apply what is already known to countries where such methods are under-developed, rather than to devote effort to minor improvements

in existing procedures. Moreover, it must be recognised that even if food spoilage by microbes were entirely prevented, the increase in total available food would be small (of the order only of a few per cent, though the benefits might be greater in some places).

5. To change the situation radically, sources of food *additional to* orthodox agricultural production must be sought for man and his domestic animals. It should be realised that microorganisms should be capable of supplying some of these; for microorganisms are able to produce edible protein, fat or carbohydrate, and vitamins, from materials entirely inaccessible to human or mammalian digestion, yet do not require agriculturally useful land.

6. As examples of microorganisms worthy of examination, the following may be suggested:

(*a*) Organisms utilising existing agricultural or industrial by-products (food yeast is the best known example).
(*b*) Fungi and bacteria decomposing cellulose or hemi-cellulose (i.e. non-woody plant tissue).
(*c*) Fungi attacking wood, especially lignin (some of these are known to be edible).
(*d*) Organisms which decompose the larger sea weeds.
(*e*) Organisms capable of multiplying in various effluents. (e.g. aquatic fungi).
(*f*) Bacteria capable of oxidising methane or other hydrocarbons.
(*g*) Photosynthetic algae or bacteria (*Chlorella* is the best investigated example).

Particular interest would attach to organisms capable at the same time of converting atmospheric nitrogen into protein, which probably exist in several of the above groups.

7. Preliminary essays in this direction, the production of food yeast and of *Chlorella*, have been discouraged by two factors; first, because insufficient attention has been paid to the preparation of sufficiently attractive materials from the crude microorganism; second, and more importantly, by the demonstration that such products do not yet compete economically with orthodox foods. But, with increasing demands on orthodox food supplies, this situation may soon change.

8. The world food shortage seems likely to become acute in the next ten or twenty years, which is not a long period for developmental research of the nature likely to be required, especially as many of the relevant microorganisms have been little studied hitherto. To permit application of such research in time, it is recommended that governments encourage it now, even though it be uneconomic at present.

ALPHABETICAL LIST OF AUTHORS

Lightning Source UK Ltd.
Milton Keynes UK
UKHW030615210722
406167UK00006B/613